D1325536

WITHDRAWN
FROM STOCK
QMUL LIBRARY

TRANSPLANTATION PATHOLOGY

TRANSPLANTATION PATHOLOGY is a specialized textbook that comprehensively covers the pathological features of all organs transplanted in clinical practice. In addition to extensive detail of morphological changes, numerous images, and the latest classification schemes, this book incorporates basic pathophysiologic mechanisms involved in the detrimental processes affecting the host and graft. Finally, there are also specialized chapters addressing the immunopathology of graft rejection, laboratory medicine and transplantation, dermatological complications in transplantation, and PTLD.

Thus, this book by renowned authors in the field provides the pathologist, clinician, clinical staff, and student a complete overview of the pathological processes and underlying mechanisms of all areas of transplantation.

Dr. Phillip Ruiz is an internationally recognized expert in transplantation pathology, immunology, and immunopathology. He received his Ph.D. in immunology from the University of Florida, his M.D. from George Washington University, and his residency (pathology)/ fellowship training at Duke University. He has been at the University of Miami since 1989, where he is a Professor of Pathology and Surgery, the Medical Director of the Transplant Laboratories, and Director of Immunopathology. His research interests include immune tolerance, subclinical rejection, and the interaction of inmate immunity with alloreactivity. He has more than 330 peer-reviewed journal articles and numerous chapters and is a frequently invited speaker at worldwide meetings. He is on the editorial board and/or a reviewer of numerous journals and a member of many professional organizations.

WO660 KUN
ORD
Daw
EGS
11/9/09
9/9/09

TRANSPLANTATION
PATHOLOGY

Edited by

Phillip Ruiz
University of Miami

CAMBRIDGE
UNIVERSITY PRESS

CAMBRIDGE UNIVERSITY PRESS
Cambridge, New York, Melbourne, Madrid, Cape Town, Singapore, São Paulo, Delhi

Cambridge University Press
32 Avenue of the Americas, New York, NY 10013-2473, USA

www.cambridge.org
Information on this title: www.cambridge.org/9780521879958

© Cambridge University Press 2009

This publication is in copyright. Subject to statutory exception
and to the provisions of relevant collective licensing agreements,
no reproduction of any part may take place without the written
permission of Cambridge University Press.

First published 2009

Printed in the United States of America

A catalog record for this publication is available from the British Library.

Library of Congress Cataloging in Publication Data
Transplantation pathology / edited by Phillip Ruiz.
p. ; cm.
Includes bibliographical references and index.
ISBN 978-0-521-87995-8 (hardback)
1. Transplantation of organs, tissues, etc. – Complications.
2. Transplantation immunology. I. Ruiz, Phillip, 1954–
[DNLM: 1. Transplantation pathology. WO 660 T7697546 2009]
RD120.78.T74 2009
617.9'54–dc22   2008025898

ISBN 978-0-521-87995-8 (hardback)

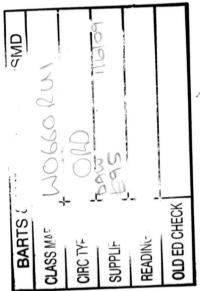

BARTS (
SMD
CLASS MA^r   WO660 RU\
CIRC TY^   OLD
SUPPLI^   DAW S
READIN^   £95
OLD ED CHECK

Every effort has been made in preparing this book to provide an accurate and up-to-date information that is in accordance with accepted standards and practice at the time of publication. Although case histories are drawn from actual cases, every effort has been made to disguise the identities of the individuals involved. Nevertheless, the authors, editors, and publishers can make no warranties that the information contained herein is totally free from error, not least because clinical standards are constantly changing through research and regulation. The authors, editors, and publishers therefore disclaim all liability for direct or consequential damages resulting from the use of material contained in this book. Readers are strongly advised to pay careful attention to information provided by the manufacturer of any drugs or equipment that they plan to use.

Cambridge University Press has no responsibility for the persistence or accuracy of URLs for external or third-party Internet Web sites referred to in this publication and does not guarantee that any content on such Web sites is, or will remain, accurate or appropriate. Information regarding prices, travel timetables, and other factual information given in this work are correct at the time of first printing, but Cambridge University Press does not guarantee the accuracy of such information thereafter.

To my wife, Cindie, to my kids, Jeffrey and Brianna, and to Mom, Dad, and my sis, Darlene.

Contents

Contributors

MANUEL CARRENO, M.D.
Department of Surgery
Transplant Laboratories
University of Miami Miller School of Medicine
Miami, Florida

ROBERT CIROCCO, M.D.
Department of Surgery
Transplant Laboratories
University of Miami Miller School of Medicine
Miami, Florida

ANTHONY J. DEMETRIS, M.D.
Department of Pathology
University of Pittsburgh School of Medicine
Pittsburgh, Pennsylvania
Division of Transplantation Pathology
University of Pittsburgh Medical Center
Pittsburgh, Pennsylvania

CINTHIA B. DRACHENBERG, M.D.
Department of Pathology
University of Maryland Medical Center
Baltimore, Maryland

MICHAEL C. FISHBEIN, M.D.
Departments of Medicine and Pathology
David Geffen School of Medicine at UCLA
Los Angeles, California

ROLANDO GARCIA-MORALES, M.D.
Department of Surgery
Transplant Laboratories
University of Miami Miller School of Medicine
Miami, Florida

ERIC D. HSI, M.D.
Section of Hematopathology
Department of Pathology
Cleveland Clinic
Lerner College of Medicine
Cleveland, Ohio

BRIAN R. KEEGAN, M.D., Ph.D.
Department of Dermatology
New York University School of Medicine
New York, New York

GARY KLEINER, M.D., Ph.D.
Department of Pediatric Allergy and Immunology
University of Miami
Miami, Florida

MICHAEL KRITZER-CHEREN, B.S.
Department of Molecular and Cell Pharmacology
University of Miami
Miami, Florida

CHI K. LAI, M.D., F.R.C.P.C.
Department of Surgical Pathology
David Geffen School of Medicine at UCLA
Los Angeles, California

EMMA L. LANUTI, M.D.
Department of Dermatology
University of Miami Miller School of Medicine
Miami, Florida

IZIDORE S. LOSSOS, M.D.
Department of Medicine
Lymphoma Program
University of Miami Miller School of Medicine
Miami, Florida

JAMES M. MATHEW, Ph.D.
Transplant Labs
Northeastern University Medical School
Chicago, Illinois

MICHAEL NALESNIK, M.D.
Division of Transplantation Pathology
Department of Pathology
University of Pittsburgh Medical Center
Montefiore University Hospital
Pittsburgh, Pennsylvania

VOLKER NICKELEIT, M.D.
Department of Pathology and Laboratory Medicine
University of North Carolina at Chapel Hill
Chapel Hill, North Carolina

ERIN OCHOA, M.D.
Division of Transplantation Pathology
Department of Pathology
University of Pittsburgh Medical Center
Montefiore University Hospital
Pittsburgh, Pennsylvania

JOHN C. PAPADIMITRIOU, M.D., Ph.D.
Division of Surgical Pathology
University of Maryland Medical Center
Baltimore, Maryland

SEONG RA, M.D.
Department of Pathology and Laboratory Medicine
David Geffen School of Medicine at UCLA
Los Angeles, California

PARMJEET RANDHAWA, M.D.
Division of Transplantation Pathology
Department of Pathology
University of Pittsburgh Medical Center
Montefiore University Hospital
Pittsburgh, Pennsylvania

MARCO ROMANELLI, M.D., Ph.D.
Department of Dermatology
University of Pisa
Pisa, Italy

PAOLO ROMANELLI, M.D.
Department of Dermatology
Division of Dermatopathology
University of Miami Miller School of Medicine
Miami, Florida

PHILLIP RUIZ, M.D., Ph.D.
Department of Surgery
Transplant Laboratories
University of Miami Miller School of Medicine
Miami, Florida

EIZABURO SASATOMI, M.D., Ph.D.
Department of Pathology
Division of Anatomic Pathology
University of Pittsburgh Medical Center
Pittsburgh, Pennsylvania

HIDENORI TAKAHASHI, M.D.
Department of Gastroenterological Surgery
Osaka University
Osaka, Japan

LAWRENCE TSAO, M.D.
Department of Clinical Pathology
Cleveland Clinic
Lerner College of Medicine
Cleveland, Ohio

ANDREAS TZAKIS, M.D.
Department of Surgery
University of Miami Miller School of Medicine
Miami, Florida

INGRID H. WOLF, M.D., Ph.D.
Division of General Dermatology
Medical University of Graz
Graz, Austria

TONG WU, M.D., Ph.D.
Department of Pathology
Division of Transplantation Pathology
University of Pittsburgh School of Medicine
Pittsburgh, Pennsylvania

HUI-MIN YANG, M.D.
Department of Pathology
UCLA David Geffen School of Medicine
Los Angeles, California
Department of Pathology
Cedars-Sinai Medical Center
Los Angeles, California

DANI S. ZANDER, M.D.
Department of Pathology
Pennsylvania State Hershey Medical Center
Hershey, Pennsylvania

Preface and Acknowledgments

The emergence of solid organ and stem cell transplantation as one of the medical miracles of the 20th century has necessitated the unending and indispensable collaboration of, among many others, basic scientists, clinicians, and physicians of all disciplines. Pathologists have been centrally poised in the development of transplantation because it is often the interpretation of the histological changes of the graft that determine whether the transplant is a success. Graft biopsies have presented a unique challenge to pathologists, because many of the morphological changes present in these cases are relatively new in their description, are often only rarely seen in general pathology practices, are constantly evolving as clinical protocols are adjusted, and often coexist with other changes that can occur in the native organ counterpart.

My interest in authoring and editing this textbook is anchored in my long-term active involvement in transplantation as an academic pathologist and in my observation of the need for a comprehensive compilation of the pathological changes present in numerous types of transplants now commonly performed. The scope of the chapters also goes beyond changes within the graft to include alterations seen in several critical native organs of the transplant patient, including skin, gastrointestinal tissue, and lymphoid organs. It is now clear that the role of the pathologist in the transplant team has evolved beyond histomorphologist and scientist. The pathologist, as those in many other areas of medicine, should have a strong working knowledge and should lead in the development of the ever-evolving clinical laboratory testing needed to monitor and evaluate the often clinically delicate transplant patient; thus, a chapter on lab medicine and transplantation has been provided. In particular, molecular biological–based testing continues to grow in importance as a means of assessing the transplant patient; numerous examples are present throughout this textbook. Finally, the pathologist must have, as with many other types of medical biopsies, a skilled understanding of the clinical features of the transplant patient – particularly in the time leading up to the biopsy – and of the patient's relevant past pre-transplant information. This latter point underscores the critical relationship that the pathologist *must* have with the transplant physicians and team to provide the most useful and accurate anatomical correlations with the ongoing clinical behavior of the patient. Relatedly, this textbook attempts to combine in many areas the clinical presentation of the patient and some current theory as to pathophysiological mechanisms with the morphological presentation in the biopsy specimen.

The production and writing of *Transplantation Pathology* would not have been possible without the contribution and cooperation of several of my esteemed friends and collaborators who are recognized experts in this subdiscipline of pathology. I am indebted to these coauthors for believing in and contributing to this endeavor and taking time from their busy schedules to provide what I consider to be excellent compilations of their particular areas of interest. This work would not have been possible without the patience and guidance of the fine people at Cambridge University Press, in particular, Marc Strauss, who first approached me about this project and who provided an abundance of ideas and suggestions that facilitated the entire process. I am deeply indebted to Cristina Hersh, Yasmine Perez, and Iliana Grana for their assistance in putting this work together and keeping it organized. I am also thankful to the many colleagues and mentors whom I have had the pleasure of working alongside over the years in the field of transplantation, most notably, Juan Scornik, Andreas Tzakis, and the late Wayne Streilein. Their dedication and enthusiasm for transplantation and immunology has always been infectious and the fuel that sustains my passion for this field. I am grateful to the dedicated group of physicians, nurses, lab technologists, and support staff comprising the outstanding transplant team at the University of Miami – their boundless energy and their compassion for our patients have always inspired me and make coming to work a labor of love. Neither this book nor my time in academia would have been possible without the continuous and loving support and sacrifices of my family, who have never questioned the long hours and who have facilitated my involvement in this rewarding field of medicine. Finally, I thank the transplant patients, who have entrusted their lives to our transplant team. The extraordinary and daily sacrifices of these remarkable individuals allow them to possess the miracle of a functioning organ from another person, and their willingness to undertake novel and often perilous new therapies or procedures permits us to acquire the necessary scientific foundation that will benefit future transplant populations.

Phillip Ruiz

CHAPTER 1

Immunopathology of Organ Transplantation

James M. Mathew, Ph.D.

Phillip Ruiz, M.D., Ph.D.

I. INTRODUCTION

i. A Historical Overview of Transplantation

The early history of transplantation is born of legends. The Saints Cosmas and Damian, who lived in the third century allegedly, treated a white patient by removing one of his legs and by grafting that of a black man who had died the same day (Figure 1.1) (1). In modern times, many experimental transplantations, mostly in dogs and cats and then in humans, were attempted in the twenties and thirties of the past century. Some of the pioneers of this era were Carrel, Jaboulay, and Voronoy. As can be expected, most of these trials ended in failures.

From the shaping work of Sir Peter B. Medawar, we now know that the failure of organ transplantation is due to immunologic reactions. Medawar et al. cited cases of patients with severe burns: autologous skin grafts healed in, but not allogeneic grafts, which were rejected, and in an accelerated fashion when taken repeatedly from the same donor (2). These observations led to extensive animal experimentations

in this area. As a result, a number of fundamental facts about organ transplantation became apparent – 1) a graft may be recognized as antigenic, and it may also be a source of immune cells; 2) this two-way immune response between recipient and donor necessitates the need for immunosuppression for the survival of the graft and the host; and 3) the ultimate goal of many of our efforts should be the induction and maintenance of immunologic tolerance.

The investigation of immunogenicity between grafts was discovered serendipitously. George Snell developed inbred mice, by consecutive brother-sister mating for studying tumor genetics. He observed that tumor grafts were accepted between inbred animals but not between animals of different strains (3). The same pattern of tissue acceptance and rejection was true for normal tissues. Snell in collaboration with Peter A. Gorer termed the underlying gene locus histocompatibility 2, or H-2. Further analysis revealed the locus to be genetically complex and the concept of the major histocompatibility complex (MHC) was born, providing the foundation for transplantation immunology

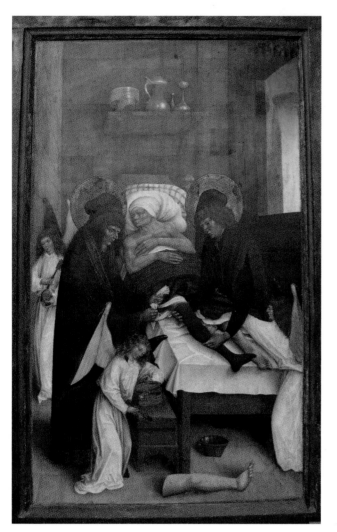

FIGURE 1.1: *Saints Cosmas and Damian. Attributed to the Master of Los Balbases (ca. 1495).*

and immunogenetics (4). The human MHC was delineated in the beginning of the fifties from a quite different discipline, that is, immunohematology. Jean Dausset observed that patients who had received many blood transfusions produced antibodies that could agglutinate white blood cells from donors but not the patient's own cells (5). Subsequent family studies indicated a genetically determined system, termed human leukocyte antigens (HLAs), and was found to be analogous with H-2 in the mouse. Research in mice and humans became mutually complementary and the Nobel Prize was awarded to Dausset in 1980, together with Snell. Further studies, mainly by Rolf Zinkernagel and Peter Doherty, revealed that MHC gene region products are vital in the regulation of immune responses: they are required for the presentation of peptide antigens to T-cell receptors (the MHC restriction) (6). However, in the context of transplantation between individuals, they became the most important markers of the biological incompatibility or main transplantation antigens.

II. BASIS OF ALLOREACTIVITY – HISTOCOMPATIBILITY ANTIGENS, NON-MHC; GRAFT IMMUNOGENICITY

The basis for alloreactive responses is genetic incompatibilities of components of tissue that are antigenic between the donor and the recipient. These moieties can be classified into three broad categories: the MHC antigens, minor histocompatibility antigens (mHags), and non-MHC or tissue-specific antigens.

i. Major Histocompatibility Antigens

The MHC of man encodes two major classes of proteins: HLA class I (HLA-A, -B, and -C) and HLA class II (HLA-DP, -DQ, and -DR) (7–11). *Class I molecules* are expressed on the surface of virtually all nucleated cells at varying densities. *Class II molecules* are expressed primarily by B lymphocytes, macrophages, and dendritic cells (DCs); however, molecules such as interferon-gamma can upregulate their expression on a variety of cell types, including endothelium, epithelium, and T lymphocytes.

The normal function of MHC molecules is to present *antigenic peptides* from proteins generated inside the cell or from an extracellular pool to T cells (12). MHC class I molecules on antigen-presenting cells (APCs) present endogenous antigens produced within the cell such as viruses and oncogenic products in the form of peptides of eight to ten amino acids long. These MHC-peptide complexes are recognized by cytotoxic CD8[+] T lymphocytes, which eliminate virally infected cells and tumor cells. Under normal circumstances, MHC class II on the APC present exogenous antigens as peptide fragments to CD4[+] helper T cells (Figure 1.2). However, a process known as cross-presentation of extracellular antigen on class I antigens to CD8[+] is also encountered (13). Two pathways for presenting peptides are determined by the mode of antigen uptake by the APC. For class I restricted presentation, surface mannose receptors route antigen to the stable early endosome compartment, where the peptides could meet MHC class I molecules. In contrast, pinocytosis of the same antigen directs it to the lysosomal compartment for presentation by class II MHC. These findings have helped to resolve questions about how APCs activate and modulate different arms of the T-cell response. Activated T helper cells produce cytokines that enhance T-cell activity and lead to the secretion of antibodies by B cells, which can eliminate extracellular antigens.

The MHC is highly *polymorphic*, enabling a species to have a greater collective immunity against pathogens, which are mutating constantly. Unfortunately, transplant rejection is a direct result of this polymorphism. The MHC molecules themselves act as primary antigens responsible for the induction of the alloimmune response.

ii. Minor Histocompatibility Antigens

Another group of antigens, the mHags, were discovered rather accidentally. The first report on the possible influence

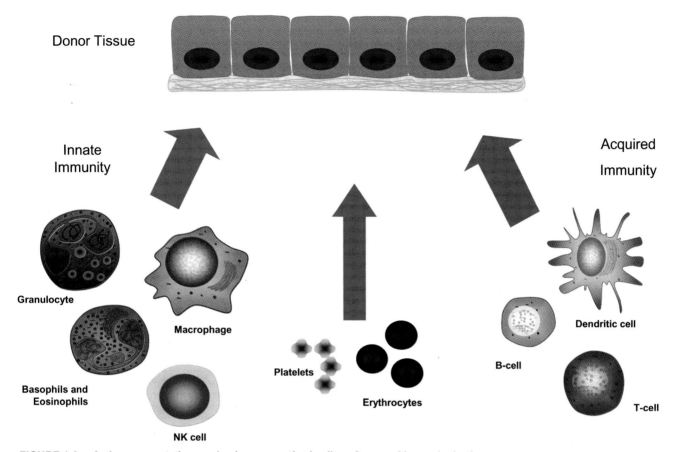

FIGURE 1.2: *Antigen presentation mechanisms operative in allograft recognition and rejection.*

of mHags on the outcome of bone marrow transplantation (BMT) was observed in a female aplastic anemia patient who rejected the bone marrow transplanted from her HLA-identical brother. Cytotoxic T cells (CTLs) isolated from the patient's blood lysed cells that were HLA matched and of male origin (14,15). The T-cell reactivity observed in the host-versus-graft (HvG) direction in this case was restricted to male cells, thus indicating that the target structures had to be encoded by a gene on the Y chromosome. Similarly, CTLs isolated from a patient suffering from severe graft-versus-host disease (GvHD) after HLA-identical BMT lysed patient's hematopoietic cells collected before BMT but not those of the donor (15). The mHag reactivity in this patient was directed against an antigen encoded by an autosomal gene. Various biochemical and molecular approaches have subsequently been used to characterize human mHags. So far more than nineteen autosomal and Y-chromosome–encoded mHags have been identified in humans (Table 1.1). The mHags are presented as peptides on the cell surface primarily by MHC class I and occasionally by class II molecules (16,17).

iii. Tissue-Specific Antigens

A third group of antigens expressed on allografts are *tissue-specific antigens*. The expressions of these antigens are restricted to various tissues and organs. There are a myriad of tissue-specific antigens that have been characterized, often through studies in cancer immunology and autoimmunity. In transplantation immunobiology, however, our understanding of these important groups of protein and glycoprotein tissue markers is very hazy and fragmented. Aside from anecdotal reports, no comprehensive study of these antigens is available mainly because of technical limitations. Most of the knowledge on this class of antigens has come from immunochemical analyses of rejected grafts from MHC-matched organs and BMT (18,19). Nevertheless, it is recognized that they exhibit some degree of polymorphism among individuals due to variations in their primary or secondary structures. These differences are the causative agents of alloreactivity.

III. IMMUNE NETWORKS INVOLVED IN ALLOREACTIVITY; HVG AND GVH, IMMUNE TOLERANCE

The MHC, mHag, and tissue-specific antigen differences between the donor and recipient result in alloreactive responses and are manifested clinically as HvG or as graft-versus-host (GvH) responses. In extreme cases, these reactions result in the loss of the graft or GvHD that can culminate in the death of the patient. However, in the

TABLE 1.1 mHags and Their Epitopes Identified at the Molecular Level

mHag*	HLA Restriction	Peptide Sequence**	mHag Gene#	References
mHags encoded by autosomal chromosome genes				
ACC1[Y]	A24	DYLQYVLQI	**BCL2A1**	245
ACC2[D]	B44	KEFEDDIINW	**BCL2A1**	245
ACC-4[R]	A*3303	WATLPLLCAR	CTSH	246
ACC-5[R]	A*3101	ATLPLLCAR	CTSH	246
ACC-6	B44	MEIFIEVFSHF	**HMSD**	247
CTL-7A7[R]	A3	RVWDLPGVLK	**PANE1**	248
DNR-7[R]	A3	SLPRGTSTPK	**SP110**	249
HA-1[H]	A*0201	VLHDDLLEA	**HMHA1**	250
HA-1[H]	A*0206	VLHDDLLEA	**HMHA1**	251
HA-1[H]	B60	KECVLHDDL	**HMHA1**	252
HA-2[V]	A*0201	YIGEVLVSV	**MYO1G**	253, 254
HA-3[T]	A1	VTEPGTAQY	AKAP13	255
HA-8[R]	A*0201	RTLDKVLEV	KIAA0020	256
HB-1[H]	B44	EEKRGSLHVV	**HMHB1**	257
HB-1[Y]	B44	EEKRGSLYVV	**HNHB1**	258
LB-ADIR-1[F]	A*0201	SVAPALALFPA	**TOR3A**	259
LRH-1	B7	TPNQRQNVC	**P2RX5**	260
RDR173[H]	B7	RPHAIRRPLAL	**ECGF1**	261
UGT2B17	A29	AELLNIPFLY	UGT2B17	262
mHags encoded by Y chromosome genes				
ACC-3	A*3303	EVLLRPGLHFR	TMSB4Y	246
DBY	DQ5	HIENFSDIDMGE	DDX3Y	263
DBY	DRB1*1501	GSTASKGRYIPPHLRNREA	DOX3Y	264
DFFRY	A*0101	IVDCLTEMY	USP9Y	265
RPS4Y	B*5201	TIRYPDPVI	RPS4Y1	266
RPS4Y	DRB3*0301	VIKVNDTVQI	RPS4Y1	16
SMCY	A*0201	FIDSYICQV	JARID1D	254
SMCY	B7	SPSVDKARAEL	JARID1D	254
UTY	B60	RESEEESVSL	UTY	267
UTY	B8	LPHNHTDL	UTY	268

* Original mHag name, if applicable, with allele as superscript.

** The polymorphic residues are underlined; in the case of Y-chromosomal mHags, amino acid difference from its X-homolog, if applicable, is underlined.

Genes expressed mainly in hematopoietic cells, potential targets for GVL effects, are shown in bold.

absence of an immune response or subsequent to overcoming one, the patient may achieve graft acceptance and true immunologic tolerance.

i. HvG Reactivity

When an organ is transplanted, the donor-derived polymorphic MHC, mHags, non-MHC, or tissue-specific molecules are recognized as foreign by the recipient. An immune response is then mounted that will destroy the transplanted organ unless effective immunosuppressive measures are taken. Organ rejection can be classified clinically as hyperacute, acute, subacute, and chronic (20). Hyperacute responses occur within minutes, are antibody mediated, and tend to be irreversible. Acute and subacute responses generally are cell mediated or antibody mediated, occur in a span of days to months, and can be reversed with a variety of immunosuppressive reagents. Chronic rejection occurs in the span of months to years,

is typically unresponsive to current therapy, and has emerged as the major problem facing transplant biologists.

It has long been observed that donor alloantigens can be presented to the recipient immune system via either the direct or the indirect antigen presentation pathways (Figure 1.2). In the *direct pathway*, intact donor class I and II MHC molecules present on the surface of *donor APC* are recognized directly *by recipient* CD8+ and CD4+ T cells, respectively. In the *indirect pathway*, donor allopeptides are taken up, processed, and presented in the context of *recipient MHC* molecules to *recipient* CD8+ and CD4+ T cells (21,22). The T-cell receptor repertoire displays a high frequency of alloreactive T cells in the direct pathway and a relatively low frequency in the indirect pathway. This suggests that direct allorecognition is responsible for early rejection episodes, while indirect allorecognition accounts for late rejection events. This is consistent with the notion that donor APC in the transplanted organ steadily disappear with time, making the direct pathway

INDIRECT

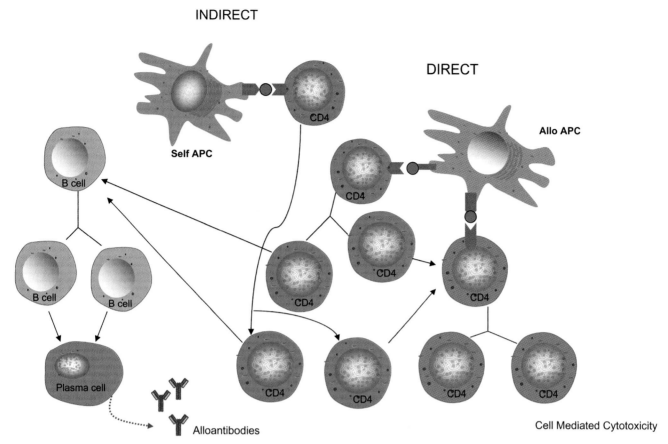

FIGURE 1.3: *Different cell types involved in allograft rejection.*

progressively inoperative. In contrast, the acquisition, processing, and presentation of donor antigens are a slower process that is more efficient during later stages after transplantation. A third pathway has also been proposed, the *semidirect pathway* (22) linking the two previous pathways. In this pathway, recipient DCs can acquire intact MHC molecules from donor cells and undertake direct presentation to recipient T cells. There is a growing body of evidence suggesting that alloreactive CD4$^+$ and CD8$^+$ T cells with specificity for both direct and indirect pathways contribute to graft rejection.

Recipient or donor T lymphocytes (CD4$^+$) recognize foreign HLA class II antigens in the allograft (Figure 1.2) and are activated to proliferate, differentiate, and secrete a variety of cytokines. These cytokines *increase* nascent expression of HLA class II antigens on engrafted tissues, such as vascular endothelium. These mediators also stimulate B lymphocytes to produce high-affinity and high-titer antibodies against the allograft, and potentiate CTLs, macrophages, and natural killer (NK) cells to develop cytotoxicity against the graft (Figures 1.2 and 1.3).

ii. GvHD

GvHD, a common complication of allogeneic hematopoietic stem cell transplantation, can also occur, albeit less frequently after solid organ transplantation. The first case was reported in 1988 (23) and the incidence of GvHD in adult liver transplant recipients is estimated to be 1–2 percent (24–27). GvHD in other (nonhepatic) solid organ transplant recipients appears somewhat less frequent although it remains a complication that should always be considered when there is a suspicious clinical presentation (see Chapter 9). Progressively lower GvHD is observed in recipients of small bowel, combined small bowel-liver allografts, or multivisceral transplants; recipients of kidney, combined kidney-pancreas, and pancreas-spleen allografts; and recipients of heart, lung, or combined heart-lung allografts (28). This profile suggests that GvHD is dependent on the transfer of a high enough "inoculum" of donor lymphocytes, probably through lymphoid tissue within and surrounding the organ being transplanted (29,30). These donor effector immune cells then mediate a vigorous and often protracted assault on host tissues. The mortality of patients diagnosed with GvHD can be very high (31–33); therefore, although GvHD affects only a relatively small number of patients, it can be a devastating complication for those who experience it. Risk factors suggested for GvHD in liver transplant recipients include close HLA match between donor and recipient (34), advanced recipient age (31,32), and underlying recipient immunodeficiency may be a contributing factor (32,33).

GvHD occurs in both *acute and chronic forms*, each with different kinetics and distinctive pathology. The principal target organs of acute GvHD are skin, liver, gut, lung, and lymphoid tissues. Much of our understanding of the GvHD process has been acquired through studies in BMT. These studies have indicated that acute GvHD can be considered in a framework of *three sequential phases*: conditioning (phase 1), donor T-cell activation (phase 2), and cellular and inflammatory effectors (phase 3) (35). Donor T cells infused into a host that has been profoundly damaged by underlying disease, infection, and the transplant-conditioning regimen result in substantial proinflammatory changes in endothelial and epithelial cells. Then antigen presentation and the subsequent activation, proliferation, and differentiation of donor T cells result in *alloreactivity* within secondary lymphoid organs (35,36). Direct and indirect antigen presentations are both involved, that is, donor T cells can be directly activated *by host-derived APCs* or *donor-derived APCs*, which cross-present host antigens (35). Changes in phase 1 dramatically influence antigen presentation. Host DCs can mature and be activated (37) by 1) inflammatory cytokines such as tumor necrosis factor-alpha (TNF-α) and interleukin-1 (IL-1), 2) microbial products such as lipopolysaccharide (LPS) and CpG oligonucleotides entering systemic circulation from intestinal mucosa damaged by conditioning, and 3) necrotic cells that were damaged by conditioning. This activation enhances the recognition of MHC antigens or mHags by mature donor T cells.

iii. Immune Tolerance

Tolerance is the *specific absence of an immune response to a given antigen* and is the ever elusive holy grail of clinical transplantation. Based upon our current approach to clinical organ transplantation, true immunologic tolerance is an infrequent occurrence whose underlying mechanisms are only partly understood. The preferred situation with tolerance in transplantation is the lack of a specific *pathogenic* response. Although tolerance can be achieved in animal models through appropriately timed disruption of numerous immune mechanisms, applications of the same methodologies to clinical organ transplantation as of yet have not led to similar success (38). Nevertheless, any meaningful discussion on tolerance can only be made based mostly on these studies in animal models. Tolerance is the default response to a multitude of self- and environmental antigens, and many of the mechanisms that maintain self-tolerance may *also* be capable of promoting allograft tolerance (39). *Tolerance mechanisms* can be broadly classified as either central or peripheral (40). Peripheral tolerance mechanisms in turn include ignorance (41,42), anergy (43–45), regulation or suppression (46–51), and apoptosis or peripheral deletion (52–55) (Table 1.2).

1. Central tolerance: Central tolerance refers to the deletion within the thymus of T cells whose affinity for self-antigens is inappropriately high and thus likely to result in autoimmunity (56–58). The tolerance displayed by neonatal mice to a transplanted organ or mice displaying mixed hematopoietic chimerism following BMT are examples of the central deletional mechanisms. In addition to central deletion, a number of mechanisms operating in the periphery have been reported to contribute to the tolerant state.

2. Ignorance: Ignorance as a mechanism mediating tolerance was demonstrated by Lakkis et al. who showed that naive mice lacking secondary lymphoid organs accepted skin or heart allografts indefinitely (59). Impaired rejection in this model resulted from the failure of T cells to be primed when they encountered donor antigens outside of lymphoid organs. However, later observations that in some settings recipient T cells can be primed by alloantigens encountered within the allograft (60) and that memory T cells can be reactivated after encountering antigen outside of secondary lymphoid organs (61,62) suggest that the role of this mechanism may be limited.

3. Suppression: Active, antigen-specific suppression of immune responses was first reported in the 1970s (63,64). Though interest in this phenomenon waned, it was rekindled by the demonstration that CD4$^+$CD25$^+$

TABLE 1.2 Tolerance Mechanisms in Transplantation

Tolerance	Mediated by	Mechanism
Central	Deletion	Reactive clones deleted in the thymus by positive or negative selection. Reviewed in [57].
Peripheral	Regulation	Regulatory cell subsets of T-cell, NK cell, DC, and B-cell lineages actively inhibiting the responses of reactive clones.
	Anergy	Incomplete activation of clones by the binding of the primary receptor (TcR or BCR) by cognate antigen in the absence of the second signal.
	Clonal exhaustion	Prolonged and sustained stimulation result in the over exertion of the clones, which in turn make them incapable of further response.
	Deletion	Removal of the reactive clones by active killing, antibody-dependent cellular cytotoxicity, apoptosis, cytokine starvation, and so forth.

FIGURE 1.4: *FoxP3+ cells in formalin-fixed human tissue (immunofluorescence microscopy, 200×).*

T cells in murine models when eliminated could result in autoimmune disorders (65,66). A growing body of experimental and clinical evidence suggests a role for regulatory T cells in the induction and maintenance of tolerance (67,68). While CD4$^+$CD25$^+$ cells constitute the most widely recognized phenotype of regulatory cells, cells of other lineages including NK1.1, C8$^+$CD28$^-$, and CD3$^+$CD4$^-$CD8$^-$ cells may display regulatory properties (69–72). Other markers of regulatory T cells may also include CD45RB (73), GITR (74,75), CTLA4 (76,77), and CD103 (78–80). However, the intracellular forkhead/winged-helix transcription factor (FoxP3) has been suggested as the default marker of true regulatory T cells (Figure 1.4) (49,81).

At least three mechanisms appear to be important for tolerance mediated by regulatory T cells. Preclinical and clinical evidence suggests that T$_R$1, T$_H$3, and NKT cells (82,83) mediate regulatory effects at least in part via production of the *cytokines* IL-10 (84) and transforming growth factor-beta (TGF-β) (85). The function of CD4$^+$ CD25$^+$ T regs also appears to be affected by the expression of the cell surface molecules GITR (74,75) and CTLA4 (76,77), which may contribute to the contact-dependent effects of regulatory cells. Finally, anergic CD4$^+$ T cells may mediate their regulatory effects by inhibiting the maturation and function of DCs (86,87).

Although regulatory T cells have been extensively studied in experimental systems, far less is known about their role in *clinical tolerance*. Salama et al. reported that CD25$^+$ regulatory cells developed as early as three months after renal transplantation and persisted for years (88). Our own studies have supported and complemented these findings (89). Additional evidence of regulation was observed in rejection-free recipients than those who had experienced rejection using ex vivo

ELISPOT analysis. Analysis of a limited number of operationally tolerant transplant recipients using the transvivo Delayed Type Hypersensitivity (DTH) assay has also suggested a role for regulation that was dependent upon the production of TGF-β (90,91) and/or IL-10 and the expression of CTLA4. Although transplant tolerance may develop as a result of spontaneous regulatory mechanisms, *clinical application* of regulation is likely to require interventions that purposely produce regulatory cells. These approaches include donor-specific transfusion (92–94), donor bone marrow cell (DBMC) (89,95,96) infusions, and clinical use of in vitro–generated regulatory T cells (97). These protocols often depend on the donor cells themselves functioning as regulatory cells and/or on the exposure to tolerogenic donor antigens to induce the recipient to develop regulatory T cells. Alternately, exposure to dominant donor antigens expressed by the transplanted organ facilitates the recipient T cells to be tolerized to most other donor antigens as well. This phenomenon is known as *linked suppression* (98,99). In rodent and large animal models, the expression of one MHC molecule recognized by regulatory T cells effectively suppresses the response to other mismatched MHC molecules. A final consideration pertinent to the clinical application of regulatory mechanisms is the possible effect of currently used immunosuppressive agents on T regs. Although still controversial, some agents such as calcineurin inhibitors may inhibit the development of tolerance by preventing the activation or function of regulatory T cells. Other agents may preferentially spare T regs when eliminating other immune cell populations.

4. Anergy and deletion: In addition to ignorance and regulation, peripheral deletion of alloreactive T cells may contribute to tolerance (52,53). This can occur in the setting of chronic alloantigen stimulation or when alloantigen is encountered under suboptimal conditions for T-cell activation. *Clonal exhaustion* has been reported after liver transplantation as an example of how chronic stimulation may induce peripheral T-cell deletion (100). Infusions of DBMC that may lack optimal antigen presentation or result in prolonged (micro) chimerism may facilitate clonal exhaustion. Alternatively, the *blockade of costimulatory signals* such as CD28 or CD154 at the time T cells encounter alloantigens has been reported to result in incomplete T-cell activation, anergy, and apoptosis (101,102). It is a distinct possibility that prolonged and sustained anergy can result in the deletion of the reactive clones. Peripheral deletion of T-cell clones can be mediated by apoptosis and this can contribute to long-term allograft acceptance (103,104). *Apoptosis* of T cells can be brought about either by cell surface death receptors or cytokine withdrawal. The death receptors mediating

TABLE 1.3 Mechanisms of Graft Injury

Deleterious Effects	Mediators	Mechanism
Innate immune activation	TLRs, inflammatory cytokines, and chemokines	Injuries, trauma of death, ischemia, and other insults result in inflammation and activation of APCs. This in turn may initiate adaptive immunity.
AR	Antibody mediated	Preformed antibodies to MHC, ABO, mHags, and tissue-specific antigens bind to their cognate receptors in the graft and activate the complement pathway.
	Cell mediated	Chemokines and cytokines attract and upregulated adhesion molecules retain immune cells, predominantly activated CD4 and CD8 T cells, and a smattering of monocytes, B cells, and NK cells, resulting in tissue damage.
Chronic rejection	Cellular infiltration, T helper 1/inflammatory cytokines secretion, and antibody deposition	The actions of the immune mediators occur late and for extended duration in the post-transplant period. May result in the fibrosis of various structures of the allograft.
Infection	Viral — CMV, EBV, polyoma, hepatitis C, and so forth	Direct pathogenic effects and indirect anti-infection immunity may cause inflammation, arteriosclerosis, or cirrhosis of the allograft.
Recurrent/de novo immune diseases	Recurrence of the original disease for which the native organ needed to be transplanted	

apoptosis comprise TNF receptor superfamily members that have a cytoplasmic death domain that binds cell-signaling proteins such as TRADD, FADD, FLICE, and caspase-3 (105–107). Cytokines promoting T-cell survival include the common [gamma] chain cytokines IL-2, IL-4, IL-7, and IL-15, and their absence predisposes cells to apoptotic death.

IV. MECHANISMS OF GRAFT INJURY

The principal causes of graft injury can be summarized as those resulting from ischemia, innate immune activation, protracted inflammation with accompanying elaboration of soluble factors, followed by acute and then chronic rejection episodes that are mediated by donor-specific antibodies, and/or active cellular infiltrations. In fact, a variety of cell types (Figure 1.3) and mediators can inflict injury to an organ allograft. Infections and recurrent/de novo immune diseases may also produce concomitant tissue damage (Table 1.3).

i. The Effects of Ischemia and Innate Immune Activation

The absence of appropriate blood flow to harvested organs (ischemia) and the return of blood supply to the allograft (reperfusion) can result in a wide variety of inflammatory and oxidative changes that can influence short- and long-term graft function (Figure 1.5). In addition to ischemia/reperfusion (I/R) injury, infections and genetic polymorphisms in the recipient can also contribute to activation of innate immune mechanisms that may then amplify antigen-specific (i.e., allospecific) acquired immune responses. Unfortunately, this may be the etiology of acute

rejection (AR) and may also contribute to long-term allograft injury through a potentiation of chronic rejection (108–110). This activation of the innate immune system by these forms of injury typically is more pronounced in cadaveric donors, although it may also be seen to a lesser degree in living donors, depending on the situation (110). The effects of I/R injury and infections in the newly transplanted organ, aside from innate immune activation, also results in the increased appearance of a variety of molecules that augment immune pathways and that likely underlies that potentiation of the acquired alloimmune response in the host. Among the molecules that are modified by early nonspecific graft injury are HLA antigens,

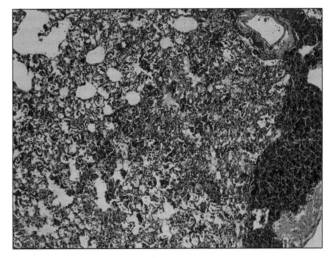

FIGURE 1.5: *Lung undergoing severe I/R injury with alveolar hemorrhage, neutrophils, necrosis, and vascular congestion (hematoxylin and eosin [H&E], 200×).*

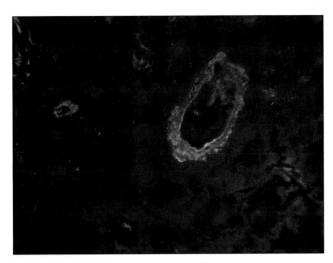

FIGURE 1.6: *C3 in kidney following I/R injury (immunofluorescence, 400×).*

adhesion molecules, various complement molecules, and molecules involved in the activation of the innate immune response (Figure 1.6); the early presence of these molecules may (111–113) identify patients at higher risk for early graft dysfunction.

There are a variety of adhesion molecules that appear altered in an allograft following nonspecific injury such as I/R injury or infection (111–113). For example, intracellular adhesion molecule 1 (ICAM-1), RANTES, vascular cell adhesion molecule 1 (VCAM-1), lymphocyte function–associated antigen (LFA-1), LFA-3, and CD40 ligand (CD40L) can be increased in organs with increased ischemic time exposure. The presence of these molecules on several cell types may contribute to delayed graft function (114–116).

Among the effects of I/R injury to the allograft has been increased expression of major and minor histocompatibility molecules in a variety of cell types in the transplant. Increased MHC class I, major histocompatibility class I–related chain A (MIC-A) and MIC-B, and de novo MHC class II have all been described to increase in allografts following ischemic injury (117–121). Allografts that have aberrant class II expression on certain parenchymal structures (e.g., tubular cells) may be predisposed to increased risk from inflammatory injury (122,123). The induction of class I or class II molecule expression in allografts has no particular pattern of expression among different types of transplants and may be difficult to predict. Certainly, the aforementioned stressors such as I/R injury can increase MHC antigen expression in the graft, depending on the procurement situation and the type of organ being harvested. The appearance of class II expression is typically immediate and associated with the initial injury, but it can also be sustained for an extended period (e.g., up to a year after transplantation) that can serve as continual source of antigenic stimulation on epithelial and endothelial structures in the graft (124–126).

Antibody-mediated allograft rejection has recently re-emerged as an important and oft underrecognized form of rejection that may be present in subclinical forms of injury to the transplant. Complement proteins are critical mediators of this and other forms of inflammatory injury to the graft, and these molecules can also be induced following nonspecific injury in the early post-transplant period (127). Biopsies taken from allografts experiencing preservation injury can demonstrate diffusely distributed C3 and other split products on many structures of the viscera. This can vary, as mentioned above with the other induced molecules, according to the extent and conditions of injury and the type of allograft being harvested (128,129). The source of the increased complement production can be intrinsic (many cell types can produce complement) and/or from infiltrating inflammatory cells (130).

Toll-like receptors (TLRs) are membrane-spanning receptors that recognize structurally conserved molecules derived from microbes; upon their recognition, these molecules may activate immune cell responses via the innate immune system. TLRs have been demonstrated on harvested organs exposed to I/R injury (131–133). In myocardial ischemia models, TLR 2 and 4 expression was found to correlate with infarct size and subsequent left ventricular dysfunction (134,135). Simultaneously, "endogenous" innate immune ligands may be released during inflammation. Such putative ligands include heat shock proteins (HSPs), uric acid, oligimers of hyaluronan, fibrinogen, and chromatin (136–142). Some of these ligands have been found to signal via TLRs, predominantly TLR 4. These studies remain controversial since the effect of confounding LPS may not have been completely excluded (136).

HSPs are cytoplasmic chaperone proteins that have a variety of functions and that are inducible under stress conditions such as heat and injury. In organ transplants, I/R injury and infections can induce the expression of this family of molecules (108–110,143–145) with variable expression according to the type of allograft and the extent of injury (144,146). Ultimately, the roles that HSPs play in graft injury remains undetermined — it is possible that these proteins may contribute to potentiating the alloimmune response and/or they may be cytoprotective and behave as chaperone proteins that allow the cells to survive biochemical insults (146–148).

All transplanted organs inherently possess a system of *innate immune defenses* and a number of the above-mentioned molecules contribute to an activation of this form of immunity. What remains uncertain is the importance of innate immunity in the context of affecting the specific adaptive immune response to the allograft. Certainly, the infiltrating inflammatory cells and the epithelial cell components of these grafts all contribute in a complex interplay to induce, perpetuate, and be affected by the activated innate immune system (149,150). Future studies will continue to address this critical relationship between these two facets of the immune system and how this contributes to graft injury or acceptance.

In addition to increased expression of various molecules, there is also an influx of various cell populations following surgery, I/R injury, and other insults in the early period, including professional antigen-presenting DCs (149), NK cells (151), and augmented resident T cells (152).

ii. Acute Rejection

The mechanisms by which allografts may experience AR are complex and can involve almost all components of the immune system. The humoral arm of the immune response (antibody mediated), the cellular or cell-mediated arm, or a combination of both processes are the general ways that alloimmune responses are manifested in the recipient toward the graft.

1. Antibody-Mediated AR

A notable proportion of AR derives from underlying anti-donor antibody that is formed de novo following the implantation of the graft or that was present before the transplant was performed. Preformed anti-HLA antibody may be present in recipients who had transfusions, pregnancies, or prior transplants (153,154). ABO antibodies can also be involved in antibody-mediated AR.

Alloantibody causes injury to the transplant via mechanisms similar to how antibody affects other pathogens (e.g., bacteria) that confront the host. The alloantibody is generally either class IgM or IgG and binds specifically to allopeptides present on the structures such as endothelium of the graft (Figure 1.7) (128,155,156). The binding may be high or low affinity in nature, and following this specific interaction, there can be fixation of complement. An intricate series of events then ensues where the complement cascade is

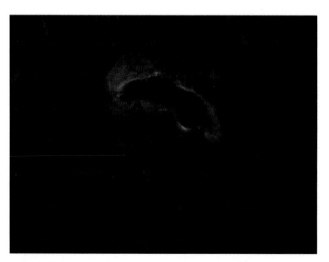

FIGURE 1.7: *IgG along vessel in kidney undergoing humoral AR (immunofluorescence, 400×).*

FIGURE 1.8: *C4d along vessel in kidney undergoing humoral AR (immunofluorescence, 400×).*

activated, releasing numerous soluble factors that can attract and activate cells of the immune system, including allospecific T cells and monocytes. This results in vascular injury (often because of endothelial cell targeting and injury), hemorrhage, and secondary inflammation throughout many areas of the allograft. Some of the complement components remain bound in covalent fashion to cell structures and this has been utilized to help identify in tissue specimens the occurrence of humoral immune processes. For example, C4d and to a lesser extent C3d are split products that have been identified in tissue sections (both paraffin and frozen sections) as "markers" of antibody-antigen interactions (157,158) (Figure 1.8). In fact, C4d staining in peritubular capillaries is now being used as one of the criteria to classify antibody-mediated rejection in kidneys, although the staining patterns may change over time (159) and there now appear to be antibody-mediated ARs that are negative for C4d in kidney and other allografts (160,161). Regardless, the presence of antibody-mediated AR in allografts, as identified by typical morphology, immunostaining, or particular cellular constituents (e.g., monocytes) (162–167) in association with peripheral donor-specific antibodies, generally correlates with reduced graft survival (153,154,168,169).

2. Cell-Mediated AR

Cell-mediated AR is the most common form of rejection in allografts and can vary notably in degrees of intensity, depending upon numerous factors such as the degree of incompatibility, the timing of the rejection, the level of immunosuppression, and the type of allograft in question (60). There are not typically pathognomonic or unique lesions but rather a constellation of morphological changes. The unifying change that most grafts demonstrate is a diffuse accumulation of chronic inflammatory cells (e.g., lymphocytes, macrophages) within the

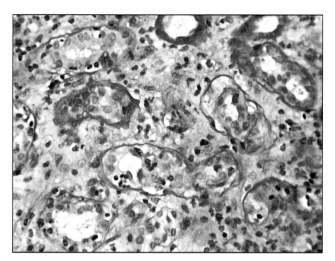

FIGURE 1.9: *Acute cellular rejection in a kidney with extensive tubulitis (periodic acid Schiff, 400×).*

interstitial spaces that contain connective tissue elements. These cells, most prominently being T cells, then infiltrate and cause injury to epithelial (e.g., kidney tubules, liver bile ducts, intestinal crypts) and vascular structures (Figure 1.9). Other cell populations, including NK/NKT cells, monocytes/macrophages, and B cells also contribute to the cell-mediated AR of transplants (60,170,171) but do not appear as critical as T cells. Among the roles of these alternate populations are antigen presentation (166,167), cell lysis, and recruitment/activation of inflammatory cells and inflammatory molecule cascades (172,173). The identification of the cells causing cell-mediated rejection can be achieved by routine histology, immunohistochemistry, cytofluorographic analysis, and molecular techniques. The relative composition of the different T-cell subtypes within rejecting allografts has been extensively examined and appears to have a relationship to the extent and severity of rejection (174–177) (Figure 1.10). There are other approaches that can also be used to examine the differentiation stage of the T cells and their level of activation (178,179); however, these more elaborate characterizations of the infiltrating T cells have for all practical purposes not yielded a higher diagnostic efficacy than routine histology and immunohistochemistry. It is hoped that characterization of cell subtypes in these organs may ultimately yield tools by which responses to therapy and the ability to be weaned from immunosuppression can be predicted.

The means by which T cells identify and localize to allografts in cell-mediated rejection is better understood although there are certainly mechanisms unique to certain organ systems. For example, CD103 appears to serve as a receptor for particular cell compartments such as epithelium of kidney transplants (180,181) (Figure 1.11). Corresponding mechanisms are almost certainly present in other solid organ allografts. Similarly, inducible lymphocyte costimulatory molecules such as CD40L and CTLA-4 are also present in the allograft cell infiltrates and are vitally important in the migration and differentiation of potent alloreactive cell populations (182,183). The means by which specific (e.g., T cells) and nonspecific (e.g., NK cells) effector cells cause injury and apoptosis to graft cells is varied but one prominent system is the perforin/granzyme family of molecules. These enzymatic molecules expressed by effector CD8+ T cells can cause lysis of cells and thus the presence of these proteins in the allograft can be indicative of an active and ongoing cell-mediated AR (184–186). The measurement of these two molecules can be performed in situ by immunohistochemistry (187,188) (Figure 1.12) or by molecular techniques such as polymerase chain reaction, where the mRNA levels of perforin and granzyme in tissue and fluids such as urine may be heralding an acute cell-mediated rejection episode.

As mentioned before, aberrant expression of histocompatibility molecules, both class I and II, occurs when there is "stress" such as I/R injury. Likewise, AR can also result in HLA class I and class II antigens to be upregulated within the allografts (189,190); this, among other changes, can help perpetuate and sustain the AR (191–193). Adhesion molecules such as the selectins, VLA4-VCAM, and LFA-1-ICAM are also influenced and affected by the presence of rejection (194–196). These latter molecules certainly contribute to the localization and binding of various immune cell populations.

Among the families of molecules appearing vital to the recruitment of leukocytes into allografts are chemokines. These molecules appear increased in concentration in various transplanted organs from experimental models and in clinical samples (175,197–199). As with most other studies of molecules involved in graft rejection, chemokines have been identified by immunohistochemical and molecular means. In particular, CXCR3 and CCR5 appear vitally important in the progression of AR (197–200) and their blockade may attenuate graft rejection (201–204). The RANTES/CCL5 protein has also been identified in several anatomical compartments of rejecting renal allografts (205,206).

iii. Chronic Rejection

Chronic rejection of organ allografts remains as the principal challenge to the successful attainment of long-term graft function and survival (109,110). In spite of the remarkable success in treating AR over the past two decades, it remains that many clinical transplants continue to experience sustained deposition of fibroelastic material in many compartments of the organ as a result of obliterative vascular injury typical of chronic rejection (Figure 1.13). The result has been that *long-term* graft survival has not notably improved as compared to twenty years ago. The underlying causes of chronic rejection are varied and appear to involve interplay of immunologic and nonimmunologic variables in the recipient (207–210). Alloimmune

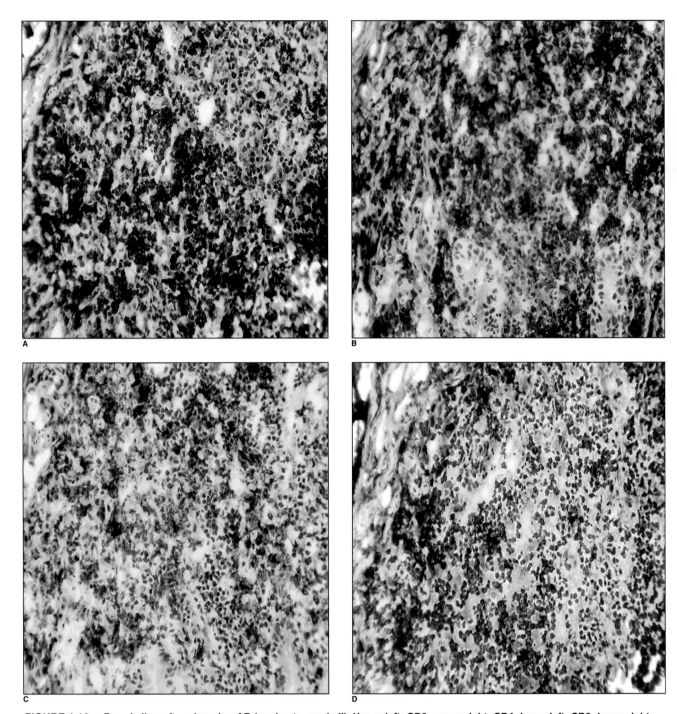

FIGURE 1.10: Bowel allograft undergoing AR (moderate, grade II). Upper left: CD3; upper right: CD4; lower left: CD8; lower right: HLA class II (200×).

processes associated with acute or subclinical rejection, I/R injury, donor and recipient variables, and as yet determined factors all simultaneously contribute to the overall injury characterized as chronic rejection.

The central and most important lesion in chronic rejection appears to be the progressive arteriopathy affecting small and large muscular arterial vessels. This lesion differs from atherosclerotic lesions in that it is diffusely distributed, has minimal lipid deposition, and has concentric lamination due to intimal hyperplasia and advential scarring. An interruption of this lesion may ultimately lead to a cessation of the downstream chronic injury in the graft that involves the interstitium and other parenchymal structures (211). Alloimmune responses appear central to the development of the graft arteriopathy since it is not seen in syngeneic models of transplantation. Antibody-mediated rejection appears to be the predominant form of alloimmunity necessary to develop this vasculopathy as based on experimental

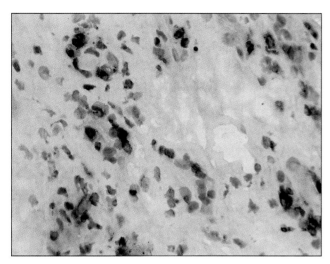

FIGURE 1.11: *CD103+ cells in kidney tubules from allograft undergoing rejection.*

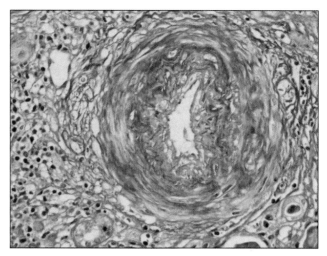

FIGURE 1.13: *Photomicrograph of kidney allograft, showing characteristic vascular lesion in chronic rejection with fibrointimal thickening and medial hyperplasia. The surrounding interstitium contains extensive fibrosis (trichrome, 400×).*

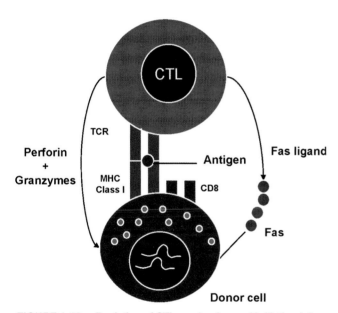

FIGURE 1.12: *Depiction of CTL mechanisms of inflicting injury on donor cells.*

and clinical evidence (212–214) although cell-mediated immunity also plays a role. Graft endothelial cells and smooth muscle cells are likely the principal target of the alloantibodies and CTLs — injury to these cells results in their undergoing apoptosis and removal, as well as proliferative changes of "repair" cell populations. There is also upregulation of molecules within the allograft and release of cytokines by injured endothelial and smooth muscle cells that facilitate the influx of cell populations such as activated macrophages and lymphocytes into the vessel (215,216). This culminates in matrix synthesis and cell proliferation. Finally, *host* precursor smooth muscle cells continue to add to the concentric lesion as it progresses (217).

The etiology of *graft fibrosis* within the interstitial regions centrally involves the inflammatory cell populations that are identifiable with AR, namely T lymphocytes and monocytes/macrophages (218,219). There is an eliciting of matrix proteins and fibrogenic factors that appears to begin in perivascular areas (220) and that culminates in the widespread diffuse fibrosis evident in end-stage chronically rejected organs. The mechanisms involved in the development of graft fibrosis are similar to fibrosis present in other disorders involving native organs, and thus, the targets for the prevention of fibrosis will ultimately be similar between transplants and native fibrogenic processes (221). There is a regenerative phase and fibroplasia phase (222) where the inflammatory, repair, and tissue remodeling processes occur simultaneously. Briefly, the injured graft tissue (likely vessels more than other components) exposes tissue determinants to platelets and an entire series of events ensue including platelet degranulation and production of matrix metalloproteinases that further compromise basement membranes and allow inflammatory cell influx with their production of cytokines and growth factors (223,224). Endothelial cells then surround the injured areas and profibrotic mediators promote differentiation of fibroblasts into myofibroblasts, which lay down extracellular matrix (ECM) components such as collagen. Unfortunately, this process is not well controlled and there is an excess ECM deposition with ineffectual remodeling, culminating in fibrosis. Chemokines can help regulate this process as well as the composition of the innate and adaptive immune cell populations involved in these pathways (223,224); TGF-β (225,226) and its isoforms appear to play a very critical role in graft fibrogenesis as well as angiotensin II (227) and plasminogen activator inhibitor (228).

iv. Infection

All transplant recipients are at an increased risk for the development of infections and this complication is not only

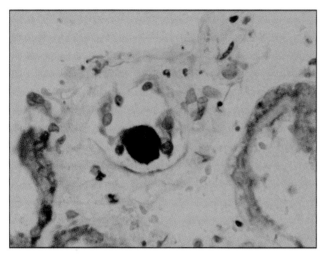

FIGURE 1.14: *CMV inclusion in crypt of bowel allograft (immunoperoxidase, 600×).*

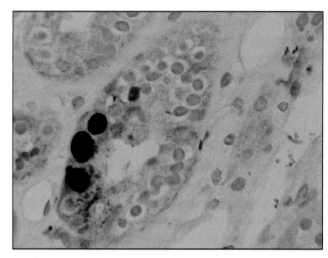

FIGURE 1.15: *Polyoma-infected tubular cells in renal allograft (immunoperoxidase, SV-40 antibody, 600×).*

the most frequent problem facing this patient population but also the most common cause of serious morbidity and mortality. Significant advances in the prophylaxis and treatment of infections following transplantation has decreased the rate of these complications (229) although the problem remains as a frequent barrier to success. The scope of infections is wide and dependent on numerous factors that include type of transplant, type of recipient, underlying coexisting disease, degree of immunosuppression, timing after transplantation, iatrogenic variables, and environmental conditions. All organ sites can be affected and the scope of infections includes bacterial, viral, protozoan, and fungal, many often in coexistence. The presence of infections aside from their direct toxicity to the host may also indirectly potentiate AR and chronic rejection processes and, on occasion, trigger autoimmune inflammation in the recipient.

Several specific infections are prominent in the transplant patient populations with some examples listed below. Cytomegalovirus (CMV) remains a frequent source of infection in transplantation (229–231) (Figure 1.14). CMV, a β-herpes-virus can have life-long latency or persistence within the host. There is a rise of CMV-specific antibodies, often within the first three months after transplantation. CMV-seronegative recipients of an organ from a CMV-seropositive donor are at highest risk for disease. Patients can present with a viral syndrome that includes fever and myalgia and organ disease can result, often within the transplanted organ but can involve many other sites (e.g., central nervous system, eye, urogenital, gastrointestinal tracts).

CMV may potentiate graft rejection by priming immune cell populations (232). Moreover, CMV also possesses the potential to augment allograft vasculopathy (233), a feature ascribed to several other viruses such as enterovirus, parvovirus, and adenovirus (234).

Polyoma BK virus (BKV) is a DNA virus in which many people (estimated 60–90 percent) are seropositive.

This virus tends to remain latent without primary symptoms and reactivation can occur in renal transplant recipients (estimated 10–68 percent) (235,236). A minor proportion (1–10 percent) of these patients with BKV reactivation progress to BKV nephropathy; the latter then can be diagnosed by histology, immunohistochemistry, and molecular means (237). The urothelium is affected by the virus and the presence of circulating virus is associated with active nephropathy because virions enter the circulation through peritubular capillaries following tubular damage (Figure 1.15).

Hepatitis B or C infection remains as one of the principal causes of end-stage liver disease and is a reason for many transplants (238). Unfortunately, hepatitis C has a very high recurrence rate in liver allografts and can often be very difficult to distinguish from AR. No reliable biomarkers exist in helping to distinguish between these two entities. Hepatitis B can also recur in allografts but the identification of this process in liver allografts is greatly assisted by the presence of specific immunoprobes (Figure 1.16).

Post-transplant lymphoproliferative disorder (PTLD) (see Chapter 10) is a common complication following organ transplantation and is often (239,240), but not exclusively, associated (241) with Epstein-Barr virus (EBV). EBV has the potential for a varied number of acute and chronic effects on the transplant recipients aside from PTLD. Aside from classical histopathological changes, immunohistochemistry, in situ hybridization, and other molecular means are utilized in helping identify and distinguish this virus from other processes (e.g., rejection) that may appear similar in presentation and appearance. Often, the therapy for EBV infection is a cessation of immunosuppression treatment; thus, careful identification of the virus (as with many other viruses in transplant patients) must be achieved from rejection processes that require additional immunosuppression.

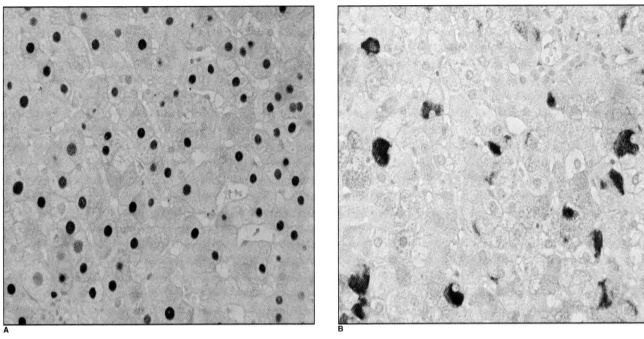

FIGURE 1.16: *Recurrent hepatitis B infection in a liver allograft. Left: hepatitis core antigen–positive cells; right: hepatitis B surface antigen–positive cells (immunoperoxidase, 400×).*

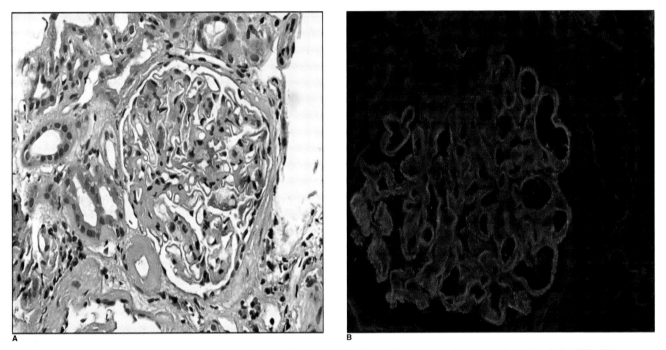

FIGURE 1.17: *Recurrent membranous glomerulonephritis in a renal allograft four years after transplantation (left: H&E, 400×; right: immunofluorescence, IgG, 400×).*

v. Recurrent/De Novo Immune Diseases

Several allografts, in particular kidney and liver, are susceptible to recurrent disease following transplantation. Among the diseases recurring with reasonably high frequency in kidney are focal segmental glomerulosclerosis, membranoproliferative glomerulonephritis, and membranous nephropathy (242–244) (Figure 1.17). Finally, as mentioned, recurrent hepatitis B and C infections of the liver allograft are commonly encountered.

V. SUMMARY

It is apparent that beginning with the trauma and injury associated with the procurement from the donor and ending with the host immune response, the organ allograft is continuously challenged for its survival. Immunosuppressive agents and other drugs that inhibit some of the above-mentioned mediators are crucial to allowing the transplant to survive. Ultimately, however, only the ability to induce donor-specific immune tolerance will allow the recipient to enjoy the benefits of the transplanted organ without the morbidity associated with current pharmaceutical therapies.

REFERENCES

1. Rinaldi, E. 1987. The first homoplastic limb transplant according to the legend of saint Cosmas and saint Damian. *Italian Journal of Orthopedics and Traumatology, 13*: 393–406.
2. Billingham, R.E., Brent, L., Medawar, P.B., Billingham, R.E., Brent, L., Medawar, P.B. 1953. Actively acquired tolerance of foreign cells. *Nature, 172*: 603–6.
3. Snell, G.D. 1957. The genetics of transplantation. *Annals of the New York Academy of Sciences, 69*: 555–60.
4. Gorer, P.A., Boyse, E.A. 1959. Pathological changes in F1 hybrid mice following transplantation of spleen cells from donors of the parental strains. *Immunology, 2*: 182–93.
5. Dausset, J., Rapaport, F.T., Colombani, J., Feingold, N. 1965. A leucocyte group and its relationship to tissue histocompatibility in man. *Transplantation, 3*: 701–5.
6. Doherty, P.C., Zinkernagel, R.M. 1975. A biological role for the major histocompatibility antigens. *Lancet, 1*: 1406–9.
7. Maiers, M., Gragert, L., Klitz, W. 2007. High-resolution HLA alleles and haplotypes in the United States population. *Human Immunology, 68*: 779–88.
8. Marsh, S.G.E. 2008. Nomenclature for factors of the HLA system, update September 2007. *International Journal of Immunogenetics, 35*: 87–8.
9. Trivedi, V.B., Dave, A.P. 2007. Human leukocyte antigen and its role in transplantation biology. *Transplantation Proceedings, 39*: 688–93.
10. Zachary, A.A., Kopchaliiska, D., Montgomery, R.A., Melancon, J.K., Leffell, M.S. 2007. HLA-specific B cells: II. Application to transplantation. *Transplantation, 83*: 989–94.
11. Marsh, S.G.E., Albert, E.D., Bodmer, W.F., Bontrop, R.E., Dupont, B., Erlich, H.A., Geraghty, D.E., Hansen, J.A., Hurley, C.K., Mach, B. et al. 2005. *Nomenclature for Factors of the HLA System, 2004.* pp. 301–69.
12. Hennecke, J., Wiley, D.C. 2001. T cell receptor-MHC interactions up close. *Cell, 104*: 1–4.
13. Burgdorf, S., Kautz, A., Bohnert, V., Knolle, P.A., Kurts, C. 2007. Distinct pathways of antigen uptake and intracellular routing in CD4 and CD8 T cell activation. *Science, 316*: 612–6.
14. Goulmy, E. 1996. Human minor histocompatibility antigens. *Current Opinion in Immunology, 8*: 75–81.
15. Goulmy, E. 2006. Minor histocompatibility antigens: from transplantation problems to therapy of cancer. *Human Immunology, 67*: 433–8.
16. Spierings, E., Vermeulen, C.J., Vogt, M.H., Doerner, L.E.E., Falkenburg, J.H.F., Mutis, T., Goulmy, E. 2003. Identification of HLA class II-restricted H-Y-specific T-helper epitope evoking CD4+ T-helper cells in H-Y-mismatched transplantation. *Lancet, 362*: 610–5.
17. van Els, C.A., Zantvoort, E., Jacobs, N., Bakker, A., van Rood, J.J., Goulmy, E. 1990. Graft-versus-host disease associated T helper cell responses specific for minor histocompatibility antigens are mainly restricted by HLA-DR molecules. *Bone Marrow Transplantation, 5*: 365–72.
18. Joyce, S., Mathew, J.M., Flye, M.W., Mohanakumar, T. 1992. A polymorphic human kidney-specific non-MHC alloantigen. Its possible role in tissue-specific allograft immunity. *Transplantation, 53*: 1119–27.
19. Mathew, J.M., Joyce, S., Lawrence, W., Mohanakumar, T. 1991. Evidence that antibodies eluted from rejected kidneys of HLA-identical transplants define a non-MHC alloantigen expressed on human kidneys. *Transplantation, 52*: 559–62.
20. Suthanthiran, M., Strom, T.B. 1994. Renal transplantation. *New England Journal of Medicine, 331*: 365–76.
21. Krensky, A.M. 1997. The HLA system, antigen processing and presentation. *Kidney International – Supplement, 58*: S2–7.
22. Jiang, S., Herrera, O., Lechler, R.I. 2004. New spectrum of allorecognition pathways: implications for graft rejection and transplantation tolerance. *Current Opinion in Immunology, 16*: 550–7.
23. Burdick, J.F., Vogelsang, G.B., Smith, W.J., Farmer, E.R., Bias, W.B., Kaufmann, S.H., Horn, J., Colombani, P.M., Pitt, H.A., Perler, B.A. et al. 1988. Severe graft-versus-host disease in a liver-transplant recipient. *New England Journal of Medicine, 318*: 689–91.
24. Chan, E.Y., Larson, A.M., Gernsheimer, T.B., Kowdley, K.V., Carithers, R.L., Jr., Reyes, J.D., Perkins, J.D. 2007. Recipient and donor factors influence the incidence of graft-vs.-host disease in liver transplant patients. *Liver Transplantation, 13*: 516–22.
25. Ghali, M.P., Talwalkar, J.A., Moore, S.B., Hogan, W.J., Menon, K.V.N., Rosen, C.B. 2007. Acute graft-versus-host disease after liver transplantation. *Transplantation, 83*: 365–6.
26. Olszewski, W.L. 2007. Donor DNA is present in recipient tissues after grafting also in graft-versus-host disease-free individuals. *Transplantation, 83*: 107–8.
27. Perri, R., Assi, M., Talwalkar, J., Heimbach, J., Hogan, W., Moore, S.B., Rosen, C.B. 2007. Graft vs. host disease after liver transplantation: a new approach is needed. *Liver Transplantation, 13*: 1092–9.
28. Assi, M.A., Pulido, J.S., Peters, S.G., McCannel, C.A., Razonable, R.R. 2007. Graft-vs.-host disease in lung and other solid organ transplant recipients. *Clinical Transplantation, 21*: 1–6.

29. Klingebiel, T., Schlegel, P.G. 1998. GVHD: overview on pathophysiology, incidence, clinical and biological features. *Bone Marrow Transplantation*, *21 Suppl. 2*: S45–9.

30. Triulzi, D.J., Nalesnik, M.A. 2001. Microchimerism, GVHD, and tolerance in solid organ transplantation. *Transfusion*, *41*: 419–26.

31. Fraser, C.J., Scott Baker, K. 2007. The management and outcome of chronic graft-versus-host disease. *British Journal of Haematology*, *138*: 131–45.

32. Holler, E. 2007. Progress in acute graft versus host disease. *Current Opinion in Hematology*, *14*: 625–31.

33. Rodriguez, V., Anderson, P.M., Trotz, B.A., Arndt, C.A.S., Allen, J.A., Khan, S.P. 2007. Use of infliximab-daclizumab combination for the treatment of acute and chronic graft-versus-host disease of the liver and gut. *Pediatric Blood and Cancer*, *49*: 212–5.

34. Petersdorf, E.W., Malkki, M. 2006. Genetics of risk factors for graft-versus-host disease. *Seminars in Hematology*, *43*: 11–23.

35. Ferrara, J.L.M., Reddy, P. 2006. Pathophysiology of graft-versus-host disease. *Seminars in Hematology*, *43*: 3–10.

36. Copelan, E.A. 2006. Hematopoietic stem-cell transplantation. *New England Journal of Medicine*, *354*: 1813–26.

37. Steinman, R.M. 2007. Dendritic cells: understanding immunogenicity. *European Journal of Immunology*, *37 Suppl. 1*: S53–60.

38. Matthews, J.B., Ramos, E., Bluestone, J.A. 2003. Clinical trials of transplant tolerance: slow but steady progress. *American Journal of Transplantation*, *3*: 794–803.

39. Lakkis, F.G. 2003. Transplantation tolerance: a journey from ignorance to memory. *Nephrology Dialysis Transplantation*, *18*: 1979–82.

40. Sykes, M. 2007. Immune tolerance: mechanisms and application in clinical transplantation. *Journal of Internal Medicine*, *262*: 288–310.

41. Anderson, C.C., Carroll, J.M., Gallucci, S., Ridge, J.P., Cheever, A.W., Matzinger, P. 2001. Testing time-, ignorance-, and danger-based models of tolerance. *Journal of Immunology*, *166*: 3663–71.

42. Perales, M.-A., Blachere, N.E., Engelhorn, M.E., Ferrone, C.R., Gold, J.S., Gregor, P.D., Noffz, G., Wolchok, J.D., Houghton, A.N. 2002. Strategies to overcome immune ignorance and tolerance. *Seminars in Cancer Biology*, *12*: 63–71.

43. Brennan, P.J., Saouaf, S.J., Greene, M.I., Shen, Y. 2003. Anergy and suppression as coexistent mechanisms for the maintenance of peripheral T cell tolerance. *Immunologic Research*, *27*: 295–302.

44. Choi, S., Schwartz, R.H. 2007. Molecular mechanisms for adaptive tolerance and other T cell anergy models. *Seminars in Immunology*, *19*: 140–52.

45. Macian, F., Im, S.-H., Garcia-Cozar, F.J., Rao, A. 2004. T-cell anergy. *Current Opinion in Immunology*, *16*: 209–16.

46. Akl, A., Luo, S., Wood, K.J. 2005. Induction of transplantation tolerance-the potential of regulatory T cells. *Transplant Immunology*, *14*: 225–30.

47. Bharat, A., Fields, R.C., Mohanakumar, T. 2005. Regulatory T cell-mediated transplantation tolerance. *Immunologic Research*, *33*: 195–212.

48. Roncarolo, M.-G., Battaglia, M. 2007. Regulatory T-cell immunotherapy for tolerance to self antigens and alloantigens in humans. *Nature Reviews Immunology*, *7*: 585–98.

49. Stephens, G.L., Shevach, E.M. 2007. Foxp3+ regulatory T cells: selfishness under scrutiny. *Immunity*, *27*: 417–9.

50. Tao, R., Hancock, W.W. 2007. Regulating regulatory T cells to achieve transplant tolerance. *Hepatobiliary and Pancreatic Diseases International*, *6*: 348–57.

51. Waldmann, H., Graca, L., Adams, E., Fairchild, P., Cobbold, S. 2005. Regulatory T cells in transplantation tolerance. *Current Topics in Microbiology and Immunology*, *293*: 249–64.

52. Chiffoleau, E., Walsh, P.T., Turka, L. 2003. Apoptosis and transplantation tolerance. *Immunological Reviews*, *193*: 124–45.

53. Sohn, S.J., Thompson, J., Winoto, A. 2007. Apoptosis during negative selection of autoreactive thymocytes. *Current Opinion in Immunology*, *19*: 510–5.

54. Fehr, T., Takeuchi, Y., Kurtz, J., Wekerle, T., Sykes, M. 2005. Early regulation of CD8 T cell alloreactivity by CD4+CD25- T cells in recipients of anti-CD154 antibody and allogeneic BMT is followed by rapid peripheral deletion of donor-reactive CD8+ T cells, precluding a role for sustained regulation. *European Journal of Immunology*, *35*: 2679–90.

55. Herndon, J.M., Stuart, P.M., Ferguson, T.A. 2005. Peripheral deletion of antigen-specific T cells leads to long-term tolerance mediated by CD8+ cytotoxic cells. *Journal of Immunology*, *174*: 4098–104.

56. Gallegos, A.M., Bevan, M.J. 2006. Central tolerance: good but imperfect. *Immunological Reviews*, *209*: 290–6.

57. Kyewski, B., Klein, L. 2006. A central role for central tolerance. *Annual Review of Immunology*, *24*: 571–606.

58. Mathis, D., Benoist, C. 2004. Back to central tolerance. *Immunity*, *20*: 509–16.

59. Lakkis, F.G., Arakelov, A., Konieczny, B.T., Inoue, Y. 2000. Immunologic 'ignorance' of vascularized organ transplants in the absence of secondary lymphoid tissue [see comment]. *Nature Medicine*, *6*: 686–8.

60. Alegre, M.-L., Florquin, S., Goldman, M. 2007. Cellular mechanisms underlying acute graft rejection: time for reassessment. *Current Opinion in Immunology*, *19*: 563–8.

61. Trambley, J., Bingaman, A.W., Lin, A., Elwood, E.T., Waitze, S.Y., Ha, J., Durham, M.M., Corbascio, M., Cowan, S.R., Pearson, T.C. et al. 1999. Asialo GM1+ CD8+ T cells play a critical role in costimulation blockade-resistant allograft rejection. *Journal of Clinical Investigation*, *104*: 1715–22.

62. Neujahr, D.C., Chen, C., Huang, X., Markmann, J.F., Cobbold, S., Waldmann, H., Sayegh, M.H., Hancock, W.W., Turka, L.A. 2006. Accelerated memory cell homeostasis during T cell depletion and approaches to overcome it. *Journal of Immunology*, *176*: 4632–9.

63. Gershon, R.K. 1975. A disquisition on suppressor T cells. *Transplantation Reviews*, *26*: 170–85.

64. Gershon, R.K., Cohen, P., Hencin, R., Liebhaber, S.A. 1972. Suppressor T cells. *Journal of Immunology*, *108*: 586–90.

65. Takahashi, T., Kuniyasu, Y., Toda, M., Sakaguchi, N., Itoh, M., Iwata, M., Shimizu, J., Sakaguchi, S. 1998. Immunologic self-tolerance maintained by CD25+CD4+ naturally anergic and suppressive T cells: induction of autoimmune

disease by breaking their anergic/suppressive state. *International Immunology*, 10: 1969–80.

66. Sakaguchi, S., Sakaguchi, N., Asano, M., Itoh, M., Toda, M. 1995. Immunologic self-tolerance maintained by activated T cells expressing IL-2 receptor alpha-chains (CD25). Breakdown of a single mechanism of self-tolerance causes various autoimmune diseases. *Journal of Immunology*, 155: 1151–64.

67. Sakaguchi, S., Powrie, F. 2007. Emerging challenges in regulatory T cell function and biology. *Science*, 317: 627–9.

68. Bopp, T., Jonuleit, H., Schmitt, E. 2007. Regulatory T cells — the renaissance of the suppressor T cells. *Annals of Medicine*, 39: 322–34.

69. Trop, S., Ilan, Y. 2002 NK 1.1+ T cell: a two-faced lymphocyte in immune modulation of the IL-4/IFN-gamma paradigm. *Journal of Clinical Immunology*, 22: 270–80.

70. Galluzzo, S., Naiyer, A.J., Manavalan, J., Scotto, L., Kim-Shulze, S., Mancini, D., Cortesini, R., Suciu-Foca, N. 2005. Generation of CD8+ CD28- T suppressor cells in heart transplant recipients. *Journal of Heart and Lung Transplantation*, 24: S106.

71. Bluestone, J.A., Abbas, A.K. 2003. Natural versus adaptive regulatory T cells. *Nature Reviews Immunology*, 3: 253–7.

72. Pillai, V., Karandikar, N.J. 2007. Human regulatory T cells: a unique, stable thymic subset or a reversible peripheral state of differentiation? *Immunology Letters*, 114: 9–15.

73. Shimada, A., Rohane, P., Fathman, C.G., Charlton, B. 1996. Pathogenic and protective roles of CD45RB (low) CD4+ cells correlate with cytokine profiles in the spontaneously autoimmune diabetic mouse. *Diabetes*, 45: 71–8.

74. Biagi, E., Di Biaso, I., Leoni, V., Gaipa, G., Rossi, V., Bugarin, C., Renoldi, G., Parma, M., Balduzzi, A., Perseghin, P. et al. 2007. Extracorporeal photochemotherapy is accompanied by increasing levels of circulating CD4+CD25+GITR+Foxp3+CD62L+ functional regulatory T-cells in patients with graft-versus-host disease. *Transplantation*, 84: 31–9.

75. Hilchey, S.P., De, A., Rimsza, L.M., Bankert, R.B., Bernstein, S.H. 2007. Follicular lymphoma intratumoral CD4+CD25+GITR+ regulatory T cells potently suppress CD3/CD28-costimulated autologous and allogeneic CD8+CD25- and CD4+CD25- T cells. *Journal of Immunology*, 178: 4051–61.

76. Ferretti, G., Felici, A., Pino, M.S., Cognetti, F. 2006. Does CTLA4 influence the suppressive effect of CD25+CD4+ regulatory T cells? *Journal of Clinical Oncology*, 24: 5469–70; author reply 5470–1.

77. Quezada, S.A., Peggs, K.S., Curran, M.A., Allison, J.P. 2006. CTLA4 blockade and GM-CSF combination immunotherapy alters the intratumor balance of effector and regulatory T cells. *Journal of Clinical Investigation*, 116: 1935–45.

78. Allakhverdi, Z., Fitzpatrick, D., Boisvert, A., Baba, N., Bouguermouh, S., Sarfati, M., Delespesse, G. 2006. Expression of CD103 identifies human regulatory T-cell subsets. *Journal of Allergy and Clinical Immunology*, 118: 1342–9.

79. Annacker, O., Coombes, J.L., Malmstrom, V., Uhlig, H.H., Bourne, T., Johansson-Lindbom, B., Agace, W.W., Parker, C.M., Powrie, F. 2005. Essential role for CD103 in the T cell-mediated regulation of experimental colitis. *Journal of Experimental Medicine*, 202: 1051–61.

80. Keino, H., Masli, S., Sasaki, S., Streilein, J.W., Stein-Streilein, J. 2006. CD8+ T regulatory cells use a novel genetic program that includes CD103 to suppress Th1 immunity in eye-derived tolerance. *Investigative Ophthalmology and Visual Science*, 47: 1533–42.

81. Kim, C.H. 2007. Molecular targets of FoxP3+ regulatory T cells. *Mini-Reviews in Medicinal Chemistry*, 7: 1136–43.

82. La Cava, A., Van Kaer, L., Fu Dong, S. 2006. CD4+CD25+ Tregs and NKT cells: regulators regulating regulators. *Trends in Immunology*, 27: 322–7.

83. Li, W., Carper, K., Perkins, J.D. 2006. Enhancement of NKT cells and increase in regulatory T cells results in improved allograft survival. *Journal of Surgical Research*, 134: 10–21.

84. Kim, H.J., Hwang, S.J., Kim, B.K., Jung, K.C., Chung, D.H. 2006. NKT cells play critical roles in the induction of oral tolerance by inducing regulatory T cells producing IL-10 and transforming growth factor beta, and by clonally deleting antigen-specific T cells. *Immunology*, 118: 101–11.

85. Carrier, Y., Yuan, J., Kuchroo, V.K., Weiner, H.L. 2007. Th3 cells in peripheral tolerance. I. Induction of Foxp3-positive regulatory T cells by Th3 cells derived from TGF-beta T cell-transgenic mice. *Journal of Immunology*, 178: 179–85.

86. Cools, N., Ponsaerts, P., Van Tendeloo, V.F.I., Berneman, Z.N. 2007. Balancing between immunity and tolerance: an interplay between dendritic cells, regulatory T cells, and effector T cells. *Journal of Leukocyte Biology*, 82: 1365–74.

87. Fujita, S., Sato, Y., Sato, K., Eizumi, K., Fukaya, T., Kubo, M., Yamashita, N., Sato, K. 2007. Regulatory dendritic cells protect against cutaneous chronic graft-versus-host disease mediated through CD4+CD25+Foxp3+ regulatory T cells. *Blood*, 110: 3793–803.

88. Salama, A.D., Najafian, N., Clarkson, M.R., Harmon, W.E., Sayegh, M.H. 2003. Regulatory CD25+ T cells in human kidney transplant recipients. *Journal of the American Society of Nephrology*, 14: 1643–51.

89. Cirocco, R.E., Carreno, M.R., Mathew, J.M., Garcia-Morales, R.O., Fuller, L., Esquenazi, V., Ciancio, G., Burke, G.W., Gaynor, J.J., Blomberg, B.B. et al. 2007. FoxP3 mRNA transcripts and regulatory cells in renal transplant recipients 10 years after donor marrow infusion. *Transplantation*, 83: 1611–9.

90. Tran, D.Q., Ramsey, H., Shevach, E.M. 2007. Induction of FOXP3 expression in naive human CD4+FOXP3 T cells by T-cell receptor stimulation is transforming growth factor-beta dependent but does not confer a regulatory phenotype. *Blood*, 110: 2983–90.

91. Wan, Y.Y., Flavell, R.A. 2007. 'Yin-Yang' functions of transforming growth factor-beta and T regulatory cells in immune regulation. *Immunological Reviews*, 220: 199–213.

92. Pearl, J.P., Xu, H., Leopardi, F., Preston, E., Kirk, A.D. 2007. CD154 blockade, sirolimus, and donor-specific transfusion prevents renal allograft rejection in cynomolgus monkeys despite homeostatic T-cell activation. *Transplantation*, 83: 1219–25.

93. Sandner, S.E., Clarkson, M.R., Salama, A.D., Sanchez-Fueyo, A., Yagita, H., Turka, L.A., Sayegh, M.H. 2005. Mechanisms of tolerance induced by donor-specific transfusion and ICOS-B7h blockade in a model of CD4+ T-cell-mediated allograft rejection. *American Journal of Transplantation*, *5*: 31–9.

94. Ruiz, P., Coffman, T.M., Howell, D.N., Straznickas, J., Scroggs, M.W., Baldwin, W.M., Klotman, P.E., Sanfilippo, F. 1988. Evidence that pretransplant donor blood transfusion prevents rat renal allograft dysfunction but not the in situ cellular alloimmune or morphologic manifestations of rejection. *Transplantation*, *45*: 1–7.

95. Ciancio, G., Burke, G.W., Moon, J., Garcia-Morales, R., Rosen, A., Esquenazi, V., Mathew, J., Jin, Y., Miller, J. 2004. Donor bone marrow infusion in deceased and living donor renal transplantation. *Yonsei Medical Journal*, *45*: 998–1003.

96. Delis, S., Ciancio, G., Burke, G.W., 3rd, Garcia-Morales, R., Miller, J. 2004. Donor bone marrow transplantation: chimerism and tolerance. *Transplant Immunology*, *13*: 105–15.

97. Chai, J.-G., Coe, D., Chen, D., Simpson, E., Dyson, J., Scott, D. 2008. In vitro expansion improves in vivo regulation by CD4+CD25+ regulatory T cells. *Journal of Immunology*, *180*: 858–69.

98. Burlingham, W.J., Jankowska-Gan, E. 2007. Mouse strain and injection site are crucial for detecting linked suppression in transplant recipients by trans-vivo DTH assay. *American Journal of Transplantation*, *7*: 466–70.

99. Kapp, J.A., Honjo, K., Kapp, L.M., Xu, X.y., Cozier, A., Bucy, R.P. 2006. TCR transgenic CD8+ T cells activated in the presence of TGFbeta express FoxP3 and mediate linked suppression of primary immune responses and cardiac allograft rejection. *International Immunology*, *18*: 1549–62.

100. Dresske, B., Lin, X., Huang, D.-S., Zhou, X., Fandrich, F. 2002. Spontaneous tolerance: experience with the rat liver transplant model. *Human Immunology*, *63*: 853–61.

101. Li, W., Zheng, X.X., Kuhr, C.S., Perkins, J.D. 2005. CTLA4 engagement is required for induction of murine liver transplant spontaneous tolerance. *American Journal of Transplantation*, *5*: 978–86.

102. Lin, H., Rathmell, J.C., Gray, G.S., Thompson, C.B., Leiden, J.M., Alegre, M.L. 1998. Cytotoxic T lymphocyte antigen 4 (CTLA4) blockade accelerates the acute rejection of cardiac allografts in CD28-deficient mice: CTLA4 can function independently of CD28. *Journal of Experimental Medicine*, *188*: 199–204.

103. Bonfoco, E., Stuart, P.M., Brunner, T., Lin, T., Griffith, T.S., Gao, Y., Nakajima, H., Henkart, P.A., Ferguson, T.A., Green, D.R. 1998. Inducible nonlymphoid expression of Fas ligand is responsible for superantigen-induced peripheral deletion of T cells. *Immunity*, *9*: 711–20.

104. Kurts, C., Heath, W.R., Kosaka, H., Miller, J.F., Carbone, F.R. 1998. The peripheral deletion of autoreactive CD8+ T cells induced by cross-presentation of self-antigens involves signaling through CD95 (Fas, Apo-1). *Journal of Experimental Medicine*, *188*: 415–20.

105. Dempsey, P.W., Doyle, S.E., He, J.Q., Cheng, G. 2003. The signaling adaptors and pathways activated by TNF superfamily. *Cytokine and Growth Factor Reviews*, *14*: 193–209.

106. Feng, X. 2005. Regulatory roles and molecular signaling of TNF family members in osteoclasts. *Gene*, *350*: 1–13.

107. Sheikh, M.S., Huang, Y. 2003. Death receptor activation complexes: it takes two to activate TNF receptor 1. *Cell Cycle*, *2*: 550–2.

108. Baluja, P., Haragsim, L., Laszik, Z. 2006. Chronic allograft nephropathy. *Advances in Chronic Kidney Disease*, *13*: 56–61.

109. Hornick, P., Rose, M. 2006. Chronic rejection in the heart. *Methods in Molecular Biology*, *333*: 131–44.

110. Nankivell, B.J., Chapman, J.R. 2006. Chronic allograft nephropathy: current concepts and future directions. *Transplantation*, *81*: 643–54.

111. Huang, Y., Rabb, H., Womer, K.L. 2007. Ischemia-reperfusion and immediate T cell responses. *Cellular Immunology*, *248*: 4–11.

112. Kupiec-Weglinski, J.W., Busuttil, R.W. 2005. Ischemia and reperfusion injury in liver transplantation. *Transplantation Proceedings*, *37*: 1653–6.

113. Ysebaert, D.K., De Greef, K.E., De Beuf, A., Van Rompay, A.R., Vercauteren, S., Persy, V.P., De Broe, M.E. 2004. T cells as mediators in renal ischemia/reperfusion injury. *Kidney International*, *66*: 491–6.

114. Dragun, D., Tullius, S.G., Park, J.K., Maasch, C., Lukitsch, I., Lippoldt, A., Gross, V., Luft, F.C., Haller, H. 1998. ICAM-1 antisense oligodesoxynucleotides prevent reperfusion injury and enhance immediate graft function in renal transplantation. *Kidney International*, *54*: 590–602.

115. Koo, D.D., Welsh, K.I., Roake, J.A., Morris, P.J., Fuggle, S.V. 1998. Ischemia/reperfusion injury in human kidney transplantation: an immunohistochemical analysis of changes after reperfusion. *American Journal of Pathology*, *153*: 557–66.

116. Herskowitz, A., Mayne, A.E., Willoughby, S.B., Kanter, K., Ansari, A.A. 1994. Patterns of myocardial cell adhesion molecule expression in human endomyocardial biopsies after cardiac transplantation. Induced ICAM-1 and VCAM-1 related to implantation and rejection. *American Journal of Pathology*, *145*: 1082–94.

117. Andersen, C.B., Ladefoged, S.D., Larsen, S. 1994. Acute kidney graft rejection. A morphological and immunohistological study on "zero-hour" and follow-up biopsies with special emphasis on cellular infiltrates and adhesion molecules. *Apmis*, *102*: 23–37.

118. Devouassoux, G., Pison, C., Drouet, C., Pin, I., Brambilla, C., Brambilla, E. 2001. Early lung leukocyte infiltration, HLA and adhesion molecule expression predict chronic rejection. *Transplant Immunology*, *8*: 229–36.

119. van der Woude, F.J., Deckers, J.G., Mallat, M.J., Yard, B.A., Schrama, E., van Saase, J.L., Daha, M.R. 1995. Tissue antigens in tubulointerstitial and vascular rejection. *Kidney International – Supplement*, *52*: S11–3.

120. Hengstenberg, C., Hufnagel, G., Haverich, A., Olsen, E.G.J., Maisch, B. 1993. De novo expression of MHC class I and class II antigens on endomyocardial biopsies from patients with inflammatory heart disease and rejection following heart transplantation. *European Heart Journal*, *14*: 758–63.

121. Farr, A.G., Mannschreck, J.W., Anderson, S.K. 1988. Expression of class II MHC antigens in murine pancreas after streptozocin-induced insulitis. *Diabetes*, *37*: 1373–9.

122. Hasegawa, S., Becker, G., Nagano, H., Libby, P., Mitchell, R.N. 1998. Pattern of graft- and host-specific MHC class II expression in long-term murine cardiac allografts: origin of inflammatory and vascular wall cells. *American Journal of Pathology, 153*: 69–79.

123. Haverty, T.P., Watanabe, M., Neilson, E.G., Kelly, C.J. 1989. Protective modulation of class II MHC gene expression in tubular epithelium by target antigen-specific antibodies. Cell-surface directed down-regulation of transcription can influence susceptibility to murine tubulointerstitial nephritis. *Journal of Immunology, 143*: 1133–41.

124. Fuggle, S.V., McWhinnie, D.L., Morris, P.J. 1987. Precise specificity of induced tubular HLA-class II antigens in renal allografts. *Transplantation, 44*: 214–20.

125. Adoumie, R., Serrick, C., Giaid, A., Shennib, H. 1992. Early cellular events in the lung allograft. *Annals of Thoracic Surgery, 54*: 1071–6; discussion 1076–7.

126. Denton, M.D., Davis, S.F., Baum, M.A., Melter, M., Reinders, M.E., Exeni, A., Samsonov, D.V., Fang, J., Ganz, P., Briscoe, D.M. et al. 2000. The role of the graft endothelium in transplant rejection: evidence that endothelial activation may serve as a clinical marker for the development of chronic rejection. *Pediatric Transplantation, 4*: 252–60.

127. Baldwin, W.M., Larsen, C.P., Fairchild, R.L. 2001. Innate immune responses to transplants: a significant variable with cadaver donors. *Immunity, 14*: 369–76.

128. Baldwin, W.M., III, Samaniego-Picota, M., Kasper, E.K., Clark, A.M., Czader, M., Rohde, C., Zachary, A.A., Sanfilippo, F., Hruban, R.H. 1999. Complement deposition in early cardiac transplant biopsies is associated with ischemic injury and subsequent rejection episodes. *Transplantation, 68*: 894–900.

129. Haas, M., Ratner, L.E., Montgomery, R.A. 2002. C4d staining of perioperative renal transplant biopsies. *Transplantation, 74*: 711–7.

130. Qian, Z., Wasowska, B.A., Behrens, E., Cangello, D.L., Brody, J.R., Kadkol, S.S., Horwitz, L., Liu, J., Lowenstein C., Hess, A.D. et al. 1999. C6 produced by macrophages contributes to cardiac allograft rejection. *American Journal of Pathology, 155*: 1293–302.

131. Kupiec-Weglinski, J.W., Busuttil, R.W. 2005. Ischemia and reperfusion injury in liver transplantation. *Transplantation Proceedings, 37*: 1653–6.

132. Lin, T., Zhou, W., Sacks, S.H. 2007. The role of complement and Toll-like receptors in organ transplantation. *Transplant International, 20*: 481–9.

133. Shigeoka, A.A., Holscher, T.D., King, A.J., Hall, F.W., Kiosses, W.B., Tobias, P.S., Mackman, N., McKay, D.B. 2007. TLR2 is constitutively expressed within the kidney and participates in ischemic renal injury through both MyD88-dependent and -independent pathways. *Journal of Immunology, 178*: 6252–8.

134. Shishido, T.M.D., Nozaki, N.M.D.P., Yamaguchi, S.M.D.P., Shibata, Y.M.D.P., Nitobe, J.M.D.P., Miyamoto, T.M.D., Takahashi, H.M.D., Arimoto, T.M.D., Maeda, K.M.D.P., Yamakawa, M.M.D.P. et al. 2003. Toll-like receptor-2 modulates ventricular remodeling after myocardial infarction. *Circulation, 108*: 2905–10.

135. Oyama, J.-i.M.D., Blais, C.J.P., Liu, X.M.D., Pu, M.M.D., Kobzik, L.M.D., Kelly, R.A.M.D., Bourcier, T.P. 2004. Reduced Myocardial ischemia-reperfusion injury in Toll-like receptor 4-deficient mice. *Circulation, 109*: 784–9.

136. Gaston, J.S.H. 2002. Heat Shock Proteins and Innate Immunity. *Clinical and Experimental Immunology, 127*: 1–3.

137. Leadbetter, E.A., Rifkin, I.R., Hohlbaum, A.M., Beaudette, B.C., Shlomchik, M.J., Marshak-Rothstein, A. 2002. Chromatin-IgG complexes activate B cells by dual engagement of IgM and Toll-like receptors. *Nature, 416*: 603–7.

138. Termeer, C., Benedix, F., Sleeman, J., Fieber, C., Voith, U., Ahrens, T., Miyake, K., Freudenberg, M., Galanos, C., Simon, J.C. 2002. Oligosaccharides of hyaluronan activate dendritic cells via toll-like receptor 4. *Journal of Experimental Medicine, 195*: 99–111.

139. Ohashi, K., Burkart, V., Flohe, S., Kolb, H. 2000. Heat shock protein 60 is a putative endogenous ligand of the toll-like receptor-4 complex. *Journal of Immunology, 164*: 558–61.

140. Johnson, G.B., Brunn, G.J., Kodaira, Y., Platt, J.L. 2002. Receptor-mediated monitoring of tissue well-being via detection of soluble heparan sulfate by toll-like receptor 4. *Journal of Immunology, 168*: 5233–9.

141. Asea, A., Kraeft, S.-K., Kurt-Jones, E.A., Stevenson, M.A., Chen, L.B., Finberg, R.W., Koo, G.C., Calderwood, S.K. 2000. HSP70 stimulates cytokine production through a CD14-dependant pathway, demonstrating its dual role as a chaperone and cytokine. *Nature Medicine, 6*: 435–42.

142. Guillot, L., Balloy, V., McCormack, F.X., Golenbock, D.T., Chignard, M., Si-Tahar, M. 2002. Cutting Edge: the immunostimulatory activity of the lung surfactant protein-A involves toll-like receptor 4. *Journal of Immunology, 168*: 5989–92.

143. Knowlton, A.A., Brecher, P., Apstein, C.S. 1991. Rapid expression of heat shock protein in the rabbit after brief cardiac ischemia. *Journal of Clinical Investigation, 87*: 139–47.

144. Ogita, K., Hopkinson, K., Nakao, M., Wood, R.F., Pockley, A.G. 2000. Stress responses in graft and native intestine after rat heterotopic small bowel transplantation. *Transplantation, 69*: 2273–7.

145. Udelsman, R., Blake, M.J., Holbrook, N.J. 1991. Molecular response to surgical stress: specific and simultaneous heat shock protein induction in the adrenal cortex, aorta, and vena cava. *Surgery, 110*: 1125–31.

146. Duquesnoy, R.J., Liu, K., Fu, X.F., Murase, N., Ye, Q., Demetris, A.J. 1999. Evidence for heat shock protein immunity in a rat cardiac allograft model of chronic rejection. *Transplantation, 67*: 156–64.

147. Hiratsuka, M., Yano, M., Mora, B.N., Nagahiro, I., Cooper, J.D., Patterson, G.A. 1998. Heat shock pretreatment protects pulmonary isografts from subsequent ischemia-reperfusion injury. *Journal of Heart and Lung Transplantation, 17*: 1238–46.

148. Squiers, E.C., Bruch, D., Buelow, R., Tice, D.G. 1999. Pretreatment of small bowel isograft donors with cobalt-protoporphyrin decreases preservation injury. *Transplantation Proceedings, 31*: 585–6.

149. Penfield, J.G., Wang, Y., Li, S., Kielar, M.A., Sicher, S.C., Jeyarajah, D.R., Lu, C.Y. 1999. Transplant surgery injury recruits recipient MHC class II-positive leukocytes into the kidney. *Kidney International, 56*: 1759–69.

150. Olszewski, W.L. 2005. Innate immunity processes in organ allografting — their contribution to acute and chronic rejection. *Annals of Transplantation*, *10*: 5–9.

151. Navarro, F., Portales, P., Candon, S., Pruvot, F.R., Pageaux, G., Fabre, J.M., Domergue, J., Clot, J. 2000. Natural killer cell and alphabeta and gammadelta lymphocyte traffic into the liver graft immediately after liver transplantation. *Transplantation*, *69*: 633–9.

152. Rabb, H. 2002. The T cell as a bridge between innate and adaptive immune systems: implications for the kidney. *Kidney International*, *61*: 1935–46.

153. Akalin, E., Watschinger, B. 2007. Antibody-mediated rejection. *Seminars in Nephrology*, *27*: 393–407.

154. Truong, L.D., Barrios, R., Adrogue, H.E., Gaber, L.W. 2007. Acute antibody-mediated rejection of renal transplant: pathogenetic and diagnostic considerations. *Archives of Pathology and Laboratory Medicine*, *131*: 1200–8.

155. Shimizu, A., Colvin, R.B. 2005. Pathological features of antibody-mediated rejection. *Current Drug Targets – Cardiovascular and Haematological Disorders*, *5*: 199–214.

156. Akalin, E., Watschinger, B., Akalin, E., Watschinger, B. 2007. Antibody-mediated rejection. *Seminars in Nephrology*, *27*: 393–407.

157. Feucht, H.E., Felber, E., Gokel, M.J., Hillebrand, G., Nattermann, U., Brockmeyer, C., Held, E., Riethmuller, G., Land, W., Albert, E. 1991. Vascular deposition of complement-split products in kidney allografts with cell-mediated rejection. *Clinical and Experimental Immunology*, *86*: 464–70.

158. Feucht, H.E., Schneeberger, H., Hillebrand, G., Burkhardt, K., Weiss, M., Riethmuller, G., Land, W., Albert, E. 1993. Capillary deposition of C4d complement fragment and early renal graft loss. *Kidney International*, *43*: 1333–8.

159. Banasik, M., Boratynska, M., Nowakowska, B., Halon, A., Koscielska-Kasprzak, K., Drulis-Fajdasz, D., Patrzalek, D., Weyde, W., Klinger, M. 2007. C4D deposition and positive posttransplant crossmatch are not necessarily markers of antibody-mediated rejection in renal allograft recipients. *Transplantation Proceedings*, *39*: 2718–20.

160. Seemayer, C.A., Gaspert, A., Nickeleit, V., Mihatsch, M.J. 2007. C4d staining of renal allograft biopsies: a comparative analysis of different staining techniques. *Nephrology Dialysis Transplantation*, *22*: 568–76.

161. Sun, Q., Liu, Z.H., Ji, S., Chen, J., Tang, Z., Zeng, C., Zheng, C., Li, L.S. 2006. Late and early C4d-positive acute rejection: different clinico-histopathological subentities in renal transplantation. *Kidney International*, *70*: 377–83.

162. Dankof, A., Schmeding, M., Morawietz, L., Gunther, R., Krukemeyer, M.G., Rudolph, B., Koch, M., Krenn, V., Neumann, U. 2005. Portal capillary C4d deposits and increased infiltration by macrophages indicate humorally mediated mechanisms in acute cellular liver allograft rejection. *Virchows Archive*, *447*: 87–93.

163. Schmidt, A., Sucke, J., Fuchs-Moll, G., Freitag, P., Hirschburger, M., Kaufmann, A., Garn, H., Padberg, W., Grau, V. 2007. Macrophages in experimental rat lung isografts and allografts: infiltration and proliferation in situ. *Journal of Leukocyte Biology*, *81*: 186–94.

164. Wyburn, K.R., Jose, M.D., Wu, H., Atkins, R.C., Chadban, S.J. 2005. The role of macrophages in allograft rejection. *Transplantation*, *80*: 1641–7.

165. Sis, B., Grynoch, R., Murray, A.G., Campbell, P., Solez, K. 2008. Antibody-mediated rejection with a striking interstitial monocyte/macrophage infiltration in a renal allograft under FTY720 treatment. *American Journal of Kidney Diseases*, *51*: 127–30.

166. Chantranuwat, C., Qiao, J.H., Kobashigawa, J., Hong, L., Shintaku, P., Fishbein, M.C. 2004. Immunoperoxidase staining for C4d on paraffin-embedded tissue in cardiac allograft endomyocardial biopsies: comparison to frozen tissue immunofluorescence. *Applied Immunohistochemistry and Molecular Morphology*, *12*: 166–71.

167. Hammond, M.E., Stehlik, J., Snow, G., Renlund, D.G., Seaman, J., Dabbas, B., Gilbert, E.M., Stringham, J.C., Long, J.W., Kfoury, A.G. 2005. Utility of histologic parameters in screening for antibody-mediated rejection of the cardiac allograft: a study of 3,170 biopsies. *Journal of Heart and Lung Transplantation*, *24*: 2015–21.

168. Nickeleit, V., Andreoni, K. 2007. The classification and treatment of antibody-mediated renal allograft injury: where do we stand? *Kidney International*, *71*: 7–11.

169. Solez, K., Colvin, R.B., Racusen, L.C., Sis, B., Halloran, P.F., Birk, P.E., Campbell, P.M., Cascalho, M., Collins, A.B., Demetris, A.J. et al. 2007. Banff '05 Meeting Report: differential diagnosis of chronic allograft injury and elimination of chronic allograft nephropathy ('CAN'). *American Journal of Transplantation*, *7*: 518–26.

170. Jukes, J.-P., Wood, K.J., Jones, N.D. 2007. Natural killer T cells: a bridge to tolerance or a pathway to rejection? *Transplantation*, *84*: 679–81.

171. Kitchens, W.H., Uehara, S., Chase, C.M., Colvin, R.B., Russell, P.S., Madsen, J.C. 2006. The changing role of natural killer cells in solid organ rejection and tolerance. *Transplantation*, *81*: 811–7.

172. Aguilar, P., Mathieu, C.P., Clerc, G., Ethevenot, G., Fajraoui, M., Mattei, S., Faure, G.C., Bene, M.C. 2006. Modulation of natural killer (NK) receptors on NK (CD3–/CD56+), T (CD3+/CD56–) and NKT-like (CD3+/CD56+) cells after heart transplantation. *Journal of Heart and Lung Transplantation*, *25*: 200–5.

173. McNerney, M.E., Lee, K.M., Zhou, P., Molinero, L., Mashayekhi, M., Guzior, D., Sattar, H., Kuppireddi, S., Wang, C.R., Kumar, V. et al. 2006. Role of natural killer cell subsets in cardiac allograft rejection. *American Journal of Transplantation*, *6*: 505–13.

174. Sanfilippo, F., Kolbeck, P.C., Vaughn, W.K., Bollinger, R.R. 1985. Renal allograft cell infiltrates associated with irreversible rejection. *Transplantation*, *40*: 679–85.

175. Azzawi, M., Hasleton, P.S., Geraghty, P.J., Yonan, N., Krysiak, P., El-Gammal, A., Deiraniya, A.K., Hutchinson, I.V. 1998. RANTES chemokine expression is related to acute cardiac cellular rejection and infiltration by CD45RO T-lymphocytes and macrophages. *Journal of Heart and Lung Transplantation*, *17*: 881–7.

176. Erren, M., Arlt, M., Willeke, P., Schluter, B., Junker, R., Deng, M.C., Assmann, G., Dietl, H.D., Senninger, N. 1999. Predictive value of the CD45RO positive T-helper

lymphocyte subset for acute cellular rejection during the early phase after kidney transplantation. *Transplantation Proceedings*, 31: 319–21.

177. Wang, P., Zhu, L., Liu, T., Zhang, X., Qiu, Y. 1999. Intragraft CD45 RO gene expression is an early marker to detect small bowel allograft rejection in rats. *Microsurgery*, 19: 348–50.

178. Seron, D., Alexopoulos, E., Raftery, M.J., Hartley, R.B., Cameron, J.S. 1989. Diagnosis of rejection in renal allograft biopsies using the presence of activated and proliferating cells. *Transplantation*, 47: 811–6.

179. Santamaria, M., Marubayashi, M., Arizon, J.M., Montero, A., Concha, M., Valles, F., Lopez, A., Lopez, F., Pena, J. 1992. The activation antigen CD69 is selectively expressed on CD8+ endomyocardium infiltrating T lymphocytes in human rejecting heart allografts. *Human Immunology*, 33: 1–4.

180. Hadley, G. 2004. Role of integrin CD103 in promoting destruction of renal allografts by CD8 T cells. *American Journal of Transplantation*, 4: 1026–32.

181. Wang, D., Yuan, R., Feng, Y., El-Asady, R., Farber, D.L., Gress, R.E., Lucas, P.J., Hadley, G.A., Wang, D., Yuan, R. et al. 2004. Regulation of CD103 expression by CD8+ T cells responding to renal allografts. *Journal of Immunology*, 172: 214–21.

182. Alegre, M., Fallarino, F., Zhou, P., Frauwirth, K., Thistlethwaite, J., Newell, K., Gajewski, T., Bluestone, J. 2001. Transplantation and the CD28/CTLA4/B7 pathway. *Transplantation Proceedings*, 33: 209–11.

183. Clarkson, M.R., Sayegh, M.H., Clarkson, M.R., Sayegh, M.H. 2005. T-cell costimulatory pathways in allograft rejection and tolerance. *Transplantation*, 80: 555–63.

184. D'Errico, A., Corti, B., Pinna, A.D., Altimari, A., Gruppioni, E., Gabusi, E., Fiorentino, M., Bagni, A., Grigioni, W.F. 2003. Granzyme B and perforin as predictive markers for acute rejection in human intestinal transplantation. *Transplantation Proceedings*, 35: 3061–5.

185. Mengel, M., Mueller, I., Behrend, M., von Wasielewski, R., Radermacher, J., Schwarz, A., Haller, H., Kreipe, H. 2004. Prognostic value of cytotoxic T-lymphocytes and CD40 in biopsies with early renal allograft rejection. *Transplant International*, 17: 293–300.

186. Wagrowska-Danilewicz, M., Danilewicz, M. 2003. Immunoexpression of perforin and granzyme B on infiltrating lymphocytes in human renal acute allograft rejection. *Nefrologia*, 23: 538–44.

187. Clement, M.V., Haddad, P., Soulie, A., Benvenuti, C., Lichtenheld, M.G., Podack, E.R., Sigaux, N., Sasportes, M. 1991. Perforin and granzyme B as markers for acute rejection in heart transplantation. *International Immunology*, 3: 1175–81.

188. Griffiths, G.M., Namikawa, R., Mueller, C., Liu, C.C., Young, J.D., Billingham, M., Weissman, I. 1991. Granzyme A and perforin as markers for rejection in cardiac transplantation. *European Journal of Immunology*, 21: 687–93.

189. Fuggle, S.V., McWhinnie, D.L., Morris, P.J. 1989. Immunohistological analysis of renal allograft biopsies from cyclosporin-treated patients. Induced HLA-class II antigen expression does not exclude a diagnosis of cyclosporin nephrotoxicity. *Transplant International*, 2: 123–8.

190. Arnaout, M.A. 1990. Structure and function of the leukocyte adhesion molecules CD11/CD18. *Blood*, 75: 1037–50.

191. Ahmed-Ansari, A., Tadros, T.S., Knopf, W.D., Murphy, D.A., Hertzler, G., Feighan, J., Leatherbury, A., Sell, K.W. 1988. Major histocompatibility complex class I and class II expression by myocytes in cardiac biopsies posttransplantation. *Transplantation*, 45: 972–8.

192. Barrett, M., Milton, A.D., Barrett, J., Taube, D., Bewick, M., Parsons, V.P., Fabre, J.W. 1987. Needle biopsy evaluation of class II major histocompatibility complex antigen expression for the differential diagnosis of cyclosporine nephrotoxicity from kidney graft rejection. *Transplantation*, 44: 223–7.

193. Belitsky, P., Miller, S.M., Gupta, R., Lee, S., Ghose, T. 1990. Induction of MHC class II expression in recipient tissues caused by allograft rejection. *Transplantation*, 49: 472–6.

194. Briscoe, D.M., Cotran, R.S. 1993. Role of leukocyte-endothelial cell adhesion molecules in renal inflammation: in vitro and in vivo studies. *Kidney International – Supplement*, 42: S27–34.

195. Heemann, U.W., Tullius, S.G., Azuma, H., Kupiec-Weglinsky, J., Tilney, N.L. 1994. Adhesion molecules and transplantation. *Annals of Surgery*, 219: 4–12.

196. Kirby, J.A. 1994. The role played by adhesion molecules during allograft rejection. *Transplant Immunology*, 2: 129–32.

197. Sekine, Y., Yasufuku, K., Heidler, K.M., Cummings, O.W., Van Rooijen, N., Fujisawa, T., Brown, J., Wilkes, D.S. 2000. Monocyte chemoattractant protein-1 and RANTES are chemotactic for graft infiltrating lymphocytes during acute lung allograft rejection. *American Journal of Respiratory Cell and Molecular Biology*, 23: 719–26.

198. Mulligan, M.S., McDuffie, J.E., Shanley, T.P., Guo, R.F., Vidya Sarma, J., Warner, R.L., Ward, P.A. 2000. Role of RANTES in experimental cardiac allograft rejection. *Experimental and Molecular Pathology*, 69: 167–74.

199. Schroppel, B., Fischereder, M., Lin, M., Marder, B., Schiano, T., Kramer, B.K., Murphy, B. 2002. Analysis of gene polymorphisms in the regulatory region of MCP-1, RANTES, and CCR5 in liver transplant recipients. *Journal of Clinical Immunology*, 22: 381–5.

200. Miura, M., Morita, K., Kobayashi, H., Hamilton, T.A., Burdick, M.D., Strieter, R.M., Fairchild, R.L. 2001. Monokine induced by IFN-gamma is a dominant factor directing T cells into murine cardiac allografts during acute rejection. *Journal of Immunology*, 167: 3494–504.

201. Schnickel, G.T., Bastani, S., Hsieh, G.R., Shefizadeh, A., Bhatia, R., Fishbein, M.C., Belperio, J., Ardehali, A. 2008. Combined CXCR3/CCR5 blockade attenuates acute and chronic rejection. *Journal of Immunology*, 180: 4714–21.

202. Merani, S., Truong, W.W., Hancock, W., Anderson, C.C., Shapiro, A.M.J. 2006. Chemokines and their receptors in islet allograft rejection and as targets for tolerance induction. *Cell Transplantation*, 15: 295–309.

203. Smith, R.N., Ueno, T., Ito, T., Tanaka, K., Shea, S.P., Abdi, R. 2007. Chemokines and chronic heart allograft rejection. *Transplantation*, 84: 442–4.

204. Stasikowska, O., Wagrowska-Danilewicz, M. 2007. Chemokines and chemokine receptors in glomerulonephritis

and renal allograft rejection. *Medical Science Monitor, 13*: RA31–6.

205. Ali, S., Malik, G., Burns, A., Robertson, H., Kirby, J.A. 2005. Renal transplantation: examination of the regulation of chemokine binding during acute rejection. *Transplantation, 79*: 672–9.

206. Racca, A., Bailat, A., Garcia, M.I., Soutullo, A., Gaite, L., Malan Borel, I. 2005. Participation of RANTES and T-cell apoptosis in human renal allograft. *Scandinavian Journal of Immunology, 61*: 157–64.

207. Afzali, B., Lechler, R.I., Hernandez-Fuentes, M.P. 2007. Allorecognition and the alloresponse: clinical implications. *Tissue Antigens, 69*: 545–56.

208. Cornell, L.D., Smith, R.N., Colvin, R.B., Cornell, L.D., Smith, R.N., Colvin, R.B. 2008. Kidney transplantation: mechanisms of rejection and acceptance. *Annual Review of Pathology, 3*: 189–220.

209. Hornick, P., Rose, M., Hornick, P., Rose, M. 2006. Chronic rejection in the heart. *Methods in Molecular Biology, 333*: 131–44.

210. Weiss, M.J., Madsen, J.C., Rosengard, B.R., Allan, J.S. 2008. Mechanisms of chronic rejection in cardiothoracic transplantation. *Frontiers in Bioscience, 13*: 2980–8.

211. Hayry, P. 1998. Chronic allograft vasculopathy: new strategies for drug development. *Transplantation Proceedings, 30*: 3989–90.

212. Lachmann, N., Terasaki, P.I., Schonemann, C., Lachmann, N., Terasaki, P.I., Schonemann, C. 2006. Donor-specific HLA antibodies in chronic renal allograft rejection: a prospective trial with a four-year follow-up. *Clinical Transplants*: 171–99.

213. Takahashi, H., Kato, T., Mizutani, K., Terasaki, P., Delacruz, V., Tzakis, A.G., Ruiz, P. 2006. Simultaneous antibody-mediated rejection of multiple allografts in modified multivisceral transplantation. *Clinical Transplants*: 529–34.

214. Terasaki, P., Lachmann, N., Cai, J., Terasaki, P., Lachmann, N., Cai, J. 2006. Summary of the effect of de novo HLA antibodies on chronic kidney graft failure. *Clinical Transplants*: 455–62.

215. Denton, M.D., Davis, S.F., Baum, M.A., Melter, M., Reinders, M.E., Exeni, A., Samsonov, D.V., Fang, J., Ganz, P., Briscoe, D.M. 2000. The role of the graft endothelium in transplant rejection: evidence that endothelial activation may serve as a clinical marker for the development of chronic rejection. *Pediatric Transplantation, 4*: 252–60.

216. Kauppinen, H., Soots, A., Krogerus, L., Brummer, T., Ahonen, J., Lautenschlager, I. 1997. Different expression of adhesion molecules ICAM-1 and VCAM-1 and activation markers MHC class II and IL-2R in acute and chronic rejection of rat kidney allografts. *Transplantation Proceedings, 29*: 3150–1.

217. Grimm, P.C., Nickerson, P., Jeffery, J., Savani, R.C., Gough, J., McKenna, R.M., Stern, E., Rush, D.N. 2001. Neointimal and tubulointerstitial infiltration by recipient mesenchymal cells in chronic renal-allograft rejection. *New England Journal of Medicine, 345*: 93–97.

218. Allan, J.S., Madsen, J.C., Allan, J.S., Madsen, J.C. 2002. Recent advances in the immunology of chronic rejection. *Current Opinion in Nephrology and Hypertension, 11*: 315–21.

219. Ozdemir, B.H., Ozdemir, F.N., Gungen, Y., Haberal, M. 2002. Role of macrophages and lymphocytes in the induction of neovascularization in renal allograft rejection. *American Journal of Kidney Diseases, 39*: 347–53.

220. Ravalli, S., Albala, A., Ming, M., Szabolcs, M., Barbone, A., Michler, R.E., Cannon, P.J. 1998. Inducible nitric oxide synthase expression in smooth muscle cells and macrophages of human transplant coronary artery disease. *Circulation, 97*: 2338–45.

221. Mannon, R.B. 2006. Therapeutic targets in the treatment of allograft fibrosis. *American Journal of Transplantation, 6*: 867–75.

222. Wynn, T.A. 2008. Cellular and molecular mechanisms of fibrosis. *Journal of Pathology, 214*: 199–210.

223. Nadeau, K.C., Azuma, H., Tilney, N.L. 1995. Sequential cytokine dynamics in chronic rejection of rat renal allografts: roles for cytokines RANTES and MCP-1. *Proceedings of the National Academy of Sciences of the United States of America, 92*: 8729–33.

224. Russell, M.E., Wallace, A.F., Hancock, W.W., Sayegh, M.H., Adams, D.H., Sibinga, N.E., Wyner, L.R., Karnovsky, M.J. 1995. Upregulation of cytokines associated with macrophage activation in the Lewis-to-F344 rat transplantation model of chronic cardiac rejection. *Transplantation, 59*: 572–8.

225. Csencsits, K., Wood, S.C., Lu, G., Faust, S.M., Brigstock, D., Eichwald, E.J., Orosz, C.G., Bishop, D.K. 2006. Transforming growth factor beta-induced connective tissue growth factor and chronic allograft rejection. *American Journal of Transplantation, 6*: 959–66.

226. Rintala, J.M., Savikko, J., Rintala, S.E., von Willebrand, E. 2006. The effect of leflunomide analogue FK778 on development of chronic rat renal allograft rejection and transforming growth factor-BETA expression. *Transplantation Proceedings, 38*: 3239–40.

227. Barocci, S., Ginevri, F., Valente, U., Torre, F., Gusmano, R., Nocera, A. 1999. Correlation between angiotensin-converting enzyme gene insertion/deletion polymorphism and kidney graft long-term outcome in pediatric recipients: a single-center analysis. *Transplantation, 67*: 534–8.

228. Ikegami, M., Nagano, T., Hara, Y., Negita, M., Imanishi, M., Ishii, T., Uemura, T., Kunikata, S., Kanda, H., Matsuura, T. et al. 1995. [Tissue type plasminogen activator (t-PA) and plasminogen activator inhibitor (PAI) in transplanted kidneys]. *Nippon Hinyokika Gakkai Zasshi – Japanese Journal of Urology, 86*: 991–5.

229. Legendre, C., Pascual, M., Legendre, C., Pascual, M. 2008. Improving outcomes for solid-organ transplant recipients at risk from cytomegalovirus infection: late-onset disease and indirect consequences. *Clinical Infectious Diseases, 46*: 732–40.

230. Egli, A., Binggeli, S., Bodaghi, S., Dumoulin, A., Funk, G.A., Khanna, N., Leuenberger, D., Gosert, R., Hirsch, H.H., Egli, A. et al. 2007. Cytomegalovirus and polyomavirus BK posttransplant. *Nephrology Dialysis Transplantation, 22 Suppl. 8*: viii72–82.

231. Steininger, C. 2007. Clinical relevance of cytomegalovirus infection in patients with disorders of the immune system. *Clinical Microbiology and Infection, 13*: 953–63.

232. Streblow, D.N., Orloff, S.L., Nelson, J.A. 2007. Acceleration of allograft failure by cytomegalovirus. *Current Opinion in Immunology, 19*: 577–82.

233. Potena, L., Valantine, H.A. 2007. Cytomegalovirus-associated allograft rejection in heart transplant patients. *Current Opinion in Infectious Diseases, 20*: 425–31.

234. Valantine, H. 2004. Cardiac allograft vasculopathy after heart transplantation: risk factors and management. *Journal of Heart and Lung Transplantation, 23*: S187–93.

235. Bonvoisin, C., Weekers, L., Xhignesse, P., Grosch, S., Milicevic, M., Krzesinski, J.-M. 2008. Polyomavirus in renal transplantation: a hot problem. *Transplantation, 85*: S42–8.

236. Dall, A., Hariharan, S. 2008. BK virus nephritis after renal transplantation. *Clinical Journal of the American Society of Nephrology: CJASN, 3 Suppl. 2*: S68–75.

237. Drachenberg, C.B., Papadimitriou, J.C., Ramos, E. 2006. Histologic versus molecular diagnosis of BK polyomavirus-associated nephropathy: a shifting paradigm? *Clinical Journal of the American Society of Nephrology: CJASN, 1*: 374–9.

238. Berenguer, M. 2007. Recurrent hepatitis C: worse outcomes established, interventions still inadequate. *Liver Transplantation, 13*: 641–3.

239. Caillard, S., Lelong, C., Pessione, F., Moulin, B. 2006. Post-transplant lymphoproliferative disorders occurring after renal transplantation in adults: report of 230 cases from the French Registry. *American Journal of Transplantation, 6*: 2735–42.

240. Cox, K.L., Lawrence-Miyasaki, L.S., Garcia-Kennedy, R., Lennette, E.T., Martinez, O.M., Krams, S.M., Berquist, W.E., So, S.K., Esquivel, C.O. 1995. An increased incidence of Epstein-Barr virus infection and lymphoproliferative disorder in young children on FK506 after liver transplantation. *Transplantation, 59*: 524–9.

241. Nelson, B.P., Nalesnik, M.A., Bahler, D.W., Locker, J., Fung, J.J., Swerdlow, S.H. 2000. Epstein-Barr virus-negative post-transplant lymphoproliferative disorders: a distinct entity? *American Journal of Surgical Pathology, 24*: 375–85.

242. Baqi, N., Tejani, A. 1997. Recurrence of the original disease in pediatric renal transplantation. *Journal of Nephrology, 10*: 85–92.

243. Choy, B.Y., Chan, T.M., Lai, K.N. 2006. Recurrent glomerulonephritis after kidney transplantation. *American Journal of Transplantation, 6*: 2535–42.

244. Newstead, C.G. 2003. Recurrent disease in renal transplants. *Nephrology Dialysis Transplantation, 18 Suppl. 6*: vi68–74.

245. Akatsuka, Y., Nishida, T., Kondo, E., Miyazaki, M., Taji, H., Iida, H., Tsujimura, K., Yazaki, M., Naoe, T., Morishima, Y. et al. 2003. Identification of a polymorphic gene, BCL2A1, encoding two novel hematopoietic lineage-specific minor histocompatibility antigens. *Journal of Experimental Medicine, 197*: 1489–500.

246. Torikai, H., Akatsuka, Y., Miyazaki, M., Warren, E.H., 3rd, Oba, T., Tsujimura, K., Motoyoshi, K., Morishima, Y., Kodera, Y., Kuzushima, K. et al. 2004. A novel HLA-A*3303-restricted minor histocompatibility antigen encoded by an unconventional open reading frame of human TMSB4Y gene. *Journal of Immunology, 173*: 7046–54.

247. Kawase, T., Akatsuka, Y., Torikai, H., Morishima, S., Oka, A., Tsujimura, A., Miyazaki, M., Tsujimura, K., Miyamura, K., Ogawa, S. et al. 2007. Alternative splicing due to an intronic SNP in HMSD generates a novel minor histocompatibility antigen. *Blood, 110*: 1055–63.

248. Brickner, A.G., Evans, A.M., Mito, J.K., Xuereb, S.M., Feng, X., Nishida, T., Fairfull, L., Ferrell, R.E., Foon, K.A., Hunt, D.F. et al. 2006. The PANE1 gene encodes a novel human minor histocompatibility antigen that is selectively expressed in B-lymphoid cells and B-CLL. *Blood, 107*: 3779–86.

249. Warren, E.H., Vigneron, N.J., Gavin, M.A., Coulie, P.G., Stroobant, V., Dalet, A., Tykodi, S.S., Xuereb, S.M., Mito, J.K., Riddell, S.R. et al. 2006. An antigen produced by splicing of noncontiguous peptides in the reverse order. *Science, 313*: 1444–7.

250. den Haan, J.M., Meadows, L.M., Wang, W., Pool, J., Blokland, E., Bishop, T.L., Reinhardus, C., Shabanowitz, J., Offringa, R., Hunt, D.F. et al. 1998. The minor histocompatibility antigen HA-1: a diallelic gene with a single amino acid polymorphism. *Science, 279*: 1054–7.

251. Torikai, H., Akatsuka, Y., Miyauchi, H., Terakura, S., Onizuka, M., Tsujimura, K., Miyamura, K., Morishima, Y., Kodera, Y., Kuzushima, K. et al. 2007. The HLA-A*0201-restricted minor histocompatibility antigen HA-1H peptide can also be presented by another HLA-A2 subtype, A*0206. *Bone Marrow Transplantation, 40*: 165–74.

252. Mommaas, B., Kamp, J., Drijfhout, J.-W., Beekman, N., Ossendorp, F., Van Veelen, P., Den Haan, J., Goulmy, E., Mutis, T. 2002. Identification of a novel HLA-B60-restricted T cell epitope of the minor histocompatibility antigen HA-1 locus. *Journal of Immunology, 169*: 3131–6.

253. den Haan, J.M., Sherman, N.E., Blokland, E., Huczko, E., Koning, F., Drijfhout, J.W., Skipper, J., Shabanowitz, J., Hunt, D.F., Engelhard, V.H. et al. 1995. Identification of a graft versus host disease-associated human minor histocompatibility antigen. *Science, 268*: 1476–80.

254. Wang, W., Meadows, L.R., den Haan, J.M., Sherman, N.E., Chen, Y., Blokland, E., Shabanowitz, J., Agulnik, A.I., Hendrickson, R.C., Bishop, C.E. et al. 1995. Human H-Y: a male-specific histocompatibility antigen derived from the SMCY protein. *Science, 269*: 1588–90.

255. Spierings, E., Brickner, A.G., Caldwell, J.A., Zegveld, S., Tatsis, N., Blokland, E., Pool, J., Pierce, R.A., Mollah, S., Shabanowitz, J. et al. 2003. The minor histocompatibility antigen HA-3 arises from differential proteasome-mediated cleavage of the lymphoid blast crisis (Lbc) oncoprotein. *Blood, 102*: 621–9.

256. Brickner, A.G., Warren, E.H., Caldwell, J.A., Akatsuka, Y., Golovina, T.N., Zarling, A.L., Shabanowitz, J., Eisenlohr, L.C., Hunt, D.F., Engelhard, V.H. et al. 2001. The immunogenicity of a new human minor histocompatibility antigen results from differential antigen processing. *Journal of Experimental Medicine, 193*: 195–206.

257. Dolstra, H., Fredrix, H., Maas, F., Coulie, P.G., Brasseur, F., Mensink, E., Adema, G.J., de Witte, T.M., Figdor, C.G., van de Wiel-van Kemenade, E. 1999. A human minor histocompatibility antigen specific for B cell acute

lymphoblastic leukemia. *Journal of Experimental Medicine*, *189*: 301–8.

258. Dolstra, H., de Rijke, B., Fredrix, H., Balas, A., Maas, F., Scherpen, F., Aviles, M.J., Vicario, J.L., Beekman, N.J., Ossendorp, F. et al. 2002. Bi-directional allelic recognition of the human minor histocompatibility antigen HB-1 by cytotoxic T lymphocytes. *European Journal of Immunology*, *32*: 2748–58.

259. van Bergen, C.A.M., Kester, M.G.D., Jedema, I., Heemskerk, M.H.M., van Luxemburg-Heijs, S.A.P., Kloosterboer, F.M., Marijt, W.A.E., de Ru, A.H., Schaafsma, M.R., Willemze, R. et al. 2007. Multiple myeloma-reactive T cells recognize an activation-induced minor histocompatibility antigen encoded by the ATP-dependent interferon-responsive (ADIR) gene. *Blood*, *109*: 4089–96.

260. de Rijke, B., van Horssen-Zoetbrood, A., Beekman, J.M., Otterud, B., Maas, F., Woestenenk, R., Kester, M., Leppert, M., Schattenberg, A.V., de Witte, T. et al. 2005. A frameshift polymorphism in P2X5 elicits an allogeneic cytotoxic T lymphocyte response associated with remission of chronic myeloid leukemia. *Journal of Clinical Investigation*, *115*: 3506–16.

261. Slager, E.H., Honders, M.W., van der Meijden, E.D., van Luxemburg-Heijs, S.A.P., Kloosterboer, F.M., Kester, M.G.D., Jedema, I., Marijt, W.A.E., Schaafsma, M.R., Willemze, R. et al. 2006. Identification of the angiogenic endothelial-cell growth factor-1/thymidine phosphorylase as a potential target for immunotherapy of cancer. *Blood*, *107*: 4954–60.

262. Murata, M., Warren, E.H., Riddell, S.R. 2003. A human minor histocompatibility antigen resulting from differential expression due to a gene deletion. *Journal of Experimental Medicine*, *197*: 1279–89.

263. Vogt, M.H.J., van den Muijsenberg, J.W., Goulmy, E., Spierings, E., Kluck, P., Kester, M.G., van Soest, R.A., Drijfhout, J.W., Willemze, R., Falkenburg, J.H.F. 2002. The DBY gene codes for an HLA-DQ5-restricted human male-specific minor histocompatibility antigen involved in graft-versus-host disease. *Blood*, *99*: 3027–32.

264. Zorn, E., Miklos, D.B., Floyd, B.H., Mattes-Ritz, A., Guo, L., Soiffer, R.J., Antin, J.H., Ritz, J. 2004. Minor histocompatibility antigen DBY elicits a coordinated B and T cell response after allogeneic stem cell transplantation. *Journal of Experimental Medicine*, *199*: 1133–42.

265. Pierce, R.A., Field, E.D., den Haan, J.M., Caldwell, J.A., White, F.M., Marto, J.A., Wang, W., Frost, L.M., Blokland, E., Reinhardus, C. et al. 1999. Cutting edge: the HLA-A*0101-restricted HY minor histocompatibility antigen originates from DFFRY and contains a cysteinylated cysteine residue as identified by a novel mass spectrometric technique. *Journal of Immunology*, *163*: 6360–4.

266. Ivanov, R., Aarts, T., Hol, S., Doornenbal, A., Hagenbeek, A., Petersen, E., Ebeling, S. 2005. Identification of a 40S ribosomal protein S4-derived H-Y epitope able to elicit a lymphoblast-specific cytotoxic T lymphocyte response. *Clinical Cancer Research*, *11*: 1694–703.

267. Vogt, M.H., Goulmy, E., Kloosterboer, F.M., Blokland, E., de Paus, R.A., Willemze, R., Falkenburg, J.H. 2000. UTY gene codes for an HLA-B60-restricted human male-specific minor histocompatibility antigen involved in stem cell graft rejection: characterization of the critical polymorphic amino acid residues for T-cell recognition. *Blood*, *96*: 3126–32.

268. Warren, E.H., Gavin, M.A., Simpson, E., Chandler, P., Page, D.C., Disteche, C., Stankey, K.A., Greenberg, P.D., Riddell, S.R. 2000. The human UTY gene encodes a novel HLA-B8-restricted H-Y antigen. *Journal of Immunology*, *164*: 2807–14.

CHAPTER 2

Dermatological Complications in Transplant Patients and Composite Tissue Allotransplant Pathology

Emma L. Lanuti, M.D.

Brian R. Keegan, M.D., Ph.D.

Ingrid H. Wolf, M.D., Ph.D.

Marco Romanelli, M.D., Ph.D.

Phillip Ruiz, M.D., Ph.D.

Paolo Romanelli, M.D.

I. INTRODUCTION

Transplant recipients are susceptible to a number of well-described complications that include drug reactions, organ rejection, organ dysfunction, infection, and cancer. The type and severity of these complications are often determined by the method and the degree of immunosuppression (1,2). The skin has long been used as a proxy for the function of the body as a whole; furthermore, it represents the primary interface between the patient and the surrounding environment. Therefore, it is useful to review the common cutaneous manifestations observed in recipients of organ transplantation and to describe several unusual observations.

II. DRUG REACTIONS IN TRANSPLANT PATIENTS

Drug rashes are common in transplant patients, given that these patients are exposed to multiple drugs including antibiotics, antiviral medications, and cytokines during immune reactions. Attributing a cutaneous drug reaction to a particular drug may be difficult due to the complexity of many immunosuppressive regimens. The drugs responsible for most cutaneous adverse drug reactions are the beta-lactams, sulfonamides, and nonsteroidal anti-inflammatory drugs. Chemotherapeutic medications reported to cause a morbilliform drug exanthem include chlorambucil, cytarabine, etoposide, 5-fluorouracil, hydroxyurea, melphalan, and procarbazine (3). Most reactions appear within a week after a drug is started, except with antibiotics and allopurinol, which can cause a reaction up to two weeks after starting the treatment. Other immunosuppressive agents associated with mucocutaneous complications include azathioprine, corticosteroids, cyclosporine, mycophenolate, rapamycin, and tacrolimus.

Although skin biopsy may clarify the type of skin reaction and the mechanism (e.g., by demonstrating immune complexes, leukocytoclastic vasculitis, or eosinophilia) they rarely, however, help to identify the causative agent. Histologically, features of drug eruptions are heterogeneous and often include interface dermatitis with basal vacuolar alteration, dyskeratotic keratinocytes, and a mild perivascular inflammatory infiltrate (4). Eosinophil counts have sensitivity ranging from 22 to 36 percent and, thus, are unlikely to be very useful for diagnosing drug reactions. Skin biopsy can differentiate skin lesions of a drug rash from a cutaneous small-vessel vasculitis since transplant patients are persistently thrombocytopenic throughout the early transplant period. *Acral erythema* is a localized cutaneous response to chemotherapeutic drugs. It presents as painful erythema mainly of palms and soles that may evolve to blistering and desquamation. Histological studies of this entity are scant, but vacuolar degeneration of the basal layer, spongiosis, dyskeratotic keratinocytes, papillary dermal edema, and a mild perivascular lymphohistiocytic infiltrate have been described (4–6).

Acne is a common skin disorder caused by immunosuppressive agents. The most prevalent cutaneous side effects of *sirolimus* are pathologies of the pilosebaceous apparatus, chronic edemas, angioedemas, and mucous membrane involvement (7–10). It has been reported that recipients of renal transplantation taking sirolimus have an unusually high frequency of acne (45 percent), erupting soon after sirolimus initiation. In sirolimus-induced acne, only inflammatory lesions have been observed (11). Sebaceous areas may be involved, but the lesions frequently extend to the forearms, internal surface of the arm, cervical area, and scalp. In some patients, severe unusual, painful, nodular, edematous lesions on the neck and face may be noted. Bacteriological and histological examinations suggest a nonspecific folliculitis (11). In patients receiving sirolimus, it is important to be aware that this drug is associated with *mucositis* that can be difficult to distinguish from herpes simplex virus (HSV) infection. Everolimus is commonly used for prophylaxis of organ rejection in adult renal and heart transplant recipients. Acne and angioedema represent typical side effects early after everolimus initiation (Figures 2.1A, 2.1B, 2.2A, 2.2B, 2.3). Everolimus acne is normally temporary and usually improves within a few weeks (12).

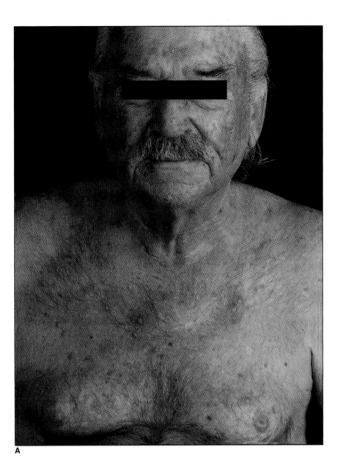

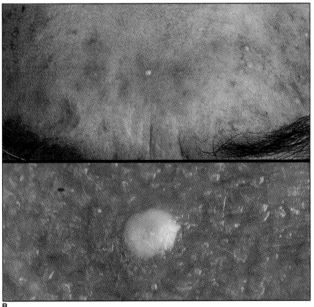

FIGURE 2.1: *(A and B) Renal transplant patient with acneiform eruption—induced by everolimus (Certican). Note erythematous papules and pustules without comedomes.*

III. NEPHROGENIC SYSTEMIC FIBROSIS

Nephrogenic systemic fibrosis is a rare condition seen in patients with renal diseases, many of whom are on hemo-

dialysis or renal transplant patients. Skin involvement is common and it was once considered a purely cutaneous disorder. Clinically, patients with skin involvement present with sclerotic induration distinguishable from

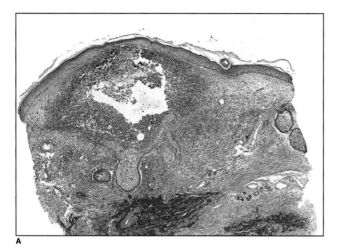
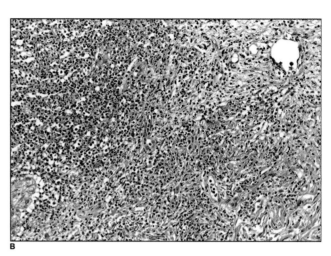

A   B

FIGURE 2.2: *(A and B) Renal transplant patient with acneiform eruption—induced by everolimus (Certican). Neutrophilic (suppurative) infiltrate (involving the follicular infundibula). Direct effect of everolimus on the follicle leads to the rupture of the follicle.*

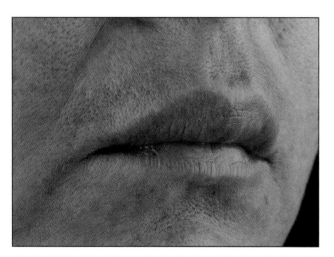

FIGURE 2.3: *Renal transplant patient. Angioedema induced by everolimus (Certican).*

scleromyxedema by its distribution pattern on the trunk and extremities and sparing of the face, absence of paraproteinemia, and absence of pools of dermal mucin and plasma cell infiltrate. Histological features include an increased number of spindle-shaped dermal fibroblast-like cells (CD34/procollagen I positive), accumulation of tissue dendritic cells, thickened collagen bundles with surrounding clefts, increased elastic fibers, and increased dermal mucin deposition. Additionally, there are increased numbers of factor XIIIa+ and CD68+ mononucleated and multinucleated cells (13). Calcification and fibrosis of the diaphragm, psoas muscle, renal tubules, and rete testes (14); a recent description of facial, pulmonary, and cardiac fibrosis (15); and the demonstration of widespread skeletal muscle involvement clearly indicate systemic involvement (16). Patients often report pruritus, causalgia, and sharp pains in the affected areas and joint contractures may develop very rapidly and be debilitating.

IV. GRAFT-VERSUS-HOST DISEASE

Graft-versus-host disease (GVHD) is a multisystem disease initiated by allogeneic T lymphocytes that recognize foreign tissue antigens in the host (see Chapter 9). As it is easily visualized, the skin is typically the first site of presentation of GVHD. It can occur after transfusion of nonirradiated blood products, transplantation of solid organs, and maternal blood transfer in an immunodeficient fetus. GVHD is divided into acute and chronic forms that have distinct disease patterns and are conventionally differentiated by whether onset is before or after 100 days following transplantation.

i. Acute GVHD

Acute GVHD follows a graft-versus-host reaction targeted against epithelia of skin, gastrointestinal tract, and liver and is manifested with rash, diarrhea, and abnormal liver function test results. *Early lesions* of acute GVHD are often folliculocentric blanching erythematous macules or papules or scarlatiniform eruption often with acral accentuation. These lesions may develop bullae and extend to erythroderma and epidermal necrosis (17,18) (Figure 2.6). Histologically, cutaneous acute GVHD is characterized by varying degrees of damage to the epidermal keratinocytes. In grade I, there is vacuolization of the basal keratinocytes (Figure 2.4A, 2.4B); in grade II, there are dyskeratotic keratinocytes and basal cell vacuolization is evident; in grade III, there are numerous necrotic keratinocytes and focal clefting of the basal layer is formed; and in grade IV, necrosis of the entire epidermis and complete separation from the dermis occurs (17) (Figure 2.5). The lymphocytic infiltration and cytopathic changes of keratinocytes are the major features of acute GVHD. Characteristically, the clustered lymphocytes around dyskeratotic and/or dead keratinocytes are referred to as *satellite cell*

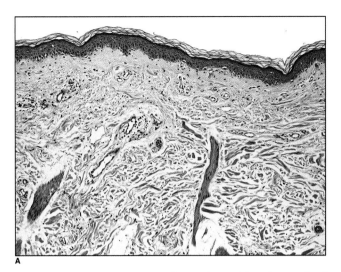
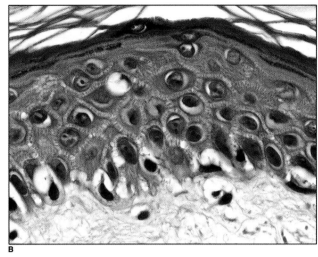

FIGURE 2.4: (A and B) Acute GVHD. Grade I: basal vacuolization. Higher magnification of A.

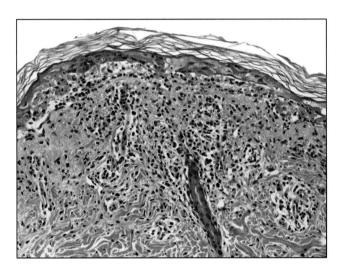

FIGURE 2.5: Acute GVDH. Grade IV: beginning separation of necrotic epidermis from dermis. Lymphocytic infiltration.

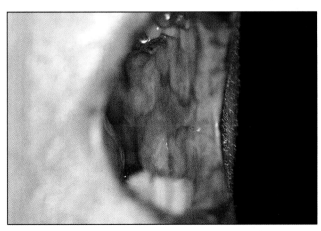

FIGURE 2.6: Acute GVHD. Erosions on lips and buccal mucosa.

necrosis. This sign usually has been considered illustrative of the pathogenesis of GVHD, with the presence of an activated donor lymphocyte recognizing a host cell. Focal or diffuse spongiosis may occur. Follicular infiltrates preferentially affect the bulge regions of anagen follicles and often precede invasion of the neighboring interfollicular dermis. Direct immunofluorescence labeling of skin biopsy specimens from patients with acute GVHD has demonstrated granular deposits of IgM and/or C3, similar to a lupus band test (19).

Many studies have been conducted to determine which lymphocyte subpopulations are found in the skin of patients with acute GVHD. The patterns can be variable. For example, the infiltrate can be composed of a mixture of CD4+ and CD8+ T cells, or with one of these subsets predominating. Two reports indicated that natural killer cells were present in acute GVHD skin lesions (20,21). B cells have not been found and cells expressing the gamma/delta T-cell receptor represent only a minority of infiltrating cells.

The diagnostic value of skin biopsies in the management of patients with a rash suspicious for GVHD is unclear. Indeed, skin biopsy findings were the reason for initiation of GVHD therapy in only 3 percent of all treated patients indicating that the biopsy seems to play only a minor role in directing a physician to initiate therapy for acute GVHD. The interpretation of the skin biopsy may be difficult because large doses of cytotoxic drugs and irradiation can produce histopathological changes that are *indistinguishable* from acute GVHD even in clinically normal skin (22–24). A likely explanation for this phenomenon is that the pathophysiology of both processes is mediated by the same effector cell, the T lymphocyte (25). HLA-DR expression on keratinocytes and on endothelial cells of the superficial vascular plexus, the presence of intraepidermal cytotoxic/suppressor T cells, and a predominance of helper/inducer T cells in the dermal inflammatory infiltrate may be seen in biopsies of both groups. Another study showed that neither skin nor rectal biopsies had a prognostic value in predicting the response to treatment (26). Despite these controversies, skin biopsies are still performed regularly on patients. To our knowledge, there have been few studies to define the role, if any, of skin biopsies in the management of such patients.

ii. Chronic GVHD

Chronic GVHD occurs in 25–50 percent of patients and is frequently preceded by the acute form of GVHD, although it may occur de novo (27,28). Chronic GVHD develops after a mean delay of onset of four months, but manifestations resembling cutaneous GVHD (cGVHD) can appear as early as day 40 following transplantation. The skin is involved in almost all cases of cGVHD and the mouth in 90 percent of patients. Both can develop spontaneously or be triggered by several events, notably UV irradiation, physical trauma, zoster, or even *Borrelia* infections. Clinically, chronic cGVHD has been classified as lichenoid or sclerodermatous lesions. Lichenoid

phase may precede the sclerodermatous phase. However, others have found that lichenoid and sclerodermatous cGVHD occur independently and dermal induration with no previous lichenoid phase may develop (29–31). The course starts as a generalized erythematous or violaceous rash, and progresses to poikiloderma with sclerotic hidebound skin (Figure 2.7A, 2.7B). Papulosquamous subtypes of GVHD have been reported including psoriasiform, keratosis pilaris–like, and asteatotic forms, and rarely, GVHD variants occur that exhibit the features of autoimmune connective tissue diseases such as dermatomyositis and lupus erythematosus (32,33). Reports cite a form of eczema-like GVHD recently referred to as eczematoid GVHD (34–36).

The so-called early phase of cGVHD is seen in lichenoid lesions. These lesions are erythematous or violaceous papules or plaques, with a squamous surface, sometimes forming larger confluent areas. These characteristic violaceous, indurated papules and plaques resemble lichen planus. The periorbital region, ears, palms, and soles are the typically affected sites (17). In some cases, lichenoid papules can occur around hair follicles or restricted to a dermatome (37). Occasionally, the center blisters leading to a vesicle, resembling dyshidrosis when present on the hands. Lichen planus–like GVHD can also affect the nails, with onychatrophia and pterygium, and the genital organs, with a risk of phimosis and vaginal strictures (17). Histologically, there is a lymphocytic infiltrate of the superficial dermis with moderate exocytosis resembling acute GVHD. In the dermis, the infiltrate is sometimes perineural (17). The epidermis is thickened with acanthosis, parakeratotic hyperkeratosis, and hypergranulosis and includes a variable degree of keratinocyte necrosis, sometimes with satellite cell necrosis (Figure 2.8A, 2.8B). It was recently shown that patients with all the histological criteria of lichenoid GVHD were more likely to die of GVHD (17).

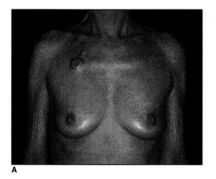 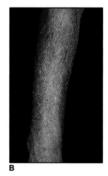

FIGURE 2.7: *(A and B) Chronic GVDH. Hyperpigmentation and scaling of the skin.*

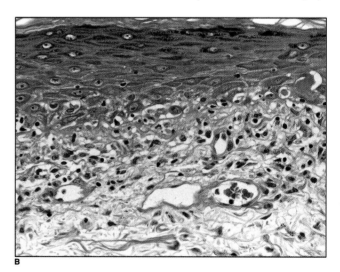

FIGURE 2.8: *(A and B) Chronic GVHD. Lichenoid interface dermatitis. Note numerous necrotic keratinocytes including satellite cell necrosis.*

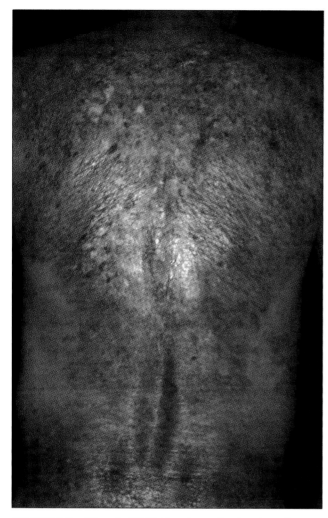

FIGURE 2.9: *Chronic GVHD. Papules and sclerodermatous changes.*

The so-called late phase corresponds to sclerodermatous lesions. Sclerodermoid GVHD (ScGVHD) has many clinicopathological patterns including cases resembling morphea, lichen sclerosus, and eosinophilic fasciitis (Figure 2.9). The diffuse form of ScGVHD is associated with deep-seated fibrosis and joint contractures. The three main histological sclerotic patterns are pandermal, patched, and deep dermal (38). Biopsies show vacuolar degeneration in the basal cell layer of the epidermis and some necrotic keratinocytes, suggestive of interface dermatitis but not enough to classify them histologically as lichenoid. Several authors have reported vacuolar degeneration as a rare finding in ScGVHD, and that when found, it may indicate an earlier lesion that is still evolving. At that time, there is marked epidermal atrophy, progressive destruction of appendageal structures, linearization of the dermoepidermal junction, and superficial collagen fibrosis. Fibrosis and destruction of adnexal structures are commonly seen in the dermis and fibrosis may extend to the subcutaneous fat (39). Keratinocytes are small, flattened, and loaded with melanin. Vacuolized or necrotic keratinocytes are few and found in the basal cell layer (Figure 2.10A, 2.10B). The dermis is the site of discrete pericapillary infiltrates. There is no pericapillary sclerosis (17). Finally, granular IgM deposits at the dermoepidermal junction may be found in biopsy specimens from patients with chronic GVHD.

In up to 75 percent of patients with ScGVHD, the skin produces a rippled fibrotic appearance similar to eosinophilic fasciitis. This sign could be a marker of the severity of the process. The presence of lichen sclerosus–like lesions, morphealike lesions, and ripply skin and the histological findings of septal fibrosis and fasciitis suggest that the sclerosis in ScGVHD can start and affect any level of the skin and can extend to involve the complete dermis, the subcutis, and even the fascia (38). Clinically, patients with hypodermic involvement often present with ripply

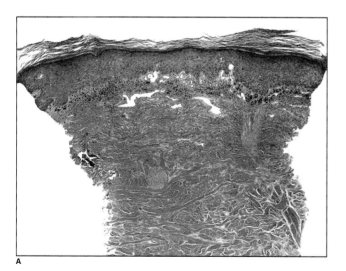

A

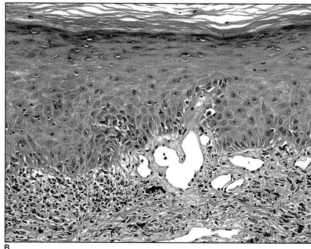

B

FIGURE 2.10: *(A and B) Chronic GVHD. Lichenoid lymphocytic infiltrate and fibrosis/sclerosis of the dermis. Note teleangiectatic vessels, melanophages, and necrotic keratinocytes.*

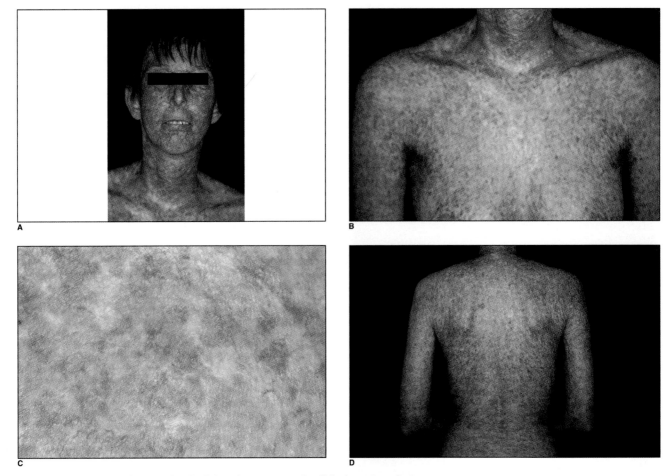

FIGURE 2.11: *(A–D) Chronic GVHD. Sclerodermatous and poikilodermatous features.*

skin, suggesting that this histological finding can be missed if the biopsies are not made deep enough.

Poikiloderma was described as a frequent finding in the first reports of cGVHD (38) (Figure 2.11A–D). Since then, it has been infrequently described, although results of ultrastructural studies showed dilated dermal capillaries. Mucin deposits within vacuolated spaces have been reported in patients with ScGVHD (38).

A *leopard-skin eruption* (widespread, well-delimited, hyperpigmented macules) may occur in patients with ScGVHD and these pigmentary changes precede, almost constantly, the development of apparent sclerosis and are very distinctive (38,40). Histology reveals sclerosis in the reticular dermis and slight vacuolar degeneration of the epidermis, with no other findings suggestive of a lichenoid eruption. Follicular involvement has been described more commonly in patients with lichenoid cGVHD but follicular keratosis can be found in the first phases of the ScGVHD. It disappears during the evolution of the disease and does not follow the pattern of the leopard-skin eruption. Histologically, follicular keratosis has a good correlation with the presence of vacuolar degeneration in the epidermis and follicular walls (38).

Oral manifestations are observed in the majority of patients with cGVHD. The mucocutaneous manifestations of cGVHD clinically resemble a wide variety of skin diseases, including lichen planus, lichenoid eruptions, sicca syndrome, morphea, scleroderma, and lichen sclerosus (41). Lichenoid lesions commonly affect all mucosal surfaces with predominant reticular and papular forms; tongue lesions usually are plaque like. Ulcerative lesions are not common, but when they appear, they are localized mainly in the buccal mucosa, palate, and dorsal part of the tongue. Atrophy of the oral mucosa also may be present, interspersed with areas of hyperkeratosis. Salivary gland involvement in cGVHD manifests as increased xerostomia, accompanied by decreased levels of salivary immunoglobulins and an increased incidence of oral infections. A *lip biopsy* specimen frequently is used to diagnose and determine the stage of the GVHD, and it has been noted that lip biopsy specimens need to include both mucosal and salivary gland tissue. Salivary gland biopsy findings have been correlated with the presence and clinical severity of GVHD, as well as being useful for evaluating the efficacy of therapeutic approaches. The qualitative and quantitative changes observed in the salivary secretions of people who have GVHD suggest suppressed local immunity that allows for the development of erosive ulcerative mucosal lesions, which may serve as a portal of entry for Candida species and of gram-negative anaerobic bacteria.

Eczematoid GVHD is an aggressive, chronic dermatosis that requires substantial immunosuppression therapy to achieve control and is associated with a poor prognosis. The histological features of GVHD coexist with the changes of dermatitis. The GVHD reaction is indicated by satellite cell necrosis, and the presence of parakeratosis, lymphocyte exocytosis, and epidermal spongiosis reflects the clinical appearance of eczema (34). The dermal changes are less marked, often showing a sparse perivascular lymphocytic infiltrate with eosinophils (34).

V. INFECTIONS IN TRANSPLANT PATIENTS

Advances in immunosuppressive medications and treatment protocols have extended the survival of transplant recipients. However, there is a close relationship between the degree of immunosuppression and the severity of infection in transplant patients. Cutaneous infections are a high cause of morbidity and mortality in transplant patients and can be caused by viruses, bacteria, or fungi. Dermatological infections after transplantation can be challenging and often need prompt treatment.

i. Viral Skin Infections in Transplant Patients

Viral skin infections are common findings in organ transplant recipients. Viral exanthems present as *macular* or *papular eruptions*. Many viral exanthems have no distinguishing histological features. Often, vacuolar alteration of the basal layer, occasional dyskeratotic keratinocytes, and a sparse lymphohistiocytic perivascular infiltrate are seen. Dermal hemorrhage is usually not seen in drug-induced reactions but may be present in some viral exanthems.

Varicella zoster virus (VZV) (a.k.a., herpes zoster) occurs in approximately 10 percent of solid organ recipients and tends to be self-limited (42). The incidence of herpes zoster in immunosuppressed patients is increased 20- to 100-fold, and the severity of the disease is also increased. In one review from a center in Canada, the overall incidence of herpes zoster following solid organ transplantation was 8.6 percent with a median time to onset of nine months; herpes zoster in these patients was also associated with high rates of cutaneous scarring (18.7 percent) and post-herpetic neuralgia (42.7 percent) (43). Reactivation of VZV is seen primarily as a vesicular infection in thoracic nerve dermatome distributions and is commonly referred to as *shingles* (Figure 2.12A, 2.12B). Histologically there are ballooned keratinocytes in the epidermis and lymphoid infiltrates in the dermis (Figure 2.13A–C). Disseminated zoster can also occur with one or multiple dermatomes with crusts and scarring (Figure 2.14A–C). Although rare, untreated primary VZV infection in transplant patients can disseminate and cause hemorrhagic pneumonia, hepatitis, or encephalitis (42). In immunocompromised patients, recurrent herpes zoster can occur. The diagnosis of VZV is made clinically, and routine laboratory tests are not useful. A Tzanck smear may be performed. Definitive diagnosis of VZV infection can be achieved through viral cultures. Immunofluorescent staining with monoclonal antibodies can also be used to confirm VZV infection or reactivation. Serological tests can provide a retrospective diagnosis of VZV infection.

Reactivation of HSV is a common problem in transplant patients. Common manifestations of HSV infection in organ transplant recipients are orolabial and anogenital lesions. HSV viral shedding can be detected within five to fourteen days after transplantation in 50–66 percent of seropositive renal allograft recipients, although symptomatic vesicles or ulcers develop in only 15–45 percent of recipients (44) (Figure 2.16). Typically, herpetic vesicles break down to

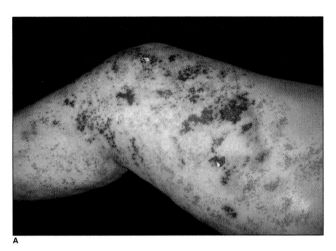

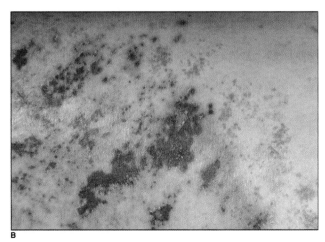

A   B

FIGURE 2.12: *(A and B) Renal transplant patient. Severe hemorrhagic zoster involving lumbar dermatomes.*

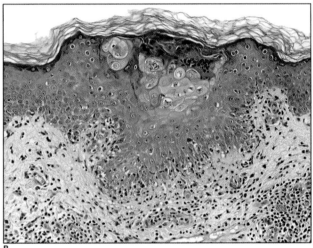

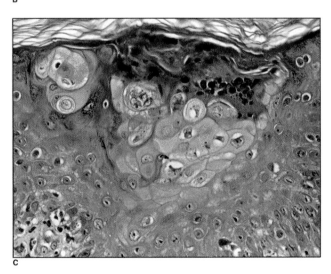

FIGURE 2.13: (A–C) Renal transplant patients. Zoster presenting ballooned keratinocytes in the epidermis. Note lymphoid infiltrates in the dermis.

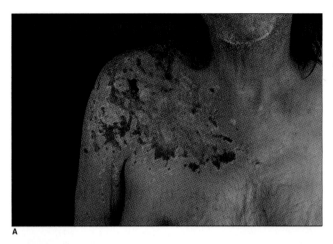

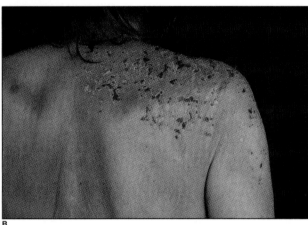

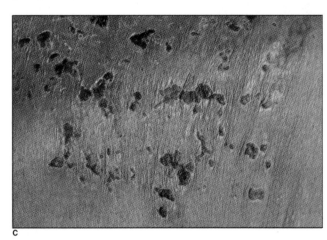

FIGURE 2.14: (A–C) Liver transplant patient. Necrotic zoster with crusts and scarring.

form shallow, grouped erosions and ulcers. In immunosuppressed patients, however, these ulcers may become large, confluent, chronic, granulating, and slow healing. Infections may be complicated by severe esophagitis, bronchopneumonia, and encephalitis. Widespread disseminated HSV infection of the skin is not common but is associated with high mortality rates. HSV infections can also trigger erythema multiforme, characterized by lesions with concentric color change (target lesions) that are symmetrically distributed predominantly over the extremities and acral areas.

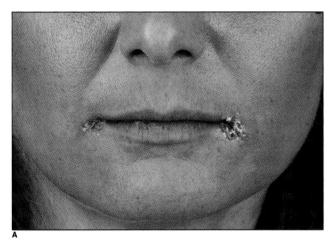
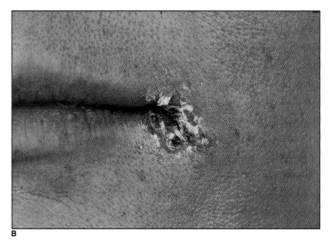

FIGURE 2.15: *(A and B) Renal transplant patient with cheilitis angularis.*

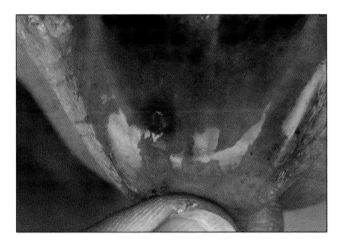

FIGURE 2.16: *Renal transplant patient. Oral herpes simplex infection.*

Diagnosis of HSV infection can usually be made by direct observation of the characteristic lesions, but the definitive diagnosis of active infection relies on culture of vesicular fluid, mucosal swabs, cerebrospinal fluid, or urine. Direct immunostaining of cells from these specimens with fluorescent dye–conjugated monoclonal antibodies specific for HSV-1 and HSV-2 antigens can be used. The Tzanck smear would show ballooned keratinocytes or giant cells but is not specific for HSV. Molecular-based techniques such as polymerase chain reaction (PCR) have been used to detect HSV in herpes encephalitis, corneal infections, and skin lesions, including HSV-associated erythema multiforme.

Sources of cytomegalovirus (CMV) infection in organ transplant recipients include reactivation of latent virus or donor-transmitted virus. Symptomatic CMV infection occurs in 20–60 percent of all transplant recipients and is a significant cause of mortality and morbidity. The patient at highest risk of symptomatic disease is a seronegative recipient matched with a seropositive donor. A primary infection or reactivation of CMV can result in asymptomatic

viral shedding to life-threatening multiorgan involvement. The patient may present with a mononucleosis-type syndrome with fever, malaise, leukopenia, and a macular rash or progress to develop pneumonia, hepatitis, gastroenteritis, and retinitis. *Cutaneous involvement* is present in 10–20 percent of patients with systemic CMV infection and is a sign of a poor prognosis. Cutaneous lesions are nonspecific and may include ulcers, morbilliform rashes, petechiae, purpuric eruptions, necrotic papules, and vesiculobullous eruptions. Chronic CMV infections are associated with risk of organ rejection, and also predispose the transplant recipient to higher risk of bacterial and fungal infections. Histology shows large intranuclear inclusions with a surrounding halo in endothelial cells. Confirmation of the diagnosis requires demonstration of the virus from skin, urine, throat washings, and buffy coat. Serologies are also helpful in determining past exposure to CMV infection, but the transplant recipient's ability to mount an increasing antibody response may be blunted. Qualitative CMV PCR assays are very sensitive in detecting CMV DNA and are used routinely in many transplant centers to diagnose active disease CMV disease, to screen patients for the use of preemptive therapy, and to monitor response to antiviral therapy.

Although transplant patients may develop a primary human herpes virus 6 (HHV-6) infection from transplanted tissue, the most common cause of active HHV-6 infection in the transplant patient is reactivation of the latent virus. It has been reported in 38–60 percent of bone marrow transplant recipients and in 31–55 percent of solid organ transplant recipients. It has been associated with *exanthem subitum* in children and is probably one of the viral causes of a mononucleosis syndrome in adults (45). One study showed that after allogeneic bone marrow transplant, there is an increased risk of developing GVHD, in which HHV-6 DNA is found in rectal and/or skin biopsy specimens (46).

Epstein-Barr virus (EBV) (HHV-4) is responsible for infectious mononucleosis, Burkitt lymphoma, oral hairy leukoplakia, and nasopharyngeal carcinoma. EBV is excreted in saliva and spread by close contact, often infecting hosts at a young age. Oral hairy leukoplakia lesions present as poorly demarcated keratotic areas with a corrugated or "hairy" appearance on the lateral borders of the tongue and are a sign of strong immunosuppression. The most severe complication of EBV is post-transplant lymphoproliferative disease (PTLD). PTLD is a well-known complication of organ transplantation (see Chapter 10). Although most post-transplant lymphomas are of B-cell origin, post-transplant primary cutaneous T-cell lymphoma has been described, presenting as tumors on the face and chest.

Human papilloma virus (HPV) is a frequent infection in transplant recipients. Verrucae can appear up to several years after transplantation and continue to grow and multiply over that time (Figure 2.17A, 2.17B). HPV infection in transplant recipients is also important because of its link to the development of certain skin cancers, in particular, *squamous cell carcinoma* (SCC). An extremely diverse group of HPV types, consisting mainly of epidermodysplasia verruciformis-associated HPV types, can be detected in benign, premalignant, and malignant skin lesions of organ transplant recipients (Figure 2.18A, 2.18B, 2.19A, 2.19B).

ii. Cutaneous Bacterial Infections in Transplant Patients

Systemic bacterial infections are a major cause of morbidity and mortality in transplant patients. Wound infections the first month after transplant are increasingly being caused by antibiotic-resistant strains (vancomycin-resistant enterococci and methicillin-resistant *Staphylococcus aureus*) (47,48). Apart from wound infections, the spectrum of clinical lesions caused by bacteria includes impetigo, folliculitis, abscesses, cellulitis, and furuncles. Group A streptococci and *Staphylococcus aureus* are the most common causative organisms, similar to normal subjects. *Staphylococcus aureus* infections can manifest as pyoderma but staphylococcal *scalded skin syndrome* (staphylogenic Lyell syndrome) as well as *toxic epidermal necrolysis* have been reported following liver transplantation (49,50).

Less commonly, *Escherichia coli*, *Legionella*, *Nocardia*, and *Salmonella* species have been reported in transplant patients (49,51,52). Atypical mycobacteria infection (*Mycobacterium kansasii*, *M. chelonae*, *M. fortuitum*, *M. marinum*) is an infrequent complication that can present months to years after transplantation with lesions affecting the skin, tenosynovium, and/or joints of the extremities (53,54). Cutaneous lesions are most common on the extremities. Symmetric subcutaneous and tenosynovial sarcoidosis in an organ transplant recipient without evidence of systemic (visceral) disease has been reported (55).

iii. Cutaneous Fungal Infections in Transplant Patients

It clearly appears that the infective risk among organ transplant recipient is higher than the general population

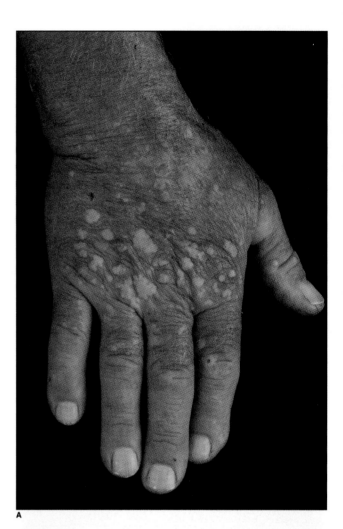

A

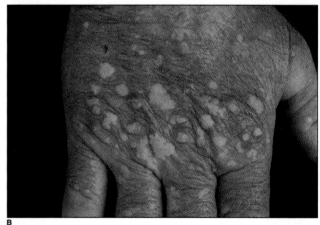

B

FIGURE 2.17: *(A and B) Large number of verrucae vulgares in a renal transplant patient.*

because of immunosuppressive therapies and possible delay in the function of the transplanted organ. Fungal infections typically develop within two months of transplantation and common sites of infection include surgical suture lines, skin, esophagus, and the urinary tract. The predominant organisms included *Candida* species and

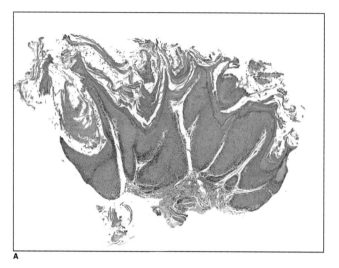
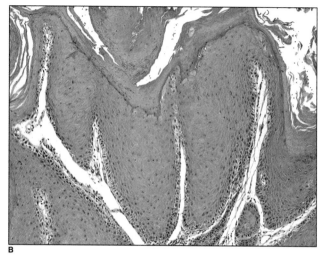

FIGURE 2.18: *(A and B) Bone marrow transplant patient. Verruca vulgaris on the tongue.*

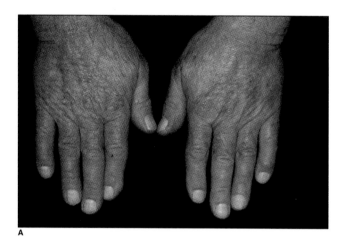
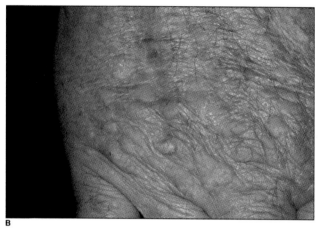

FIGURE 2.19: *(A and B) Renal transplant patient. Actinic keratoses and HPV-induced plane warts.*

Aspergillus species. Although fungal infections are decreasing with the practice of prophylaxis, they are still are a large cause of morbidity and mortality.

The incidence of invasive candidiasis has declined, but *Candida* species remains the most frequent cause of fungal infections, with *Candida albicans* accounting for most cases (48). Oral candidal infections may appear in one of several forms, most frequently as pseudomembranous candidacies (removable white plaques). Other less common clinical presentations include chronic hyperplastic candidacies (leukoplakia-like plaques that do not rub off), erythematous candidiasis (patchy or diffuse erythema), and angular cheilitis (Figure 2.15A, 2.15B). Skin lesions, usually erythematous and maculopapular in nature, can be the first evidence of disseminated candidiasis.

After *C. albicans*, *Aspergillus* species are the second most common cause of opportunistic fungal infections in humans (56). The lungs are the predominant site of infection and cutaneous aspergillosis may be primary or secondary. Secondary cutaneous aspergillosis occurs as a result of hematogenous dissemination or by extension to skin from contiguous anatomic structure and presents as eruptive maculopapules, whereas the rare type, primary cutaneous aspergillosis, manifestations are hemorrhagic bullae or an indurated, erythematous, violaceous plaque that progresses to a necrotic ulcer with a black eschar. The emergence of a new opportunistic *Aspergillus* infection, *A. ustus*, in solid organ transplant recipients has recently been reported (57–59).

Only rarely have cutaneous manifestations of other fungi such as *Cryptococcus neoformans*, *Exophiala jeanselmei*, *Wangiella dermatitidis*, or *Alternaria* species been reported (49). In organ transplant recipients, cutaneous cryptococcosis most commonly presents as bacterial cellulitis (60). Cutaneous cryptococcosis represents disseminated infection and may also present itself as erythematous swellings, nodular firm, cystic-appearing excrescences, granulomas, acneiform papules or pustules, crusted or infiltrating plaques, or ulcers. Organ recipients living in areas of endemic histoplasmosis, coccidiomycosis, and blastomycosis infections are at risk of primary infection or reactivation following immunosuppression. Cutaneous involvement is most often a sign of *dissemination* and should be treated promptly in these patients.

Dermatophytes can cause several skin lesions in transplant recipients including *Tinea corporis*, *T. pedis*, scalp infections, and nail infections. Localization is commonly on the face and buttock. Fingernail infections and involvement of multiple nails have been seen more commonly in immunocompromised patients than in other subjects. *Pityriasis versicolor* also has higher rates of infection in transplant patients (61).

VI. SKIN CANCER

The increased incidence of skin cancers in transplant patients is well documented (1,62), with SCC, basal cell carcinoma (BCC), melanoma, Kaposi's sarcoma (KS), and PTLD being the most commonly identified malignancies. In addition, it has been shown that these malignancies have more aggressive profiles in immunosuppressed patients leading to more morbidity (63). This increase in rate and aggressiveness of cutaneous malignancy is due in part to

infection by oncogenic organisms, loss of immune surveillance, and direct damage of DNA (64,65).

A notable proportion (25 percent) of patients will develop their first SCC within five years of transplantation and usually in sun-exposed areas of the body with an increase in incidence of 60- to 100-fold over nontransplanted patients (66) (Figure 2.20A–B). The transplant patients at the highest risk are heart, kidney, and liver recipients (64). Risk factors for development of SCC include history of SCC; Fitzpatrick skin type I, II, or III; increased age; HPV infection (HPV-5, HPV-8, HPV-16, and HPV-18); and history of UV exposure (1). It is interesting to note that there may be some negative interaction between these last two factors as UV exposure has been shown to inactivate the E6 protein of HPV, thus limiting its oncogenic potential (67), an interesting observation that requires more research. Given the time required to progress to SCC (68), it is, therefore, likely that the chain of events is initiated soon after transplantation. Histologically, SCC in organ transplant patients is similar to other SCC as they demonstrate nests of squamous epithelial cells arising from the epidermis and extending into the dermis. Minor differences that have been

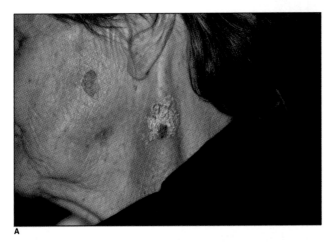
A

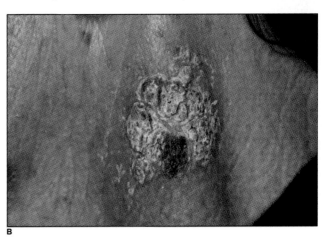
B

FIGURE 2.20: *(A and B) Renal transplant patient. Actinic keratoses and progression into invasive SCC.*

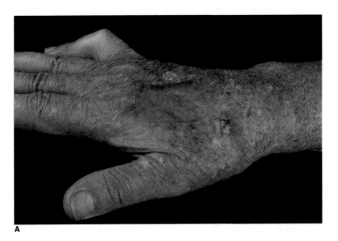
A

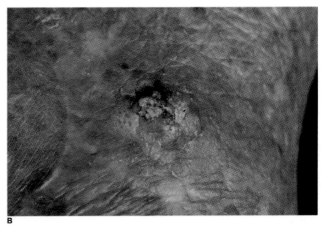
B

FIGURE 2.21: *(A and B) Renal transplant patient. SCC on sun-exposed skin.*

reported include an increase in spindle cell morphology, acantholytic changes, early dermal invasion, an infiltrative growth pattern with or without desmoplasia, Bowen's disease with carcinoma, and a deeper invasion at diagnosis. Higher rates of metastasis to the parotid gland have been blamed on the combination of high incidence on the head and neck region, deeper invasion, and immunologic suppression. The management of SCC in organ transplant patients has been described in detail, with the emphasis being a requirement for more aggressive treatment, more frequent examinations, lower thresholds for biopsy, and the addition of imaging studies.

The rate of BCC formation is about tenfold higher in transplantation recipients (69). This increase is not as substantial as some of the other cutaneous malignancies leading the authors to suggest that the immune system is not as essential in regulation of this malignancy. One difference that was recently described demonstrated that there is an increased superficial component to BCC in transplant patients (70). Histopathologically, there are few differences in the presentation, as the basal cell carcinomas are composed of nests or islands of basaloid cells with periphery of palisading cells (71). The nuclei are hyperchromatic and sometimes atypical with numerous mitotic figures and little cytoplasm. A high rate of apoptosis and cell death is also noted. As with SCC, the management of BCC is generally more aggressive in organ transplant patients.

A 3.8- to 8-fold increase in the incidence of melanoma has been described in transplant patients (72). It is interesting to note that a higher than expected proportion of these cancers developed in dysplastic nevi, which leads to the postulation that this was primarily a function of loss of immune suppression. The histopathological diagnosis of melanoma is both complex and evolving and differences in melanoma histology have not been specifically described in organ transplant patients; a detailed review of melanoma is provided by van Dijk et al. (73). Reducing the degree of immunosuppression has been suggested in the management of melanoma in organ transplant patients (74); however, this is a complex clinical question requiring extensive analysis and discussion with the patient.

KS is associated with HHV-8 infection and is a relatively common malignancy after kidney transplantation, with a recent report showing incidence nearly 500–1,000 times higher than the nontransplanted patients (75) often developing approximately sixteen months after transplantation. This is classified as iatrogenic KS and is thought to be secondary to the choice of immunosuppressive regimen (76). Histopathologically, iatrogenic KS is not significantly different than other forms of KS consisting of interwoven bands of vascular cleft–like spaces between spindle cells in a network of collagen fibers (77). Extravasated erythrocytes and hemosiderin-laden macrophages are commonly present. Patients with superficial disease respond to withdrawal of immunosuppression without serious renal dysfunction (78).

PTLD is a known complication of solid organ and bone marrow transplantation. The overall incidence of PTLD in allograft recipients varies depending on the type of organ transplanted, the degree of immunosuppressive therapy, and the age of the patient (see Chapter 10). *Cutaneous lesions*, which have a relatively better prognosis than internal lesions, may present as ulcers, nodules, or erythematous plaques. Most commonly, PTLD manifesting itself in the skin represent an EBV-driven proliferation of B lymphocytes, which histologically is represented as hyperplasia or malignant lymphoma (79–81). Although most PTLD results from an abnormal growth of EBV-transformed B cells, EBV-negative PTLD and PTLD of T cell origin (82) do occur, particularly in PTLD that develops more than one year after transplantation.

Merkel cell carcinoma (83), angiosarcoma (84), fibroxanthoma (85), verrucous carcinoma (86), and metastatic disease have also been reported in transplant patients; however, since large-scale studies have not been performed so we will only mention their observation.

VII. PATHOLOGY OF COMPOSITE TISSUE ALLOTRANSPLANTATION

Composite tissue allotransplantation (CTA) is a relatively new area of allotransplantation (87) that encompasses surgical therapy of a variety of severe tissue or limb defects, including hand transplantation (88), abdominal wall transplantation (89), and face transplants (90). CTAs typically include skin, which is utilized to monitor signs of graft dysfunction and/or rejection. The skin may display erythema, edema, rash, desquamation, ulceration, or necrosis. Skin biopsies are utilized to monitor *acute cellular rejection* and to date there have been several grading schemes that have been proposed to assess this complication (91–93). At the 2007 Banff Conference in La Coruna, Spain, a worldwide consortium of pathologists and clinicians with experience in clinical CTA met to define a universally accepted histological classification (Table 2.1) (94). Histologically, the skin

TABLE 2.1 The Banff 2007 Working Classification of Skin-Containing Composite Tissue Allograft Pathology (94)

Grade 0: No or rare inflammatory infiltrates.

Grade I: Mild. Mild perivascular infiltration. No involvement of the overlying epidermis.

Grade II: Moderate. Moderate to severe perivascular inflammation with or without mild epidermal and/or adnexal involvement (limited to spongiosis and exocytosis). No epidermal dyskeratosis or apoptosis.

Grade III: Severe. Dense inflammation and epidermal involvement with epithelial apoptosis, dyskeratosis, and/or keratinolysis.

Grade IV: Necrotizing acute rejection. Frank necrosis of epidermis or other skin structures.

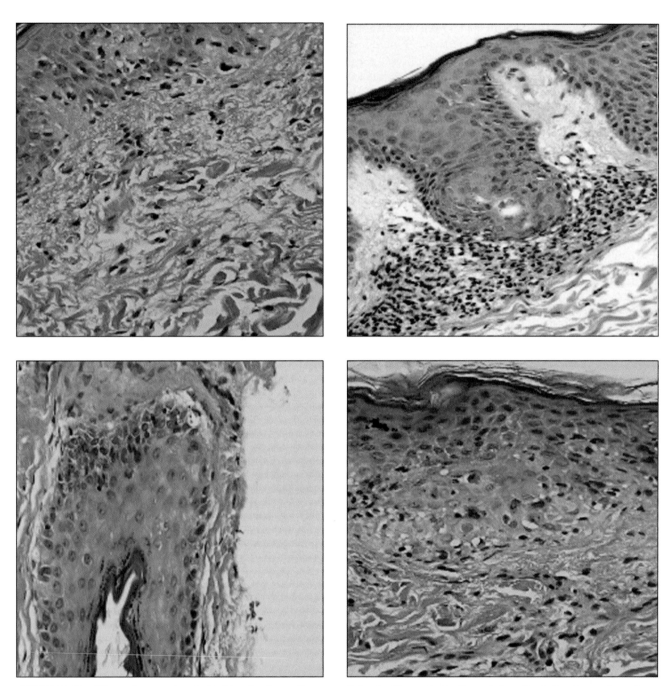

FIGURE 2.22: *Photomicrographs of skin biopsies from allogeneic abdominal transplants. Upper left: patient showing early acute cellular rejection (grade 1, mild) with mild lymphocytic infiltrate; patient showing grade 2 (moderate) acute rejection with more intense infiltrate in subepidermal region (upper right) with appendage involvement (lower left); patient with focal necrosis of keratinocytes (lower right) – acute rejection (grade 3, severe). Hematoxylin and eosin, 200×.*

biopsies demonstrate mononuclear cell (small or large lymphocytes, macrophages) infiltration often with neutrophils (Figure 2.22). The infiltrate may involve epidermis, adnexal structures, and dermis in a perivascular and/or interstitial pattern of involvement (Figure 2.22). There may also be spongiosis, keratinocyte apoptosis, dyskeratosis, and necrosis (Figure 2.22). Eosinophils may be present but this cell population is not considered

in grading. *Acute humoral rejection* as of yet has not been consistently described in CTA rejection and is thus not present in the Banff classification. Cases with donor-HLA-specific antibodies and histological evidence of vasculitis, neutrophilic margination, and necrosis should be evaluated for the presence of C4d deposition.

Chronic rejection is not currently defined in CTA. To date, chronic injury to skin and appendages in skin of

CTA has been observed but the underlying causes of the fibrotic changes, injury, and atrophy to the allograft are not well defined or readily distinguishable. Concurrent immune and nonimmune etiologies overlap in causing chronic injury to the skin. Changes that may be seen are fibrosis of dermis and subcutaneum, vascular narrowing with myointimal proliferation, loss of adnexa, muscle atrophy, and nail changes.

REFERENCES

1. Kuijken I, BBJ. 2000. Skin cancer risk associated with immunosuppressive therapy in organ transplant recipients: epidemiology and proposed mechanisms. *BioDrugs 14(5)*: 319–29.
2. Ulrich C, Hackethal M, Meyer T, Geusau A, Nindl I, Ulrich M, Forschner T, Sterry W, Stockfleth E. 2008. Skin infections in organ transplant recipients. *JDDG 6*: 98–104.
3. Mays SR, KJ, Truong E, Kontoyiannis DP, Hymes SR. 2007. Approach to the morbilliform eruption in the hematopoietic transplant patient. *Seminars in Cutaneous Medicine and Surgery 26*: 155–162.
4. Kohler S, HM, Chao NJ, Smoller BR. 1997. Value of skin biopsies in assessing prognosis and progression of acute graft-versus-host disease. *American Journal of Surgical Pathology 21*: 988–96.
5. Baack BR, BW. 1991. Chemotherapy-induced acral erythema. *Journal of American Academy of Dermatology 24*: 457–61.
6. Bauer DJ, HA, Horn TD. 1993. Histologic comparison of autologous graft-vs-host reaction and cutaneous eruption of lymphocyte recovery. *Archives of Dermatology 129*: 855–8.
7. Aboujaoude W, MM, Govani MV. 2004. Lymphedema associated with sirolimus in renal transplant recipients. *Transplantation 77(7)*: 1094–6.
8. Mahé E, ME, Lechaton S, Sang KH, Mansouri R, Ducasse MF, Mamzer-Bruneel MF, de Prost Y, Kreis H, Bodemer C. 2005. Cutaneous adverse events in renal transplant recipients receiving sirolimus-based therapy. *Transplantation 79(4)*: 476–82.
9. Mohaupt MG, VB, Frey FJ. 2001. Sirolimus-associated eyelid edema in kidney transplant recipients. *Transplantation 72(1)*: 162–4.
10. van Gelder T, tMC, Hené R, Weimar W, Hoitsma A. 2003. Oral ulcers in kidney transplant recipients treated with sirolimus and mycophenolate mofetil. *Transplantation 75(6)*: 788–91.
11. Mahé E, ME, Lechaton S, Drappier JC, de Prost Y, Kreis H, Bodemer C. 2006. Acne in recipients of renal transplantation treated with sirolimus: clinical, microbiologic, histologic, therapeutic, and pathogenic aspects. *Journal of American Academy of Dermatology 55(1)*: 139–42.
12. Lehmkuhl H, RH, Eisen H, Valantine H. 2005. Everolimus (Certican) in heart transplantation: optimizing renal function through minimizing cyclosporine exposure. *Transplantation Proceedings 37(10)*: 4145–9.
13. Cowper SE, SL, Bhawan J, Robin HS, LeBoit PE. 2001. Nephrogenic fibrosing dermopathy. *American Journal of Dermatopathology 23(5)*: 383–93.
14. Ting WW, SM, Madison KC, Kurtz K. 2003. Nephrogenic fibrosing dermopathy with systemic involvement. *Archives of Dermatology 139*: 903–6.
15. Jimenez SA, AC, Sandorfi N, Derk C, Latinis K, Sawaya H, Haddad R, Shanahan JC. 2004. Dialysis-associated systemic fibrosis (nephrogenic fibrosing dermopathy): study of inflammatory cells and transforming growth factor beta1 expression in affected skin. *Arthritis and Rheumatism 50(8)*: 2660–6.
16. Levine JM, TR, Elman LB, Bird SJ, Lavi E, Stolzenberg ED, McGarvey ML, Asbury AK, Jimenez SA. 2004. Involvement of skeletal muscle in dialysis-associated systemic fibrosis (nephrogenic fibrosing dermopathy). *Muscle Nerve 30(5)*: 569–77.
17. Aractingi S, CO. 1998. Cutaneous graft-versus-host disease. *Archives of Dermatology 134(5)*: 602–12.
18. Johnson ML, FE. 1998. Graft-versus-host reactions in dermatology. *Journal of American Academy of Dermatology 38(3)*: 369–92.
19. Tsoi MS, SR, Jones E, Weiden PL, Shulman H, Witherspoon R, Atkinson K, Thomas ED. 1978. Deposition of IgM and complement at the dermoepidermal junction in acute and chronic cutaneous graft-vs-host disease in man. *Journal of Immunology 120(5)*: 1485–92.
20. Gilliam A, W-MD, Korngold R, Murphy G. 1996. Apoptosis is the predominant form of epithelial target cell injury in acute experimental graft versus host disease. *Journal of Investigative Dermatology 107*: 377–83.
21. Leskinen R, TE, Volin L, Ruutu T, Häyry P. 1992. Immunohistology of skin and rectum biopsies in bone marrow transplant recipients. *APMIS 100*: 1115–22.
22. Drijkoningen M, DW-PC, Tricot G, Degreef H, Desmet V. 1988. Drug-induced skin reactions and cutaneous graft-versus-host reaction: a comparative immunohistochemical study. *Blut 56*: 69–73.
23. Sale GE, LK, Barker EA, Shulman HM, Thomas ED. 1977. The skin biopsy in the diagnosis of acute graft-versus-host disease in man. *American Journal of Pathology 89(3)*: 621–35.
24. Zhou Y, BM, Rivers JK. 2000. Clinical significance of skin biopsies in the diagnosis and management of graft-vs-host disease in early postallogeneic bone marrow transplantation. *Archives of Dermatology 136(6)*: 717–21.
25. Ferrara JL, LR, Chao NJ. 1999. Pathophysiologic mechanisms of acute graft-vs.-host disease. *Biology of Blood and Marrow Transplantation 5(6)*: 347–56.
26. Sviland L, OA, Eastham EJ, Hamilton PJ, Proctor SJ, Malcom AJ. 1988. Histological features of skin and rectal biopsy specimens after autologous and allogeneic bone marrow transplantation. *Journal of Clinical Pathology 41*: 148–54.
27. Atkinson K. 1990. Chronic graft-versus-host disease. *Bone Marrow Transplantation 5(2)*: 69–82.
28. Rouquette-Gally AM, BD, Gluckman E, Abuaf N, Combrisson A. 1987. Autoimmunity in 28 patients after allogeneic bone marrow transplantation: comparison with Sjögren syndrome and scleroderma. *British Journal of Haematology 66(1)*: 45–7.
29. Andrews ML, RI, Weedon D. 1997. Cutaneous manifestations of chronic graft-versus-host disease. *Australasian Journal of Dermatology 38(2)*: 53–62.

30. *Farmer E.* 1985. Human cutaneous graft-versus-host disease. *Journal of Investigative Dermatology 85(1 Suppl.)*: 124S–8S.

31. White JM, CD, du Vivier AW, Pagliuca A, Ho AY, Devereux S, Salisbury JR, Mufti GJ. 2007. Sclerodermatous graft-versus-host disease: clinical spectrum and therapeutic challenges. *British Journal of Dermatology 156(5)*: 1032–8.

32. Leber B, WI, Rodriguez A, McBride JA, Carter R, Brain MC. 1993. Reinduction of remission of chronic myeloid leukemia by donor leukocyte transfusion following relapse after bone marrow transplantation: recovery complicated by initial pancytopenia and late dermatomyositis. *Bone Marrow Transplantation 12(4)*: 405–7.

33. Ollivier I, WP, Gherardi R, Wechsler J, Kuentz M, Cosnes A, Revuz J, Bagot M. 1998. Dermatomyositis-like graft-versus-host disease. *British Journal of Dermatology 138(3)*: 558–9.

34. Creamer D, M-SC, Osborne G, Kenyon M, Salisbury JR, Devereux S, Pagliuca A, Ho AY, Mufti GJ, du Vivier AW. 2007. Eczematoid graft-vs-host disease: a novel form of chronic cutaneous graft-vs-host disease and its response to psoralen UV-A therapy. *Archives of Dermatology 143(9)*: 1157–62.

35. Sloane JP, TJ, Imrie SF, Easton DF, Powles RL. 1984. Morphological and immunohistological changes in the skin in allogeneic bone marrow recipients. *Journal of Clinical Pathology 37(8)*: 919–30.

36. Tanasescu S, BX, Thomine E, Boullie MC, Vannier JP, Tron P, Joly P, Lauret P. 1999. Eczema-like cutaneous graft versus host disease treated by UV-B therapy in a 2-year-old child [in French]. *Annals of Dermatology and Venereology 126(1)*: 51–3.

37. Beers B, KR, Kaye V, Dahl M. 1993. Unilateral linear lichenoid eruption after bone marrow transplantation: an unmasking of tolerance to an abnormal keratinocyte clone? *Journal of American Academy of Dermatology 28*: 888–92.

38. Peñas PF, J-CM, Aragüés M, Fernández-Herrera J, Fraga J, García-Díez A. 2002. Sclerodermatous graft-vs-host disease: clinical and pathological study of 17 patients. *Archives of Dermatology 138(7)*: 924–34.

39. Chosidow O, BM, Vernant JP, Roujeau JC, Cordonnier C, Kuentz M, Wechsler J, André C, Touraine R, Revuz J. 1992. Sclerodermatous chronic graft-versus-host disease. Analysis of seven cases. *Journal of American Academy of Dermatology 26(1)*: 49–55.

40. Roujeau JC, RJ, Touraine R. 1980. Graft versus host reactions. In: Rook A, Savin J, eds. *Recent Advances in Dermatology 5*: 131–57.

41. Eggleston TI, ZV, Lumerman H. 1998. Graft-versus-host disease. Case report and discussion. *Oral Surgery Oral Medicine Oral Pathology Oral Radiology and Endodontics 86(6)*: 692–6.

42. Rubin R. 1994. *Clinical Approach to Infection in the Compromised Host*, 3rd ed. Plenum Medical Book Company, New York, NY.

43. Gourishankar S, MJ, Jhangri GS, Preiksaitis JK. 2004. Herpes zoster infection following solid organ transplantation: incidence, risk factors and outcomes in the current immunosuppressive era. *American Journal of Transplantation 4(1)*: 108–15.

44. Smith SR, BD, Alexander BD, Greenberg A. 2001. Viral infections after renal transplantation. *American Journal of Kidney Diseases 37*: 659–76.

45. LaRocco MT, BS. 1997. Infection in the bone marrow transplant recipient and role of the microbiology laboratory in clinical transplantation. *Clinical Microbiology Reviews 10(2)*: 277–97.

46. Appleton AL, SL, Peiris JS, Taylor CE, Wilkes J, Green MA, Pearson AD, Kelly PJ, Malcolm AJ, Proctor SJ, et al. 1995. Human herpes virus-6 infection in marrow graft recipients: role in pathogenesis of graft-versus-host disease. *Bone Marrow Transplantation 16(6)*: 777–82.

47. Bakir M, BJ, Newell KA, Millis JM, Buell JF, Arnow PM. 2001 Epidemiology and clinical consequences of vancomycin-resistant ente-rococci in liver transplant patients. *Transplantation 72(6)*: 1032–7.

48. Singh N, PD, Chang FY, Gayowski T, Squier C, Wagener MM, Marino IR. 2000. Methicillin-resistant Staphylococcus aureus: the other emerging resistant Gram-positive coccus among liver transplant recipients. *Clinical Infectious Disease 30(2)*: 322–7.

49. Schmied E, DJ, Euvrard S. 2004. Nontumoral dermatologic problems after liver transplantation. *Liver Transplantation 10(3)*: 331–9.

50. Strauss G, MA, Rasmussen A, Kirkegaard P. 1997. Staphylococcal scalded skin syndrome in a liver transplant patient. *Liver Transplantation Surgery 3(4)*: 435–6.

51. Fishman JA, RR. 1998. Infection in organ-transplant recipients. *New England Journal of Medicine 338(24)*: 1741–51.

52. Varon NF, AG. 2004. Emerging trends in infections among renal transplant recipients. *Expert Review of Anti-Infective Therapy 21*: 95–109.

53. Nathan DL, SS, Kestenbaum TM, Casparian JM. 2000. Cutaneous Mycobacterium chelonae in a liver transplant patient. *Journal of American Academy of Dermatology 43*: 333–6.

54. Patel R, RG, Keating MR, Paya CV. 1994. Infections due to nontuberculous mycobacteria in kidney, heart, and liver transplant recipients. *Clinical Infectious Disease 19*: 263.

55. Carlson JA, W-LH, Kutzner H, Jones DM, Tobin E. 2007. Sarcoidal granulomatous tenosynovitis of the hands occurring in an organ transplant patient. *Journal of Cutaneous Pathology 34(8)*: 658–64.

56. Paya C. 1993. Fungal infections in solid-organ transplantation. *Clinical Infectious Disease 16(5)*: 677–88.

57. Panackal A, IA, Hanley EW, Marr KA. 2006. Aspergillus ustus infections among transplant recipients. *Emerging Infectious Diseases 12(3)*: 403–8.

58. Stiller MJ, TL, Rosenthal SA, Riordan A, Potter J, Shupack JL, Gordon MA. 1994. Primary cutaneous infection by Aspergillus ustus in a 62-year-old liver transplant recipient. *Journal of American Academy of Dermatology 31(2 Pt. 2)*: 344–7.

59. Vagefi PA, Cosimi AB, Ginns LC, Kotton CN. 2008. Cutaneous Aspergillus Ustus in a lung transplant recipient: emergence of a new opportunistic fungal pathogen. *The Journal of Heart and Lung Transplantation 27*: 131–4.

60. Husain S, Wagener MM, Singh N. 2001. Cryptococcus neoformans infection in organ transplant recipients: variables

influencing clinical characteristics and outcome. *Emerging Infectious Diseases* 7: 375–81.
61. Virgili A, ZM, La Malfa V, Strumia R, Bedani PL. 1999. Prevalence of superficial dermatomycoses in 73 renal transplant recipients. *Dermatology 199(1)*: 31–4.
62. Greenlee RT, Murray T, Bolden S, Wingo PA. 2000. Cancer statistics, 2000. *CA: A Cancer Journal for Clinicians 50*: 7–33.
63. Ulrich C, ST, Nindl I, Meyer T, Sterry W, Stockfleth E. 2003 Cutaneous precancers in organ transplant recipients: an old enemy in a new surrounding. *British Journal of Dermatology 149(66 Suppl.)*: 40–2.
64. Berg D, Otley CC. 2002. Skin cancer in organ transplant recipients: Epidemiology, pathogenesis, and management. *Journal of the American Academy of Dermatology 47*: 1–17; quiz 18–20.
65. Herman S, Rogers HD, Ratner D. 2007. Immunosuppression and squamous cell carcinoma: a focus on solid organ transplant recipients. *SKINmed 6*: 234–8.
66. Perrem K, LA, Conneely M, Wahlberg H, Murphy G, Leader M, Kay E. 2007. The higher incidence of squamous cell carcinoma in renal transplant recipients is associated with increased telomere lengths. *Human Pathology 38(2)*: 351–8.
67. Dang C, Koehler A, Forschner T, Sehr P, Michael K, Pawlita M, Stockfleth E, Nindl I. 2006. E6/E7 expression of human papillomavirus types in cutaneous squamous cell dysplasia and carcinoma in immunosuppressed organ transplant recipients. *British Journal of Dermatology 155*: 129–36.
68. Fuchs A, Marmur E. 2007. The kinetics of skin cancer: progression of actinic keratosis to squamous cell carcinoma. *Dermatologic Surgery 33*: 1099–101.
69. Boukamp P. 2005. Non-melanoma skin cancer: what drives tumor development and progression? *Carcinogenesis, 26(10)*: 1657–67.
70. Harwood CA, PC, McGregor JM, Sheaff MT, Leigh IM, Cerio R. 2006. Clinicopathologic features of skin cancer in organ transplant recipients: a retrospective case-control series. *Journal of American Academy of Dermatology 54(2)*: 290–300.
71. McGibbon, D. 1985. Malignant epidermal tumours. *Journal of Cutaneous Pathology 12(3–4)*: 224–38.
72. Penn I. 1996. Malignant melanoma in organ allograft recipients. *Transplantation, 61(2)*: 274–8.
73. van Dijk MC AK, van Hees F, Klaasen A, Blokx WA, Kiemeney LA, Ruiter DJ. 2008. Expert review remains important in the histopathological diagnosis of cutaneous melanocytic lesions. *Histopathology, 52(2)*: 139–46.
74. Neuburg M. 2007. Transplant-associated skin cancer: role of reducing immunosuppression. *Journal of the National Comprehensive Cancer Network 5*: 541–9.
75. Marcelin AG, CV, Dussaix E. 2007. KSHV after an organ transplant: should we screen?. *Current Topics in Microbiology and Immunology 312*: 245–62.
76. Campistol JM, Schena FP. 2007. Kaposi's sarcoma in renal transplant recipients – the impact of proliferation signal inhibitors. *Nephrology Dialysis Transplantation 22* (Suppl. 1): i17–22.
77. Chow JW, LS. 1990. Endemic and atypical Kaposi's sarcoma in Africa—histopathological aspects. *Clinical and Experimental Dermatology 15(4)*: 253–9.
78. Nagy S, GR, Kemeny L, Szenohradszky P, Dobozy A. 2000. Iatrogenic Kaposi's sarcoma: HHV8 positivity persists but the tumors regress almost completely without immunosuppressive therapy. *Transplantation 69(10)*: 2230–1.
79. Gonthier DM, Hartman G, Holley JL. 1992. Posttransplant lymphoproliferative disorder presenting as an isolated skin lesion. *American Journal of Kidney Diseases 19*: 600–3.
80. Schumann KW, Oriba HA, Bergfeld WF, Hsi ED, Hollandsworth K. 2000. Cutaneous presentation of posttransplant lymphoproliferative disorder. *Journal of the American Academy of Dermatology 42*: 923–6.
81. Takahashi S, Watanabe D, Miura K, Ozawa H, Tamada Y, Hara K, Matsumoto Y. 2007. Epstein-Barr virus-associated post-transplant lymphoproliferative disorder presenting with skin involvement after CD34-selected autologous peripheral blood stem cell transplantation. *European Journal of Dermatology 17*: 242–4.
82. Coyne JD, Banerjee SS, Bromley M, Mills S, Diss TC, Harris M. 2004. Post-transplant T-cell lymphoproliferative disorder/T-cell lymphoma: a report of three cases of T-anaplastic large-cell lymphoma with cutaneous presentation and a review of the literature. *Histopathology 44*: 387–93.
83. Dreno B, Mansat E, Legoux B, Litoux P. 1998. Skin cancers in transplant patients. *Nephrology Dialysis Transplantation 13*: 1374–79.
84. O'Connor JP, Quinn J, Wall D, Petrie JJ, Hardie JR, Woodruff PW. 1986. Cutaneous angiosarcoma following graft irradiation in a renal transplant patient. *Clinical Nephrology 25*: 54–5.
85. Kanitakis J, Euvrard S, Montazeri A, Garnier JL, Faure M, Claudy A. 1996. Atypical fibroxanthoma in a renal graft recipient. *Journal of the American Academy of Dermatology 35*: 262–4.
86. Kolker AR, Wolfort FG, Upton J, Tahan SR, Hein KD, Zewert TE. 1998. Plantar verrucous carcinoma following transmetatarsal amputation and renal transplantation. *Annals of Plastic Surgery 40*: 515–9.
87. Lanzetta M, Petruzzo P, Dubernard JM, Margreiter R, Schuind F, Breidenbach W, Nolli R, Schneeberger S, van Holder C, Gorantla VS, et al. 2007. Second report(1998–2006) of the International Registry of Hand and Composite Tissue Transplantation. *Transplant Immunology 18*: 1–6.
88. Gabl M, Pechlaner S, Lutz M, Bodner G, Piza H, Margreiter R. 2004. Bilateral hand transplantation: bone healing under immunosuppression with tacrolimus, mycophenolate mofetil, and prednisolone. *Journal of Hand Surgery – American Volume 29*: 1020–7.
89. Levi DM, Tzakis AG, Kato T, Madariaga J, Mittal NK, Nery J, Nishida S, Ruiz P. 2003. Transplantation of the abdominal wall. *Lancet 361*: 2173–6.
90. Devauchelle B, Badet L, Lengele B, Morelon E, Testelin S, Michallet M, D'Hauthuille C, Dubernard J-M. 2006. First human face allograft: early report. *Lancet 368*: 203–9.
91. Kanitakis J, Petruzzo P, Jullien D, Badet L, Dezza MC, Claudy A, Lanzetta M, Hakim N, Owen E, Dubernard J-M. 2005. Pathological score for the evaluation of allograft

rejection in human hand (composite tissue) allotransplantation. *European Journal of Dermatology 15*: 235–8.

92. Cendales LC, Kirk AD, Moresi JM, Ruiz P, Kleiner DE. 2006. Composite tissue allotransplantation: classification of clinical acute skin rejection. *Transplantation 81*: 418–22.

93. Bejarano PA, Levi D, Nassiri M, Vincek V, Garcia M, Weppler D, Selvaggi G, Kato T, Tzakis A. 2004. The pathology of full-thickness cadaver skin transplant for large abdominal defects: a proposed grading system for skin allograft acute rejection. *American Journal of Surgical Pathology 28*: 670–5.

94. Cendales LC, KJ, Schneeberger S, Burns C, Ruiz P, Landin L, Remmelink M, Hewitt CW, Landgren T, Lyons B, Drachenberg CB, Solez K, Kirk AD, Kleiner DE, Racusen L. 2008. The Banff 2007 working classification of skin-containing composite tissue allograft pathology. *American Journal of Transplantation, 8*: 1396–400.

CHAPTER 3

The Pathology of Kidney Transplantation

Volker Nickeleit, M.D.

I. INTRODUCTION

At present, kidney transplants are the most common solid organ grafts worldwide. Ever since the fundamental surgical and immunological problems were mastered years ago, renal grafting has subsequently evolved into a cost effective, "routine" therapy that improves not only the quality of life but also the survival of patients with various etiologies of end-stage kidney disease (1,2,3).

Due to the introduction of new, potent immunosuppressive drugs into the clinical management of renal allograft recipients, starting with cyclosporine-A (CsA) almost three decades ago, graft and patient survival have constantly improved, in particular, during the first year after transplantation with a lower frequency of acute rejection episodes and a good response rate to antirejection therapy (2,4). Graft survival at one year [living (L) and standard deceased (D) donor organs] has improved from (L) 91.3, (D) 80.5 percent (transplant year 1990) to (L) 94.2, (D) 89.3 percent (transplant year 2000); improvement between 2.9 (L) and 8.8 percent (D) over a ten-year time span (5). Unfortunately, however, specific improvements in long-term allograft survival have only been modest with largely unchanged curves of late graft survival (6). Graft survival at five years has improved from (L) 76.1, (D) 58.8 percent (transplant year 1990) to (L) 79.4, (D) 68.2 percent (transplant year 2000); improvement between 3.3 (L) and 9.4 percent (D) over a ten-year time span (largely as a reflection of the improved one-year transplant survival) (2,5). The reason for the discrepancy between "early" and "late" improvement of graft survival are multifactorial and influenced not only by the degree of immunosuppression but also by major histocompatibility complex (MHC) matching; the source (cadaver versus living) and age of the donor organs, the occurrence of de novo lesions (e.g., hypertension-induced arterionephrosclerosis, calcineurin inhibitor–induced drug toxicity), and recurrent kidney disease (e.g., glomerulonephritides, diabetic nephropathy). In addition, the number and types of acute rejection episodes, donor recipient age and race, and recipient compliance with drug therapy are important factors influencing long-term outcome (7). To optimize the management of renal allografts, the expert evaluation of renal biopsy samples plays a crucial role.

The targeted therapy of allograft dysfunction is a challenging task requiring special expertise. Clinical signs of allograft "failure", that is, the elevation of serum creatinine and BUN levels, hematuria, or proteinuria, often inadequately reflect intragraft pathology. To render a specific diagnosis and to initiate effective treatment, a renal allograft biopsy is commonly regarded as the diagnostic gold standard. Previous studies have demonstrated that renal allograft biopsies modified the clinical diagnoses in 27–46 percent of cases, changed therapy in 42–83 percent of patients, and prevented additional immunosuppression in 19–30 percent of graft recipients, underscoring the clinical significance of a morphological diagnosis (8–15). Since kidney transplants are placed into the iliac fossa, needle core biopsies are usually easily collected. For proper interpretation by light and immunofluorescence (IF) microscopy, biopsy samples should be adequate in size. The so-called *Banff '97 adequacy criteria* (16) should only be regarded as the minimum standard for rendering meaningful interpretations—in my mind they do not constitute best practice guidelines. Morphological biopsy diagnoses are clinically most useful during early/acute phases of

allograft dysfunction when disease processes are active and respond to therapeutic intervention. Late graft biopsies in patients with creeping deterioration of graft function are least informative and frequently only reveal signs of sclerosis.

Renal pathologists interpreting allograft biopsies, often on an expedited basis, face complex challenges: several diseases may affect the transplanted organ simultaneously; suboptimal tissue collection and preservation can impair the decision-making process; and patients may be treated with a wide range of potent, sometimes toxic treatment modalities, the selection of which firmly rests on the accuracy of the histological diagnosis. The whole spectrum of diseases known to occur in native kidneys has been observed in renal transplants and disorders other than rejection may arise de novo or as recurrent disease in the grafted organ, occasionally even superimposed on rejection episodes. Since renal transplants have already had a "first life" as native kidneys in the donors, renal disease can already be present in the kidney graft at the time of transplantation.

This chapter will focus on the most important transplant-specific morphological changes and disease entities. Non-transplant–specific diseases including recurrent and de novo glomerulonephritides show identical changes in native and transplanted kidneys. The reader is referred to standard text books of renal pathology for in-depth descriptions of all non-transplant–specific alterations.

II. BIOPSIES AND HISTOLOGICAL EVALUATIONS OF ALLOGRAFTS

A renal biopsy—native or transplant—is an invasive procedure that is clinically used in a targeted fashion to obtain a morphological diagnosis, to get prognostic information, and to guide treatment. Thus, once a patient is "put at risk" by an invasive biopsy, the goal should be to collect sufficient tissue and to render the best possible diagnosis. Often, also immunohistochemical and electron microscopical analyses are needed in addition to light microscopic and IF studies, to render a definitive histological interpretation. If a biopsy is indicated, the most appropriate needle size should be used (in my experience fourteen or fifteen gauge) and two to three tissue cores of 1–1.5 cm in length should be collected. Sampling results are best when the biopsies are performed by experienced nephrologists or radiologists. Needle core biopsies can also be successfully obtained at the time of grafting in the operating room by the transplant surgeons.

At present, the vast majority of percutaneous renal allograft biopsies are done under ultrasound guidance with a biopsy gun. Biopsy guns have an excellent record of safety that is largely independent of the needle size (fourteen versus eighteen gauge) when common contraindications are considered (17–21). In a large multicenter study of

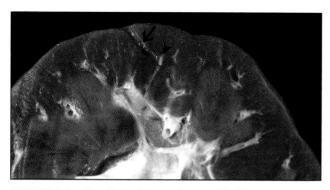

FIGURE 3.1: *Needle track (arrow) caused by biopsy sampling with a spring loaded "gun" using a fifteen-gauge needle. The needle went tangentially into the cortex and outer medulla. The sample contained a "large" arcuate caliber vessel (arrow head) that would not have been collected in a wedge biopsy.*

TABLE 3.1 "Chapel Hill" Criteria for Assessing the Diagnostic Adequacy of Renal Allograft Biopsies

1. At least two biopsy cores available for standard light microscopic evaluation
2. $\geq$12 glomeruli (located in the deep cortex)
3. $\geq$2 large interlobular arteries/branches of arcuate arteries (with at least 2–3 layers of medial smooth muscle cells)
4. Portion of medulla

more than 2,000 protocol biopsies, no patient death and only one potentially avoidable graft loss was reported (22). Similar results were more recently published from a large single center in Germany (23). Ultrasound guidance increases the probability of obtaining cortex from 75 percent to more than 90 percent; guidance by on-site examination with a dissecting microscope increases tissue adequacy to nearly 100 percent (24). Of note, small eighteen-gauge needles render insufficient samples in a high percentage of renal allograft biopsies (up to 47 percent at Hannover Hospital in Germany) (23), and in contrast to common belief, smaller needle sizes are not associated with a lower rate of complications (18–21). Larger biopsy needles (fourteen or fifteen gauge) provide more tissue and, thus, they are diagnostically more useful, in particular when evaluating graft biopsies that require careful analysis of the arterial tree (Figure 3.1) (18). Although modern biopsy guns produce long tissue cores seemingly demonstrating the presence of abundant material, this impression is misleading since approximately half the cores generally consist of medulla that is of only limited diagnostic value. If biopsy guns are employed on exposed renal transplants in the operating room, the entire tissue core may contain medulla. Open-wedge biopsies typically require anesthesia and are not commonly taken after transplantation. Wedges are more frequently obtained during organ procurement to access the suitability for transplantation, that is, harvest biopsies, or at time of grafting, that is, implantation zero-hour biopsies. Surgeons often prefer wedge biopsies since bleeding can be better controlled and sampling seems to generate large tissue fragments. Wedge biopsies, however, are not ideal since they are obtained from outer cortical zones that lack large interlobular arteries (25) and do not allow adequate insight into the arterial tree. In addition, subcapsular areas can show marked, 1- to 2-mm–wide zones of interstitial fibrosis and global glomerulosclerosis resulting in an overestimation of "chronic injury." The latter aspect may even be further enhanced by nonrepresentative "wedge" biopsy sampling from regions of parenchymal scarring that attract the surgeon's attention in the operating room.

Two previous studies indicated that the sensitivity to diagnose rejection is 90 percent in a single biopsy core (26,27); accordingly two cores should have a predicted sensitivity of 99 percent, supporting the notion that two biopsy cores are required to make a definitive histological diagnosis of rejection.

I recommend that as a standard operating procedure two to three biopsy cores are collected with a fourteen- or fifteen-gauge needle. The cores should be divided for light and IF microscopy. Electron microscopical studies are typically limited to cases in which a glomerulonephritis or glomerulopathy is suspected, that is, clinical evidence of hematuria and/or proteinuria, or older grafts in order to evaluate glomerular and peritubular capillary wall remodeling [reviewed in (28)]. I perform ultrastructural studies on all grafts after transplantation year 1. The largest tissue portions should always be processed for light microscopical studies. Routinely, my laboratory prepares ten slides, each carrying three 2- to 3-μm–thick tissue sections, stained with hematoxylin and eosin (H&E, three levels), periodic acid Schiff (PAS, three levels), trichrome (three levels), and elastic tissue stains (one level). We also prepare three extra glass slides with unstained sections for potential additional studies to avoid tissue loss caused by readjusting paraffin blocks on the microtomes. Further step sections into the paraffin blocks are obtained if no conclusive diagnosis can be rendered. Chapel Hill (University of North Carolina) standards for tissue adequacy (Table 3.1) are as follows: 1) at least two biopsy cores are available for standard light microscopic studies, 2) twelve or more glomeruli are found (away from the subcapsular region that often shows nonspecific sclerosis), 3) two or more "large" interlobular arteries/branches of arcuate caliber vessels are sampled (i.e., vessels with at least two to three layers of medial smooth muscle cells), 4) a portion of medulla is present (to rule out polyomavirus nephropathy).

Tissue for IF microscopy can be collected by cutting off one half of one (fresh) biopsy core, that is, approximately 7 mm, and monitoring under a dissecting scope for the presence of renal cortex. The longitudinal splitting of entire biopsy cores is strongly discouraged since it can cause severe squeezing artifacts. Renal tissue for IF studies is best embedded in optimum cutting temperature (O.C.T.) medium and frozen in precooled isopentane; freezing in liquid nitrogen is too harsh and freezing in a cryostat too slow, resulting in severe preservation artifacts. If fresh tissue cannot be expeditiously frozen in isopentane, then alternatively a sample may be transported in Michel's medium that preserves antigens for up to several days. Michel's can, however, cause marked distortion of the tubulo-interstitial compartment, thereby limiting some IF studies, such as the evaluation of C4d or tubular MHC class II staining patterns. I recommend that all allograft biopsies, including zero-hour implantation biopsies, are routinely stained by IF for IgG, IgA, IgM, complement factor C3, fibrinogen, kappa, and lambda light chains, and the complement degradation product C4d. I additionally stain all biopsies for the expression of MHC class II (HLA-DR). Since IF studies only provide a somewhat limited insight into structural changes and frozen tissue cores represent additional diagnostic material that can harbor diagnostic lesions not found elsewhere, additional sections should be taken from the frozen tissue block and analyzed in H&E and PAS incubations. Instead of IF studies some centers, especially in Europe, perform immunohistochemistry on formalin-fixed and paraffin-embedded tissue sections with good results.

If tissue is needed for electron microscopy (EM) it can be obtained by cutting off small portions of the fresh biopsy cores (approximately 1–2 mm of cortex). Of note, only very limited tissue samples with approximately three glomeruli are needed for ultrastructural analysis. "Thick" sections stained with toluidine blue can be prepared from the Epon-embedded material for additional (standard) light microscopic evaluation of the tissue sample collected for EM studies.

The diagnostic "rush" interpretation of frozen renal allograft biopsies is generally discouraged since freezing (with the exception of freezing in precooled isopentane) often introduces artifacts impairing the histological evaluation, such as widening of the interstitium mimicking edema. No diagnosis in renal transplantation, with the exception of harvest evaluations, has to be made within minutes. Thus, time can be taken to produce tissue sections of high quality, thereby enabling the best diagnostic interpretation. At the University of North Carolina, all tissue is typically conventionally processed. Initial H&E and IF sections are made available to the transplant pathologists within four to five hours post biopsy.

III. DONOR ORGANS AND IMPLANTATION BIOPSIES

All transplants had already a "previous life" before transplantation, in particular those cadaveric organs originating from the so-called expanded donor pool [accounting for approximately 15 percent of cadaveric transplants in the United States; reviewed in (29)]. Thus, besides pediatric

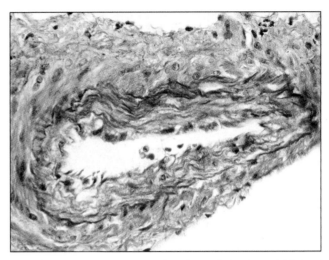

FIGURE 3.2: *Moderate to marked donor derived arterial intimal fibroelastosis was detected eleven days after transplantation in an organ of cadaveric origin with delayed graft function. The elastic tissue stain high lights the multilayering of elastic lamellae in the thickened intima; a characteristic sign of hypertension-induced damage (compare with Figure 3.21). 80× original magnification.*

and adolescent donor organs, practically all others come with varying degrees of preexisting, clinically silent "chronic" injury, commonly arterionephrosclerosis (Figure 3.2) (30). Active renal diseases, such as glomerulonephritides, are rarely transmitted with the graft and can resolve after transplantation (31–37). Donor-derived glomerular IgA deposits, noted in mesangial regions in approximately 2 percent of implantation biopsies at Chapel Hill, 14 percent [Santiago, Chile (38)], 19 percent [Brussels, Belgium (32)], and 24 percent [Nanjing, China (39)] usually disappear within a few months after surgery (32,39–41); they rarely persist without apparent impact on graft survival (32,39). In the Chinese series from Nanjing, IgA deposits were associated with significant mesangial proliferations, mostly transient proteinuria, hematuria, and hypertension, and an increased rate of acute rejection episodes; three-year graft survival, however, did not differ from controls (39).

The contributions pathologists can make during organ harvesting and surgery are two-fold: 1) determination of the suitability of donor organs for transplantation, and 2) recording of preexisting donor lesions for subsequent comparative analyses during the post-transplantation time course. The extent to which preexisting chronic lesions predict inferior outcome or potentially even mark unsuitability of an organ for grafting have not been systematically studied in controlled trials. No study has established conclusive criteria of glomerular, interstitial, and arterial sclerosis beyond which a donor organ must not be used. A great concern of setting largely arbitrary criteria is that precious donor organs will be discarded needlessly, when programs such as "old for old" may utilize such kidneys. Of note, the practice to use the percentage of globally sclerosed glomeruli as a guideline for organ transplant suitability has not been determined in multicenter prospective studies. One seminal retrospective analysis suggested a 20 percent cutoff for global glomerulosclerosis to separate grafts with generally favorable versus unfavorable outcome [graft loss 7 versus 38 percent (30)]. Similar observations were subsequently reported by some (42,43) but not all investigators (44,45). Even marked arteriosclerosis was not associated with increased graft failure rates in one series (46), and "only" impacted long-term transplant survival (mean: fifty-month follow-up) in another study (29).

It is important to consider the observation that despite substantial sclerosis, the majority of organs described in the aforementioned studies functioned and could therefore be of benefit to some patients with end-stage renal disease. Based on the inborn limitations of wedge biopsies and frozen section evaluations and the largely undefined histological criteria for identifying organs unsuited for transplantation, fibrosis, and glomerulosclerosis should *not* be the sole parameters used for discarding organs. Consequently the histopathologist's role during organ harvesting is only limited. Yet, harvest biopsies provide important data on preexisting donor lesions and can amend or even replace zero-hour implantation biopsies.

Implantation biopsies taken before or after reperfusion provide a unique view of renal lesions in individuals without apparent renal disease. These biopsies should be large enough to provide adequate insight into the arterial tree. They require a complete histological workup, that is, full light microscopic evaluation including special stains, and particularly in presensitized and retransplant recipients, IF studies with C4d staining (47). In case "harvest biopsies" are used for scoring purposes, frozen tissue blocks have to be reprocessed for standard light microscopic analysis. Most relevant for subsequent studies and the proper evaluation of de novo, post-transplant changes is the careful scoring of chronic injury, that is, arterial intimal fibroelastosis (in large interlobular arteries and branches of arcuate caliber vessels), arteriolosclerosis with hyalinosis, interstitial fibrosis and tubular atrophy, and global glomerulosclerosis. To be consistent, scoring can be performed according to the Banff '97 criteria (16); the results might be designated with a prefix "D" (for preexisting <u>d</u>onor disease) for clear subsequent distinction from de novo changes.

We have found hyaline arteriolosclerosis and/or arterial intimal fibroelastosis in 68 percent of living and conventional cadaveric donor organs. Moderate or marked vascular sclerosis was noted in 18 percent of cases. It was associated with increased baseline serum creatinine levels three and six months after transplantation (six months post-transplantation serum creatinine 1.55 versus 1.22 mg/dl in donor organs with no or minimal vascular sclerosis; p < 0.02). At Chapel Hill moderate or marked arteriolosclerosis in donor organs was not associated with increased graft failure rates. Similar observations were

reported by others including one series from a pool of extended cadaveric donor organs (46,48). In our patient population in Chapel Hill, neither global glomerulosclerosis nor interstitial fibrosis or tubular atrophy was significant, and histological changes did not correlate with delayed graft function. However, other centers reported that severe arterial sclerosis was, associated with a high risk of delayed graft function in recipients of marginal donor organs (29,46).

Occasionally scattered rare polymorphonuclear leukocytes are found in glomerular capillaries of post-perfusion implantation biopsies. Such changes are mostly caused by ischemic endothelial cell injury; they are—if focal and without concurrent C4d deposits—of no prognostic significance. Focal and segmental, small intraglomerular fibrin thrombi may contribute to delayed function, however, they do not predict poor outcome (49), presumably due to rapid lysis by the normal host fibrinolytic system. In one report, minute "foreign carbohydrate appearing" particles were observed in rare intraglomerular and peritubular capillaries in 11 percent of post-perfusion cadaveric implantation biopsies. The polarizable particles were not apparent in standard H&E incubations but stained strongly with PAS stains. They were believed to originate from surgical gloves and to be carried into the microvasculature by means of machine perfusion; the particles did not indicate adverse outcome (50). We have not detected such particles.

IV. ISCHEMIA REPERFUSION INJURY

If dialysis is required after surgery, the term "delayed graft function" is used, whereas "primary nonfunction" defines that a graft never produced urine. In particular, organs originating from cadaveric and non-heart–beating donors experience delayed graft function due to extended cold and warm ischemia times (51–53). Kidneys of non-heart–beating donor origin showed delayed graft function in 33–84 percent of cases, and primary nonfunction in 7–18 percent (29,54–57). In contrast, in standard cadaveric donor organs, the incidence of delayed graft function was between 15 and 23 percent (29,58); 19 percent in our series at the University of North Carolina in Chapel Hill (in comparison to 2 percent in organs of living donation). The average reported duration of delayed graft function was ten to fifteen days (59). Approximately 95–98 percent of grafts functionally recover; 50 percent within ten days, 83 percent within twenty days after surgery, and 93–98 percent long term [reviewed in (51)]. Organs of living and standard cadaveric origin only seldom present with primary nonfunction (2–3 percent) (55,57). Of note, delayed graft function is a clinical term describing a symptom. The *differential diagnosis* includes (alone or in combination) ischemic tubular injury, surgical complications, calcineurin inhibitor–induced toxicity, hyperkalemia, rapamycin therapy, antibody- or cellular-mediated

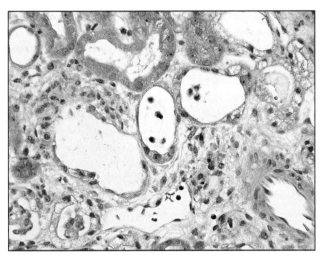

FIGURE 3.3: *The biopsy was obtained from a graft with delayed function eight days after transplantation (organ of living unrelated origin with prolonged warm ischemia time). Marked ischemic tubular injury was apparent with tubular dilatation and flattening of the epithelial cells. Two tubular cross sections contained scattered inflammatory cells. The interstitium revealed moderate edema, scattered mononuclear inflammatory cells, and focal dilatation of peritubular capillaries. There was no evidence of rejection including absent staining of C4d, and no tubular expression of MHC class II (HLA-DR). This histological pattern of ischemic injury has to be distinguished from pyelonephritis (compare with Figure 11.53) and antibody-mediated allograft rejection (compare with Figure 11.32). H&E stain, 150× original magnification.*

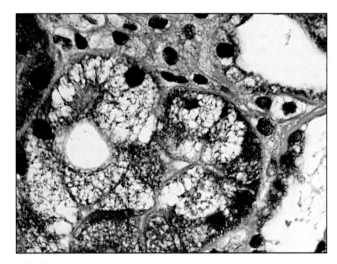

FIGURE 3.4: *Ischemic tubular epithelial cell injury commonly results in nonisometric vacuolization of the cytoplasm. This pattern of injury has to be distinguished from isometric vacuolization, that is, so-called osmotic nephrosis, induced by drugs including calcineurin inhibitors (compare with Figure 3.35). Same case as illustrated in Figure 3.3, trichrome stain, 400× oil original magnification.*

TABLE 3.2 **Common Causes of Tubular Vacuolization**

Ischemia	nonisometric
Calcineurin inhibitor–induced toxic tubulopathy	isometric
Sucrose	isometric
Hydroxyethyl starch	isometric
Dextran	isometric
Mannitol	isometric
Radiocontrast media	isometric
Intravenous immunoglobulins	isometric

rejection (the latter seen as early as five days after transplantation), and severe preexisting donor organ arterionephrosclerosis. For diagnostic and therapeutic purposes, a graft biopsy is often required.

Most allografts with delayed function show acute ischemic injury that is proportionate to the ischemia time. The histological changes are similar to so-called *acute tubular injury* (ATI) observed in native kidneys and include tubular dilatation, loss of the apical tubular brush border, flattening of epithelial cells, mitotic figures, and intratubular proteinaceous debris. In some cases, intratubular proteinaceous casts and scattered interstitial polymorphonuclear and eosinophilic leukocytes can be conspicuous (Figure 3.3); the differential diagnosis includes ascending pyelonephritis (see Infections) and C4d-positive antibody-mediated graft rejection (see Rejection). Ischemic tubular injury is commonly associated with nonisometric vacuolization of the cytoplasm that can be further intensified by drug administration before, during, or after transplantation (Figure 3.4; Table 3.2). One recent report described a case of prolonged tubular vacuolization of more than five months duration (60). In ATI, the interstitium may show focal minimal edema and inflammatory cell infiltrates (mononuclear cells, rare polymorphonuclear and even eosinophilic leukocytes). ATI and delayed graft function can be associated with dilatation of peritubular capillaries filled with mononuclear and polymorphonuclear leukocytes (Figure 3.3). Such capillary changes are secondary to poor function and parenchymal injury; they can also be seen in native kidneys and do not indicate an antibody-mediated rejection episode (unless C4d is diffusely detected along peritubular capillaries). Arteritis is limited to cases with concurrent rejection. In some cases of ATI and marked, preexisting arterionephrosclerosis, fibrosed arterial intimal layers can show edema and striking enlargement of myofibroblasts and endothelial cells. This histological finding is of no significance; it is not associated with C4d positivity and should not be mistaken for rejection (Figure 3.5). Although severe ischemia-reperfusion injury, such as seen in organs from non-heart–beating donors, may result in the activation of the mannose-binding lectin pathway of complement activation, ischemic injury is typically not associated with the accumulation of the complement degradation product C4d along peritubular capillaries (47,61,62). If C4d is found in the

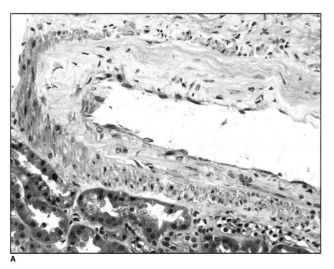 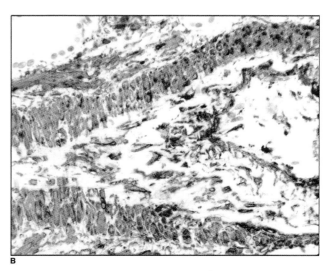

A B

FIGURE 3.5: *The biopsy was obtained from a graft with poor function eleven days after transplantation (organ of cadaveric origin). An arcuate caliber artery with preexisting moderate to severe intimal fibroelastosis showed peculiar activation of endothelial cells and enlargement of intimal myofibroblasts. There was no evidence of rejection including transplant endarteritis, that is, no intimal inflammation, no CD3- or CD68-positive cells, and C4d was absent. The tubulo-interstitial compartment revealed ischemic injury. The arterial changes are of no diagnostic significance; they should not be misinterpreted as rejection. (A) H&E stain, and (B) immunohistochemistry on formalin-fixed and paraffin-embedded tissue to detect alpha smooth muscle–specific antigen myofibroblasts, both 100× original magnification.*

setting of ischemia-reperfusion injury, a "pure" antibody-mediated rejection episode has to be considered as the primary cause for graft dysfunction.

There is mounting evidence that T cells, in particular CD4+ lymphocytes, natural killer cells, and interferon-γ (rather than polymorphonuclear leukocytes) play a crucial role in the development of ischemia reperfusion injury likely due to direct "cross-talk" of activated T lymphocytes with the endothelium of the microvasculature and upregulation of adhesion molecules (63,64). T-cell activation and the upregulation of adhesion molecules could also explain the association between tubular injury and tubular MHC expression. In the mouse unilateral, transient clamping of the native renal artery resulted in increased tubular expression of MHC class I (up to 3.6 folds) within 3 days after injury and class II (between 1.5 and 3 folds) within 7 days (65). These experiments provide a possible explanation for how ischemia can promote acute rejection. Whether typical ischemia reperfusion injury (i.e., excluding other causes of delayed graft function such as early rejection episodes, surgical complications, and censoring data for preexisting donor disease) predicts inferior long-term graft survival as an independent risk factor remains to be proven. By multivariate analysis, delayed graft function by itself is not a significant risk factor for graft loss (58). Rather, it appears that the adverse prognosis associated with delayed graft function is related to an increased incidence of rejection (58,66). The frequency of acute rejection in protocol biopsies taken during the first month after transplantation has reportedly been signifi-

cantly higher in patients with delayed graft function than those without (66).

V. REJECTION

i. Background and Classification

Numerous different injuries can affect renal allografts and besides rejection-induced inflammation, practically all other diseases affecting native kidneys can also be found in transplants. It is incumbent on the pathologist to render a specific diagnosis and to properly guide therapy.

The major risk factors for rejection are the degree of histocompatibility between recipient and graft, recipient presensitization, the immunosuppressive drug regimen, recipient age, sex, race, and importantly patient compliance (7,67). Modern, third-generation immunosuppressive drug regimens including tacrolimus, mycophenolate-mofetil, and sirolimus, as well as potent induction protocols have reduced the frequency of clinically apparent acute rejection episodes considerably. At present, so-called acute rejection episodes affect 12–18 percent of living donor kidneys and 14–30 percent of cadaveric organs during the first six months after grafting. Acute rejection currently accounts for 11–16 percent of graft losses in the first year (68,69).

Rejection episodes can be classified according to different schemes that guide therapeutic decisions and influence outcome analyses of multicenter studies including drug trials. All classification schemes are, however, only dynamic makeshift constructs. They are heavily influenced not only by available knowledge, experience, and technology but also by tradition, trends, and opinions.

Frequently, transplant physicians prefer a "simple" classification approach that is mainly based on the temporal occurrence of a rejection episode following surgery. According to this concept, "hyperacute" or "accelerated acute" rejection implies a very early event (within hours or days after transplantation), "acute" rejection is diagnosed within days or weeks, and "chronic" rejection is considered to be a late event occurring months or years after grafting. However, these general clinical terms are imprecise and not suited to categorize rejection-induced graft injury and tissue remodeling, to guide therapy, or to render prognostic information. For example, on histological grounds acute and chronic changes are often not sharply separated entities but rather represent a continuum (70,71). "Acute" rejection may involve the tubulo-interstitial compartment and/or arteries, it may be cell mediated and/or antibody driven, it occurs as early as few days or as late as decades after transplantation, and it can be superimposed on other types of graft injury, such as preexisting donor disease, or calcineurin inhibitor toxicity, with different therapeutic and prognostic implications. Similarly, problematic are two other commonly used classifiers: cellular- and humoral/antibody-mediated rejection. "Acute cellular" rejection has been a trendy term over the past thirty years being used as caption for 1) tubulo-interstitial rejection, 2) transplant endarteritis, and 3) transplant glomerulitis (72,73). In contrast, antibody-mediated injury, often due to preformed antibodies, was believed to cause fibrinoid arterial wall necrosis, and rare forms of hyperacute and accelerated acute rejection (72,74). In the recent past, however, due to the introduction of C4d staining into the evaluation of transplant biopsies, we have learned that antibodies contribute to graft injury and rejection more frequently than traditionally believed and that the conventional sharp separation between "cellular" and "humoral" rejection is not appropriate (62,75–79).

Standard clinical parameters, in particular serum creatinine and BUN levels, only poorly reflect intragraft disease. Graft injury including rejection can occur without significant renal dysfunction, that is, so-called subclinical rejection, and vice versa a rise in serum creatinine does not necessarily indicate transplant rejection. Some rejection episodes can smolder and do not rapidly progress to severe graft injury and failure.

A renal allograft biopsy is generally considered to be the gold standard for the evaluation of clinical or subclinical graft injury and for the classification and typing of rejection episodes (see Biopsies and Histological Evaluations of Allografts). Two classification schemes, *Banff* (80,81) and *CCTT* (collaborative clinical trials in transplantation) (26), combine histological, clinical, and pathophysiological parameters of rejection, and they define specific disease categories. Most widely used and accepted is the so-called Banff system (named after a small resort town in the Canadian Rocky Mountains), introduced in 1993 (80). Over the

TABLE 3.3 2007 Update of the Banff Classification Scheme (81)

1. Normal
2. Antibody-mediated changes (may coincide with categories 3, 4, 5, and 6), due to documentation of circulating anti-donor antibody, C4d, and allograft pathology
   C4d deposition without morphological evidence of active rejection

C4d+, presence of circulating anti-donor antibodies, no signs of acute or chronic TCMR or ABMR (i.e., g0, cg0, ptc0, no ptc lamination). Cases with simultaneous borderline changes or acute tubular necrosis are considered as indeterminate

   Acute antibody-mediated rejection

C4d+, presence of circulating anti-donor antibodies, morphological evidence of acute tissue injury, such as (type/grade):
   I. ATN-like minimal inflammation
   II. Capillary and or glomerular inflammation (ptc/g >0) and/or thromboses
   III. Arterial – v3

   Chronic active antibody-mediated rejection

C4d+, presence of circulating anti-donor antibodies, morphological evidence of chronic tissue injury, such as glomerular double contours, peritubular capillary basement membrane multilayering, interstitial fibrosis/tubular atrophy, and/or fibrous intimal thickening in arteries

3. Borderline changes: "suspicious" for acute T-cell–mediated rejection (may coincide with categories 2, 5, and 6). This category is used when no intimal arteritis is present, but there are foci of tubulitis (t1, t2, or t3) with minor interstitial infiltration (i0 or i1) or interstitial infiltration (i2, i3) with mild (t1) tubulitis.

4. T-cell–mediated rejection (TCMR, may coincide with categories 2 and 5)

   Acute T-cell–mediated rejection (type/grade):

IA. Cases with significant interstitial infiltration (>25% of parenchyma affected, i2 or i3) and foci of moderate tubulitis (t2)
IB. Cases with significant interstitial infiltration (>25% of parenchyma affected, i2 or i3) and foci of severe tubulitis (t3)
IIA. Cases with mild to moderate intimal arteritis (v1)
IIB. Cases with severe intimal arteritis comprising >25% of the luminal area (v2)
III. Cases with "transmural" arteritis and/or arterial fibrinoid change and necrosis of medial smooth muscle cells with accompanying lymphocytic inflammation (v3)

   Chronic active T-cell–mediated rejection, "chronic allograft arteriopathy" (arterial intimal fibrosis with mononuclear cell infiltration in fibrosis, formation of neo-intima)

5. Interstitial fibrosis and tubular atrophy, no evidence of any specific etiology (may include nonspecific vascular and glomerular sclerosis, but severity graded by tubulo-interstitial features)

   Grade

 I. Mild interstitial fibrosis and tubular atrophy (<25% of cortical area)
 II. Moderate interstitial fibrosis and tubular atrophy (26–50% of cortical area)
 III. Severe interstitial fibrosis and tubular atrophy/loss (>50% of cortical area)

6. Other: changes not considered to be due to acute or chronic rejection

years, it has undergone several changes [see Table 3.3 for the most recent version (81)] and significantly impacted the standardization of the classification of kidney transplant rejection. Banff has facilitated comparative studies and is used in the vast majority of published reports including practically all pharmaceutical drug trials requiring the analysis of allograft biopsies. Over the years, Banff has increasingly strived after providing an "etiology-based" categorization of renal allograft rejection; an ultimately desirable but currently problematic approach. Thus, not surprisingly, Banff, like many other multidisciplinary consensus classifications, has weaknesses:

1. The threshold levels to diagnose tubulo-interstitial cellular rejection (Banff category 4, type 1) are set high, resulting in the potential for under diagnosis of rejection episodes (26,82,83).

2. The Borderline category (Banff category 3) is unsatisfactory. It is often used as a "waste basket" that may even contain unrecognized severe rejection episodes, such as "unrecognized" transplant endarteritis.

3. Preexisting donor disease, such as arterionephrosclerosis, remains unclassified. All changes listed in Banff categories 2–6 can be superimposed on "donor disease" with currently undetermined clinical significance.

4. Although much emphasis is placed on the C4d staining status of graft biopsies, surprisingly little knowledge and guidance exist on how to best evaluate C4d staining (frozen tissue samples and IF microscopy versus formalin-fixed material and immunohistochemistry), and how to adequately incorporate focal C4d positivity into the Banff system. Moreover, C4d-negative antibody-mediated rejections are certainly a possibility but have thus far not been adequately characterized.

5. The histological subtypes listed under "acute antibody-mediated" rejection (category 2) are of no prognostic significance, and they are not specific for antibody-mediated graft injury [including inflammation of peritubular capillaries (84)]. Arterial v3 lesions are classified twice: in category 2 and category 4, type 3. Rejection episodes with massive intravascular thrombosis due to preformed antibodies (so-called hyperacute rejection) are no longer specifically recognized.

6. The classification and scoring of mixed antibody/C4d-positive and cellular rejection episodes is not adequately emphasized (79).

7. The category of so-called chronic active antibody-mediated rejection (category 2) is poorly understood, and its introduction appears to be premature. Future studies have to aim at carefully analyzing the timely relationship of cell- and antibody-mediated graft injury and potential causes of sclerosis.

8. If "chronic active" rejection exists (categories 2 and 4), then "chronic inactive/burnt-out/scarred" rejection must exist as well. This entity is, however, not defined in the Banff scheme.

9. The various etiologies of so-called transplant glomerulopathy with duplication of glomerular capillary walls are inadequately defined.

10. Recommendations on tissue sampling should be definitive; "minimal adequacy" criteria and "standard adequacy" criteria should not be used side by side (74).

I prefer a primarily histology-based, dynamic classification of rejection (85). In the following paragraphs, I will illustrate rejection-induced changes in the three major anatomic tissue compartments—arteries (vessels), glomeruli, and the tubulo-interstitial space, with a highlighting of important diagnostic and clinical aspects. Rejection-induced tissue injury and inflammation can affect the interstitium/tubules, glomeruli, and arteries either alone or in combination. Rejection may be found in primarily unaltered parenchyma or it can be superimposed on preexisting lesions, such as donor-derived arterionephrosclerosis. Depending on the time of diagnosis, the natural progression, and the response to therapy, rejection can be seen in an early exudative/infiltrative/proliferative, or smoldering/sclerosing, or burnt-out/scarred stage. Rejection, in particular in the infiltrative inflammatory disease phase, can heal with complete functional and morphological restitution (i.e., restitutio ad integrum). Tissue remodeling and sclerosis are particularly stimulated during smoldering rejection episodes and the increased recruitment of "nonclassical" inflammatory cell elements such as myofibroblasts (71,86). The end result of severe or protracted rejection is sclerosis with varying degrees of scar formation (see Sclerosing/Sclerosed Transplant Arteriopathy) (70).

Rejection-induced graft fibrosis should be diagnosed and its etiology separated from other types of graft injury and scar formation, for example, preexisting donor disease, de novo hypertension–induced arterionephrosclerosis, calcineurin inhibitor–induced structural toxicity, and various recurrent or de novo kidney diseases. If the likely cause of graft sclerosis cannot be determined, then the descriptive term "interstitial fibrosis and tubular atrophy, not otherwise specified" seems to be the most appropriate. The "waste-basket" Banff term "chronic allograft nephropathy (CAN)" has recently been abandoned (87).

A histology-based classification of rejection-induced graft injury can be further amended by diagnostic classifiers, such as C4d staining results (marking antibody-mediated tissue injury) or others. A histology-based diagnosis could read: "Transplant endarteritis (mild) superimposed on moderate donor-derived arteriosclerosis. Concurrent focal tubulo-interstitial rejection; C4d positive. Comment: The pattern of changes suggests a mixed antibody and cellular rejection episode; circulating donor-specific antibodies should be searched for." I think that such a cautious classification approach is robust, detailed, flexible, and reflects key events of tissue injury. It provides all therapeutically and prognostically relevant information, and largely avoids misleading categories, such as acute or chronic, cellular or humoral. In the future, even transcriptomic and gene chip analyses may be utilized "as classifiers" to amend histological criteria and to provide specific biological, clinical, and prognostic information (88–90).

ii. Tubulo-interstitial Rejection

Commonly used synonyms: Acute cellular rejection (Banff category 4, type 1; CCTT type 1).

Definition: Inflammatory cell infiltrates (mainly mononuclear cells) in the interstitial compartment (mainly cortical) accompanied by edema and tubulitis (i.e., infiltration of mononuclear cells into nonatrophic tubules).

Gross pathology: The kidney is enlarged and pale, yellowish brown. On cross section, the medulla is slightly darker, especially along the corticomedullary junction (so-called white graft rejection). Current patient management strategies have made graft loss secondary to pure tubulointerstitial cellular rejection episodes exceptionally rare events.

Histology: Focal or diffuse mononuclear inflammatory cell infiltrates, characteristically accompanied by mild to moderate edema, are typically seen in the renal cortex, whereas the medulla is commonly spared (Figure 3.6); it

is only involved in marked rejection episodes. The inflammatory cells are activated, can show rare mitotic figures, and express markers of cell proliferation, such as Ki-67 (Figure 3.7). The inflammatory cells loosely aggregate without distinct borders and typically surround nonatrophic tubules in nonfibrotic areas in a fingerlike fashion (Figure 3.8). The inflammatory infiltrate is primarily composed of activated T-lymphocytes (CD3, CD4, CD8), abundant and sometimes dominant macrophages/histiocytes (CD68) (91–95),

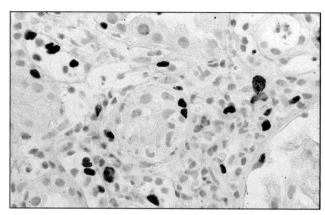

FIGURE 3.7: *Tubulo-interstitial rejection. The infiltrating mononuclear cells are activated and express nuclear antigens related to DNA replication and phases of the cell cycle. Note the tubular cross section in the middle of the field with tubulitis and nuclear expression of MIB-1/Ki-67 in the invading inflammatory cell nuclei in the absence of marked tubular necrosis. This presentation is typical for tubulo-interstitial rejection. Immunohistochemical incubation to detect MIB-1/Ki-67 nuclear antigens in formalin-fixed and paraffin-embedded tissue sections, 160× original magnification.*

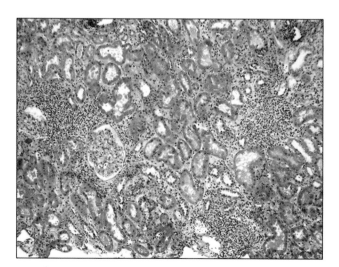

FIGURE 3.6: *Tubulo-interstitial rejection. About 2.5 months after transplantation, the patient presented with an elevation of serum creatine levels from baseline 1.2 to 1.8 mg/dl. The tubulo-interstitial compartment showed diffuse predominantly mononuclear inflammatory cell infiltrates and moderate focally accentuated edema. Tubules diffusely expressed MHC class II (HLA-DR); C4d was not detected. H&E stain, 40× original magnification.*

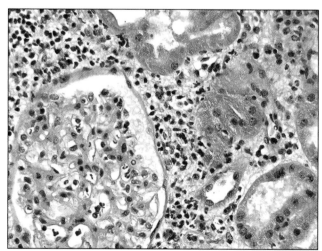

FIGURE 3.8: *Tubulo-interstitial rejection (same case as Figure 3.6). Higher magnification demonstrates a mixed inflammatory cell infiltrate containing eosinophilic leukocytes and scattered rare plasma cells in the edematous interstitium. Tubulitis is unimpressive and a glomerulus unremarkable. H&E stain, 100× original magnification.*

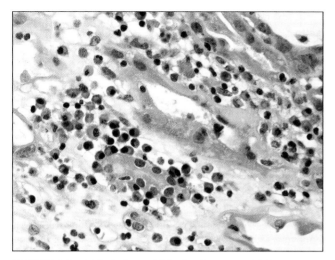

FIGURE 3.9: *Tubulo-interstitial rejection, very rich in plasma cells. Eight years after transplantation, a noncompliant patient, who had experienced prior rejection episodes, presented with a rise in serum creatinine from baseline 1.1 to 13 mg/dl. The interstitium was edematous and contained eosinophilic leukocytes and abundant plasma cells that surrounded, that is, "hugged," injured tubules without causing tubulitis. Tubules diffusely expressed MHC class II (HLA-DR); C4d was not detected. There was no evidence of an infection including CMV, EBV, and polyomaviruses. H&E stain, 200× oil original magnification.*

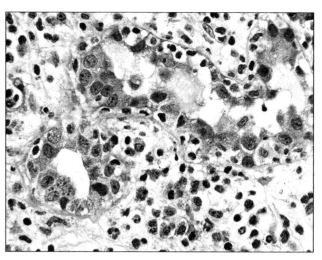

FIGURE 3.10: *Tubulo-interstitial rejection. This field shows prominent tubulitis. The invading mononuclear cells, predominantly lymphocytes, are located under activated and injured tubular epithelial cells and line the inner aspect of the tubular basement membranes. The presence of a perinuclear halo serves as a helpful diagnostic clue to distinguish lymphocytes from tubular epithelial cells. The interstitium is edematous and contains mononuclear inflammatory cells, eosinophilic leukocytes, and plasma cells. Trichrome stain, 200× original magnification.*

as well as varying numbers of plasma cells (CD138) sometimes mounting "plasma cell–rich" rejection episodes (Figure 3.9) (96,97). In addition, CD20-positive B cells, eosinophilic leukocytes, and polymorphonuclear leukocytes can be detected. CD20-positive lymphocytes can infiltrate the cortex diffusely, form small nodules, and occasionally even germinal centers. They typically account for less than 50 percent of the inflammatory reaction (92,98–101). Scattered polymorphonuclear leukocytes are commonly seen in or adjacent to severely injured tubules; they can be abundant adjacent to infarcts. Eosinophils (and edema) mark the "active and acute" phase of an inflammatory reaction; their presence should not be misinterpreted as evidence of an allergic etiology/allergic interstitial nephritis (Figures 3.8 and 3.9) (102). In areas of inflammation, peritubular capillaries are dilated and can contain numerous lymphocytes and monocytes (84,103) that migrate from the capillaries into the interstitium and ultimately into tubules. Inflammatory cell migration from the capillaries takes place without destruction of the capillary endothelial cells and interstitial hemorrhage is uncommon.

Nonatrophic tubules, most frequently distal segments, show varying degrees of tubulitis, typically as a focal phenomenon. Diffuse tubulitis is uncommon. Tubulitis is characterized by mononuclear cells (one or more T lymphocytes and/or macrophages) located inside the basement membrane and under or inbetween epithelial cells. It is best recognized in PAS-stained tissue sections. The invading T lymphocytes can usually be distinguished from the

surrounding activated tubular epithelial cells by their very dark nucleus and a perinuclear halo (differential diagnosis: apoptotic bodies). Tubular epithelial cell nuclei are typically larger than the infiltrating inflammatory cells, often contain small nucleoli, and show a less dense and finely granular chromatin structure (Figure 3.10). Rejection-induced tubulitis is practically never caused by eosinophilic and polymorphonuclear leukocytes, or plasma cells, and significant tubular cell necrosis is uncommon. The lack of severe tubular destruction is an important feature since it might provide an explanation for the reversibility of tubulo-interstitial rejection (Figures 3.6–3.10). In rare instances, tubular rupture occurs that can be associated with small, nonnecrotizing, histiocytic granulomas, or Tamm-Horsfall protein exudation into the interstitial compartment. Diffuse cases of tubulo-interstitial rejection can involve Bowman's capsule and result in small, segmental inflammatory "pseudocrescents," that is, "tubulitis of Bowman's capsule."

In pure tubulo-interstitial cellular rejection, without accompanying vascular or glomerular rejection, the glomeruli and vessels are unchanged except for an increased number of circulating intraglomerular mononuclear cell elements (differential diagnosis: transplant glomerulitis, see Transplant Glomerulitis). Tubulo-interstitial rejection can be associated with rejection phenomena in other tissue compartments, first and foremost transplant endarteritis (see Transplant Endarteritis).

Besides typical morphological changes, many renal allografts show lesions currently considered to be nondiagnostic: sharply demarcated, densely packed lymphocytic aggregates without interstitial edema and tubulitis adjacent to sclerotic glomeruli, in the adventitial layer of medium size arteries, and at the corticomedullary junction, that is, in places of lymphocytic recirculation. Lymphocytes are often found in areas of interstitial fibrosis and tubulitis may be seen in atrophic tubules with thickened basement membranes. At present, these changes are considered to be nondiagnostic for rejection. However, there is mounting concern that such lesions may be harmful for long-term graft function, and our diagnostic criteria may change in the future (81,99,104).

Besides "classical" inflammatory cell elements mentioned above, many other cell types contribute to the inflammatory response in tubulo-interstitial cellular rejection, such as natural killer cells, mast cells, or dendritic cells (105–107); they are of no direct diagnostic significance at the present time.

Immunohistology: In typical cases of interstitial rejection, immunohistological incubations to detect immunoglobulins or complement factors are unrevealing. The interstitial edema usually contains abundant fibrin and atrophic tubular basement membranes in areas of tissue remodeling typically show nondiagnostic complement factor C3 and C4d deposits. The immunohistochemical detection of HLA-DR and ICAM-1 in tubular epithelial cells as markers of "activation" may be helpful to confirm the diagnosis of rejection (Figure 3.11) (82,108,109).

Approximately 20–65 percent of tubulo-interstitial rejection episodes show C4d deposits along peritubular capillaries. These cases represent mixed cellular- and antibody-mediated graft injury (62,110–113) with increased numbers of intracapillary CD68-positive monocytes (103).

Differential diagnosis: The differential diagnosis mainly includes drug-induced allergic interstitial nephritides that can present with identical histological changes (see Drug-Induced Acute Tubulo-interstitial Nephritis). Allergic nephritides are often, but not always, most pronounced at the corticomedullary junction and characteristically C4d negative. However, a clear distinction between "tubulo-interstitial rejection" and "allergic interstitial nephritis" can sometimes not be made. Since both disease entities respond to steroid therapy, the pathologist, if in doubt, best errors on the side of "rejection." Of note, B cells including CD20-positive lymphocytes, sometimes forming nodules and lymphoid follicles, are a prominent part of interstitial nephritides found in native kidneys; they are not specific for inflammatory conditions seen in allografts (114). B-cell–rich rejection episodes containing abundant plasma cells or CD20-positive lymphocytes have to be distinguished from post-transplant lymphoproliferative disorders (PTLD, see EBV/Post-Transplant Lymphoproliferative Disorders) that commonly express abundant Epstein-Barr virus (EBV) – related antigens and mRNAs.

Comment: Tubulo-interstitial rejection is cell mediated, mainly driven by T-lymphocytes and macrophages. It responds well to bolus steroid therapy and renal function typically returns to baseline levels if the biopsy samples are large enough to exclude concurrent transplant endarteritis, glomerulitis, and C4d positivity (76,111,115,116). C4d-positive tubulo-interstitial rejection episodes, that is, mixed cellular- and antibody-mediated graft injury (combined Banff category 4, type 1, and category 2 rejection) are clinically more severe, they more frequently result in graft failure, and require targeted and aggressive therapy (76,111,113). The presence of concurrent transplant endarteritis has specific therapeutic and prognostic implications (see Transplant Endarteritis). Whether the predominant infiltrating cell type, that is, T cells, CD20-positive B cells, plasma cells, macrophages, or eosinophilic leukocytes, significantly and independently impacts long-term graft function and survival is unclear and currently controversially debated (93,96,97,100–102,117–123). The predominant inflammatory cell type may, however, influence the response to antirejection treatment [bolus steroids, antilymphocytic sera, rituximab (100,124,125)].

The extent of tubulo-interstitial inflammation, defined by the degree of parenchymal inflammation and tubulitis, neither directly correlates with the presence of transplant endarteritis nor with poor outcome (116,126–128). This observation is of particular importance since it challenges the common clinical practice of simply grading the severity of rejection episodes based on the extent of cortical inflammation. It also questions the concept of "borderline" rejection advocated in the Banff classification scheme (16,81,129–131).

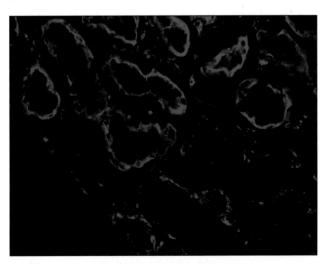

FIGURE 3.11: *A case of tubulo-interstitial cellular rejection with typical focal expression of MHC class II (HLA-DR) in the cytoplasm of tubular epithelial cells (upper portion of the image). In contrast, most tubules in the lower part of the field do not express class II antigens. Tubular MHC class II expression is an indicator of epithelial cell activation that can serve as an ancillary marker of cell-mediated rejection. Direct IF microscopy with a fluorescein conjugated anti-MHC class II antibody, 200× original magnification.*

In my practice, I avoid the diagnosis "borderline." If biopsies show minimal tubulo-interstitial inflammation in the presence of transplant glomerulitis, endarteritis, or C4d positivity, a diagnosis of "rejection" can easily be rendered. In order to establish the diagnosis of (pure) tubulo-interstitial cellular rejection, I use criteria and cutoff levels initially defined in the CCTT classification scheme (Table 3.4) (26): at least 5 percent of the cortex must have interstitial mononuclear cell infiltrates associated with edema and tubulitis (defined as one or more infiltrating mononuclear cells in a nonatrophic tubular cross section) in three or more tubules in inflamed areas. In rejection, tubules typically express MHC class II (additional immunohistochemical diagnostic classifier). If tubulo-interstitial cellular rejection is considered in my differential diagnosis and if the above-mentioned histological cutoff values are not reached (after leveling through the block), then I suggest rejection in the setting of marked concurrent tubular class II expression (82). This diagnostic approach has proven to be of great value in my practice. Possibly in the future, other (tubular) markers may further help to diagnose rejection-induced tubulo-interstitial injury more accurately (132).

Tubulo-interstitial rejection is best characterized and identified in the early infiltrative and proliferative, that is, "inflammatory" disease phase that typically responds well to antirejection therapy (115), often with histological clearance (133). Likely persistent and smoldering rejection episodes can lead to increasing levels of interstitial fibrosis and tubular atrophy (99,134,135). However, many different disease entities alone or in combination can result in the common pathway of "interstitial scarring," and lymphocytic infiltrates are common in areas of fibrosis in native and transplant kidneys. Thus, in contrast to "vascular" and "glomerular" rejection that can show distinct "chronic rejection–induced tissue remodeling," chronic rejection limited to the tubulo-interstitial compartment cannot be easily diagnosed.

TABLE 3.4 Minimal Histological Criteria to Diagnose (Pure) Tubulo-interstitial Cellular Rejection – "Chapel Hill Standards"

1. Cortical mononuclear cell inflammation ≥5% of nonscarred parenchyma

2. Mild to moderate interstitial edema

3. Tubulitis (≥1 infiltrating mononuclear cell) in ≥3 nonatrophic tubules in most inflamed areas

- Scattered eosinophilic leukocytes and ATI are commonly detected
- MHC class II is typically expressed in tubular epithelial cells
- If criteria 1–3 are not fulfilled, but tubules strongly express MHC class II, then the presence of a rejection episode is suggested
- If criteria 1–3 are not fulfilled but transplant endarteritis, transplant glomerulitis, or C4d positivity is noted, a diagnosis of rejection must be rendered and accordingly defined

iii. Arterial/Vascular Rejection

The term arterial or vascular rejection is used descriptively to define rejection-related changes in the arterial tree: arterioles, small, and large arteries. It does not imply a specific etiology and should not be mistaken for "humoral or antibody mediated rejection." Inflammation and rejection associated lesions can also be seen in venules and lymphatics (136). They are considered to be nondiagnostic and often related to inflammatory cell trafficking and recirculation (137,138). Rejection-related changes in glomerular or peritubular capillaries will be discussed separately.

Marked arterial rejection is commonly associated with impaired blood flow and varying degrees of ischemic injury predominately affecting the tubulo-interstitial compartment: ischemic injury, marked intra cytoplasmic protein reabsorption droplets in tubular epithelial cells (in the absence of nephrotic range proteinuria), marked interstitial edema and scleredema, and increased numbers of interstitial eosinophilic leucocytes. On occasion, "glomerular low flow" can result in tuft collapse mimicking "collapsing focal and segmental glomerulosclerosis". The described changes can serve as helpful clues to "suspect" vascular rejection and to initiate a targeted search by step sectioning through all remaining tissue blocks.

1. Transplant Arteriopathy with Massive Thrombosis

Commonly used synonyms: Hyperacute rejection (Banff category 2 acute antibody-mediated rejection, not further specified).

Definition: Occlusive thrombi in all caliber arteries and capillaries due to deposition of preformed antibodies and severe endothelial injury.

Gross pathology: Typically during surgery the grafts swell, turn reddish-blue, mottled, and develop infarcts. Current patient management strategies have made graft loss secondary to transplant arteriopathy with massive thrombosis exceptionally rare events.

Histology: Characteristic for "transplant arteriopathy with massive thrombosis" is the formation of fibrin thrombi in large and small caliber arteries as well as glomerular capillaries (Figure 3.12). Arterial thrombi can show a polymorphonuclear leukocyte reaction along the endothelial cell surface, a "nonspecific" change that should not be misinterpreted as an "antibody-mediated type of injury." Despite thrombosis, vascular walls often remain viable, even in areas of infarction. If renal allografts survive, then subsequent biopsies may show surprisingly few remaining thrombi. This focality is due to the unaltered fibrinolytic activity in the recipient resulting in thrombolysis in the allograft. Thrombus formation causes severe acute ischemic injury, focal hemorrhage, polymorphonuclear leukocyte infiltration, and in most severe cases frank infarcts. Polymorphonuclear leukocytes are found in the interstitium either as a demarcation phenomenon between viable

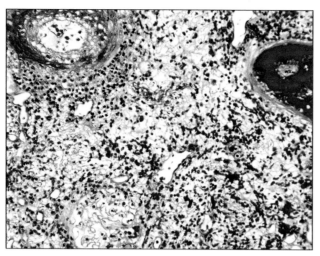

FIGURE 3.12: *Transplant arteriopathy with massive thrombosis. Two months after transplantation, graft nephrectomy was performed due to anuria, pain, and infarction. Most arteries contained partially occlusive recent thrombi. The interstitium was severely edematous and infarcted. Due to severe necrosis, C4d staining could not be adequately interpreted. Trichrome stain, 80× original magnification.*

and infarcted areas or adjacent to tubules with severe ischemic injury. Significant lympho-histiocytic infiltrates, that is, signs of cellular rejection in the interstitium and arteries, are generally lacking, although they can evolve if grafts survive for a few weeks. Of note, as a general rule if conspicuous thrombi are found in areas of parenchymal infarction, then they should be interpreted as causative events—and not—as secondary, reactive phenomena.

Immunohistology: During the early phases of rejection, linear deposits of IgG and IgM together with complement factors including C4d are present along the vascular endothelium of arteries, glomeruli, and peritubular capillaries. In nephrectomy specimens with complete necrosis, immunoglobulin deposits may be scant or even lacking. Transplant arteriopathy with massive thrombosis is generally C4d positive (in particular in the renal medulla since capillaries in the cortex may be severely damaged).

Differential diagnosis: The differential diagnosis mainly includes surgical complications or underlying, and unnoticed coagulopathies. While transplant arteriopathy with massive thrombosis characteristically affects the entire arterial tree including large hilar vessels and glomerular capillaries, with C4d deposits along peritubular capillaries, surgical complications, and "clotting" disorders on the other hand are C4d negative and largely limited to arteries and veins near the anastomotic site.

Comment: Since the introduction of effective cross matching, rejection episodes with widespread thrombi have become exceptionally rare events (139). At present, ABO incompatible grafting is one clinical scenario that can still lead to massive thrombus formation in some instances. Such rejection episodes typically occur immediately after

transplantation (minutes > hours > days). Preformed circulating recipient antibodies bind to the endothelium of arteries and capillaries in the graft and rapidly lead o massive thrombosis and infarction. Transplant arteriopathy with massive thrombosis is the "prototype" for an antibody-mediated rejection phenomenon. Outcome in fully developed cases is generally ominous. Plasmapheresis may be tried in more protracted cases.

2. Necrotizing Transplant Arteriopathy

Commonly used synonyms: Accelerated acute rejection (Banff category 4, type 3, or category 2 acute antibody-mediated rejection, type 3; CCTT type 3).

Definition: Trans- or intramural "fibrinoid" arterial wall necrosis affecting all caliber arteries (interlobar, arcuate, interlobular) in association with varying degrees of arterial inflammation.

Gross pathology: The kidneys are usually swollen with hemorrhagic and anemic infarcts side by side (mottled appearance). In the most severe cases, the nephrectomy specimens have a dark red, edematous appearance, closely resembling cases of transplant arteriopathy with massive thrombosis.

Histology: Lesions are typically focal and only involve some segments of the arterial tree. Fibrinoid arterial wall necrosis can be transmural (from the intimal to the adventitial layer) or intramural (involving only the media with or without destruction of the internal elastic lamina), circumferential or segmental. Arterial necrosis is frequently associated with varying degrees of intimal or transmural inflammation, ranging from minimal to marked (Figure 3.13). Despite severe changes in the vascular walls, intimal surfaces can still be covered by endothelial cells and occlusive thrombi are uncommon, although small intimal fibrin or platelet aggregates may occur. If the rejection episodes respond to treatment, then necrotic vascular walls may fibrose with occasional formation of microaneurysms. In the assessment of arterial wall necrosis and "chronic" scarring, elastic tissue stains and the demonstration of marked destruction of the internal elastic laminae are diagnostically most useful.

Often the interstitium shows cellular rejection (including edema and foci of tubulitis) and in severe cases patchy hemorrhage or infarction. Glomeruli can appear normal, show capillary collapse due to "low flow," contain fibrin thrombi, or present with more typical rejection-induced transplant glomerulitis. Concurrent transplant endarteritis is common. The differential diagnosis includes other vasculitides, such as antineutrophilic cytoplasmic antibody disease/ANCA, induced injury or in cases with scant inflammation and necrosis of small vessel athrombotic microangiopathy.

Immunohistology: In typical cases immunohistological incubations to detect immunoglobulins or complement factors are unrevealing. Fibrin can be found in necrotic arterial walls, in the edematous interstitium, and in foci of

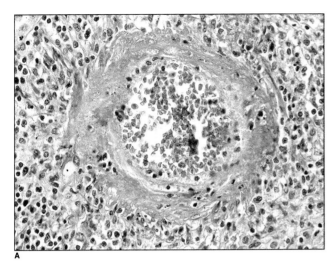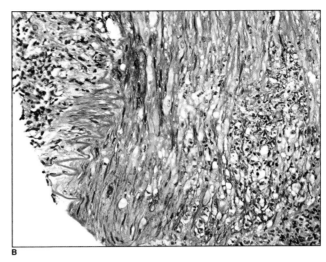

FIGURE 3.13: *Necrotizing transplant arteriopathy (A, B). (A) The interlobular artery shows circumferential, transmural fibrinoid necrosis of the medial smooth muscle layer. Note scattered intramural inflammatory cells. The arterial lumen is patent and contains red blood cells. Diffuse inflammation is seen in the interstitium. Graft nephrectomy twenty-two days after transplantation. (B) Two months after transplantation of a cadaveric organ, the patient presented with an increase in the serum creatinine from baseline 2.1 to 3.1 mg/dl. The arcuate artery demonstrated not only marked intimal inflammation (on the left) but also intramural inflammatory cell aggregates with focal fibrinoid necrosis. Tubulo-interstitial rejection was also present, C4d was not detected. (A) H&E stain, 100× original magnification. (B) Trichrome stain, 100× original magnification.*

hemorrhage or recent infarction. In my experience, approximately 50 percent of cases with necrotizing transplant arteriopathy demonstrate C4d deposits along peritubular capillaries (62).

Differential diagnosis: The differential diagnosis mainly includes thrombotic microangiopathies (TMAs) with marked arterial wall necrosis. Although a distinction between rejection and TMAs can sometimes be difficult, significant vascular wall inflammation, involvement of large caliber arteries, rejection-induced changes in the tubulo-interstitial or glomerular compartments, and C4d positivity along peritubular capillaries usually help to render a diagnosis of rejection and to rule out "TMAs." Rare cases, such as those induced by antibodies directed against angiotensin receptors may present with overlapping histological features (140).

Comment: Necrotizing transplant arteriopathy is typically seen within the first weeks after grafting, however, it can also be found in failed transplants off immunosuppression years after surgery. It is an uncommon form of rejection (seen in approximately 1–4 percent of all rejection episodes occurring within the first weeks after grafting). The specific etiology of fibrinoid arterial wall necrosis is undetermined. Antibodies (de novo ?) likely cause injury in C4d-positive cases, whereas cellular rejection including transplant endarteritis may induce vascular wall necrosis in others (113,141,142). Outcome is generally poor; most grafts are lost within weeks after biopsy (113,116,142).

3. Transplant Endarteritis

Commonly used synonyms: Infiltrative and proliferative transplant vasculopathy, acute transplant vasculitis, endo-

vasculitis, endothelialitis, intimal arteritis (Banff category 4, type 2; CCTT, type 2).

Definition: Subendothelial/intimal inflammation (lymphocytes and macrophages) in all caliber arteries without thrombosis and without de novo intimal sclerosis. The medial smooth muscle layers are unaltered.

Gross pathology: Failed grafts exhibit small anemic infarcts, foci of hemorrhage, and often parenchymal fibrosis. Graft loss is commonly caused by a combination of concurrent severe transplant endarteritis, sclerosing transplant arteriopathy, and tubulo-interstitial rejection.

Histology: Transplant endarteritis can affect all caliber arteries in the renal parenchyma as well as (grafted) extra-renal vessels in the hilar adipose tissue and along the ureters (71). In renal biopsies, typically only few arteries are involved either in a circumferential or in a segmental fashion, preferentially at branching points. Arcuate caliber vessels are "hot spots." Unaffected arteries are either normal, show nondiagnostic changes, such as endothelial cell activation (including the formation of so-called arches), or contain increased numbers of circulating lymphocytes (Figure 3.14). Transplant endarteritis, like all (vascular) changes seen in rejection, can be superimposed on preexisting donor lesions, such as arterionephrosclerosis (see Figure 3.20 in Sclerosing/Sclerosed Transplant Arteriopathy).

Transplant endarteritis progresses through different "inflammatory phases." *Infiltrative phase*: The earliest nondiagnostic changes are detected along the luminal surface with endothelial cell activation including nuclear enlargement, cytoplasmic swelling, and vacuolization (Figure 3.14). This activation (including the expression of adhesion molecules (109,143,144) facilitates the transmigration of

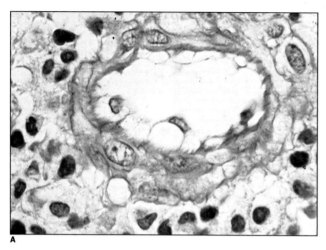
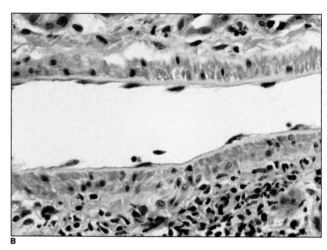

A   **B**

FIGURE 3.14: *Endothelial cell activation—nondiagnostic changes (A, B). (A) A small interlobular artery shows marked activation of the endothelial cell layer including the formation of so-called arches. (B) This artery reveals enlargement of endothelial cell nuclei and rare intraluminal mononuclear cells. Subendothelial inflammatory cells are not present and a diagnosis of "transplant endarteritis" cannot be rendered (compare with Figure 3.15). (A and B) H&E stain, 160× original magnification.*

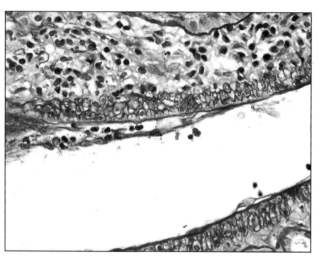

FIGURE 3.15: *Transplant endarteritis. Eight days after transplantation, a renal biopsy showed inflammatory cells in between and under activated endothelial cells along one segment of an interlobular artery. The medial smooth muscle layer was unremarkable. The interstitium revealed tubulo-interstitial rejection, C4d was not detected. PAS stain, 200× oil original magnification.*

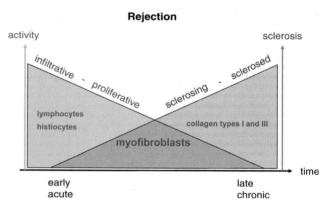

FIGURE 3.16: *Schema of rejection. Active/infiltrative/ proliferative—sclerosing—inactive/scarred rejection phenomena commonly form a continuum rather than sharply separated disease entities. Myofibroblasts are crucial cell elements that are already recruited during the early, infiltrative stages of rejection. They promote sclerosis by synthesizing collagens. The described changes are most easily appreciated in vascular rejection episodes (71).*

lymphocytes and macrophages. Transplant endarteritis is defined as the subendothelial/intimal accumulation of one or more lymphocytes or histiocytes. The invading mononuclear inflammatory cells are often arranged in small clusters and associated with edema (Figure 3.15). In addition, scattered rare eosinophilic leukocytes may occasionally be found, whereas lymphocytes of B-cell lineage are exceptionally rare. Endothelial cells overlying pockets of inflammation are typically activated; conspicuous endothelial cell necrosis or occlusive thrombus formation are lacking. During persistent intimal inflammation, histiocytes can transform into foam cells. *Proliferative phase:* The infiltrative stage imperceptibly evolves into the proliferative stage characterized not only by increasing numbers of subendothelial mononuclear cell elements but additionally also by increasing numbers of spindle-shaped cells, that is, myofibroblasts, and a high proliferative activity based on Ki-67/ MIB-1 expression (71,145). While the number of myofibroblasts increases over time, the number of lymphocytes and to a lesser extent histiocytes usually decreases (71,145). Foam cells typically persist. The accumulation of myofibroblasts is associated with the deposition of "early" extracellular matrix proteins, in particular fibronectins and collagen type IV. Of note, "scar" collagens 1 and 3 are absent; their deposition marks the transformation of transplant endarteritis into sclerosing transplant arteriopathy (see Sclerosing/Sclerosed

Transplant Arteriopathy, Figure 3.16) (71). Since the inflammatory process is limited to the intima, both the internal elastic lamina and the media remain unchanged.

Transplant endarteritis is commonly accompanied by tubulo-interstitial rejection that can be rich in eosinophilic leukocytes and show pronounced edema (102,128,146). Rejection-induced inflammation is limited to arteries in approximately 5–10 percent of cases. Glomeruli can be normal or show transplant glomerulitis in approximately 30 percent of patients (see Transplant Glomerulitis).

Immunohistology: Many cells infiltrating the intima of arteries are CD68-positive monocytes/macrophages. In addition, T lymphocytes are detected among which CD8 cells are more common than CD4 cells (about 2:1) (71,145). Even during the early infiltrative stages of transplant endarteritis, scattered alpha smooth muscle actin–positive myofibroblasts are found that tend to form clusters close to the internal elastic lamina in the proliferative phase. The intimal inflammatory process typically lacks a B-cell component (very rarely, individual CD20-positive cells or CD138-positive plasma cells are seen). Activated endothelial cells and infiltrating mononuclear cells upregulate MHC class II (HLA-DR) and adhesion molecules such as ICAM or VCAM. IF microscopy with a standard panel of antibodies does not reveal a significant and diagnostic staining pattern in arteries or glomeruli.

A significant percentage of rejection episodes with transplant endarteritis shows a concurrent antibody-mediated component of graft injury based on the detection of C4d along peritubular capillaries (30–70 percent of patients, see Antibody-Mediated Rejection and C4d Staining, Figures 3.17 and 3.18) (62,110,111,147,148).

Differential diagnosis: Transplant endarteritis is highly suggestive of rejection-induced graft injury. Similar vascular changes can occasionally be seen in other types of vasculitides, such as lupus nephritis or ANCA-induced small vessel vasculitis. However, these latter cases are typically accompanied by glomerulonephritides or marked immune complex deposits. If many B cells, that is, CD20-positive cells, are found in inflamed intimal layers, then a diagnosis of PTLD should be considered (see Infections/Epstein-Barr virus).

Comment: Transplant endarteritis is a cell-mediated type of injury, driven by T cells and macrophages (71,145,149). C4d-positive cases represent *mixed* "cellular" and "humoral" rejection that should be specifically diagnosed (Banff category 4, type II and category II rejection, see Antibody-Mediated Rejection and C4d Staining). Transplant endarteritis is a common phenomenon, seen in approximately 30 percent of rejection episodes occurring during the first year. I have diagnosed it as early as six days and as late as seventeen years after transplantation. It may often be underdiagnosed due to small (inadequate) biopsy samples lacking sufficient interlobular arteries/branches of arcuate vessels.

The diagnosis of transplant endarteritis carries great prognostic and therapeutic significance. Patients usually do not benefit from conventional bolus steroid therapy but rather require potent treatment with antilymphocytic sera (115,116,127,150,151). Transplant endarteritis has a less favorable long-term prognosis than tubulo-interstitial rejection (126–128); the difference becomes already apparent after one year of follow-up (116) and is most pronounced in cases with severe intimal inflammation (151). C4d-positive transplant endarteritis, that is, cellular and concurrent antibody-mediated graft injury, is clinically more severe than corresponding C4d-negative cases and frequently results in graft failure (76,111).

Treatment is most effective during the early, infiltrative phase of intimal inflammation when lympho-histocytic infiltrates are limited and myofibroblasts are largely absent (115,151). However, even aggressive antirejection therapy often does not result in the complete histological clearance of intimal inflammation (133), which persists and smolders in approximately 20 percent of my cases in which repeat biopsies were available for review. "Smoldering" intimal inflammation and myofibroblast activation result in progressive intimal sclerosis, that is, sclerosing transplant arteriopathy. In this regard, myofibroblasts are of utmost importance since they serve as machineries for collagen type 1 and 3 production and intimal scar formation (71,86). The origin of myofibroblasts is undetermined (86); they may potentially originate from circulating recipient progenitor cells (152).

4. Sclerosing/Sclerosed Transplant Arteriopathy

Commonly used synonyms: Chronic vascular rejection, chronic transplant vasculopathy, Banff category 4 chronic active T-cell–mediated rejection or Banff category 2 chronic active antibody-mediated rejection, not classified according to CCTT.

Definition: Rejection-induced arterial intimal thickening due to de novo collagen types I and III deposition; no intimal elastosis; varying degrees of concurrent intimal inflammation ranging from absent to marked.

Gross pathology: Failed grafts are commonly shrunken and scarred; they can rarely be calcified. Graft loss is usually caused by a combination of concurrent severe transplant endarteritis, and marked, sclerosing and sclerosed transplant arteriopathy. Small hemorrhagic infarcts may be seen (Figure 3.19).

Histology: Sclerosing/sclerosed transplant arteriopathy represents inflammation, that is, transplant endarteritis, induced concentric or eccentric intimal scar formation which is often pronounced at arterial branching points. It is histologically characterized by several features: 1) varying degrees of intimal sclerosis with deposition of fibrillary collagens types 1 and 3; 2) lack of elastic lamellae, that is, no

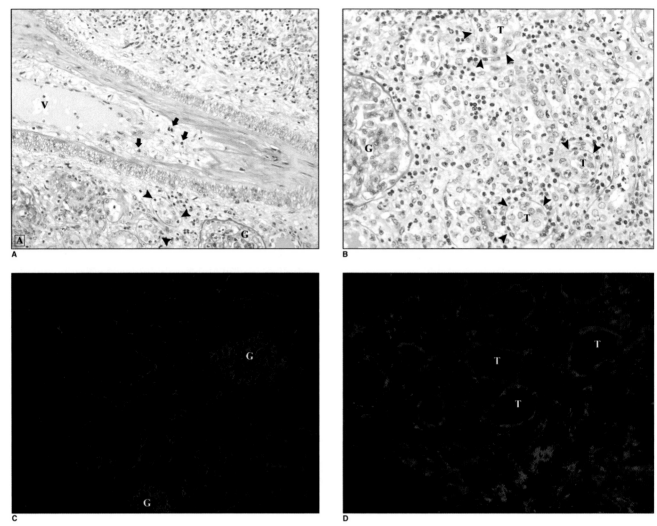

FIGURE 3.17: *Transplant endarteritis and tubulo-interstitial rejection, C4d positive (so-called mixed cellular and antibody-mediated rejection, A–D). The patient presented with deterioration of graft function eighteen days after transplantation. At time of biopsy, high titers of anti-donor class I antibodies were found. (A and B) An intraparenchymal artery (V) showed marked transplant endarteritis (bold arrows; note: intimal inflammation was superimposed on donor arteriosclerosis). The interstitium revealed pronounced, diffuse predominantly mononuclear inflammatory cell infiltrates and tubulitis (T = tubulus; the arrowheads in A and B mark the tubular basement membranes of severely inflamed tubular cross sections). Glomeruli (G) were without significant changes. PAS stains, (A) 200× and (B) 300× original magnification. (C) C4d was diffusely found along peritubular capillaries marking an additional antibody-mediated injury (G = glomerulus). Indirect IF microscopy with a monoclonal antibody directed against the complement degradation product C4d on fresh frozen tissue, 200× original magnification. (D) MHC class II (HLA-DR) was expressed by tubular epithelial cells (T = tubulus), direct IF microscopy with a fluorescein-conjugated anti-MHC class II antibody, 300× original magnification.*

significant intimal fibroelastosis; 3) varying numbers of randomly arranged myofibroblasts with enlarged nuclei; 4) scattered mononuclear inflammatory cells that can form small clusters in some cases; 5) occasional foam cells; 6) rudimentary neo-media formation under the endothelial layer in few instances; and 7) enlargement and hyperchromasia of endothelial cells. The inner elastic lamina usually remains intact; it is only disrupted as a consequence of severe medial inflammation and necrosis (70,71).

Typical for intimal scarring secondary to inflammation and endothelial cell injury is the absence of elastosis. This

feature can easily be demonstrated with elastic tissue stains (Figures 3.20 and 3.21). Of note, the elastic stains have to be adequately titered in order to demonstrate thin internal elastic laminae of interlobular arteries; aortic walls are often inadequate positive control samples due to the abundance of "thick" elastic lamellae.

In some patients intimal scarring can be an active, and progressive disease process promoted by inflammation (Figure 3.16). In these cases, varying numbers of lymphocytes, histocytes, and often abundant myofibroblasts are found in the thickened intima (Figure 3.22). Potentially even eosinophilic leukocytes may play a significant role in

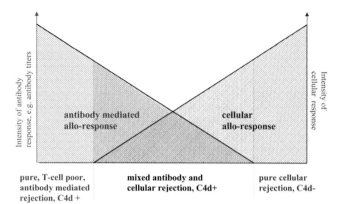

FIGURE 3.18: *Schema of rejection. Active rejection episodes can either be "pure" antibody or pure cellular-mediated events or represent mixed rejection with varying degrees of humoral and cellular components.*

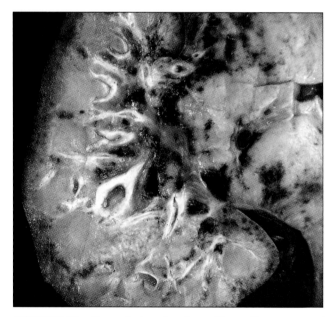

FIGURE 3.19: *Transplant nephrectomy. The graft was removed ten years after transplantation due to severe (active) sclerosing transplant arteriopathy with focal occlusive thrombosis, transplant glomerulopathy, and marked parenchymal fibrosis. Note multiple foci of hemorrhage due to severe vascular rejection in intra- and extraparenchymal arteries in the cortex and perihilar fat. C4d was not detected. The clinical suspicion of a "mass lesion" consistent with an "extranodal lymphoma" had resulted in the surgical removal of the graft, which showed no tumor growth but rather extensive, rejection-related perihilar fat necrosis.*

the development of intimal sclerosis (153). Inflammatory cells occasionally form small aggregates close to the internal elastic lamina or under the endothelium (Figure 3.20B, C).

I use the term "sclerosing arteriopathy" to emphasize the active and progressive component of fibrous remodeling driven by inflammation. Of note, the presence of foam cells should not be used as sole indicator of "activity." At present, it is undetermined how many inflammatory cells

are needed in the intima in order to designate a case as "active." At minimum I require the presence of clusters of two or more lymphocytes before rendering the diagnosis of "sclerosing arteriopathy." I tend to diagnostically ignore very rare scattered mononuclear inflammatory cells.

If the sclerosed intima lacks signs of inflammation, I consider the arteriopathy to be inactive, with burnt-out scar formation (Figures 3.16 and 3.21). I use the term "sclerosed arteriopathy" to emphasize this aspect (Figure 3.23).

Frequently, sclerosing or sclerosed transplant arteriopathy is superimposed on varying degrees of preexisting donor disease, that is, hypertension-induced arterionephrosclerosis (Figure 3.20). In these cases, remote, dense fibro-elastosis is detected along the outer aspect of the thickened intima with superimposed typical sclerosing/ sclerosed arteriopathy comprising the inner intimal zones.

Cases of sclerosing or sclerosed transplant arteriopathy are often associated with transplant glomerulopathy and glomerulitis, that is, signs of glomerular rejection (in my experience in approximately 40 percent of biopsies) and possible tubulo-interstitial rejection. Severe transplant arteriopathy can result in arterial stenosis, ischemia, tubular atrophy, and interstitial fibrosis. On occasion, so-called scleredema is found, that is, a glassy appearing interstitial fibrosis that develops in cases of persistent and severe interstitial edema.

Immunohistology: Immunohistology is unrevealing (145). In some cases, deposits of IgM, complement factor C3, C4d, and C5b-9 are present in arterial walls (nondiagnostic observation). C4d can be found along peritubular capillaries in cases of sclerosing arteriopathy in approximately 30–60 percent of biopsies (147). C4d deposits are uncommon in burnt-out sclerosed transplant arteriopathies.

Differential diagnosis: The major differential diagnosis of sclerosed transplant arteriopathy includes arterio (nephro) sclerosis induced by hypertension. Arterio (nephro) sclerosis typically shows a hypocellular intima with only rare, small, spindle-shaped fibrocytes embedded in a dense, fibrotic intima rich in elastic lamellae, that is, marked fibroelastosis. The accumulation of foam cells or neo-media formation are not features of arterio (nephro) sclerosis but rather mark "rejection." Of note, rejection-induced arteriopathies can be superimposed on (preexisting) arterio (nephro) sclerosis.

Occasionally, sclerosing phases of thrombotic micro-angiopathies (TMAs) may mimic rejection-induced transplant arteriopathies. In both cases, marked myofibroblastic proliferations lacking fibroelastosis are seen in the intimal layers. A definitive diagnosis can usually be rendered since TMAs primarily affect very small arteries, arterioles and glomerular vascular poles, whereas rejection-induced changes are predominantly found in arcuate caliber vessels. Furthermore, in contrast to rejection-induced

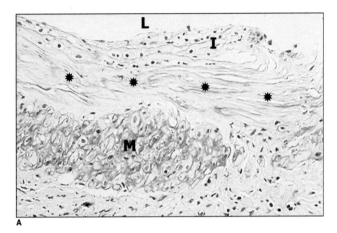

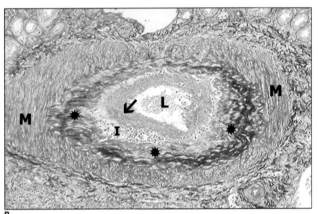

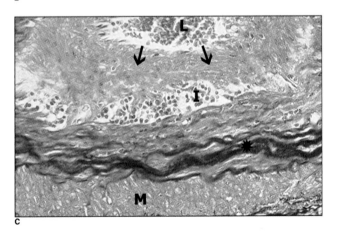

◄ *FIGURE 3.20:   Transplant endarteritis superimposed on preexisting donor arteriosclerosis: from early infiltrative endarteritis to subsequent sclerosing arteriopathy (A–C): (A) An arcuate caliber artery showed twelve days after transplantation marked transplant endarteritis with mononuclear inflammatory cell infiltrates superimposed on preexisting intimal fibroelastosis (asterisks: donor-derived intimal fibroelastosis, L = arterial lumen, I = mononuclear cell infiltrates in intima, M = medial smooth muscle layer). (B and C) Five months later, a repeat biopsy revealed (active) sclerosing transplant arteriopathy with aggregates of mononuclear inflammatory cells located deep in the intimal layer adjacent to donor derived remote fibroelastosis. As a consequence of protracted intimal inflammation, subendothelial sclerosis had developed, which was free of elastic lamellae (small arrows in B and C). (A) PAS stain, 80× original magnification; (B) trichrome stain, 40× original magnification; (C) elastic tissue stain, 80× original magnification.*

factor stimulate the proliferation of myofibroblasts and the synthesis of extracellular matrix proteins, in particular fibrillary scar collagens types 1 and 3. In addition to "cell-mediated arterial rejection/inflammation" likely, also circulating donor-specific antibodies play a currently poorly defined role in the pathogenesis of intimal sclerosis (149), at least in C4d-positive cases. Since myofibroblasts are not resident cells in normal intimal layers they have to be recruited during endarteritis and sclerosis.

Sclerosed, inactive, transplant arteriopathy does not respond to treatment (burnt-out intimal scar). However, if signs of concurrent active rejection are noted in the biopsy sample (Figure 3.23), that is, sclerosing transplant arteriopathy, tubulo-interstitial or glomerular rejection, or potentially C4d positivity along peritubular capillaries, specific anti rejection therapy can be beneficial (antilymphocytic preparations, high dose tacrolimus or mycophenolate-mofetil, IVIG, etc.). Although mild focal sclerosed transplant arteriopathy may be without significant detrimental impact on graft survival, most cases present with concentric intimal thickening, stenosis, and graft loss often occurs within months.

iv. Glomerular Rejection

Similar to the term "arterial or vascular rejection," the category "glomerular rejection" is also solely descriptive and defines rejection related changes in the glomerular compartment. It does not indicate a specific underlying etiology and should not be mistaken for humoral or antibody-mediated injury. Rejection-induced glomerular inflammation and remodeling has to be distinguished from other potential glomerular diseases, such as immune complex–mediated glomerulonephritides or thrombotic microangiopathies. A definitive diagnosis can usually be rendered based on clinical findings including abnormalities of the urine sediment (hematuria, red blood cell casts, and proteinuria), careful IF and electron microscopical analyses searching for immune complex

fibrous intimal remodeling, myofibroblastic proliferations in cases of sclerosing TMAs tend to be regular without significant inflammation and C4d deposits along peritubular capillaries are typically absent.

Comment: Sclerosing and sclerosed transplant arteriopathy is an immune-mediated type of injury, that is, it represents the scarring stage of transplant endarteritis (70,71,145). It can develop within few weeks (71). Intimal inflammation and the release of various cytokines and growth factors including platelet-derived growth factor, transforming growth factor beta, basic fibroblast growth

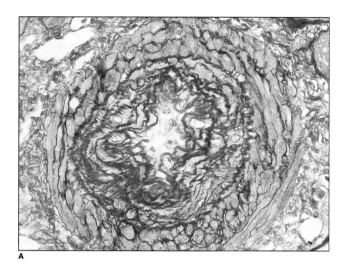

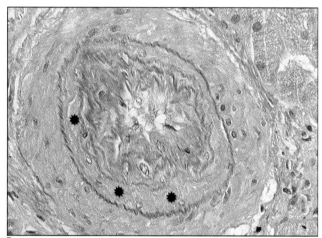

◄ **FIGURE 3.21:** *Sclerosed transplant arteriopathy compared to hypertension-induced arteriosclerosis (A–C). (A and B) A branch of an arcuate caliber artery shows marked intimal fibrosis with scattered myofibroblasts. Endothelial cells are enlarged. There is no sign of intimal inflammation. Note the lack of significant elastic lamellae in the widened intimal zone (asterisks in B). This is a typical picture of burnt-out and inactive intimal scar formation subsequent to preceding intimal inflammation, that is, transplant endarteritis (compare with Figure 3.20). The biopsy was taken 7.3 years after grafting in a patient with transplant endarteritis four months after transplantation. (C) Sclerosed transplant arteriopathy has to be distinguished from "ordinary" hypertension-induced arterial intimal fibroelastosis illustrated in C. Due to protracted endothelial cell activation and injury induced by high blood pressure, multiple layers of elastic lamellae were deposited and formed the basis for intimal fibroelastosis. (L = arterial lumen, M = medial smooth muscle layer). (A) Trichrome and (B) elastic tissue stain, 180× original magnification. (C) Elastic tissue stain, 300× original magnification.*

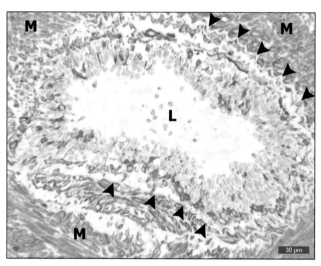

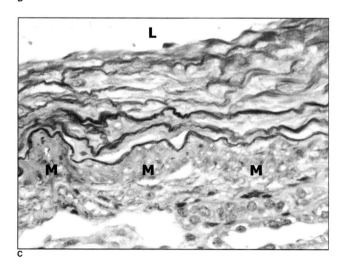

FIGURE 3.22: *In a non-human primate model of sclerosing transplant arteriopathy, abundant myofibroblasts can be seen in the thickened and inflamed intimal layer (arrow heads mark the internal elastic lamina, M = medial smooth muscle layer, L = arterial lumen). Additional stains demonstrated de novo deposition of collagens types 1 and 3. The changes were observed forty-five days after induction of transplant endarteritis (71). Immunohistochemical incubation to detect alpha smooth muscle actin with a polyclonal antibody on formalin-fixed and paraffin-embedded tissue section, 200× original magnification.*

1. Transplant Glomerulitis

Commonly used synonyms: Acute transplant glomerulopathy.

Definition: Endocapillary hypercellularity with mononuclear and/or polymorphonuclear cells filling dilated capillary loops.

Histology: Transplant glomerulitis is an endocapillary form of inflammation with "infiltration and proliferation." It usually affects capillary tufts in a focal and segmental pattern; diffuse and global lesions are less

deposits, and the overall histological "gestalt." Of note, the significance of transplant glomerulitis and glomerulopathy are often not fully appreciated. Both lesions are scored in the Banff system but remain without much diagnostic consideration in the final categorization of rejection (74,81).

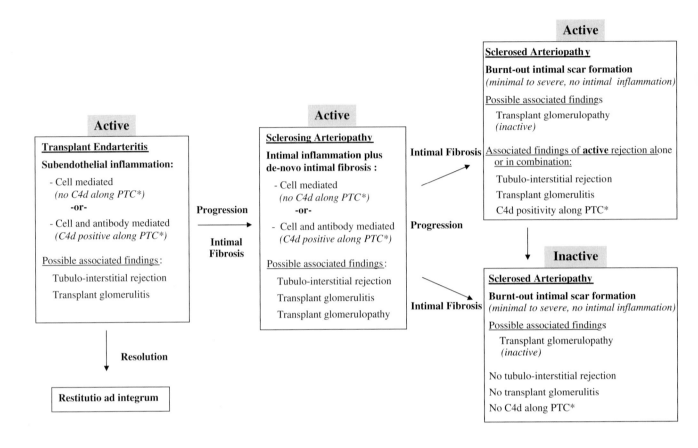

Active

Transplant Endarteritis

Subendothelial inflammation:

- Cell mediated
  (no C4d along PTC*)
  -or-
- Cell and antibody mediated
  (C4d positive along PTC*)

Possible associated findings:

Tubulo-interstitial rejection

Transplant glomerulitis

Progression

Intimal Fibrosis

Resolution

Restitutio ad integrum

Active

Sclerosing Arteriopathy

Intimal inflammation plus de-novo intimal fibrosis :

- Cell mediated
  (no C4d along PTC*)
  -or-
- Cell and antibody mediated
  (C4d positive along PTC*)

Possible associated findings:

Tubulo-interstitial rejection

Transplant glomerulitis

Transplant glomerulopathy

Intimal Fibrosis

Progression

Intimal Fibrosis

Active

Sclerosed Arteriopathy

Burnt-out intimal scar formation
(minimal to severe, no intimal inflammation)

Possible associated findings

Transplant glomerulopathy
(inactive)

Associated findings of **active** rejection alone or in combination:

Tubulo-interstitial rejection

Transplant glomerulitis

C4d positivity along PTC*

Inactive

Sclerosed Arteriopathy

Burnt-out intimal scar formation
(minimal to severe, no intimal inflammation)

Possible associated findings

Transplant glomerulopathy
(inactive)

No tubulo-interstitial rejection

No transplant glomerulitis

No C4d along PTC*

* *linear C4d deposits along peritubular capillaries (PTC)*
as sign of antibody mediated graft injury / rejection

FIGURE 3.23: **The progression of rejection episodes with transplant endarteritis: from active, via sclerosing, to inactive and burnt out.**

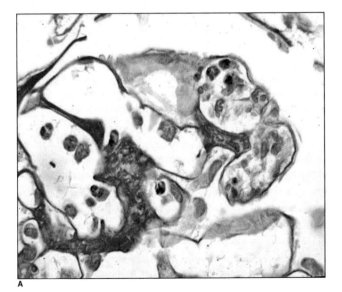

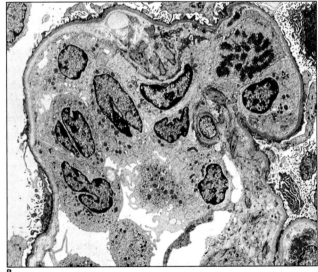

A   B

FIGURE 3.24: **Transplant glomerulitis (A, B). (A) The patient presented thirty-five days after transplantation with allograft dysfunction and minimal proteinuria. Dilated glomerular capillaries were segmentally occluded by inflammatory cells, that is, the glomeruli showed transplant glomerulitis. In addition, tubulo-interstitial rejection and transplant endarteritis were noted; C4d was not found. (B) Electron microscopy from the same case demonstrated abundant intracapillary mononuclear cells with one mitotic figure (upper right corner). Peripheral capillary basement membranes were unremarkable. (A) PAS stain, 200× oil original magnification; (B) electron microscopy, 6,000× original magnification.**

common. The affected glomerular loops are typically dilated and filled/occluded with three or more activated and sometimes mitotically active mononuclear cells—lymphocytes, monocytes, endothelial cells; occasionally polymorphonuclear leukocytes are seen as well (Figure 3.24) (154). Minute fibrin accumulations or microthrombi can be found, in particular in C4d-positive biopsies with antibody-mediated graft injury. Global and diffuse glomerular capillary thrombosis, however, is not a feature of "transplant glomerulitis" but rather limited to cases of concurrent "transplant arteriopathy with massive thrombosis." Transplant glomerulitis, in particular severe cases, can occasionally present with segmental mesangiolysis as a sign of pronounced endocapillary inflammation and glomerular tuft injury. Despite glomerular inflammation, however, fibrinoid tuft necrosis, extracapillary crescent formations, mesangial proliferations, and structural irregularities of peripheral glomerular basement membranes (GBMs) are usually absent. If GBM duplications are noted, they mark the development of "transplant glomerulopathy" (see Transplant Glomerulopathy) (154,155).

Transplant glomerulitis is hardly ever seen as an isolated event (less than 3 percent of cases in my practice), but it is rather commonly associated with tubulo-interstitial and vascular rejection (71,154). In my experience—if biopsies are adequate (see section 2)—transplant glomerulitis (as defined above) is statistically significantly associated with transplant endarteritis or necrotizing transplant arteriopathy (concurrence rate approximately 60 percent at Chapel Hill). This association has also been reported by others (71,154,156,157). Of note, the degree of transplant glomerulitis does not correlate with the degree of tubulo-interstitial or vascular rejection (154).

Immunohistology: The most common antigens found in the glomeruli are C4d, IgM, and complement factor C3 followed by minute fibrin deposits and rarely other immunoglobulins. The IF staining profile is largely interpreted to be nondiagnostic and due to capillary wall injury (154,158). Typically, staining is transient and detected in a linear fashion along GBMs, especially in those capillary tufts affected by endocapillary inflammation. Significant granular immune complex–type deposits are absent (differential diagnosis: immune complex–type glomerulonephritis). Approximately 60 percent of cases with transplant glomerulitis show C4d deposits along peritubular capillaries (62,103,159) Transplant glomerulitis shows increased numbers of monocytes and T lymphocytes, in particular CD8-positive cytotoxic cell elements (91,156). In cases with peritubular capillary C4d staining and an antibody-mediated alloresponse, transplant glomerulitis is dominated by CD68-positive monocytes (103,160,161).

Differential diagnosis: Transplant glomerulitis has to be distinguished from various types of recurrent or de novo immune complex–mediated glomerulonephritides

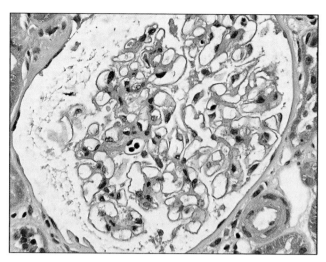

FIGURE 3.25: *Glomerular changes—nondiagnostic. This glomerulus shows two circulating inflammatory cells in a capillary loop that is not dilated and not occluded. These changes are insufficient for rendering a diagnosis of "transplant glomerulitis." H&E stain, 100× original magnification.*

that usually present with an active urine sediment (hematuria, proteinuria), diffuse and global mesangio- and endocapillary proliferations, and significant immune complex type deposits by IF and electron microscopy. In comparison, transplant glomerulitis is usually associated with other morphological signs of tubulo-interstitial and/or vascular rejection, thereby facilitating the diagnostic decision-making process. Original reports suggesting a direct causative association between transplant glomerulitis and cytomegalovirus (CMV) infections (158) could not be substantiated in subsequent studies (91,154,162,163).

When establishing a diagnosis of glomerular rejection with transplant glomerulitis adherence to the above-mentioned definitions is crucial, that is, glomerular capillaries have to be dilated and occluded by mononuclear cells or polymorphonuclear leukocytes. Transplant glomerulitis has to be clearly distinguished from nondiagnostic changes with scattered circulating inflammatory cell elements in the glomerular capillaries (Figure 3.25).

Comment: At present, transplant glomerulitis is an infrequent finding, that is detected in only approximately 15 percent of biopsies with signs of tubulo-interstitial rejection. It was more prevalent in the 1970s and 1980s (154). Transplant glomerulitis is primarily a cell-mediated type of injury, driven by T cells and macrophages (71,161). Donor-specific antibodies contribute to glomerular rejection in approximately 60 percent of cases that show C4d positivity along peritubular capillaries (62,103,159,161). The alloresponse in transplant glomerulitis is directed against unknown (glomerular) endothelial cell antigens. It causes endothelial cell activation and injury and ultimately

TABLE 3.5 Transplant Glomerulopathy: Etiologic Factors to be Considered in the Differential Diagnosis

A. Conditions resulting in a prototypic type of glomercular remodeling/glomerulopathy

1. Rejection: pure cell mediated	(C4d negative)	- common
2. Rejection: mixed cell and antibody mediated	(C4d positive)	- common
3. Rejection: pure antibody mediated	(C4d positive)	- infrequent
4. Thrombotic microangiopathy (recurrent, de-novo) (HUS/TTP)	(C4d negative)	- infrequent
5. Calcineurin inhibitor induced toxicity	(C4d negative)	- infrequent

B. Conditions mimicking transplant glomerulopathy

6. Immune complex mediated membranoproliferative glomerulonephritis (MPGN type 1) (C4d negative) - infrequent

glomerular wall remodeling, that is, transplant glomerulopathy (see Transplant Glomerulopathy). The common pathway of injury endothelial cell damage is not unique but rather shared with other diseases, such as thrombotic microangiopathies (Table 3.5). Since endothelial cells are major targets of the alloresponse not only in transplant glomerulitis but also in all vascular rejection episodes including transplant endarteritis, the close association between "glomerular" and "vascular" rejection is not surprising (156). Consequently, the detection of transplant glomerulitis should always trigger an intensive search for concurrent vascular rejection including multiple additional step sections into the paraffin blocks.

Like all other forms of rejection-induced infiltrative and proliferative inflammatory conditions, transplant glomerulitis is also primarily seen within the first weeks or months after grafting (103,154,157). In my practice, the median time of diagnosis is sixty days after surgery with a wide range of presentation spanning ten days to eleven years.

No general recommendations are available on how to treat rejection episodes with transplant glomerulitis most effectively. I usually regard glomerular rejection as "more severe" and consider it to be a sign of vascular rejection/transplant endarteritis that commonly requires therapy with anti lymphocytic sera such as thymoglobulin. Two recent reports suggest that transplant glomerulitis rich in monocytes indicates poor outcome (160,164). C4d-positive cases may require additional treatment aiming at decreasing circulating donor-specific antibody titers. Whether isolated cases of transplant glomerulitis not associated with other signs of rejection benefit from specific therapy is undetermined.

2. Transplant Glomerulopathy

Commonly used synonyms: Chronic transplant glomerulopathy.

Definition: Minimal to marked duplication of GBMs without significant cell interpositions, that is, TMA-like glomerular remodeling.

Histology: Transplant glomerulopathy represents inflammation-induced (i.e., transplant glomerulitis) capillary wall remodeling (70,71,154,155). In PAS-, trichrome-, or silver-stained sections, peripheral GBM segments are characteristically thickened with duplications ranging from focal and segmental minimal to global and diffuse marked (Figure 3.26) (165). Significant, so-called mesangial cell interpositions are generally absent. The changes closely resemble glomerular remodeling seen in protracted

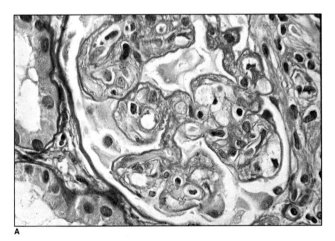

A

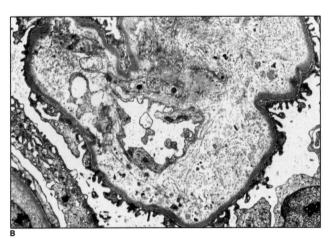

B

FIGURE 3.26: *Transplant glomerulopathy (A, B). (A) The glomerulus shows global duplication of capillary walls without significant hypercellularity or cell interposition, that is, "thrombotic-microangiopathy-like" changes. (B) Electron microscopy from a different case demonstrates activation of capillary endothelial cells and very marked widening of the lamina rara interna. The artificially created subendothelial compartment contains rudimentary, thin lamellae of lamina densa like material. These ultrastructural changes represent the early phase of basement membrane remodeling in transplant glomerulopathy. (A) Trichrome stain, 160× original magnification; (B) electron microscopy, 5,000× original magnification.*

cases of thrombotic microangiopathies including mesangiolysis. Mesangial regions are commonly expanded due to matrix deposition. Significant mesangial proliferations or crescent formations are not, however, defining features of transplant glomerulopathy. Ultimately, remodeling and injury of capillary tufts lead to segmental glomerulosclerosis, that is, secondary "FSGS," global glomerular obsolescence, and nephron loss.

Electron microscopy reveals the earliest signs of transplant glomerulopathy with endothelial cell activation including translocation of nuclei toward peripheral capillary wall segments, loss of fenestration, and minimal widening of the lamina rara interna. These early changes are reversible. They are not apparent by standard light microscopy, and are generally not considered during the diagnostic decision making process commonly lacking ultrastructural studies. Persistent endothelial cell activation and injury, such as driven by protracted transplant glomerulitis, leads to the deposition of subendothelial basement membrane/lamina densa—like material and GBM duplication (Figures 3.26B and 3.27) (166) that is easily noted by standard microscopy. Since endothelial cells may undergo phases of activation followed by quiescent intervals, the subendothelial accumulation of new densa like material can occasionally be wavy with a vaguely layered appearance (167). Scattered, small, ill-defined, and "loose appearing" electron dense deposits may be found in the mesangium or along the lamina rara interna, often associated with the interposition of small, endothelial cell processes. These latter changes should not be misinterpreted as evidence of a membranoproliferative, immune complex–mediated glomerulonephritis (167).

Similar to glomerular capillary wall abnormalities defining transplant glomerulopathies also peritubular capillaries can show basement membrane laminations that are most

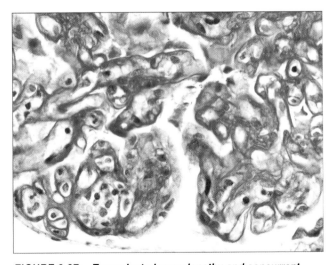

FIGURE 3.27: *Transplant glomerulopathy and concurrent transplant glomerulitis. Peripheral GBMs are globally thickened and segmentally duplicated. One dilated capillary loop is occluded by inflammatory cells. PAS stain, 200× oil original magnification.*

likely also induced by endothelial cell injury. The peritubular capillary thickening may in very severe cases already be seen in PAS stained sections, however, it is usually best appreciated by electron microscopy (168). I consider more than 5 circumferential basement membrane layers in peritubular capillaries suggestive of "rejection induced" remodeling.

In my experience transplant glomerulopathy shows evidence of persistent activity, i.e. glomerulitis and/or interstitial rejection, in approximately 50% of biopsies (Figure 3.27). Similar observations have been reported by others (71,165). A tight association is seen between glomerulopathy and vascular rejection, that is, transplant endarteritis, sclerosing or sclerosed arteriopathy (71,155,166) (concurrence rate of 60 percent at Chapel Hill).

Immunohistology: The immunohistological findings vary from glomerulus to glomerulus and from one glomerular segment to another. The most common antigens are C4d, IgM, and complement factor C3, followed by usually very scant deposits of IgG or fibrin. C4d, limited to the glomerular compartment and not accompanied by peritubular deposits, is often found with moderate to strong linear staining intensity along duplicated and severely altered peripheral glomerular capillary walls (an observation of undetermined diagnostic significance). In addition, approximately 50 percent of biopsies with transplant glomerulopathy (and in particular those with concurrent transplant glomerulitis) reveal C4d accumulations along peritubular capillaries (62,147). If concurrent transplant glomerulitis is noted, immunophenotyping shows increased numbers of endocapillary T lymphocytes and macrophages; polymorphonuclear leukocytes are, uncommon.

Differential diagnosis: The differential diagnosis of transplant glomerulopathy includes various diseases and etiologies listed in Table 3.5. It is important to remember that glomerular capillary wall remodeling, that is, transplant glomerulopathy, is not caused by a single etiological factor. Rather, GBM duplication represents a common final pathway of various forms of endothelial cell injury induced by different "TMA-like" insults, among which cellular and antibody-mediated/C4d-positive allograft rejection episodes are the most common forms. In order to identify the most likely underlying cause of transplant glomerulopathy concurrent histological changes need to be assessed: transplant glomerulitis or endarteritis (indicating a cell-mediated rejection process), C4d positivity along peritubular capillaries (marking an antibody-mediated type of graft injury), calcineurin inhibitor–induced toxicity in afferent arterioles (favoring a toxic variant of glomerulopathy), or significant immune complex–type deposits in the setting of urine sediment abnormalities (suggesting an immune complex–mediated type of injury). If HUS/TTP was the underlying disease that had caused chronic renal failure, then disease recurrence should be considered. IF/immunohistochemical and electron microscopical studies are adjunct methods to render a specific diagnosis (28).

Comment: Transplant glomerulopathy is an infrequent finding, seen in approximately 5 percent of all graft biopsies (169). It is uncommon during the first months after transplantation but subsequently shows an increasing prevalence reaching 25 percent in kidney transplants older than 10 years in one series (155). Transplant glomerulopathy represents rejection-induced glomerular injury (165), and closely resembles TMAs with GBM duplications (70,71,155). In my experience, approximately 50 percent of cases show signs of activity with persistent transplant glomerulitis and/or an antibody-mediated type of injury based on C4d deposits along peritubular capillaries (62, 159); other groups detected concurrent transplant glomerulitis and HLA antibodies in up to 76 percent of patients (165). Circulating donor-specific antibodies were closely linked to the development of transplant glomerulopathy in a non-human primate model (170). Similar to transplant glomerulitis, transplant glomerulopathies are also associated with vascular rejection episodes (166), most commonly sclerosing or sclerosed arteriopathies (155).

Transplant glomerulitis and in particular transplant glomerulopathy can clinically mimic primary glomerulonephritides or glomerulopathies, such as "focal and segmental glomerulosclerosis (FSGS)," since patients usually present with varying degrees of hematuria and proteinuria that can reach nephrotic range in cases of marked GBM duplication (155).

lation of C4d along the walls of peritubular capillaries in the renal cortex and medulla is "transplant specific," and it is reasonable to conclude that the immunohistochemical detection of C4d in renal allografts can be considered as a "footprint" of an antibody response (62,148,174–176,181). The C4d observation has served as a vital tool to detect donor-specific antibodies in tissue sections since previous attempts during humoral rejection episodes had largely been unsuccessful, likely due to the rapid shedding and endocytosis of immunoglobulins from endothelial cell surfaces (72,182,183). Consequently, many rejection episodes with an antibody component remained undiagnosed in the past. The introduction of C4d into the evaluation of renal allograft biopsies has helped to address this shortcoming.

In C4d-positive cases circulating donor-specific antibodies against MHC class I or class II can often be detected, that is, in approximately 90 percent of patients. In approximately 10 percent of C4d-positive allograft recipients, the search for antibodies yields no results, potentially due to technical limitations of the applied assays or the presence of unusual antibodies, such as those directed against angiotensin II type 1—receptor-related antigens (Figure 3.28) (140,148,181). In a high percentage of patients, circulating antibodies can also be found *without* corresponding C4d deposits in renal biopsies (181); reaching up to 70–90 percent in a recent study (184). The clinical significance of this observation is currently undetermined.

v. Antibody-Mediated Rejection and C4d Staining

1. Background

Stimulated by the pioneering work by H. Feucht et al. more than a decade ago, the immunohistochemical detection of the complement degradation product C4d in renal allografts has led to major changes in our understanding (and classification) of kidney transplant pathology (75,112,171–177).

C4d is the degradation product of the activated complement factor C4, a component of the classical complement cascade that is typically initiated by binding of antibodies to specific target molecules. Following the activation and degradation of C4, thio-ester groups are exposed which allow transient, covalent binding of the degradation product C4d to endothelial cell surfaces and extracellular matrix components of vascular basement membranes near the sites of C4 activation. C4d is also found in intracytoplasmic vacuoles of endothelial cells (159). An alternative, antibody-independent pathway of C4 activation has been described, that is, the mannan-binding lectin pathway (178–180); however, this mechanism does not seem to play a significant role in renal allograft injury and rejection. Since C4d is only very rarely observed along peritubular capillaries in native kidneys, such as exceptional cases of systemic lupus erythematosus or anti-GBM disease (personal observation), the accumu-

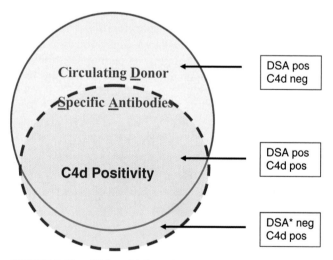

FIGURE 3.28: *C4d positivity only marks a subgroup of complement activating donor-specific antibodies that bind to antigens in the renal microvasculature. It is currently undetermined whether the inability to detect circulating antibodies in the setting of C4d positivity in approximately 10 percent of cases reflects their nonexistence or a technical problem of assay sensitivity, for example, unusual antibodies that escape common detection, low antibody titers, and so forth. The clinical significance of noncomplement activating antibodies in the absence of C4d deposits is only incompletely understood; they appear to be of minor clinical significance.*
DSA: Donor Specific Antibody

2. C4d and Histology

In my experience, based on a largely nonsensitized standard patient population, C4d is detected in approximately 30 percent of all diagnostic graft biopsies corresponding to approximately 35 percent of all biopsied patients. However, the incidence of C4d positivity varies greatly and is transplant center dependent. C4d is typically found early after transplantation (median thirty-five days, range: 7–5646 days), and it has occasionally even been detected at time of grafting in post-perfusion implantation biopsies (47). C4d has a dynamic pattern of deposition; it can accumulate within four days and disappear within eight days (62). In some patients, C4d can persist after anti-rejection therapy with potentially detrimental impact on long-term graft function and survival. C4d has also been found in rare protocol biopsies of stable grafts (185), and it is a common finding in ABO incompatible organ transplant recipients (186).

C4d is scored in renal allograft biopsies based on immunohistochemical or IF studies using either formalin-fixed and paraffin-embedded biopsy samples or alternatively fresh frozen tissue. A strong, diffuse, and circumferential staining of peritubular capillaries in nonfibrotic and nonnecrotic cortical and/or medullary regions is generally considered to be diagnostic (Figure 3.29) (62,81,148,187,188). Rare cases with marked cortical edema and fibrosis may only reveal diagnostic peritubular staining in the medulla. C4d deposits in other locations, including vessels with arteriolosclerosis, atrophic tubular basement membranes, endothelial surfaces of large arteries, and glomerular basement membranes are currently considered to be nondiagnostic (Figure 3.30) and should not be used during the clinical decision making process.

Despite the tremendous interest in C4d staining results, surprisingly little conformity exists on how to best evaluate and interpret findings. One recent study suggests that IF microscopy with a monoclonal antibody is superior to immunohistochemistry on formalin fixed tissue samples utilizing a polyclonal antibody (189). No uniform recommendations and guidelines exist on how to report focal C4d positivity, where there is staining of less than 50 percent of peritubular capillary walls.

The updated Banff classification scheme of renal allograft rejection has introduced a scoring scheme for C4d staining results (Table 3.6) that seems to be useful for everyday practice considering our current limited knowledge base (81). If possible I prefer C4d analyses on frozen tissue sections and I report the degree/percentage of positivity in my diagnoses as a "classifier". As illustrated in (Figure 3.31) many histological changes can be seen in concurrence with circulating donor-specific antibodies and C4d positivity that should be reflected in the final diagnosis. Some aspects were already discussed in paragraphs v.i–v.iv of note, only few rejection episodes with primary injury of

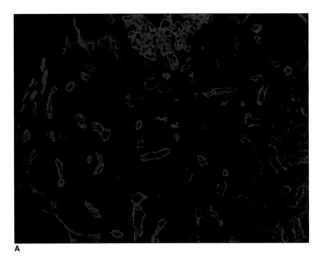

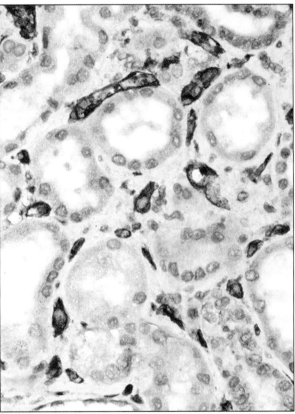

FIGURE 3.29: *C4d staining—diagnostic pattern (A, B). (A) C4d is detected with strong, linear staining intensity along the walls of peritubular capillaries in nonfibrotic areas. This capillary staining pattern is considered to be diagnostic. It is frequently accompanied by C4d positivity along glomerular basement membranes (considered to be nondiagnostic). Indirect IF microscopy with a monoclonal antibody directed against the complement degradation product C4d on fresh frozen tissue, 100× original magnification. (B) Staining for C4d along peritubular capillaries on formalin-fixed and paraffin-embedded tissue sections can give a crisp positive reaction. However, formalin fixation and paraffin embedding results in decreased sensitivity to detect C4d, and IF studies illustrated in (A) are regarded to be the "gold standard." Indirect immunohistochemistry with a polyclonal antibody directed against C4d on formalin-fixed and paraffin-embedded tissue sections, 200× original magnification.*

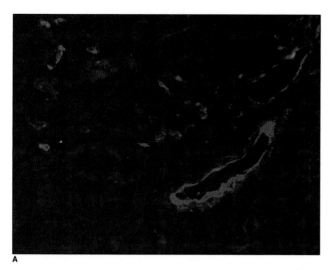
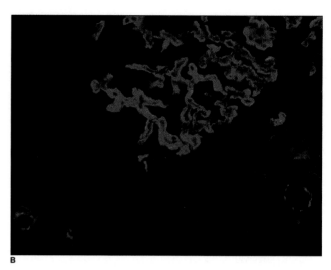

A   B

FIGURE 3.30: C4d staining—nondiagnostic changes (A, B). (A) C4d can be detected as a nondiagnostic finding in sclerosed walls of small arteries, in foci of arteriolar hyalinosis, and along internal elastic lamellae in vascular walls. Illustrated in the middle of the field is a very small caliber interlobular artery with nonspecific intramural C4d accumulations. In addition, C4d is noted along some atrophic tubular basement membranes. (B) This case of tacrolimus-induced structural glomerular toxicity demonstrated global duplication of capillary walls and intense basement membrane (GBM) staining for C4d (linear, granular, and lumpy). C4d was not detected along peritubular capillaries and there was no clinical evidence of circulating donor-specific antibodies. Such isolated glomerular C4d staining reflects severe GBM remodeling and should not be interpreted as a sign of an antibody-mediated alloresponse. (A and B) Indirect IF microscopy with a monoclonal antibody directed against the complement degradation product C4d on fresh frozen tissue, 200× original magnifications.

TABLE 3.6 Scoring of C4d Staining (81)

C4d0	Negative	0%
C4d1	Minimal C4d stain/detection	1–10%
C4d2	Focal C4d stain/positive	10–50%
C4d3	Diffuse C4d stain/positive	>50%

capillary endothelial cells, that is, capillary transplant vasculopathy, represent pure T-cell poor antibody-mediated graft injury (Figures 3.18 and 3.31).

a. Capillary Transplant Vasculopathy, C4d

Positive Commonly used synonyms: Acute, T-cell poor, pure humoral rejection (Banff category II, types I and II, acute rejection; not classified according to CCTT).

Definition: Diffuse capillary injury with intracapillary accumulation of polymorphonuclear leukocytes and mononuclear cell elements, occasional microthrombus formation, strong C4d positivity; presence of circulating donor-specific antibodies in the plasma; absence of tubulo-interstitial rejection and transplant endarteritis.

Gross pathology: Grafts are swollen, hemorrhagic, and infarcted. The appearance is identical to "transplant arteriopathy with massive thrombosis" (see Transplant Arteriopathy with Massive Thrombosis).

Histology: In typical cases, focal or diffuse injury of peritubular capillaries is noted in the cortex. The capillaries are dilated and filled with polymorphonuclear leukocytes and/or monocytes, and can occasionally contain fibrin thrombi (112,161,190). Capillary leakage results in interstitial hemorrhage and edema with rare inflammatory cells, including lymphocytes, histiocytes, and polymorphonuclear leukocytes (Figure 3.32). The impaired capillary blood flow causes acute ischemic tubular injury (AIN), and sometimes even frank necrosis. Signs of cellular rejection with conspicuous tubulitis are lacking. Arteries are generally uninvolved and lack thrombus formation. Rare cases can present with fibrinoid arterial wall necrosis. Transplant endarteritis or marked transmural inflammation, however, are characteristically absent. Vascular injury with TMA-like changes has been reported, but it is uncommon (191,192).

Often capillary injury involves not only peritubular but also glomerular capillaries, which contain mononuclear and polymorphonuclear inflammatory cells, that is, signs of transplant glomerulitis, and fibrin thrombi. Mesangiolysis and segmental tuft necrosis are limited to very severe cases.

Immunohistology: The most characteristic finding, which led to the recognition of this entity, is the strong and diffuse linear accumulation of C4d along peritubular capillaries. In addition—although it is not considered to be of additional diagnostic significance—C3d is found (192). The detection of linear immunoglobulin deposits (IgG, IgM) along capillary walls is an exceptionally rare event. In areas of hemorrhage and necrosis, fibrin deposits are conspicuous. Glomerular C4d deposits with linear staining along peripheral basement membranes are frequently seen, however, they remain without direct diagnostic significance.

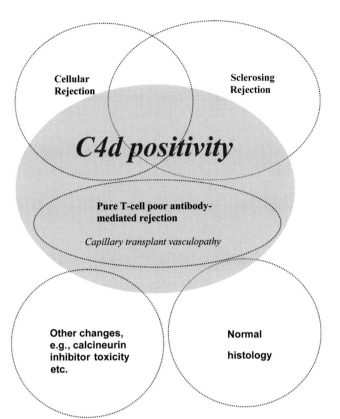

FIGURE 3.31: *Donor-specific antibodies and histological changes. Donor-specific antibodies (C4d positivity) can be found in association with different histological changes and even in the setting of normal histology. Only a minority of acute rejection episodes represent "pure" T-cell poor, antibody-mediated acute rejection, that is, capillary transplant vasculopathy. The immune status, antibody titers, and antibody specificity influence the histological phenotype and clinical dominance.*

Comment: C4d-positive capillary transplant vasculopathy is caused by circulating donor-specific anti-class I or frequently anti-class II antibodies, however, also other currently poorly defined antibodies may be involved in the pathogenesis (140). In contrast to transplant vasculopathy with massive intravascular thrombosis the donor-specific antibodies are often formed "de novo" after transplantation with largely undetermined antigen specificity along endothelial surfaces.

C4d-positive capillary transplant vasculopathy, or acute pure humoral rejection, is a newly recognized entity and much remains to be learned. It is an infrequent phenomenon that accounts for less than 5 percent of all rejection episodes in my experience. The incidence is much higher in pre-sensitized patient populations and ABO incompatible graft recipients. Acute pure humoral rejection is typically diagnosed within the first weeks after transplantation. Therapeutic attempts are made with high-dose IVIG treatment and/or plasmapheresis or immunoabsorption. Graft survival varies. It seems to be poor in cases with marked capillary thrombosis and parenchymal necrosis. However,

clinical experience with this form of rejection is currently still limited.

In my opinion, C4d-positive capillary transplant vasculopathy has to be clearly separated from other histological changes associated with C4d deposits, in particular, C4d-positive cellular rejection episodes (tubulo-interstitial rejection and transplant endarteritis). From a pathophysiological point of view, the latter rejection phenomena reflect a mixed cellular and humoral etiology that should be studied and potentially also treated separately (62,77,112). This sharp distinction, however, is not always made, thereby contributing to unclear terminology and confusing literature reports (113).

VI. CALCINEURIN INHIBITOR AND OTHER DRUG-INDUCED TOXIC CHANGES

i. Calcineurin Inhibitors

1. Background

Calcineurin inhibiting drugs, mainly cyclosporine A (CsA) and tacrolimus (FK506), have tremendously improved outcome in organ transplantation. With the introduction of CsA into patient management in the early 1980s, one-year survival of deceased donor kidney grafts increased from less than 60 percent prior to CsA to 82 percent by 1993 (193) (UNOS data). CsA, the prototypic calcineurin inhibitor, is a cyclic, lipophilic undecapeptide isolated from a soil fungus (Tolypocladium inflatum Gams) (194). Tacrolimus (FK506), a macrolide isolated from the fungus *Streptomyces tsukubaensis* in Japan, was introduced into clinical transplantation in the early 1990s. Tacrolimus does not share any structural similarities with CsA, however, both drugs are remarkably similar with regard to mechanisms of action, therapeutic and adverse effects (195–200).

CsA and tacrolimus bind to intracytoplasmic receptor proteins, the immunophilins (201–206). The immunophilin/CsA or tacrolimus complexes bind to and inhibit a phosphatase, calcineurin. Calcineurin dephosphorylates intracytoplasmic nuclear regulatory proteins in lymphocytes and facilitates their translocation into the nucleus and activation as intranuclear factors for various mediators (e.g., IL-2, IL-4, interferon gamma, and tumor necrosis factor alpha) (207). Calcineurin typically promotes T-cell activation. In therapeutic doses, CsA and tacrolimus block approximately 50 percent of the calcineurin activity.

Calcineurin inhibitors play a major role in the immunosuppression of allograft recipients (208,209). Currently, in the United States, tacrolimus is administered more often than CsA (67 percent of renal transplant recipients in 2003) (210). Tacrolimus is favored by many physicians because it reduces the incidence of acute rejection episodes and improves outcome including cosmetic problems such as hirsutism or gingival hyperplasia. CsA, on the other hand,

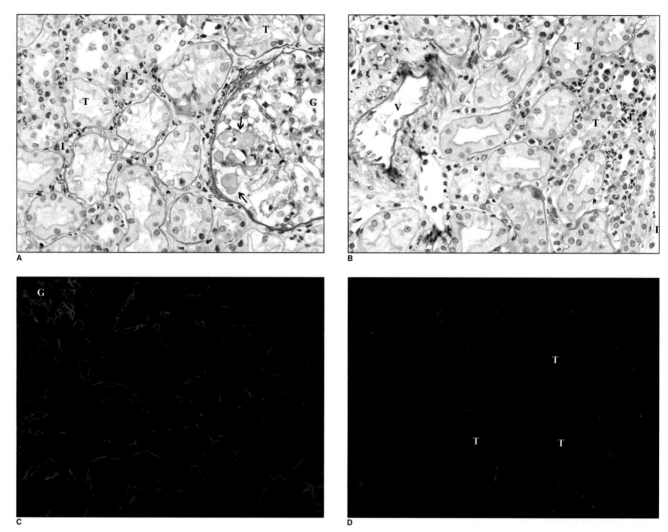

FIGURE 3.32: *Capillary transplant vasculopathy, C4d positive (so-called pure, T-cell poor, antibody-mediated acute rejection, (A–D). The patient presented with abrupt, severe deterioration of renal function seven days after transplantation. At time of biopsy, high titers of anti-donor class II antibodies were found and panel reactive antibody titers had risen from 0 percent at the time of grafting to 45 percent. (A and B) The interstitial compartment (I) showed focal edema and mixed inflammatory cell infiltrates with polymorphonuclear leukocytes surrounding tubules (T) in a finger-like fashion. Some tubules demonstrated signs of acute epithelial cell injury; tubulitis was not detected. Small fibrin thrombi were noted in glomerular capillaries (G, arrows), but not in an intraparenchymal artery (V). (C) C4d was diffusely found along peritubular capillaries (G = glomerulus). (D) MHC class II (HLA-DR) was not expressed by tubular epithelial cells (T = tubulus). (A and B) PAS-stained sections, 250× original magnification. (C) Indirect IF microscopy with a monoclonal antibody directed against the complement degradation product C4d on fresh frozen tissue, 200× original magnification. (D) Direct IF microscopy with a fluorescein-conjugated anti-MHC class II antibody, 300× original magnification.*

induces hyperglycemia less frequently (199,211–213). Some studies seem to demonstrate equal efficacy of both CsA and tacrolimus in suppressing acute rejection episodes and improving long-term graft outcome under current, optimized dosing regimens (214,215).

Unfortunately, calcineurin inhibitor therapy is associated with a nephrotoxic side effect, which can be seen in two major forms: 1) as functional toxicity (with vasospasms lacking morphological changes) and 2) as structural toxicity (with various early or late histological alterations, typically associated with functional toxicity) Figures 3.33 and 3.34). Side effects are dose dependent and most often seen

with high trough levels; however, they can also occur with optimal therapeutic concentrations, implying idiosyncratic reactions in certain individuals. CsA and tacrolimus both demonstrate identical structural toxicity primarily involving tubules, arterioles, and glomeruli in native and transplanted kidneys that will be referred to as "calcineurin inhibitor–induced toxicity (CNIT)" (199,200,216,217). Here I will largely follow M.J. Mihatsch's pioneering classifications of CNIT toxicity (218–221).

Although CsA and tacrolimus can contribute to the slow deterioration of renal function over years [likely in association with other contributing factors such as

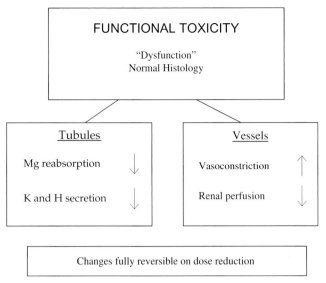

FUNCTIONAL TOXICITY

"Dysfunction"
Normal Histology

Tubules		Vessels	
Mg reabsorption	↓	Vasoconstriction	↑
K and H secretion	↓	Renal perfusion	↓

Changes fully reversible on dose reduction

FIGURE 3.33: *Schematic listing of some functional calcineurin inhibitor–induced changes.*

hypertension or hyperlipidemia (217,222)], end-stage renal failure primarily caused by calcineurin inhibitors is uncommon [reported with a prevalence of 3.2 percent in 125 pediatric heart transplant recipients years after surgery (223)]. Ojo et al. found end-stage renal disease in 4.8 percent of patients with nonrenal transplants under calcineurin inhibitor therapy (often associated with other risk factors such as age, race, sex, hypertension, diabetes mellitus, hepatitis C infections) (222). In a series of transplant nephrectomies M.J. Mihatsch attributed allograft failure solely caused by calcineurin inhibitor toxicity to only 1 percent of cases and allograft failure caused by toxicity plus co-factors to 6 percent (personal communication). The current consensus is that allografts on the whole still do very well under calcineurin inhibitor therapy and that end-stage renal disease due to toxic side effects constitutes only a minimal risk.

2. Functional Toxicity (Figure 3.33)

Patients treated with calcineurin inhibitors and in particular those displaying "functional toxicity" commonly show a markedly decreased glomerular filtration rate (due to arteriolar vasospasms) and evidence of arterial hypertension. Most pronounced cases of "functional CNIT" clinically present with acute renal failure and oliguria. Morphologically, allograft biopsies are normal in appearance. The diagnosis "functional CNIT" is made by exclusion only after having step sectioned through the entire tissue blocks and excluded other causes of kidney graft dysfunction, including isolated episodes of "transplant endarteritis." More severe and protracted cases of functional CNIT, especially in ischemically (pre)injured grafts early after transplantation,

can show signs of ATI, edemo, and congestion of peritubular capillaries containing mononuclear cell elements, (221,224). Functional toxicity reverses upon dose reduction, and even toxicity with protracted oliguria usually resolves (225).

3. Structural Toxicity (Figure 3.34)

Structural changes induced by calcineurin inhibitors can primarily be seen in tubules, arterioles, and glomeruli. "Striped" interstitial fibrosis on the other hand is a non-diagnostic secondary phenomenon reflecting nephron loss. Structural toxicity is generally associated with a component of functional toxicity, that is, a rise in serum creatinine due to vasospasms.

a. **Tubules** The proximal tubules generally show the greatest morphological changes, whereas ducts in the medulla typically remain unaffected. Three morphological changes in the tubular compartment have been linked to CNIT: 1) isometric vacuolization, 2) tubular calcifications, and 3) giant mitochondria. They may occur alone or in combination in the same biopsy sample and can be detected by light and electron microscopy. Immunohistochemistry or IF microscopy is noncontributory. The interstitium is often normal or demonstrates focal minimal edema. Only cases with toxic tubulopathies superimposed on preexisting ischemic injury may show marked edema and ischemic type ATI. Interstitial inflammatory cell infiltrates are characteristically very sparse and tubulitis is absent (224,226). If marked mononuclear inflammatory cells and tubulitis are found, a concurrent acute cellular rejection episode has to be considered.

Isometric clear vacuolization, defined as cells filled with uniformly sized small vacuoles, is found in the cytoplasm of tubular epithelial cells, sometimes associated with loss of the brush border. It is said to predominate in the straight portion of the proximal tubule (227), although in my experience it also occurs in the convoluted portion and might occasionally even be seen in parietal epithelial cells lining Bowman's space. The vacuoles, much smaller than the nucleus, contain clear aqueous fluid (Figure 3.35). They are due to dilated and empty appearing portions of the endoplasmic reticulum that can easily be detected by electron microscopy (227). Under current therapeutic dose regimens, isometric cytoplasmic vacuolization is mostly patchy, involving only scattered tubular segments. Although typically the entire cytoplasm of an affected tubular cell is vacuolated, changes may be less pronounced during early toxic injury. Of note, the degree of vacuolization does not directly correlate with calcineurin inhibitor trough levels. Among over 1000 diagnostic renal transplant biopsies examined in Basel, Switzerland, in the 1980s, isometric tubular vacuolization was found in 40 percent of biopsies in the first two weeks, in 30 percent at six

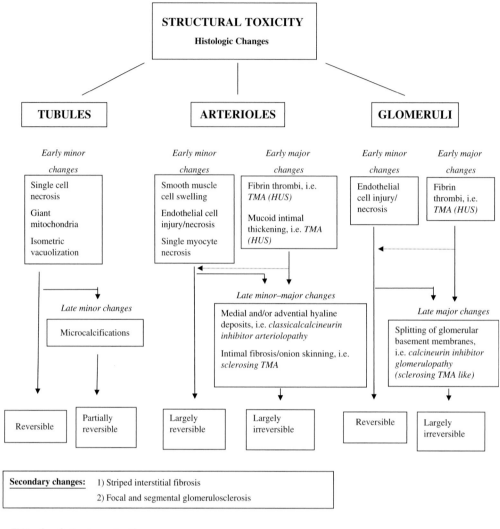

FIGURE 3.34: *Schematic listing of structural calcineurin inhibitor–induced toxic changes [modified from (425)].*

months, in 18 percent at one year, and in about 8 percent at three years (221). Currently, the prevalence of toxic tubulopathy has significantly decreased. Giant mitochondria and small, egg-shell–shaped dystrophic tubular calcifications that have been also been described as signs of CNIT (221) do not appear to have any diagnostic significance under modern drug dosing regimens. CNIT tubulopathies are of no profound long-term clinical significance; both isometric vacuolizations and giant mitochondria are fully reversible while dystrophic calcifications likely persist.

Differential diagnosis: The rough and smooth endoplasmic reticulum can show a tendency to dilate and form vacuoles, even in patients with stable function (228). Isometric vacuolization of tubular epithelial cells is not pathognomonic for CNIT since identical light microscopic changes can be seen in a variety of diseases, including fatty changes in the setting of the nephrotic syndrome or cases of "osmotic nephrosis" following therapy with mannitol, dextran, radiolabeled contrast media or sucrose rich hyperimmune globulin and IVIG solutions (Table 3.2) (229–231). In contrast to CNIT tubulopathy, however, these cases typically demonstrate dilated lysosomes by electron microscopy. Nonisometric and irregular intracytoplasmic tubular vacuoles of different sizes should not be misinterpreted as evidence of toxic tubulopathy (Figure 3.4). They are commonly seen in various forms of tubular injury, mainly ischemia. Vacuolization may also be seen in scattered atrophic tubules located in zones of fibrosis. These changes are of undetermined therapeutic significance.

b. **Blood Vessels** arterioles and glomerular capillaries: Structural CNIT in arterioles and glomeruli is best categorized as "TMA" displaying different patterns and degrees

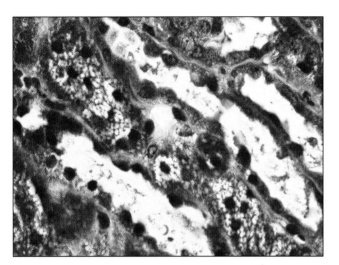

FIGURE 3.35: *Calcineurin inhibitor–induced early tubulopathy. The patient presented eight days after transplantation on tacrolimus based immunosuppression with slow improvement of graft function. Tubular epithelial cells showed "osmotic nephrosis," that is, isometric vacuolization of the cytoplasm suggestive of calcineurin inhibitor–induced toxic changes. C4d was not detected (compare with Figure 3.4). Trichrome stain, 200× oil original magnification.*

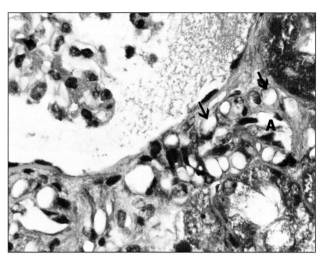

FIGURE 3.36: *Calcineurin inhibitor–induced early arteriolopathy. An afferent arteriole demonstrates marked swelling, that is, so-called ballooning, of medial smooth muscle cells (arrows). Such changes are suggestive of very early calcineurin inhibitor–induced arteriolopathies (A = arteriolar lumen). Same case as illustrated in figure 35. Trichrome stain, 200× oil original magnification.*

of severity (220). The thrombotic-microangiopathy–like toxic changes range from common, very mild and limited variants (i.e., CNIT arteriolopathies or glomerulopathies) to infrequent fully developed forms of the hemolytic uremic syndrome. Mild thrombotic-microangiopathy–like toxic changes are without great clinical significance; they are fully or partially reversible on dose reduction. Severe variants with fully developed, systemic TMAs/hemolytic uremic syndrome can result in graft failure.

Arterioles: CNIT is found in small vessels, most characteristically in afferent "renin-producing" arterioles. The arteriolar lesions can extend in severe cases downstream into the glomerulus and upstream into small arteries with up to two layers of smooth muscle cells. Larger arteries are characteristically spared (232–234).

1. Arteriolar medial smooth muscle swelling—early minor changes. Occasionally in afferent arterioles marked swelling, so-called ballooning, of many medial smooth muscle cells is seen that can obscure the normal vascular architecture. The cytoplasm of the medial cells contains very large, clear vacuoles ("empty" appearance), caused by marked dilatation of the endoplasmic reticulum (Figure 3.36). These changes are early, fully reversible signs of toxic cell injury; they rarely progress to CNIT arteriolopathy with hyaline deposits. Of note: Arteriolar medial smooth muscle cell swelling should only be diagnostically considered as a sign of CNIT in parenchymal zones lacking pronounced ATI since ischemia can induce similar histological changes.

2. Arteriolar medial hyaline deposits (classical CNIT arteriolopathy)—late changes. The classical morphology of

structural CNIT arteriolopathy has been described as "nodular protein deposits (hyaline deposits) replacing (individual) necrotic smooth muscle cells of the media" (220), "occasionally in a pearl-like pattern" (233). Hyaline nodules can be most pronounced along the adventitial layer; they stain intensely with PAS incubations (Figure 3.37). Although individual myocyte necrosis is a feature of structural calcineurin inhibitor toxicity, extensive fibrinoid arteriolar wall necrosis or transmural inflammation is typically not found (differential diagnosis: florid TMA, small vessel vasculitis, or vascular rejection with fibrinoid arterial necrosis).

The severity of CNIT arteriolopathy varies considerably, even in the same biopsy. Some vessels may show only mild changes with few intramural/adventitial hyaline nodules whereas others demonstrate advanced arteriolopathies with segmental or circumferential, transmural hyalinosis, complete loss of medial smooth muscle cells, and stenosis. The endothelial cell layers remain typically intact, even in severe cases, and fibrin thrombi are absent. IF microscopy is rather nonspecific with the accumulation of IgM and the complement factors C1q, C3, C5b-9, and C4d in foci of hyaline deposits (C4d is, however, not detected along peritubular capillaries). There is no widely accepted scheme for scoring the severity and degree of CNIT arteriolopathies. The Banff '97 classification system and "ah" scoring are not well suited for this purpose (16). Recently, the updated Banff '07 system (81) has introduced an alternative quantitative scoring scheme of CNIT arteriolopathies that may prove to be clinically useful (Table 3.7).

CNIT arteriolopathy with hyalinosis can develop quickly and may be detected soon after transplantation (in my experience as early as fifteen days after surgery).

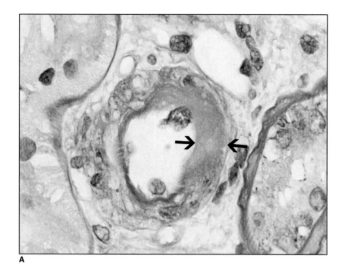

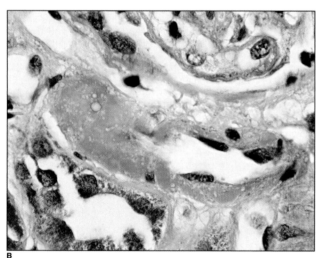

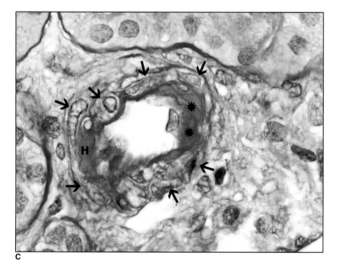

◄ **FIGURE 3.37:** *Calcineurin inhibitor–induced late/classical arteriolopathy compared to hypertension-induced arteriolar hyalinosis (A–C). (A, B) In CNIT the afferent arterioles show segmental transmural hyaline deposits replacing medial smooth muscle cells (aah2, arrows in A). (C) Calcineurin inhibitor–induced structural arteriolopathies have to be distinguished from "ordinary" hypertension-induced lesions with arteriolosclerosis and hyalinosis illustrated in C. Hypertension most often induces subendothelial hyaline deposits (asterisks) that can occasionally protrude into the medial layer (H). However, significant replacement of smooth muscle cells is typically lacking (arrows illustrate the intact smooth muscle cells). (A) Trichrome stain, and (B, C) PAS stains; 350× oil original magnification.*

TABLE 3.7 Scoring of Classical Calcineurin Inhibitor–Induced Toxic Arteriolopathies with Intramural Hyaline Deposits [according to (81)]

aah	0	No CNIT arteriopathy
aah	1	Hyaline deposits in the media present in one arteriole (no circumferential involvement)
aah	2	Hyaline deposits in the media present in more than one arteriole (no circumferential involvement)
aah	3	Transmural and circumferential hyaline deposits replacing the entire arteriolar wall, independent of the number of involved vessels

deposits replacing necrotic smooth muscle cells in the afferent arteriole," increased from 5 percent at six months (percent of all examined arterioles) to 9 percent at one year, and 12 percent at two years (235). Similarly, in renal transplant patients on CsA, 15 percent of protocol biopsies at six months showed CNIT arteriolopathies, which increased to 45 percent in protocol biopsies eighteen months after grafting (236). The cumulative prevalence of CNIT arteriolopathy reaches 100 percent at ten years, that is, all transplants are affected (216). Under modern low doses of calcineurin inhibitors, however, the overall prevalence of CNIT arteriolopathy has decreased as illustrated by Mihatsch and colleagues. In 1981, 70 percent of all biopsies in Basel, Switzerland, demonstrated toxic vascular lesions whereas in 1990 the prevalence had decreased to 40 percent; the average percentage of affected arterioles decreased from 17 to 7 percent (235).

Depending on the clinical situation and the immunosuppressive drug regimens, CNIT arteriolopathies can progress, stabilize or even regress over time. Progression affects arterioles with marked transmural and circumferential hyalinosis, resulting in vascular occlusion and nephron loss (216,221). Regression of toxic arteriolopathies has been reported in small series of diagnostic repeat allograft biopsies on dose reduction or discontinuation in the setting of mild to moderate CNIT arteriolopathies (Figure 3.38)

Typically, only a minority of arterioles are affected and the lesions can easily be overlooked (235). In one carefully analyzed series of renal transplants from Basel, Switzerland, the percentage of arterioles affected by "protein

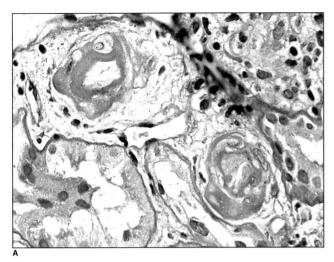
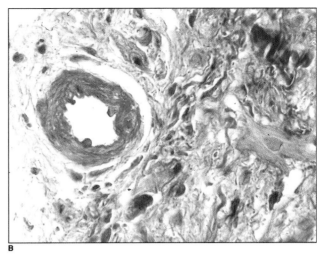

A

B

FIGURE 3.38: Resolution of calcineurin inhibitor–induced late structural arteriolopathy (A, B). (A) Fifty-four weeks after transplantation, moderate (aah2) toxic arteriolopathy was seen under CsA therapy. (B) Discontinuation of the calcineurin inhibitor resulted in complete resolution of the intramural hyaline deposits observed in a repeat biopsy after one year. (A) PAS stain, 180× original magnification. (B) Trichrome stain, 180× original magnification. (Courtesy of Michael J. Mihatsch, Basel, Switzerland.)

(216,237,238). CNIT regression is histologically characterized by the resolution of hyaline deposits and arteriolar wall remodeling. Medial smooth muscle layers show structural irregularities including increased amounts of basement membrane–like material (unorganized appearance) (238). Even circumferential arteriolar hyaline deposits may sometimes undergo resolution and repair (237). "Healing" of CNIT arteriolopathy was also found in a rat model following the discontinuation of CsA for two months (239).

In general, the detection of CNIT arteriolopathies does not necessarily indicate poor long-term prognosis. Serum creatinine levels improve in most patients on dose reduction (likely in part due to the clinical correction of functional toxicity and vasoconstriction), and drastic changes to the immunosuppressive drug regimens are not always required.

Differential diagnosis: Arteriolar hyalinosis not only is induced by calcineurin inhibitors but can frequently be seen in patients suffering from long-standing arterial hypertension or diabetes mellitus. Arteriolosclerosis in the setting of arterial hypertension differs from CNIT arteriolopathy since it presents predominantly with subendothelial hyaline deposits that are commonly covered by an intact, although sometimes atrophic medial smooth muscle layer (Figure 3.37C). Medial and transmural hyaline deposits are less common. Arteriolar hyalinosis in cases of diabetic nephropathy, in native or transplanted kidneys, is very similar to CNIT arteriolopathy and a distinction cannot be easily made based on morphological grounds (221).

While some overlap between CNIT and hypertensive arteriolopathies undoubtedly exists, when the hyalinosis has multiple, discrete nodules the size and location of the medial smooth muscle cells, classical CNIT should be diagnosed. Of note, since kidney transplant recipients treated with calcineurin inhibitors frequently suffer from arterial hypertension, CNIT and hypertensive arteriolopathies can concur, in particular years after grafting. Mihatsch refers to these "late" lesions as "arteriolopathies of the mixed conventional hypertensive and CNIT types."

Glomeruli: 1. Glomerular fibrin thrombi and endothelial swelling—early minor and major changes. Intraglomerular fibrin thrombi (typically in a focal and segmental distribution pattern) are most often found in cases of calcineurin inhibitor–induced TMAs, and may be associated with arteriolar changes and mesangiolysis (see below). Sometimes, however, intraglomerular thrombi may occur as isolated events (240). Glomerular endothelial cell injury and activation, without fibrin thrombi, are frequently seen and commonly not associated with characteristic morphological changes appreciated by standard light microscopic examination.

2. GBM duplication (CNIT glomerulopathy)—late changes. CNIT glomerulopathy histologically presents as "thrombotic-microangiopathy–like" glomerular remodeling. Repetitive, often sublethal, calcineurin inhibitor–induced glomerular endothelial cell injury, that is, early minor or major CNIT glomerular toxicity, can lead to structural changes. They are characterized by widening of the lamina rara interna and subendothelial new basement membrane formation resulting in the duplication of capillary walls, that is, CNIT glomerulopathy (Figure 3.39). The splitting of GBMs is commonly seen in a focal and segmental distribution pattern and not associated with prominent cell interpositions. Mesangial regions can be mildly expanded

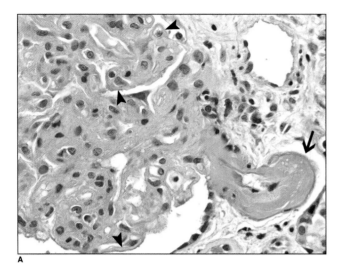

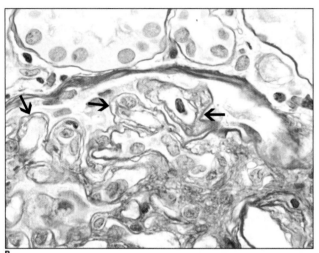

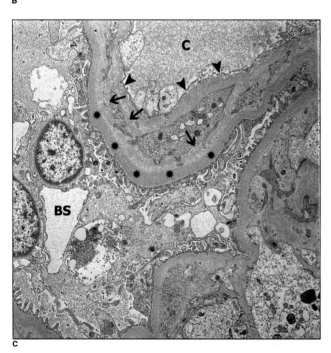

◀ *FIGURE 3.39:   Calcineurin inhibitor–induced late glomerulopathy (A–C). The patient presented six years after transplantation on tacrolimus monotherapy with elevated serum creatinine levels of 1.6 mg/dl, baseline 1.0 mg/dl. (A, B) The glomeruli showed global marked thickening of capillary walls with duplications (arrow heads in A and arrows in B). Significant glomerular hypercellularity and cell interpositions were not present. An afferent arteriole demonstrated characteristic marked structural toxic changes, that is, aah3 (arrow in A). C4d was not detected, and there was no evidence of tubulo interstitial or vascular rejection. (C) Electron microscopy demonstrated structural remodeling with subendothelial formation of a partially wavy (small arrows) rudimentary new basement membrane layer (arrow heads along the endothelial lining). Such changes are caused by repetitive calcineurin inhibitor–induced injury to glomerular endothelial cells, usually without evidence of preceding florid TMAs. Interposition of mostly endothelial cell processes can occur and should not be misinterpreted as a sign of a "membranoproliferative glomerulonephritis." C = glomerular capillary lumen, BS = Bowman's space, asterisks = original GBM. (A) H&E-stained section 180× original magnification, (B) PAS stain, 250× oil original magnification, (C) electron photomicrograph, 7,500× original magnification.*

due to matrix deposition. In some cases, glomerular capillary lumens contain scattered mononuclear cell elements including lymphocytes. Conspicuous capillary dilatation with occlusive clustering of inflammatory cells is typically absent; its presence should raise the possibility of rejection-induced transplant glomerulopathy and glomerulitis.

By IF microscopy, glomeruli show only nondiagnostic IgM and complement factor C1q, C3 C4d, and C5b-9 deposits. On rare occasions, CNIT glomerulopathy is associated with focal and segmental minimal to mild (nondiagnostic) granular IgG, IgA, or light chain accumulations along peripheral basement membranes. Electron microscopy demonstrates widening of the rara interna and subendothelial rudimentary new basement membrane formation, sometimes with a layered appearance due to repetitive endothelial cell injury and basement membrane production. The newly formed subendothelial compartment can contain cell processes and occasional small (nondiagnostic) electron dense deposits (Figure 3.39C).

CNIT glomerulopathies are characteristically associated with CNIT arteriolopathies that are often most severe in arterioles feeding the affected glomeruli (Figure 3.39A). Mihatsch reported CNIT glomerulopathy in 65 percent of biopsies with severe, in 25–45 percent with mild to moderate, and none without evidence of CNIT arteriolopathy (221,241).

No detailed outcome studies are available from CNIT glomerulopathies with duplication of basement membranes. Based on my very limited personal experience, GBM duplication appears to persist for long periods of time, even after discontinuation of calcineurin inhibitor therapy. FSGS often develops as a secondary phenomenon due to glomerular injury and "overload nephropathy." In very rare cases, I have also observed collapsing variants of

FSGS in the setting of severe, stenosing CNIT arteriolopathies. Other nonspecific glomerular changes include global atrophy or sclerosis, typically due to severely stenosed afferent arterioles and ischemia (242).

Differential diagnosis: The detection of duplicated peripheral GBMs in renal transplants raises three major differential diagnoses: 1) late phase of a TMA not induced by calcineurin inhibitors (e.g., recurrent disease), 2) membranoproliferative glomerulonephritides (MPGN), and 3) transplant glomerulopathy induced by cellular and/or antibody-mediated rejection (see Transplant Glomerulopathy, Table 3.5). TMAs of other causes can only be diagnosed on clinical grounds including detailed knowledge of the underlying native kidney disease that had resulted in renal failure. MPGN are characterized by glomerular hypercellularity, an accentuation of the tuft lobulation including conspicuous cell interpositions, and the accumulation of immune complex type deposits. Patients often present with active urine sediments and low serum complement levels. Transplant glomerulopathies in the setting of rejection are histologically very similar to CNIT changes. Several clues help to distinguish "rejection related" from "CNIT" glomerulopathies: the former typically show evidence of concurrent rejection—transplant endarteritis and/or sclerosing allograft arteriopathy, transplant glomerulitis, or C4d deposits along peritubular capillaries. These rejection-related changes are typically lacking in CNIT glomerulopathies that rather show marked CNIT arteriolopathies.

c. **TMA—Early Major Changes** A florid TMA (hemolytic uremic syndrome) with thrombi in arterioles and glomerular capillaries represents the most severe form of CNIT. Arterioles are typically focally affected and often contain at the glomerular vascular poles fibrin and platelet thrombi, which can extend distally into glomerular capillaries (often in a segmental pattern) and proximally into pre-arterioles. Medial smooth muscle layers frequently show single cell necrosis (Figure 3.40A). Rare cases present with thrombus formation that is limited to glomeruli (240). Arteriolar mucoid intimal thickening and edematous swelling are uncommon changes. Similar to other forms of a TMA, vascular lesions can occasionally resolve or undergo remodeling with intimal sclerosis, sometimes concentric with an "onion-skin" appearance. Glomerular remodeling following the lysis of thrombi and endothelial cell injury can result in mesangiolysis and segmental duplication of peripheral basement membranes, that is, CNIT glomerulopathy identical to other late stages of a TMA.

IF microscopy is rather nonspecific with focal fibrin deposits; IgM and the complement factors C3, C5b-9, and C4d are found in foci of arteriolar hyalinosis as well as in a linear fashion along GBMs. C4d is not detected along peritubular capillaries. If peritubular C4d is found (and/or other histological evidence of acute rejection such as typical transplant endarteritis), a diagnosis of acute rejection has to be rendered.

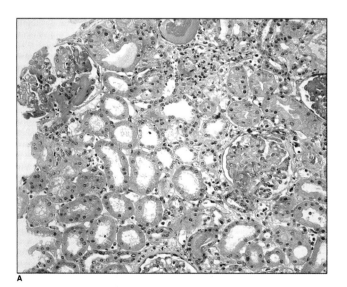

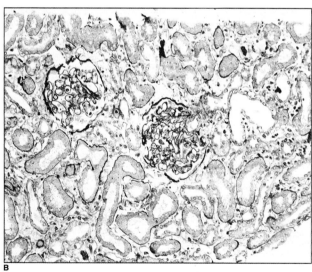

A   B

FIGURE 3.40: *Florid TMA due to calcineurin inhibitor–induced toxicity with resolution during follow-up (A, B). The patient received cyclosporine-based immunosuppression after transplantation of a cadaveric allograft and presented on postoperative day 6 with new onset oliguria, a sudden rise in serum creatinine levels, and anemia. (A) The initial biopsy showed recent, occlusive fibrin thrombi in many glomerular capillaries and segmental fibrinoid necrosis of an afferent arteriolar wall in the glomerulus on the left. (B) A repeat allograft biopsy following the discontinuation of cyclosporine illustrated complete resolution with "restitutio ad integrum." Renal allograft function was normal seven months after transplantation. (A) H&E stain, and (B) methenamine silver stain, 100× original magnification. (Courtesy of Alenka Vizjak and Dusan Ferluga, Ljubljana, Slovenia.)*

The central event in TMAs induced by calcineurin inhibitors is endothelial injury, sometimes further enhanced by the activation of the clotting system. Calcineurin inhibitor–induced TMA is generally an early event occurring within the first few weeks to months after grafting (240,243–245) with only sporadic cases seen later (246,247). In kidney transplant recipients, the TMA may be limited to the renal allograft without systemic symptoms (243,248). Such limited form was observed in 38 percent of cases (8/21) in one series and associated with 100 percent graft survival (249). Severe forms of CNIT-induced TMA show typical systemic signs with thrombocytopenia, microangiopathic hemolytic anemia, elevated lactic dehydrogenase, and hyperbilirubinemia. Schwimmer and colleagues reported that 62 percent of their patients (13/21) with CNIT-induced TMA presented with generalized, systemic symptoms, 38 percent of whom lost their kidney transplants (249). The incidence of TMA has been diminishing since CsA was initially introduced. It caused graft loss in 8 percent of 200 consecutive renal allografts in the early 1980s (accounting for 40 percent of those that failed) (250). Series of patients from the past twenty years reported an incidence of 0.9–14.1 percent (240,243,245,248,249,251–253), representing 26 percent of all cases of TMA after renal transplantation (251). The treatment of calcineurin inhibitor–induced TMAs includes the discontinuance or reduction of CsA/tacrolimus (sometimes with switch to sirolimus), and occasionally plasmapheresis, intravenous immunoglobulin, or thrombolytic agents (244,245,253,254), with an overall graft salvage rate of approximately 80–90 percent (240,244,254). In one study of repeat biopsies, histological resolution with lysis of fibrin thrombi was found in 27 percent of grafts (Figure 3.40B) (240). If outcome is stratified into "renal limited forms of a TMA" and "systemic generalized variants," graft survival rates were 100 percent in the former group (with reduction, temporary discontinuation, or conversion of calcineurin inhibitor therapy) and 62–90 percent in the latter cohort (including plasmapheresis as a treatment option) (249,253). Other studies, however, reported less favorable outcome (even in renal limited forms) with an overall graft survival rate of only 69 percent (248).

Differential diagnosis: TMAs/the hemolytic uremic syndrome induced by CNIT has to be distinguished from other causes based on clinical grounds; a distinction cannot be rendered morphologically.

d. **Interstitial Fibrosis and Tubular Atrophy** In general, calcineurin inhibitor therapy contributes to interstitial scarring. However, the patchy/striped fibrotic interstitial changes observed by the histopathologist in renal biopsies are often nonspecific phenomena simply indicating nephron loss. They lack diagnostic specificity (255).

ii. Drug-Induced Acute Tubulo-interstitial Nephritis

Allergic types of interstitial nephritides induced by various drugs can cause problems for the histopathologist since the morphological changes are identical to those seen in cases of tubulo-interstitial rejection. Overall acute allergic interstitial nephritides seem rare after kidney transplantation (256), possibly due to steroid based immunosuppression preventing the development of interstitial inflammation in many cases.

Tubulo-interstitial rejection and allergic type interstitial nephritides can similarly demonstrate patchy mononuclear cell infiltrates, often with small clusters of plasma cells, eosinophils in variable numbers, edema, focal tubulitis, and tubular injury. Acute rejection occasionally has a prominent eosinophilic infiltrate (122,257–261), and drug-induced interstitial nephritis on the other hand may have no eosinophils (262). If the inflammatory cells predominate at the cortico-medullary junction/outer medulla and spare the cortex, a diagnosis of allergic interstitial nephritis is most likely (256). The additional detection of ill-formed, small, nonnecrotizing granulomas may serve as a further diagnostic clue in some cases. As in native kidneys, outcome of allergic interstitial nephritides is good following drug discontinuance (256). Of note, often it is impossible to make a clear distinction based on morphological criteria. In those cases, it seems best to error on the side of rejection and initiate antirejection therapy with bolus steroids that will help to decrease all tubulo-interstitial inflammatory cell infiltrates.

iii. Sirolimus

Sirolimus (rapamycin, Rapamune) is a new class of drugs with immunosuppressive properties and additional inhibitory effects on cell proliferation. It is a macrolide that binds to a protein named mTOR (mammalian target of rapamycin), a kinase that controls the phosphorylation of proteins and thereby blocks mRNA translation of cell cycle regulators (263). It also blocks via mTOR the production of vascular endothelial growth factor and can induce endothelial cell death and thrombosis in tumor vessels (264–266). In theory, sirolimus may prevent the development of graft sclerosis (267–269). Some toxic side effects have been described that should be recognized by histopathologists. Of note, CsA can increase sirolimus blood levels by 80–230 percent compared to the administration of sirolimus alone (270). Vice versa, sirolimus can increase toxic side effects of calcineurin inhibitors and the coadministration of both drugs requires careful dose adaptation (271–273).

Sirolimus can show various side effects, including cytopenia of myeloid, erythroid, and platelet cell elements, hyperlipidemia, gastrointestinal intolerance with diarrhea, mouth ulcers, cardiac arrhythmias, and impaired wound

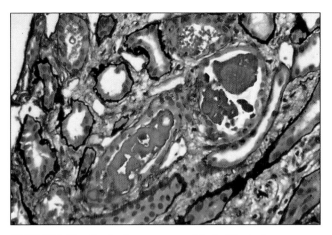

FIGURE 3.41: *Toxic changes associated with sirolimus therapy. The tubules show acute injury and contain amorphous, proteinaceous material (granular or casts with fracture ligns). Methenamine silver, 160× original magnification. (Courtesy of Kelly Smith, Seattle, WA.)*

healing (267,274,275). Sirolimus appears to increase the incidence (59) and particularly the duration of delayed graft function (276–278) (alone or in combination with calcineurin inhibitors) in a dose-dependent manner (59). Mostly transient acute renal failure was also observed in patients treated for various native kidney diseases (279). Early after transplantation tubules can show "myeloma-cast–like" changes with fractured, amorphous, eosinophilic, proteinaceous material, influx of histiocytes, and formation of multinucleated giant cells (Figure 3.41). Smith et al. described the changes as most pronounced in biopsies taken more than two weeks into the course of delayed graft function from patients treated with sirolimus and often a calcineurin inhibitor. Resolution of the casts and functional recovery were noted after two weeks in three of three patients (59). In my practice, I have not yet seen such dramatic histological changes induced by sirolimus.

Sirolimus additionally seems to injure small vessels (280–283). Thrombotic microangiopathies were observed in four renal allografts from patients on sirolimus containing calcineurin inhibitor free immunosuppressive drug protocols. In three of the four patients, the histological diagnosis of a TMA and concurrent cellular rejection was made within the first three months after grafting and in the remaining patient after many years in association with chronic rejection (283). In one series a renal function improved in three of four patients with a TMA following the discontinuation of sirolimus (284).

Sirolimus also promotes *proteinuria* and potentially the development of focal and segmental glomerulosclerosis (285–288).

VII. INFECTIONS

Many infections can affect immunosuppressed renal allograft recipients either as systemic events or as limited diseases. Some infections are restricted to the allograft. Here, I will discuss the most important, clinically and diagnostically challenging infections found in kidney transplants, most importantly polyoma BK virus nephropathy and PTLDs. Table 3.8 lists morphological clues that help to diagnose some of the most common viral infections.

i. Polyoma BK Virus Nephropathy

1. Background

The polyomavirus family consists of different viral strains, among which the BK and JC virus strains are pathogenic in humans and can cause renal allograft infections (the SV-40 strain only seems to play a very minor role). Polyomaviruses are double stranded, nonencapsulated DNA viruses of approximately 5,300 base pairs with substantial gene

TABLE 3.8 Histological Changes Induced by Intrarenal Viral Replication—Diagnostic Clues [modified from (1)]

	Adenovirus	Polyomavirus	CMV	EBV PTLD
Viral inclusion types				
Nuclear: ground glass, homogeneous	+++	++	±	–
Nuclear: with halo	±/+	±/+	+++	–
Nuclear: uncommon (granular/clumped)	±	+/++	–	–
Cytoplasmic	–	–	+	–
Sites of viral replication				
Tubular epithelial cells	+++	+++	+++	–
Endothelial cells	–	–	++	–
Mononuclear cells	±	–	+	+++
ATI	+++	±/+++	±/++	±
Focal parenchymal necrosis	±/+++	–	+	±
Interstitial hemorrhage	+/++	–	–	±
Granuloma formation	+/++	±	±	–
Interstitial inflammation	++	+/++	+/++	+++

TABLE 3.9 Polyomavirus Infections [modified from (357)]

Primary infection	Initial infection with viremic spread to permissive tissues (e.g., kidneys, urothelium); minor clinical symptoms
Latent infection	Dormant, persistent, asymptomatic infections of permissive cells (e.g., renal tubular, transitional cells) following primary infections; virus detection only with molecular techniques
Serological evidence of infection	Varying antibody titer levels found in nearly all healthy children and 60–90% of asymptomatic adults; no correlation with latent viral load levels; weak correlation with viral disease (PVN, PML)
Viral activation	Evidence of polyomavirus replication: 1) decoy cells or free virions in the urine and 2) viral detection by PCR in the urine, serum, or cerebrospinal fluid. Often seen as a transient, asymptomatic event; always part of viral disease
Viral disease (PVN, PML, hemorrhagic cystitis)	Histological evidence of viral activation in organs associated with varying tissue injury and clinical symptoms*

PML, progressive multifocal leukoencephalopathy.

* PVN stage A shows only minimal ATI and often no renal dysfunction.

homology. Polyomaviruses are ubiquitous and have specifically adapted to their hosts during evolution. They are of no clinical significance in immune competent individuals. Disease caused by polyomaviruses is only seen in patients with pronounced and persistent immunosuppression (Table 3.9).

Polyomavirus allograft nephropathy (PVN) following kidney transplantation was first described by the pathologist Mackenzie nearly three decades ago in a kidney transplant recipient (289). It was not, however, until the introduction of potent third-generation immunosuppressive drugs into clinical practice, mainly high-dose tacrolimus and mycophenolate mofetil, that transplant centers experienced "an epidemic" of PVN as a mostly iatrogenic complication due to "overimmunosuppression" (290–296). In contrast, specific risk factors of disease are only poorly defined (297,298). Currently, PVN has a prevalence of 1–10 percent and a reported graft failure rate of more than 50 percent in some series (295,299–304). It vastly exceeds the prevalence of productive CMV graft infections. It is likely that the incidence of PVN will decrease in the future under altered and optimized immunosuppression. A recent encouraging report from the Mayo Clinic found a highly significant reduction in the incidence of PVN from 10.5–2.5 percent following the clinical introduction of "low-dose" maintenance tacrolimus immunosuppression (295). At present, however, PVN still constitutes a major clinical challenge. Specific and potent antiviral drugs to treat productive polyomavirus infections are not available.

Consequently, much emphasis is placed on patient screening and a diagnosis of PVN at an early disease stage that often responds favorably to our limited therapeutic options mainly consisting of a reduction of maintenance immunosuppression. Pathologists play a crucial role in risk assessment, diagnosis, and patient monitoring.

Infections with polyomaviruses and PVN are characterized by several key features (Table 3.9):

1. PVN is caused by the re-activation of latent intrarenal/intragraft, donor derived, polyomaviruses under long-lasting and intense immunosuppression.
2. Slight changes in the immune status can lead to transient, mostly asymptomatic, and self-limiting activation of latent polyomaviruses (305), especially in the urothelium, which harbors latent BK virus infections in 43 percent of individuals (306). Such activation is characterized by the detection of free viral particles in the urine (by electron microscopy or PCR techniques) and viral inclusion bearing cells, so-called decoy cells in urine cytology specimens. Signs of transient, asymptomatic viral activation are occasionally detected in serum samples by PCR. Such polyomavirus (re)activation is commonly not accompanied by PVN. PVN, however, is always associated and typically preceded by the activation of polyomaviruses (307–313).
3. PVN is typically diagnosed ten to fourteen months after transplantation with only anecdotal cases reported as early as six days or as late as six years after grafting (302,314). Depending on the extent of virally induced tubular injury, patients clinically present with varying degrees of allograft dysfunction.
4. PVN is best diagnosed histologically in a graft biopsy, which additionally provides prognostically relevant information on the disease stage or concomitant rejection. Since PVN affects the kidney in a *focal* fashion, adequate samples are needed to guarantee an optimal diagnostic yield (see Biopsies and Histological Evaluations of Allografts). The diagnosis may be missed in 25–37 percent of cases if only one small core of renal cortex is sampled (301,315); occasionally, multiple-step sections have to be studied with ancillary techniques (immunohistochemistry, in situ hybridization) in order to establish a definitive diagnosis (316).
5. PVN is nearly always caused by a productive infection with the BK virus strain. Only a minority of cases (approximately 20–30 percent) show activation of polyoma BK and JC viruses simultaneously with, as yet, undetermined biological significance (316–318). Polyomavirus nephropathies that are only induced by a productive JC virus infection are rare and SV-40 virus infections are exceptional (316,319,320). PVN is hardly ever seen in association with a concurrent second viral infection (303,321). Morphological changes induced by productive BK, JC, or SV-40 polyomavirus infections

are identical; ancillary techniques such as immunohisto-chemistry, in situ hybridization, or PCR are required for the exact identification of viral strains.

6. In general, PVN persists for months or even years (more than two years in one of our patients). Rapid disease resolution within three to four weeks is rarely seen.

7. PVN is typically limited to the transplant and the worst case scenario is graft failure. Thus, patients are usually not at risk for a generalized infection.

The definitive diagnosis of PVN ideally requires a kidney biopsy and the detection of characteristic histological changes.

2. Morphological Changes and Diagnosis

PVN is defined as an intrarenal, productive polyomavirus infection (BK virus greater than JC virus) involving the renal medulla and/or cortex with light microscopic *and/or* immunohistochemical *or* in situ hybridization evidence of viral replication accompanied by varying degrees of parenchymal damage ranging from minimal to marked (Table 3.9).

Gross pathology: Transplant nephrectomy specimens from patients with PVN show uncharacteristic changes closely resembling fibrotic lesions seen in other chronic diseases leading to graft failure. In PVN, the removed allografts are generally slightly decreased in size, firm, with an ill-defined cortico-medullary junction and thinned, sclerosed cortex. The renal surface is either smooth or granular. Infarction and/or large scar formation are not features of PVN.

Histology: Histological signs caused by a productive polyomavirus infection of the kidney are characteristically found in *epithelial cells* lining collecting ducts, tubules, and Bowman's capsule (parietal epithelial cells). Viral

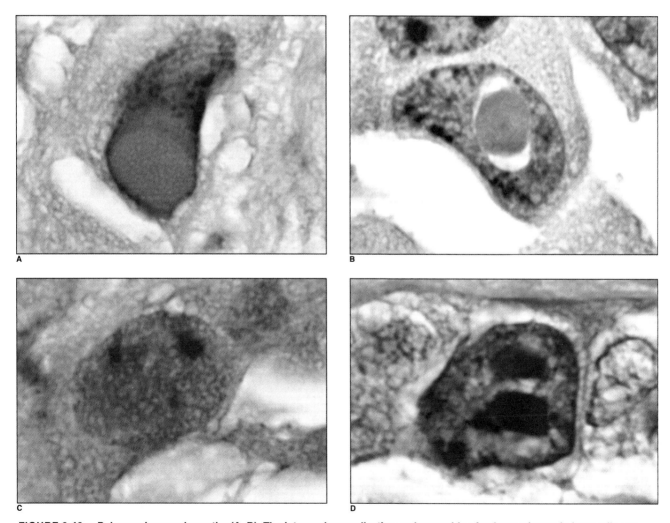

FIGURE 3.42: *Polyomavirus nephropathy (A–D). The intranuclear replication and assembly of polyomaviruses in host cells can induce different nuclear alterations: (A) an amorphous, ground-glass type of inclusion body (type 1); (B) a central intranuclear inclusion body surrounded by a halo (type 2); (C) nuclear enlargement and finely granular changes (type 3); (D) vesicular, clumped changes (type 4). H&E stain, 400× oil original magnification.*

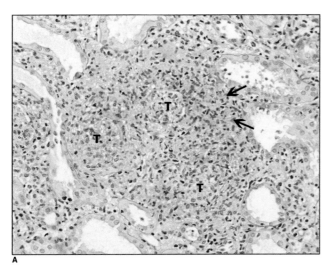
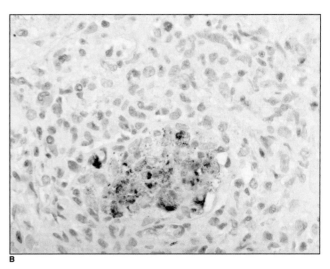

FIGURE 3.43: *Polyomavirus nephropathy (A, B). (A) This case shows ill defined, tubulo-centric, epithelioid granulomas (arrows; T = dilated tubular cross section). (B) Immunohistochemical incubation illustrating virions in the center of a small granuloma. H&E stain (A) 80× original magnification, and (B) immunohistochemical incubation to detect viral capsid proteins, 180× original magnification.*

replication and the assembly of daughter virions result in the formation of intranuclear inclusion bodies, cell injury, and lysis (291,293,308,309,311). The replication of polyomaviruses does not induce any histologically discernible cytoplasmic inclusions. Four types of virally induced nuclear changes exist and hybrid forms are common (Figure 3.42) (311,322,323): *type 1* (the most frequent form)—an amorphous, basophilic ground-glass inclusion body; *type 2*—a central, eosinophilic, granular inclusion surrounded by a mostly incomplete halo (CMV like); *type 3*—a finely granular variant without a halo; and *type 4*—a vesicular variant with clumped, irregular chromatin and large viral aggregates; nucleoli may be found. These nuclear changes are (at least in part) due to different patterns of viral aggregation, that is, evenly dispersed virions cause type 1 inclusions and large, crystalloid aggregates type 4 changes. Most easily discernible are type 1 and 2 inclusions. Type 3 and 4 changes are least specific and may be mimicked by ATI and cell regeneration. Rarely (in my experience in approximately 5 percent of PVN cases), virally induced nuclear changes are absent and viral replication can only be demonstrated by immunohistochemistry or in situ hybridization (representing very early phases of polyomavirus replication; disease stage A). PVN typically involves renal tubules and collecting ducts in a focal fashion. Severely injured tubules containing many inclusion bearing epithelial cells are typically located adjacent to normal ducts. Especially in disease stage A, viral inclusion bodies are often most abundant in the renal medulla. Glomerular capillary tufts, blood vessels, inflammatory and mesenchymal cells are typically nonpermissive for the replication of BK/polyomaviruses.

Uncommon histological features of PVN include: pseudo-crescents in glomeruli [due to marked, virally induced injury of parietal epithelial cells (322,324,325)], nonnecrotizing small epithelioid granulomas in and adjacent to severely injured tubules (326), and immune complex–type deposits in tubular basement membranes (Figures 3.43 and 3.44) (327). These changes do not appear to carry any independent prognostic significance exceeding the staging of PVN. Viral inclusion bodies are also found in the transitional cell layer lining the renal pelvis, the (graft) ureter and potentially even the recipient's urinary bladder (322,328). Polyomavirus replication in the urothelium, however, is not a defining histological feature characterizing PVN since it can also be seen in patients without viral nephropathy as a transient and asymptomatic sign of viral activation or in the setting of hemorrhagic cystitis (without PVN) following bone marrow transplantation (329,330).

Ancillary diagnostic techniques: In tissue specimens, polyomavirus replication is readily detected with commercially available antibodies directed against the SV-40 T antigen (large T antigen) that cross-react with all polyomaviruses pathogenic in humans (i.e., BK, JC, and SV-40) and give a crisp, purely intranuclear staining signal (Figures 3.45–3.47). The expression of the T antigen marks the initial phase of polyomavirus replication and precedes the formation of intranuclear viral inclusion bodies in some infected cells. Thus, intense staining signals may be seen in normal nuclei/tissue (292,311,322,331) as the earliest morphological evidence of viral replication and PVN. Polyomaviruses can also be identified by in situ hybridization or with antibodies directed against viral capsid proteins (Figure 3.43B). These latter techniques mostly detect "mature" virions and, therefore, not only mark intranuclear but additionally also dense intratubular viral aggregates. Strain-specific antibodies directed against BK, JC, or

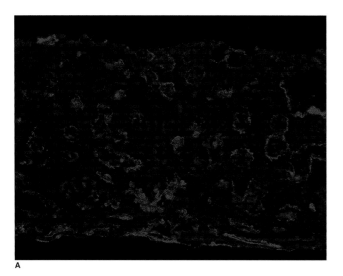

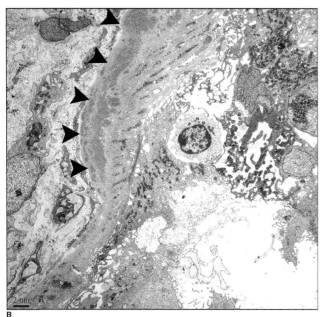

FIGURE 3.44: *Polyomavirus nephropathy (A, B) presenting with immune complex type deposits along tubular basement membranes in a patient in disease stage C. (A) IF microscopy employing an antibody directed against IgG shows diffuse, granular deposits along most tubular basement membranes, 60× original magnification. (B) Electron microscopy from the same case demonstrates immune complex–type deposits along the outer aspect of a thickened tubular basement membrane (arrow heads). Transmission electron microscopy, 7,000× original magnification.*

SV-40 viruses exist, although most of them are primarily used by the research community; their use for diagnostic clinical purposes does not carry any advantage over antibodies to SV-40 T antigen since PVN is nearly always driven by the replication of BK viruses. Of note, depending on the technique used, staining results may vary greatly. Suboptimal staining protocols can result in an artificially low number of "positive signals" rather than a marked decrease of the overall staining intensity. Sometimes, diffuse artifactual nuclear staining is encountered with mild to moderate signals in practically all nuclei. Strain-specific antibodies directed against the BK virus T antigen (clone BK.T-1) cross-react with unrelated nuclear proteins (Ku86) and may give nonspecific results (332). Epithelial cells with signs of polyomavirus replication express p53 tumor suppressor proteins (333) and the proliferation marker Ki-67as signs of altered (viral) DNA assembly.

PCR techniques may also be utilized to demonstrate viral DNA or RNA in tissue samples and to confirm the diagnosis of PVN (334–336). However, PCR results must be interpreted with great caution. Only very strong amplification signals of viral DNA (greater than ten viral copies per cell equivalent), in the setting of histologically or immunohistochemically demonstrable virally induced cytopathic changes, can be used to confirm the diagnosis of PVN, to identify the viral strain, and to distinguish clinically significant productive from clinically insignificant latent polyomavirus infections (334,335,337–341). The detection of viral RNA in renal biopsy cores by PCR clearly indicates viral replication/PVN. RNA extraction and amplification methods, however, are challenging techniques susceptible to error, and do not provide information exceeding the results obtained with standard immunohistochemistry (such as the detection of the SV-40 T antigen) (335,336).

In PVN, standard IF microscopy with a common panel of antibodies directed against IgG, IgA, IgM, kappa and lambda light chains, fibrinogen, and complement factor C3 generally does not show any diagnostic staining pattern in tubules, glomeruli, or blood vessels. In some patients, PVN is associated with a type III hypersensitivity reaction, resembling "anti-TBM disease" in native kidneys. These cases are characterized by granular, immune deposits along thickened tubular basement membranes that are easily discernible by IF microscopy (using various antibodies directed against immunoglobulins and complement factors) or by electron microscopy (Figure 3.44) (342).

PVN and virally induced tubular injury are not associated with marked and diffuse upregulation of MHC class II (i.e., HLA-DR) in tubular epithelial cells or with the deposition of the complement degradation product C4d along peritubular capillaries (62,300,343). Both the detection of C4d and tubular HLA-DR expression can help to establish a diagnosis of (concurrent) allograft rejection (344).

By electron microscopy, polyomaviruses present as viral particles of 30–50 nm in diameter that occasionally form crystalloid aggregates (308,312). Polyomaviruses are ultrastructurally identified by size and their icosahedral capsid structure; polyomavirus strains cannot be distinguished. Virions are primarily found in the nucleus, rarely in the cytoplasm.

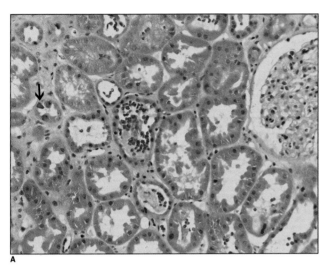
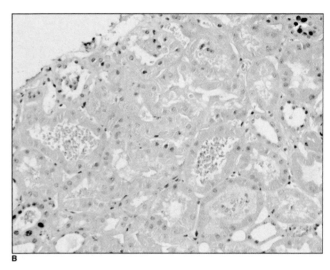

FIGURE 3.45: *Polyomavirus nephropathy (A, B)—early histological disease stage A. (A) During the early phase of polyomavirus replication, alterations are only found in few nuclei containing inclusion bodies (arrow) and (B) demonstrating immunohistochemical evidence of a productive infection. (A) H&E stain, and (B) immunohistochemical incubation to detect the SV-40T antigen, 100× original magnification.*

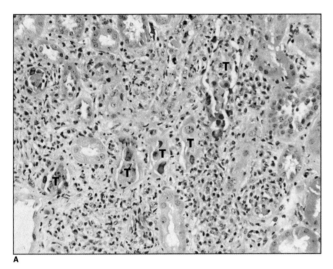
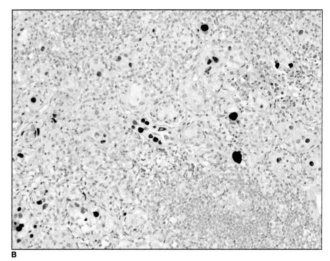

FIGURE 3.46: *Polyomavirus nephropathy (A, B)—fully developed histological disease stage B. (A) During the florid phase of polyomavirus replication, conspicuous tubular injury caused by viral replication and host cell lysis is seen (T = severely injured tubular cross sections containing intranuclear inclusion bearing epithelial cells). The interstitium is severely inflamed. (B) Immunohistochemical incubations to demonstrate the expression of the SV-40T antigen show intranuclear staining signals in many tubular cells. (A) H&E stain, and (B) immunohistochemical incubation to detect the SV-40T antigen (B), 100× original magnification.*

Morphological staging of PVN (Table 3.10): The severe tubular changes represented by virally induced tubular injury and the denudation of tubular basement membranes can not only cause dysfunction but also lead to atrophy and fibrosis—these changes are the most important for the clinical presentation and course of PVN. Based on the degree of tubulo-interstitial damage, PVN is subgrouped into *four disease stages*: early "A," fully developed "B," fibrosing "C," and burnt-out "D" (301,308,315,331,345–348). Pertinent to staging are the severity of virally induced epithe-

lial cell injury, interstitial fibrosis, and tubular atrophy rather than the extent of interstitial inflammation. Progression from one disease stage to another can occur within a few months (300,347). *PVN stage A* (Figure 3.45) represents the earliest disease phase with only focal "nonlytic" viral replication and inconspicuous denudation of tubular basement membranes; it is often limited to the renal medulla. The interstitium is normal or only shows minimal inflammation and fibrosis. The detection of one intranuclear viral inclusion body or alternatively a crisp

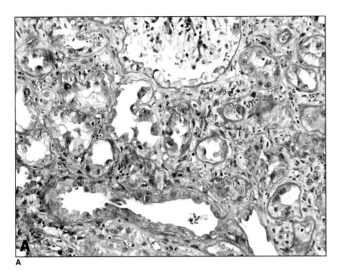
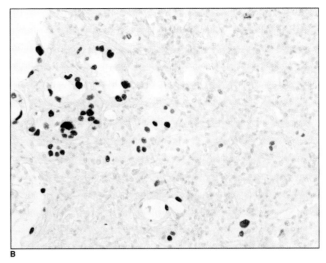

FIGURE 3.47: Polyomavirus nephropathy (A, B)—fibrosing histological disease stage C. (A) The interstitium shows diffuse, pronounced fibrosis and tubular atrophy with mild inflammation; a glomerulus is without significant abnormalities. (B) Immunohistochemical incubations to demonstrate the expression of the SV-40T antigen show intranuclear staining signals in many tubular cells. (A) Trichrome stain, and (B) immunohistochemical incubation to detect the SV-40T antigen, 100× original magnification.

TABLE 3.10 PVN: Disease Stages [modified from (357)]

Stage A* (early phase)
  Viral activation in cortex and/or medulla with intranuclear inclusion bodies and/or positive immunohistochemical or in situ hybridization signals
  No or minimal tubular epithelial cell necrosis/lysis
  No or minimal denudation of tubular basement membranes
  No or minimal interstitial inflammation in foci with viral activation
  No or minimal tubular atrophy and interstitial fibrosis (≤10%)

Stage B* (fully developed phase)
  Pronounced viral activation in cortex and/or medulla
  Marked virally induced tubular epithelial cell lysis
  Denudation of tubular basement membranes
  Interstitial inflammation** (mild to marked)
  Interstitial fibrosis and tubular atrophy

    Stage B1 – ≤25% of specimen involved
    Stage B2 – >25% and <50% of specimen involved
    Stage B3 – ≥50% of specimen involved (and ≤50% fibrosis)

Stage C* (fibrosing phase)
  Viral activation in cortex and medulla (minimal to marked)
  Per definition: interstitial fibrosis and tubular atrophy >50% of sample
  Tubular epithelial cell lysis and basement membrane denudation (minimal to marked)
  Interstitial inflammation (minimal to marked)

Stage D (burnt-out phase)***
  No viral replication (by light microscopy, immunohistochemistry, in situ hybridization)
  Varying degrees of interstitial fibrosis and tubular atrophy (minimal to marked)

---

*   Concurrent signs of BK virus activation: 1) urine: decoy cells, free virions, high PCR readings; 2) plasma: detectable BK virus DNA by PCR.

**   Interstitial inflammation and tubulitis can in some cases mark concurrent cellular rejection; rejection-induced changes are not part of PVN staging.

*** The burnt-out stage of PVN only shows uncharacteristic changes that cannot be distinguished from nonspecific graft fibrosis; the diagnosis can only be suspected based on the patient's history.

staining signal in one nucleus (with or without an inclusion body) suffices for proving "active" viral replication and rendering the diagnosis of PVN stage A. *Fully developed PVN* (stage B; Figure 3.46) is characterized by marked virally induced tubular injury and epithelial cell lysis, conspicuous denudation of tubular basement membranes, and interstitial edema with a mixed, mild to marked inflammatory cell infiltrate (B and T lymphocytes, plasma cells, and histiocytes). *PVN stage C* (Figure 3.47) shows marked interstitial fibrosis and tubular atrophy involving more than 50 percent of the tissue sample. Stage C is associated with varying degrees of inflammation and viral replication. *The burnt-out stage of PVN* (stage D) following the resolution of viral replication demonstrates nonspecific chronic changes falling into the spectrum of so-called chronic allograft nephropathy: varying degrees of interstitial fibrosis and tubular atrophy (ranging from minimal to marked), and occasionally mild lymphocytic inflammation in areas of parenchymal scarring. Any signs of polyomavirus replication by light microscopy and immunohistochemistry/in situ hybridization are, by definition, no longer detectable.

PVN and inflammation: PVN is associated with varying degrees of interstitial inflammation. The inflammatory cell infiltrate can represent "virally induced" interstitial nephritis with polymorphonuclear leukocytes located adjacent to severely injured tubules, plasma cells, and rarely plasma cell tubulitis (292,308,314,348). In particular, patchy inflammatory cell infiltrates primarily located in the medulla and associated with "tubular epithelial cell atypia/injury" should raise the level of suspicion for PVN (potentially lacking easily discernible viral inclusion bodies). In some cases, mononuclear cell

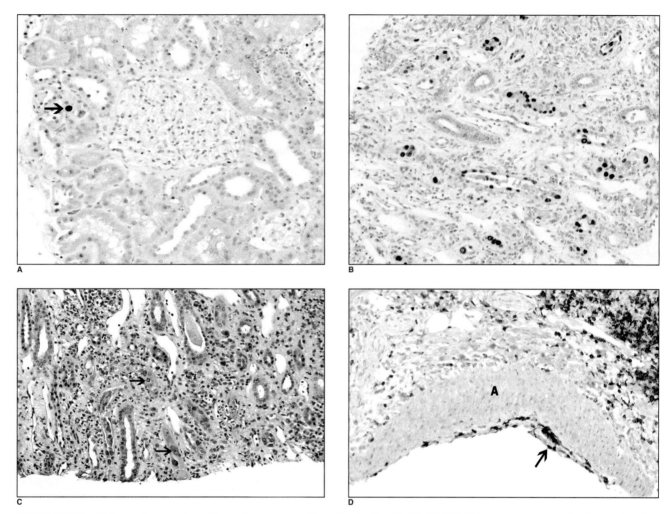

FIGURE 3.48: *Polyomavirus nephropathy and concurrent allograft rejection (A–D). (A) Initial biopsy approximately six months after transplantation: in this patient, immunohistochemistry showed a single nucleus with strong staining for the SV-40T antigen. The biopsy was interpreted to be "nondiagnostic." The correct diagnosis of PVN, disease stage A, was not rendered, and no changes were made in the immunosuppressive drug regimen. Immunohistochemical incubation to detect the SV-40T antigen, 80× original magnification. (B–D) Follow-up biopsy approximately eight months after transplantation: Polyomavirus replication had progressed and presented in the florid disease stage B. Many tubules and nuclei showed injury (arrows in C) including signs of intranuclear viral replication (B and C). (D) In addition, concurrent rejection was diagnosed with conspicuous evidence of transplant endarteritis in an arcuate caliber artery (A = arterial wall; arrow marks intimal inflammation). (B) Immunohistochemical incubation to detect the SV-40T antigen; (C) H&E stain; (D) immunohistochemical incubation to detect CD3-positive lymphocytes in the inflamed intimal layer; all 80v original magnifications.*

infiltrates rich in lymphocytes and a lymphocytic tubulitis can be found representing concurrent acute allograft rejection. The diagnosis of acute rejection and PVN is challenging. It can be facilitated by the detection of transplant endarteritis, transplant glomerulitis, as well as the tubular expression of MHC class II (HLA-DR) and/or the deposition of the complement degradation product C4d along peritubular capillaries (Figure 3.48) (62,292,307,314,344,349,350). Of note, PVN stage A lacks a significant inflammatory cell infiltrate. If only focal signs of polyomavirus replication are detected without significant epithelial cell lysis (i.e., disease stage A) in the setting of marked interstitial inflammation, then PVN and a concurrent cellular tubulo-interstitial rejection episode (Banff

category 4, type 1) has to be considered (344). The immunohistochemical phenotyping of the inflammatory cells in PVN has shown plasma cell (CD138) as well as B (CD20) or T cell (CD3) dominant infiltrates with currently undetermined pathophysiological significance. Immunophenotyping for that is, the detection of CD20 (B cells) versus CD3 (T-cell)–rich lymphocytic infiltrates, is diagnostically *not helpful* for distinguishing viral nephritis from concurrent acute allograft rejection (344, 351–353). If concurrent rejection is diagnosed in the setting of PVN, anecdotal reports indicate that patients benefit from transient antirejection therapy before, in a second phase, therapeutic attempts are initiated to treat PVN (307,311,323,344,346,354).

3. Clinical Screening Assays for PVN

The optimal timing of a diagnostic transplant biopsy becomes a clinical challenge, in particular in disease stage A that can present with stable graft function (298,355). Overall improved graft survival has been reported from centers with vigorous patient screening programs that facilitate an early intervention (307,311,323,346,354,356–358).

Renal allograft recipients at risk for PVN and in whom a diagnostic graft biopsy is indicated can be clinically identified by detecting signs of polyomavirus activation. Commonly used "BK virus activation assays" include quantitative PCR tests (best performed on plasma or alternatively urine samples), urine cytology, and urine electron microscopy (292,313,346,347,357). Patients with PVN typically present with large numbers of polyomavirus inclusion bearing epithelial cells in the urine, so-called *decoy cells* (ten or more decoy cells per ThinPrep slide; positive and negative predictive values for PVN: 27 and 100 percent, respectively) (Figure 3.49) (290,291,307,312,322,323,347,359,360). Similar predictive values are found for quantitative PCR assays on voided urine samples with cutoff levels of 1×10^7 or greater BK virus copies/ml used as an indication for positive PVN. All patients with viral nephropathy shed abundant free virions in the urine detectable by negative staining electron microscopy (294,313,361). Among all BK virus activation assays, quantitative *plasma* PCR tests (cutoff 1×10^4 BK virus copies/ml) predict disease best with 74 percent probability (negative predictive value: 87 percent).

At Chapel Hill, we often use an alternative, new noninvasive method to accurately diagnose PVN in urine samples. The urine test is not based on general signs of BK virus activation but rather targets three-dimensional, cast-like polyomavirus clusters as specific disease markers (Figure 3.50). Dense aggregates of polyomaviruses (so-called Haufen a German term for "stack" or "heap") form in virally injured nephrons, are flushed into the urine, and can easily be detected by standard negative staining electron microscopy in voided urine samples. Urinary Haufen, in sharp contrast to all BK virus activation assays including the detection of free, nonclustered virions in the urine, are specific for viral nephropathy. In our experience, the qualitative detection of Haufen in voided urine samples predicts PVN with greater than 95 percent positive and negative predictive values (362).

Thus, pathologists can play a crucial role in the risk assessment for PVN. One voided urine sample can be analyzed by cytology (to search for decoy cells) and potentially also by negative staining electron microscopy [to search for Haufen; for technical details see (313)]. If both tests are positive, the diagnosis of PVN is established. A renal biopsy may still be obtained for disease staging and to rule out concurrent rejection. In general, all screening test results should be made available to histopathologists at time of

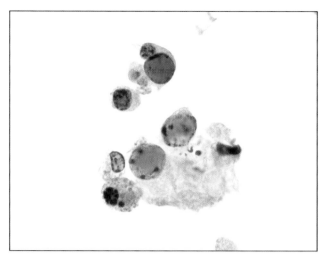

FIGURE 3.49: *Polyomavirus inclusion bearing decoy cells in a voided urine sample. Decoy cells most frequently show glassy appearing intranuclear viral inclusion bodies. They are a morphological sign of polyomavirus activation and likely mostly originate from the transitional cell layers of the bladder and ureters. Liquid-based urine cytology preparation, Papanicolaou stain, 600× oil original magnification.*

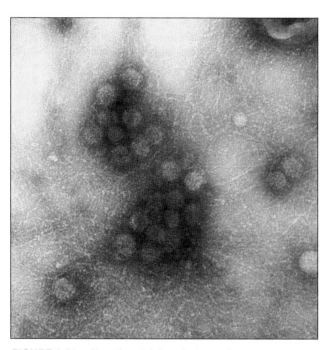

FIGURE 3.50: *Negative staining electron microscopy on a voided urine sample to detect polyomaviruses. Patients with PVN characteristically shed large, three-dimensional viral aggregates, so-called Haufen; 80,000× original magnification.*

graft biopsy; positive tests should trigger an intensive search for morphological signs of polyomavirus replication (including the analysis of multiple step sections and ancillary immunohistochemical or in situ hybridization studies).

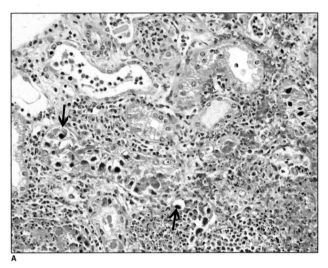
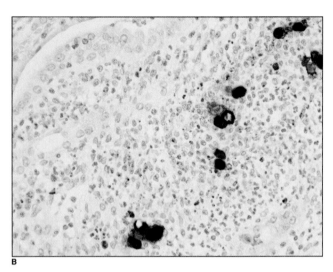

FIGURE 3.51: *Productive adenovirus graft infection (A, B). (A) Adenovirus replication is characterized by severe, necrotizing interstitial inflammation, interstitial hemorrhage, tubular injury, and ground-glass type of intranuclear viral inclusion bodies in epithelial cells (arrows). (B) Immunohistochemistry to detect adenovirus antigens shows viral particles predominantly in epithelial cell nuclei. (A) H&E stain, 25× original magnification, and (B) immunohistochemistry to detect adenoviruses, 100× original magnification.*

If kidney allografts are lost due to progressive viral nephropathy, re-transplantation is an option. Small case series have provided encouraging results: recurrent PVN was only observed in approximately 12 percent of all repeat allografts (304,363–365).

ii. Adenovirus

Adenovirus infections of renal allografts are very *infrequent* complications after transplantation (366,367). Morphological changes caused by productive infections are summarized in Table 3.8; they include 1) intranuclear viral inclusions in epithelial cells, 2) severe tubular destruction with rupture of basement membranes and focal necrosis, 3) marked interstitial inflammation, and 4) focal interstitial hemorrhage and intratubular red blood cell casts (Figure 3.51) (1,368). The replication of adenoviruses induces cytopathic intranuclear changes in *tubular cells* and occasionally also in *parietal epithelial cells* lining Bowman's capsule with mostly smudgy, "ground-glass" type of inclusion bodies (similar to polyomavirus type 1 changes). Rarely, viral inclusion bodies are surrounded by a halo (i.e., CMV like) (321,369). Nodular and granulomatous inflammatory cell infiltrates are found in areas with marked viral replication. They are primarily composed of mononuclear and plasma cells. Foci of necrosis and tubular disruption show abundant polymorphonuclear leukocytes. On occasion, necrotic regions can be large and wedge shaped. Glomeruli and blood vessels are generally not affected. Common ancillary diagnostic techniques include immunohistochemistry and electron microscopy. Immunohistochemistry with antibodies directed against outer viral antigens shows strong nuclear and less intense cytoplasmic staining

in epithelial cells (Figure 3.51 B). Ultrastructurally, virions of approximately 75–80 nm are found in nuclei and the cytoplasm. Free viral particles can typically also be detected in the urine by negative staining electron microscopy. In contrast to PVN, however, dense viral aggregates, that is, Haufen, or abundant decoy cells are not seen in voided urine samples. IF microscopy with a standard panel of antibodies directed against immunoglobulins and complement factors is unrevealing. In my experience, adenovirus infections are not associated with the deposition of the complement degradation product C4d along peritubular capillaries.

The differential diagnosis includes other types of viral infections, mainly PVN. Adenovirus replication can usually be suspected by light microscopy based on 1) frank tubular destruction with foci of necrosis, 2) granulomatous inflammation with palisading of macrophages around severely injured tubules, and 3) interstitial hemorrhage. A superimposed second viral kidney infection in cases of adenovirus-induced nephritis seems to be rare; in one series only one of fourteen patients demonstrated concurrent focal PVN and zero of fourteen had signs of CMV replication (321).

Adenovirus infections are most often caused by subgroup B, serotypes 7, 11, 34, and 35. Serotypes 34, 35, and, most frequently, 11 have been associated with hemorrhagic cystitis and necrotizing interstitial nephritis (321,369–372). Infections can be asymptomatic; cause localized disease such as enteritis, cystitis, or nephritis; or present as disseminated severe illness. Patients suffering from adenovirus-induced nephritis most often present within the first three months after transplantation with renal failure, hematuria, sometimes dysuria and hemorrhagic cystitis, and often (but not always) with evidence of a generalized infection including fever. Although treatment strategies for adenovirus allograft infections are not well defined [they include the reduction of the immunosuppression, IVIG, intravenous ribavirin, and ganciclovir (367,370–374)], most patients nevertheless recover surprisingly rapidly with profound improvement of renal function and long-term graft survival (367,371,373–375). In one patient, viral clearance from the kidney transplant could be documented in a repeat graft biopsy within four weeks (372). Disseminated adenovirus infections can be fatal (321,369,376–378).

iii. Cytomegalovirus

CMV, a herpesvirus, is one of the most common pathogens in renal transplant recipients. CMV can cause a symptomatic infection during the first months after transplantation, generally characterized by fever, leukopenia, hepatitis, or pneumonitis, and viremia (379). The kidneys are infrequently affected in only approximately 25 percent of patients suffering from "CMV disease" (380,381). In the Western world, effective patient screening and clinical management strategies have made productive CMV infections of renal transplants exceedingly rare. This observation contrasts a recent study from India reporting a prevalence of CMV renal allograft infections of 1.9 percent (382).

Lesions induced by the replication of CMV in the kidneys have been described both in native organs and transplants (Table 3.8) (380,381). Cytopathic changes are typically very focal and most often seen in the nuclei and cytoplasm of *tubular epithelial cells*, sometimes in *endothelial cells*, and only occasionally in *mononuclear inflammatory cells* (380,381). CMV-infected cells are enlarged with nuclei containing a central round inclusion body surrounded by a circumferential halo, that is, the typical "owls-eye" appearance. Also, homogenous smudgy appearing intranuclear inclusions are occasionally observed. Small basophilic "lumpy" cytoplasmic viral inclusions are frequently (but not always) detected in cells with virally induced intranuclear changes (380). The replication of CMV in the tubular compartment can be associated with a nodular, occasionally granulomatous appearing mononuclear inflammatory cell infiltrate. Interstitial inflammation was absent in two of six cases of CMV nephropathy in one series (381). Foci of necrosis and microabscesses can occur, but are uncommon (381). Rarely, CMV infects *glomerular cells* and causes an acute glomerulonephritis with crescents (383–386); in one exceptional case, CMV replication was limited to glomerular endothelial cells and not accompanied by inflammation (385).

Ancillary diagnostic techniques to confirm the diagnosis of a productive CMV infection include immunohistochemistry (e.g., best with an antibody directed against the immediate early antigen), in situ hybridization or by electron microscopy. Ultrastructurally, virions of approximately 150 nm are found in nuclei and the cytoplasm. IF microscopy with a standard panel of antibodies detecting immunoglobulins and complement factors is unrevealing (380). Whether a productive intragraft CMV infection is associated with the accumulation of the complement degradation product C4d along peritubular capillaries is unknown, but it seems to be unlikely.

CMV DNA is found in the absence of cytopathic changes, and consequently, PCR studies for viral DNA do not clearly distinguish between productive and latent infections (387). Thus, it remains unclear whether the use of highly sensitive techniques (such as tissue CMV PCR) really demonstrates a higher prevalence of "CMV disease" as suggested (388). The minimal criteria to establish the diagnosis of CMV nephritis include the demonstration of cytopathic changes, CMV proteins, or mRNA. This diagnostic strategy is not unique to CMV infections but similar to other potentially pathogenic DNA viruses that establish latency in humans, such as polyomaviruses. The differential diagnosis of CMV nephropathy includes other types of viral infections, mainly caused by polyomaviruses or adenovirus. Since CMV (in contrast to polyomavirus and adenovirus) often replicates in endothelial and inflammatory cells, a distinction between rejection-induced changes and infection driven inflammation is difficult. Some original reports had described a "CMV glomerulopathy" (158); this lesion is now classified as rejection-induced transplant glomerulitis.

CMV infections can stimulate indirect effects on the kidney graft by modulating the immune response and *promoting rejection episodes* (379). The most convincing evidence that CMV indirectly causes graft injury was reported by Reinke, who showed that 85 percent of patients with "late-acute rejection" responded to ganciclovir therapy (389).

iv. Epstein Barr Virus (EBV)/PTLDs

1. Background

According to the 2001 WHO definition, "post-transplant lymphoproliferative disorder is a lymphoid proliferation or lymphoma that develops as a consequence of immunosuppression in a recipient of a solid organ or bone marrow allograft. PTLDs comprise a spectrum ranging from early, Epstein-Barr virus (EBV) driven polyclonal proliferations resembling infectious mononucleosis to EBV positive or EBV negative lymphomas of predominantly B-cell or less often T-cell type" (see chapter 10) (Table 3.11) (390). Molecular studies have shown a *progression* from polymorphism, to clonality and subsequent oncogene mutations (391). percent (392).

A prerequisite for the development of PTLD is intense immunosuppression targeting T cells. Generally, the higher the dose of immunosuppression, the more rapid the onset of PTLD, which can arise as soon as one month after

TABLE 3.11 Post-Transplant Lymphoproliferative Disease (PTLD)*

Early lesions

  Reactive plasmacytic hyperplasia
  Infectious mononucleosis like
PTLD polymorphic
  Poly-/oligoclonal (rare)
  Monoclonal
PTLD monomorphic
  B-cell neoplasms
    Diffuse large B-cell lymphoma (immunoblastic, centroblastic, anaplastic)
    Burkitt's/Burkitt's-like lymphoma
    Plasma cell myeloma
    Plasmacytoma-like B-cell lymphoma
  T-cell neoplasms
    Peripheral T-cell lymphoma (NOS)
    Other
  Hodgkin and Hodgkin-like lymphoma

---

* WHO classification of PTLD (390).

transplantation. The intensity of the immunosuppression probably also accounts for the difference in the prevalence of PTLD in heart and kidney transplant recipients. The risk for developing lymphoid neoplasias is estimated to be 20 times that of the normal population for renal allograft and 120 times normal for cardiac transplant recipients (390). Another major risk factor is the constellation of the recipient's and donor's EBV serostatus, that is, transplantation from a sero-positive donor into a sero-negative recipient is associated with a high risk for PTLD (393).

PTLD (limited for study purposes to cases of "developing non-Hodgkin lymphomas") has been reported with a prevalence of 1.4 percent among 25,127 renal allograft recipients transplanted in the United States in the late 1990s (394). A similar prevalence was reported from the transplant center in Pittsburgh [1.2 percent in adults and 10.1 percent in pediatric kidney transplant recipients on tacrolimus therapy (395)]. PTLDs may be less common in other parts of the world (396).

Overall, more than 80 percent of the tested PTLD cases are *EBV positive* (390,397,398). EBV-negative cases are more frequent among renal allograft recipients and in patients presenting with T-cell lymphomas (390,399,400). B cells are the origin of more than 85 percent of PTLDs in organ transplant recipients (401,402). In contrast to non-PTLD B-cell lymphomas, clonality of the neoplastic cells is not always demonstrable, in particular in "early" and "polymorphic" PTLD variants. T-cell lymphomas comprise approximately 15 percent and null cells less than 1 percent of PTLDs (401). The majority (90 percent) of PTLDs in solid organ recipients are of *host origin* (393); only rare PTLDs arise from the transplanted donor lymphocytes. Donor origin PTLD was reported in six patients (four

kidney and two liver recipients); in all cases, the neoplasm was limited to the transplanted organ and/or regional lymph nodes and outcome was good (403,404).

In general, EBV-positive PTLDs arise within the first two post-transplant years, whereas EBV-negative cases have a median onset of fifty to sixty months after grafting (405,406). PTLD rarely involves the peripheral blood and more often extranodal sites (396). The distribution of EBV-positive PTLDs was documented in a series of nine non-human primate research animals with kidney transplants that showed involvement of lymph nodes (100 percent of cases), liver (56 percent), lung (44 percent), heart (44 percent), renal allograft (44 percent), and native kidneys (22 percent) (407). In humans, *PTLDs involve the renal allograft* in approximately 14–30 percent of patients (396,408,409); they were restricted to the kidney transplant in 12 percent of cases in one series (409). PTLDs restricted to the kidney transplant often occur early (on average five months) after surgery, are more frequently of donor cell origin, and fare favorably (393). The overall five-year adult patient and graft survival in PTLD was 86 and 60 percent in Pittsburgh (395); patient survival was reportedly less favorable in high-grade, lymphomatous PTLD variants (393,394). In particular, polymorphic PTLDs respond to antiviral therapy and a reduction in immunosuppression, whereas monomorphic, monoclonal PTLDs that show mutations of the bcl-6 gene require specific antitumor therapy (393). Surgical resection has been performed for localized disease (limited to the allograft or ureters) with good success (403,410,411). Recent successful therapeutic attempts were made with the anti CD20 antibody rituximab in patients with monomorphic and polymorphic PTLDs, resulting in complete remission in more than 50 percent of patients (412,413). PTLDs of T-cell lineage have a poor prognosis (393).

Monoclonal gammopathies have a prevalence of about 30 percent in sera from renal transplant patients (fairly even distribution from one to more than fourteen years after transplantation); most monoclonal gammopathies are transient, but were persistent in 26 percent; 33 percent of those with persistent gammopathy had multiple myeloma (414).

The clinical presentation is heterogenous and dependent upon the location and extent of the disease. Patients with kidney transplant involvement typically present with graft dysfunction and may sometimes show a "mass lesion" in imaging studies. The histological diagnosis of PTLD in a renal allograft is challenging, in particular, in unsuspected cases limited to the transplant.

2. Morphological Changes and Diagnosis

Gross pathology: Most nephrectomies show diffuse involvement by PTLDs. The organs are swollen with an ill-defined cortico-medullary junction and can demonstrate petechiae. Macroscopic changes are identical to cases of acute, predominantly tubulo-interstitial cellular rejection.

Histology: Most cases of PTLD involving the kidneys are of the polymorphic variant (408,409) and can, therefore, mimic cellular rejection (403,404,409,415–424). The interstitial compartment typically shows vaguely nodular, expansile aggregates of mononuclear cell elements containing plasma cells and varying numbers of activated lymphocytes admixed with "blastoid" cell elements containing prominent nucleoli. Mitotic figures can usually be found and occasionally foci of serpiginous necrosis. The neoplastic mononuclear cells often invade tubules (i.e., tubulitis); they can also penetrate into arterial intimal layers (i.e., transplant endarteritis) (Figure 3.52). Transplant glomer-

ulitis, however, is uncommon. The replication of EBV does not induce any viral inclusion bodies.

The major differential diagnosis of PTLD involving renal allografts is acute rejection (398,417) that would be treated with an increase in immunosuppression. Both in rejection and PTLD the mononuclear cells have enlarged nuclei with nucleoli, and they can show mitotic activity (although "blasts" and mitoses are more common in PTLD). In addition, tubulitis and endarteritis may be found in PTLD (Figure 3.52D). Several features should raise the suspicion of PTLD. The most helpful clue in my experience is the presence of dense, vaguely nodular, expansile sheets of activated lymphoid cell elements without an admixture of granulocytes or macrophages.

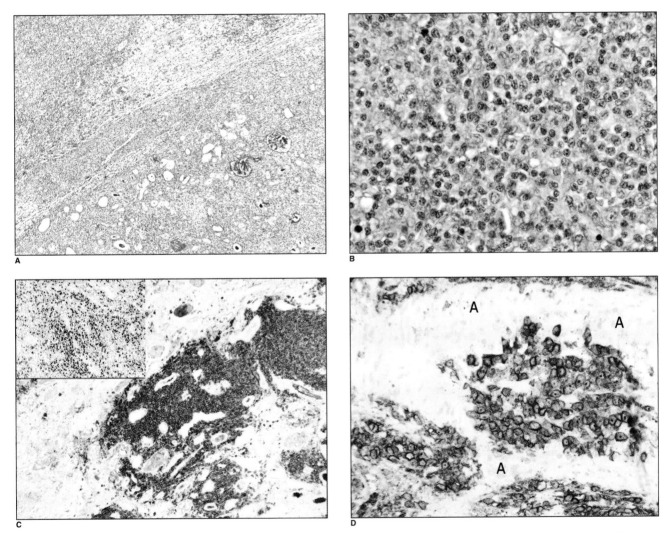

FIGURE 3.52: PTLD, polymorphic variant (A–D). (A) Low magnification reveals a diffuse mononuclear inflammatory cell infiltrate, involving not only the renal parenchyma but also the perirenal soft tissue. (B) High-power examination shows a diffuse, mononuclear cell infiltrate containing several activated lymphoid cell elements with enlarged nuclei and prominent nucleoli, that is, blasts. (C) An immunohistochemical stain identifies the vast majority of mononuclear cell elements as CD20 expressing B lymphocytes; most of them also express EBER (blue intranuclear staining reaction; insert). (D) CD20-positive B lymphocytes can also be detected in an artery (A = arterial wall) mimicking rejection-induced transplant endarteritis. (A and B) PAS stains, (A) 6× original magnification, and (B) 180× original magnification; (C and D) immunohistochemical incubation to detect CD20, (A) 100× original magnification, and (D) 140× original magnification. (Insert) In situ hybridization to detect EBER, 180× original magnification.

Tubules often seem to be "pushed apart." In comparison to cellular rejection that typically presents with conspicuous interstitial edema, neoplastic infiltrates in PTLD are commonly rather densely packed with only minimal edematous fluid. PTLDs, but not cellular rejection, commonly involve the renal capsule and perirenal adipose tissue. The presence of serpiginous necrosis is also a sign of PTLD (409), although its absence is not helpful, nor is interstitial hemorrhage that can be seen in severe rejection episodes. To make things worse, it has been suggested that rejection can co-exist with PTLD (409).

Ancillary diagnostic techniques: Immortalized B cells express six nuclear antigens (e.g., EBNA-2), two EBV-encoded nuclear RNAs (EBERs), and three membrane proteins (e.g., latent membrane protein, LMP-1) that are of diagnostic value during the histological work up of renal biopsies [reviewed in (420)]. Since the vast majority of PTLDs are of B-cell lineage and driven by the replication of EBV, diagnostic confirmation can generally be achieved by immunohistochemistry (demonstrating abundant CD20-, CD19-, and/or CD79a-positive cells of B lineage) as well as in situ hybridization for EBER (revealing strong and diffuse staining signals; the detection of rare EBER-positive cells should not be considered diagnostic for PTLD (390). CD3- and CD68-positive cells, hallmarks of cellular rejection, are generally relatively sparse, that is, accounting for less than 50 percent of the inflammatory cell infiltrates. In contrast to cellular rejection, B cells in PTLD are also found in foci of tubulitis and endothelialitis.

Immunohistochemical stains for LMP-1 and usually EBNA can be focal and scattered making them less reliable markers in the diagnostic decision making process. The number of positive cells is variable, even within the same tumor, and positivity can be increased around areas of necrosis. Tests to detect clonality (e.g., immunoglobulin gene rearrangement) help to confirm the presence of a monomorphic PTLD; polyclonality, however, does not exclude early and polymorphic PTLD variants. Additional clinical information (such as preceding rejection episodes treated with ATG or OKT3) and significantly elevated plasma EBV viral load levels (by PCR) may further help to confirm the diagnosis of PTLD. Rare forms of T-cell–mediated PTLDs may cause diagnostic problems since they are often EBER negative (390); these latter tumors, however, commonly present as high grade neoplasms that can be easily distinguished from acute cellular rejection.

v. Pyelonephritis

The pathogenesis of acute bacterial pyelonephritis is identical in native and transplanted kidneys, although the diagnosis in kidney transplants can be more challenging (Figure 3.53). Features distinguishing pyelonephritis include densely packed intratubular polymorphonuclear

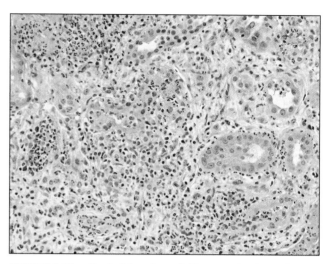

FIGURE 3.53: *Bacterial pyelonephritis occurring in an allograft two years after transplantation. The interstitium is edematous and contains a diffuse inflammatory cell infiltrate very rich in polymorphonuclear leukocytes that surround and focally invade injured tubules. One tubular cross section on the left contains a densely packed cellular cast composed of polymorphonuclear leukocytes. In the right clinical setting, the histological differential diagnosis (theoretically) includes ischemia/reperfusion injury and "pure" antibody-mediated C4d-positive rejection, which characteristically do not show parenchymal destruction and microabscess formation. H&E stain, 120× original magnification.*

leukocyte casts associated with polymorphonuclear leukocytes in the interstitium and between tubular epithelial cells. Pyelonephritis is typically a patchy disease process that may be most pronounced in the medulla. In very severe cases, often associated with bacteremia or urosepsis, microabscesses can be seen. The complement degradation product C4d is characteristically absent and not detected along peritubular capillaries. The differential diagnosis includes acute ischemic tubular injury (ATI), such as reperfusion injury following the grafting of a cadaveric donor organ, or an antibody-mediated rejection episode. In contrast to a pyelonephritis, ATI typically reveals marked and diffuse tubular injury with vacuolization of epithelial cells and only scattered polymorphonuclear leukocytes. Ischemic infarcts, seen in cases of severe ATI, are not found in pyelonephritides. A pure antibody-mediated rejection episode can look very similar to "conventional" ATI; however, it characteristically shows strong C4d positivity.

VIII. SUMMARY

Kidney transplantation has developed into a very effective way to treat patients with endstage renal disease and to not only improve morbidity and mortality but also quality of life. Modern immunosuppressive drug regimens have substantially reduced acute rejection episodes and made long-term graft survival possible. At present, the half life for all types of kidney transplants exceeds ten years. In the improved management of renal allograft recipients, transplant pathologists have played a major role. Kidney pathology, the fundamental backbone of all allograft-related science, has provided crucial insights into pathobiological key events causing rejection and graft loss, and morphological studies have fostered our basic understanding of graft injury. For example, polyoma-BK virus nephropathy, a major complication following kidney transplantation, was first described by a pathologist thirty years ago. Subsequently, fifteen years later it was a second-generation transplant pathologist who rediscovered the disease and identified it as a major cause of graft loss in modern days.

When evaluating renal allografts, a "look through the microscope" gives many important pieces of information on "primary" and "secondary" disease processes as well as insights into disease "activity" and "chronicity" at one glance, thereby making pathology a very powerful tool with unsurpassed informative yields. In the future, the introduction of new immunohistochemical and molecular markers into the evaluation of transplant pathology, the intelligent adaptation of classification schemes of renal allograft rejection, and the design and interpretation of new animal models will aid in the diagnostic interpretation of graft biopsies. This will require major contributions from dedicated and highly experienced transplant pathologists. In this regard, I hope that this chapter on kidney transplant pathology can provide some useful insights and food for thought for all pathologists and researchers interpreting renal allografts. But be aware: much remains to be learned and discovered in the future!

REFERENCES

1. Singh HK, Nickeleit V. Kidney disease caused by viral infections. *Curr Diag Pathol* 2004; **10**: 11–21.
2. Andreoni KA, Brayman KL, Guidinger MK, Sommers CM, et al. Kidney and pancreas transplantation in the United States, 1996–2005. *Am J Transplant* 2007; **7**: 1359–1375.
3. Evans RW, Kitzmann DJ. An economic analysis of kidney transplantation. *Surg Clin North Am* 1998; **78**: 149–174.
4. Excerpts from the United States renal data system 2007 annual data report atlas of chronic kidney disease & end-stage renal disease in the United States. *Am J Kid Dis* 2008; **51**.
5. Health Resources and Services Administration HSB, Division of Transplantation: 2006 Annual Report of the U.S. Organ Procurement and Transplantation Network and the Scientific Registry of Transplant Recipients: Transplant Data 1996-2005. Rockville, MD, 2006; http://www.optn.org/AR2006/survival_rates.htm
6. Meier-Kriesche HU, Schold JD, Kaplan B. Long-term renal allograft survival: have we made significant progress or is it time to rethink our analytic and therapeutic strategies? *Am J Transplant* 2004; **4**: 1289–1295.
7. Cecka JM. The OPTN/UNOS Renal Transplant Registry. *Clin Transpl* 2005: 1–16.
8. Waltzer WC, Miller F, Arnold A, Jao S, et al. Value of percutaneous core needle biopsy in the differential diagnosis of renal transplant dysfunction. *Journal of Urology* 1987; **137**: 1117–1121.
9. Matas AJ, Tellis VA, Sablay L, Quinn T, et al. The value of needle renal allograft biopsy. III. A prospective study. *Surgery* 1985; **98**: 922–926.
10. Parfrey PS, Kuo YL, Hanley JA, Knaack J, et al. The diagnostic and prognostic value of renal allograft biopsy. *Transplantation* 1984; **38**: 586–590.
11. Kiss D, Landman J, Mihatsch M, Huser B, et al. Risks and benefits of graft biopsy in renal transplantation under cyclosporin-A. *Clin Nephrol* 1992; **38**: 132–134.
12. Manfro RC, Lee JY, Lewgoy J, Edelweiss MI, et al. The role of percutaneous renal biopsy in kidney transplant. *Revista Da Associacao Medica Brasileira* 1994; **40**: 108–112.
13. Kon SP, Templar J, Dodd SM, Rudge CJ, et al. Diagnostic contribution of renal allograft biopsies at various intervals after transplantation. *Transplantation* 1997; **63**: 547–550.
14. Pascual M, Vallhonrat H, Cosimi AB, Tolkoff-Rubin N, et al. The clinical usefulness of the renal allograft biopsy in the cyclosporine era: a prospective study. *Transplantation* 1999; **67**: 737–741.
15. Al-Awwa IA, Hariharan S, First MR. Importance of allograft biopsy in renal transplant recipients: correlation between clinical and histological diagnosis. *Am J Kidney Dis* 1998; **31**: S15–18.
16. Racusen LC, Solez K, Colvin RB, Bonsib SM, et al. The Banff 97 working classification of renal allograft pathology. *Kidney International* 1999; **55**: 713–723.
17. Webb NJ, Pereira JK, Chait PG, Geary DF. Renal biopsy in children: comparison of two techniques. *Pediatric Nephrology* 1994; **8**: 486–488.
18. Nicholson ML, Wheatley TJ, Doughman TM, White SA, et al. A prospective randomized trial of three different sizes of core-cutting needle for renal transplant biopsy. *Kidney Int* 2000; **58**: 390–395.
19. Jennette JC, Kshirsagar AV. How can the safety and diagnostic yield of percutaneous renal biopsies be optimized? *Nat Clin Pract Nephrol* 2008; **4**: 126–127.
20. Manno C, Strippoli GF, Arnesano L, Bonifati C, et al. Predictors of bleeding complications in percutaneous ultrasound-guided renal biopsy. *Kidney Int* 2004; **66**: 1570–1577.
21. Song JH, Cronan JJ. Percutaneous biopsy in diffuse renal disease: comparison of 18- and 14- gauge automated biopsy devices. *J Vasc Interv Radiol* 1998; **9**: 651–655.
22. Furness PN, Philpott CM, Chorbadjian MT, Nicholson ML, et al. Protocol biopsy of the stable renal transplant: a multicenter study of methods and complication rates. *Transplantation* 2003; **76**: 969–973.
23. Schwarz A, Gwinner W, Hiss M, Radermacher J, et al. Safety and adequacy of renal transplant protocol biopsies. *Am J Transplant* 2005; **5**: 1992–1996.
24. Beckingham IJ, Nicholson ML, Kirk G, Veitch PS, et al. Comparison of three methods to obtain percutaneous

needle core biopsies a renal allograft. *Br J Surgery* 1994; **81**: 898–899.

25. Haas M, Segev DL, Racusen LC, Bagnasco SM, et al. Arteriosclerosis in kidneys from healthy live donors: comparison of wedge and needle core perioperative biopsies. *Arch Pathol Lab Med* 2008; **132**: 37–42.

26. Colvin RB, Cohen AH, Saiontz C, Bonsib S, et al. Evaluation of pathologic criteria for acute renal allograft rejection: reproducibility, sensitivity, and clinical correlation. *J Am Soc Nephrol* 1997; **8**: 1930–1941.

27. Sorof JM, Vartanian RK, Olson JL, Tomlanovich SJ, et al. Histopathological concordance of paired renal allograft biopsy cores. Effect on the diagnosis and management of acute rejection. *Transplantation* 1995; **60**: 1215–1219.

28. Herrera GA, Isaac J, Turbat-Herrera EA. Role of electron microscopy in transplant renal pathology. *Ultrastruct Pathol* 1997; **21**: 481–498.

29. Saidi RF, Elias N, Kawai T, Hertl M, et al. Outcome of kidney transplantation using expanded criteria donors and donation after cardiac death kidneys: realities and costs. *Am J Transplant* 2007; **7**: 2769–2774.

30. Gaber LW, Moore LW, Alloway RR, Amiri MH, et al. Glomerulosclerosis as a determinant of posttransplant function of older donor renal allografts. *Transplantation* 1995; **60**: 334–339.

31. Kiser RL, Thomas DB, Andreoni K, Klemmer PJ. Preexisting crescentic glomerulonephritis in the renal allograft. *Am J Kidney Dis* 2003; **42**: E20–E26.

32. Cosyns JP, Malaise J, Hanique G, Mourad M, et al. Lesions in donor kidneys: nature, incidence, and influence on graft function. *Transpl Int* 1998; **11**: 22–27.

33. Parker SM, Pullman JM, Khauli RB. Successful transplantation of a kidney with early membranous nephropathy. *Urology* 1995; **46**: 870–872.

34. Nakazawa K, Shimojo H, Komiyama Y, Itoh N, et al. Preexisting membranous nephropathy in allograft kidney. *Nephron* 1999; **81**: 76–80.

35. Lipkowitz GS, Madden RL, Kurbanov A, Mulhern JG, et al. Transplantation and 2-year follow-up of kidneys procured from a cadaver donor with a history of lupus nephritis. *Transplantation* 2000; **69**: 1221–1224.

36. Brunt EM, Kissane JM, Cole BR, Hanto DW. Transmission and resolution of type I membranoproliferative glomerulonephritis in recipients of cadaveric renal allografts. *Transplantation* 1988; **46**: 595–598.

37. Mizuiri S, Shigetomi Y, Sugiyama K, Miyagi M, et al. Successful transplantation of a cadaveric kidney with postinfectious glomerulonephritis. *Pediatr Transplant* 2000; **4**: 56–59.

38. Rosenberg HG, Martinez PS, Vaccarezza AS, Martinez LV. Morphological findings in 70 kidneys of living donors for renal transplant. *Pathol Res Pract* 1990; **186**: 619–624.

39. Ji S, Liu M, Chen J, Yin L, et al. The fate of glomerular mesangial IgA deposition in the donated kidney after allograft transplantation. *Clin Transplant* 2004; **18**: 536–540.

40. Silva FG, Chandler P, Pirani CL, Hardy MA. Disappearance of glomerular mesangial IgA deposits after renal allograft transplantation. *Transplantation* 1982; **33**: 214–216.

41. Sanfilippo F, Croker BP, Bollinger RR. Fate of four cadaveric donor renal allografts with mesangial IgA deposits. *Transplantation* 1982; **33**: 370–372.

42. Randhawa PS, Minervini MI, Lombardero M, Duquesnoy R, et al. Biopsy of marginal donor kidneys: correlation of histologic findings with graft dysfunction. *Transplantation* 2000; **69**: 1352–1357.

43. Escofet X, Osman H, Griffiths DF, Woydag S, et al. The presence of glomerular sclerosis at time zero has a significant impact on function after cadaveric renal transplantation. *Transplantation* 2003; **75**: 344–346.

44. Pokorna E, Vitko S, Chadimova M, Schuck O, et al. Proportion of glomerulosclerosis in procurement wedge renal biopsy cannot alone discriminate for acceptance of marginal donors. *Transplantation* 2000; **69**: 36–43.

45. Edwards EB, Posner MP, Maluf DG, Kauffman HM. Reasons for non-use of recovered kidneys: the effect of donor glomerulosclerosis and creatinine clearance on graft survival. *Transplantation* 2004; **77**: 1411–1415.

46. Karpinski J, Lajoie G, Cattran D, Fenton S, et al. Outcome of kidney transplantation from high-risk donors is determined by both structure and function. *Transplantation* 1999; **67**: 1162–1167.

47. Haas M, Ratner LE, Montgomery RA. C4d staining of perioperative renal transplant biopsies. *Transplantation* 2002; **74**: 711–717.

48. Oda A, Morozumi K, Uchida K. Histological factors of 1-h biopsy influencing the delayed renal function and outcome in cadaveric renal allografts. *Clinical Transplantation* 1999; **13 Suppl. 1**: 6–12.

49. Gaber LW, Gaber AO, Tolley EA, Hathaway DK. Prediction by postrevascularization biopsies of cadaveric kidney allografts of rejection, graft loss, and preservation nephropathy. *Transplantation* 1992; **53**: 1219–1225.

50. Guarrera JV, Nasr SH, Reverte CM, Samstein B, et al. Microscopic intrarenal particles after pulsatile machine preservation do not adversely affect outcomes after renal transplantation. *Transplant Proc* 2006; **38**: 3384–3387.

51. Perico N, Cattaneo D, Sayegh MH, Remuzzi G. Delayed graft function in kidney transplantation. *Lancet* 2004; **364**: 1814–1827.

52. Dittrich S, Groneberg DA, von Loeper J, Lippek F, et al. Influence of cold storage on renal ischemia reperfusion injury after non-heart-beating donor explantation. *Nephron Exp Nephrol* 2004; **96**: e97–e102.

53. Arias-Diaz J, Alvarez J, del Barrio MR, Balibrea JL. Non-heart-beating donation: current state of the art. *Transplant Proc* 2004; **36**: 1891–1893.

54. Renkens JJ, Rouflart MM, Christiaans MH, van den Berg-Loonen EM, et al. Outcome of nonheart-beating donor kidneys with prolonged delayed graft function after transplantation. *Am J Transplant* 2005; **5**: 2704–2709.

55. Rudich SM, Kaplan B, Magee JC, Arenas JD, et al. Renal transplantations performed using non-heart-beating organ donors: going back to the future? *Transplantation* 2002; **74**: 1715–1720.

56. Sanchez-Fructuoso A, Prats Sanchez D, Marques Vidas M, Lopez De Novales E, et al. Non-heart beating donors. *Nephrol Dial Transplant* 2004; **19 Suppl. 3:** iii26–iii31.

57. Nicholson ML, Metcalfe MS, White SA, Waller JR, et al. A comparison of the results of renal transplantation from non-heart-beating, conventional cadaveric, and living donors. *Kidney Int* 2000; **58:** 2585–2591.

58. Troppmann C, Gillingham KJ, Gruessner RW, Dunn DL, et al. Delayed graft function in the absence of rejection has no long-term impact. A study of cadaver kidney recipients with good graft function at 1 year after transplantation. *Transplantation* 1996; **61:** 1331–1337.

59. Smith KD, Wrenshall LE, Nicosia RF, Pichler R, et al. Delayed graft function and cast nephropathy associated with tacrolimus plus rapamycin use. *J Am Soc Nephrol* 2003; **14:** 1037–1045.

60. Ebcioglu Z, Cohen DJ, Crew RJ, Hardy MA, et al. Osmotic nephrosis in a renal transplant recipient. *Kidney Int* 2006; **70:** 1873–1876.

61. de Vries B, Walter SJ, Peutz-Kootstra CJ, Wolfs TG, et al. The mannose-binding lectin-pathway is involved in complement activation in the course of renal ischemia-reperfusion injury. *Am J Pathol* 2004; **165:** 1677–1688.

62. Nickeleit V, Zeiler M, Gudat F, Thiel G, et al. Detection of the complement degradation product C4d in renal allografts: diagnostic and therapeutic implications. *J Am Soc Nephrol* 2002; **13:** 242–251.

63. Molitoris BA, Sutton TA. Endothelial injury and dysfunction: role in the extension phase of acute renal failure. *Kidney Int* 2004; **66:** 496–499.

64. Bonventre JV, Zuk A. Ischemic acute renal failure: an inflammatory disease? *Kidney Int* 2004; **66:** 480–485.

65. Shoskes DA, Parfrey NA, Halloran PF. Increased major histocompatibility complex antigen expression in unilateral ischemic acute tubular necrosis in the mouse. *Transplantation* 1990; **49:** 201–207.

66. Howard RJ, Pfaff WW, Brunson ME, Scornik JC, et al. Increased incidence of rejection in patients with delayed graft function. *Clinical Transplantation* 1994; **8:** 527–531.

67. Takemoto SK, Pinsky BW, Schnitzler MA, Lentine KL, et al. A retrospective analysis of immunosuppression compliance, dose reduction and discontinuation in kidney transplant recipients. *Am J Transplant* 2007; **7:** 2704–2711.

68. Kasiske BL, Gaston RS, Gourishankar S, Halloran PF, et al. Long-term deterioration of kidney allograft function. *Am J Transplant* 2005; **5:** 1405–1414.

69. Cecka JM. The OPTN/UNOS Renal Transplant Registry. *Clinical Transplants 2003.* UCLA Immunogenetics Center: Los Angeles, CA, 2004, p. 1.

70. Mihatsch MJ, Nickeleit V, Gudat F. Morphologic criteria of chronic renal allograft rejection. *Transplant Proc* 1999; **31:** 1295–1297.

71. Wieczorek G, Bigaud M, Menninger K, Riesen S, et al. Acute and chronic vascular rejection in nonhuman primate kidney transplantation. *Am J Transplant* 2006; **6:** 1285–1296.

72. Colvin RB. Kidney. In: Colvin RB, and Bhan AK, McCluskey RT (eds). *Diagnostic Immunopathology*, 2nd edn. Raven Press: New York, 1995, pp. 329–365.

73. Mauiyyedi S, Colvin RB. Pathology of kidney transplantation. In: Morris PJ (ed). *Kidney Transplantation*, 5th edn. W.B. Saunders Co.: Philadelphia, PA, 2001, pp. 243–376.

74. Racusen LC, Solez K, Colvin RB, Bonsib SM, et al. The Banff 97 working classification of renal allograft pathology. *Kidney Int* 1999; **55:** 713–723.

75. Feucht HE, Schneeberger H, Hillebrand G, Burkhardt K, et al. Capillary deposition of C4d complement fragment and early renal graft loss. *Kidney International* 1993; **43:** 1333–1338.

76. Nickeleit V, Mihatsch MJ. Kidney transplants, antibodies and rejection: is C4d a magic marker? *Nephrol Dial Transplant* 2003; **18:** 2232–2239.

77. Nickeleit V, Andreoni K. The classification and treatment of antibody-mediated renal allograft injury: where do we stand? *Kidney Int* 2007; **71:** 7–11.

78. Sun Q, Liu ZH, Cheng Z, Chen J, et al. Treatment of early mixed cellular and humoral renal allograft rejection with tacrolimus and mycophenolate mofetil. *Kidney Int* 2007; **71:** 24–30.

79. Al-Aly Z, Reddivari V, Moiz A, Balasubramanian G, et al. Renal allograft biopsies in the era of C4d staining: the need for change in the Banff classification system. *Transplant Int* 2008; **21:** 268–275.

80. Solez K, Axelsen RA, Benediktsson H, Burdick JF, et al. International standardization of criteria for the histologic diagnosis of renal allograft rejection: the Banff working classification of kidney transplant pathology. *Kidney Int* 1993; **44:** 411–422.

81. Solez K, Colvin R, Racusen L, Haas M, et al. Banff 07 Classification of Renal Allograft Pathology: Updates and Future Directions. *Am J Transplant* 2008; **8:** 753–760.

82. Nickeleit V, Zeiler M, Gudat F, Thiel G, et al. Histological characteristics of interstitial renal allograft rejection. *Kidney Blood Press Res* 1998; **21:** 230–232.

83. Saad R, Gritsch HA, Shapiro R, Jordan M, et al. Clinical significance of renal allograft biopsies with "borderline changes," as defined in the Banff Schema. *Transplantation* 1997; **64:** 992–995.

84. Gibson IW, Gwinner W, Brocker V, Sis B, et al. Peritubular Capillaritis in Renal Allografts: Prevalence, Scoring System, Reproducibility and Clinicopathological Correlates. *Am J Transplant* 2008; **8(4):** 819–25.

85. Mihatsch MJ, Nickeleit V. [Dynamic and flexible classification of transplant rejection]. *Verh Dtsch Ges Pathol* 2002; **86:** 19–27.

86. Schuerich W, Seemayer TA, Hinz B, Gabbiani G. Myofibroblast. In: Mills SE (ed). *Histology for pathologists*, 3rd edn. Lippincott Williams&Wilkins: Philadelphia, PA, 2007, pp. 123–164.

87. Solez K, Colvin RB, Racusen LC, Sis B, et al. Banff '05 Meeting Report: differential diagnosis of chronic allograft injury and elimination of chronic allograft nephropathy ('CAN'). *Am J Transplant* 2007; **7:** 518–526.

88. Mueller TF, Einecke G, Reeve J, Sis B, *et al.* Microarray analysis of rejection in human kidney transplants using pathogenesis-based transcript sets. *Am J Transplant* 2007; **7:** 2712–2722.

89. Famulski KS, Broderick G, Einecke G, Hay K, *et al.* Transcriptome analysis reveals heterogeneity in the

injury response of kidney transplants. *Am J Transplant* 2007; **7**: 2483–2495.

90. Mengel M, Sis B, Halloran PF. SWOT analysis of Banff: strengths, weaknesses, opportunities and threats of the international Banff consensus process and classification system for renal allograft pathology. *Am J Transplant* 2007; **7**: 2221–2226.

91. Hiki Y, Leong AS, Mathew TH, Seymour AE, et al. Typing of intraglomerular mononuclear cells associated with transplant glomerular rejection. *Clin Nephrol* 1986; **26**: 244–249.

92. Bishop GA, Hall BM, Duggin GG, Horvath JS, et al. Immunopathology of renal allograft rejection analyzed with monoclonal antibodies to mononuclear cell markers. *Kidney Int* 1986; **29**: 708–717.

93. Zhang PL, Malek SK, Prichard JW, Lin F, et al. Monocyte-mediated acute renal rejection after combined treatment with preoperative Campath-1H (alemtuzumab) and postoperative immunosuppression. *Ann Clin Lab Sci* 2004; **34**: 209–213.

94. Hancock WW, Thomson NM, Atkins RC. Composition of interstitial cellular infiltrate identified by monoclonal antibodies in renal biopsies of rejecting human renal allografts. *Transplantation* 1983; **35**: 458–463.

95. Hancock WW, Atkins RC. Immunohistological analysis of sequential renal biopsies from patients with acute renal rejection. *J Immunol* 1985; **136**: 2416–2420.

96. Charney DA, Nadasdy T, Lo AW, Racusen LC. Plasma cell-rich acute renal allograft rejection. *Transplantation* 1999; **68**: 791–797.

97. Meehan SM, Domer P, Josephson M, Donoghue M, et al. The clinical and pathologic implications of plasmacytic infiltrates in percutaneous renal allograft biopsies. *Hum Pathol* 2001; **32**: 205–215.

98. Martins HL, Silva C, Martini D, Noronha IL. Detection of B lymphocytes (CD20+) in renal allograft biopsy specimens. *Transplant Proc* 2007; **39**: 432–434.

99. Mengel M, Gwinner W, Schwarz A, Bajeski R, et al. Infiltrates in protocol biopsies from renal allografts. *Am J Transplant* 2007; **7**: 356–365.

100. Bagnasco SM, Tsai W, Rahman MH, Kraus ES, et al. CD20-positive infiltrates in renal allograft biopsies with acute cellular rejection are not associated with worse graft survival. *Am J Transplant* 2007; **7**: 1968–1973.

101. Hippen BE, DeMattos A, Cook WJ, Kew CE, 2nd, et al. Association of CD20+ infiltrates with poorer clinical outcomes in acute cellular rejection of renal allografts. *Am J Transplant* 2005; **5**: 2248–2252.

102. Meleg-Smith S, Gauthier PM. Abundance of interstitial eosinophils in renal allografts is associated with vascular rejection. *Transplantation* 2005; **79**: 444–450.

103. Fahim T, Bohmig GA, Exner M, Huttary N, et al. The cellular lesion of humoral rejection: predominant recruitment of monocytes to peritubular and glomerular capillaries. *Am J Transplant* 2007; **7**: 385–393.

104. Colvin RB. Eye of the needle. *Am J Transplant* 2007; **7**: 267–268.

105. Loverre A, Capobianco C, Stallone G, Infante B, et al. Ischemia-reperfusion injury-induced abnormal dendritic cell traffic in the transplanted kidney with delayed graft function. *Kidney Int* 2007; **72**: 994–1003.

106. Woltman AM, de Fijter JW, Zuidwijk K, Vlug AG, et al. Quantification of dendritic cell subsets in human renal tissue under normal and pathological conditions. *Kidney Int* 2007; **71**: 1001–1008.

107. Lajoie G, Nadasdy T, Laszik Z, Blick KE, et al. Mast cells in acute cellular rejection of human renal allografts. *Mod Pathol* 1996; **9**: 1118–1125.

108. Hall BM, Bishop GA, Duggin GG, Horvath JS, et al. Increased expression of HLA-DR antigens on renal tubular cells in renal transplants: relevance to the rejection response. *Lancet* 1984; **2**: 247–251.

109. Nickeleit V, Miller M, Cosimi AB, Colvin RB. Adhesion molecules in human renal allograft rejection: Immunohistochemical analysis of ICAM-1, ICAM-2, ICAM-3, VCAM-1, and ELAM-1. In: Lipsky PE, Rothlein R,, Kishimoto TK, Faanes RB, et al. (eds). *Structure, Function, and Regulation of Molecules Involved in Leukocyte Adhesion.* Springer-Verlag: New York, 1993, pp. 380–387.

110. Wang X, Smith KD, Nicosia RF, Alpers CE, et al. Associations of C4d deposition, transplant glomerulopathy and rejection in renal allograft biopsies performed 10 or more years after transplantation. *Modern Path* 2008; **21 Suppl. 1:** 296A (abstract).

111. Herzenberg AM, Gill JS, Djurdjev O, Magil AB. C4d deposition in acute rejection: an independent long-term prognostic factor. *J Am Soc Nephrol* 2002; **13**: 234–241.

112. Nickeleit V, Mihatsch MJ. Kidney transplants, antibodies and rejection: is C4d a magic marker? *Nephrol Dial Transplant* 2003; **18**: 2232–2239.

113. Mauiyyedi S, Crespo M, Collins AB, Schneeberger EE, et al. Acute humoral rejection in kidney transplantation: II. Morphology, immunopathology, and pathologic classification. *J Am Soc Nephrol* 2002; **13**: 779–787.

114. Heller F, Lindenmeyer MT, Cohen CD, Brandt U, et al. The contribution of B cells to renal interstitial inflammation. *Am J Pathol* 2007; **170**: 457–468.

115. Gaber LW, Moore LW, Alloway RR, Flax SD, et al. Correlation between Banff classification, acute renal rejection scores and reversal of rejection. *Kidney Int* 1996; **49**: 481–487.

116. Nickeleit V, Vamvakas EC, Pascual M, Poletti BJ, et al. The prognostic significance of specific arterial lesions in acute renal allograft rejection. *J Am Soc Nephrol* 1998; **9**: 1301–1308.

117. Sarwal M, Chua MS, Kambham N, Hsieh SC, et al. Molecular heterogeneity in acute renal allograft rejection identified by DNA microarray profiling. *N Engl J Med* 2003; **349**: 125–138.

118. Eikmans M, Roos-van Groningen MC, Sijpkens YW, Ehrchen J, et al. Expression of surfactant protein-C, S100A8, S100A9, and B cell markers in renal allografts: investigation of the prognostic value. *J Am Soc Nephrol* 2005; **16**: 3771–3786.

119. Croker BP, Clapp WL, Abu Shamat AR, Kone BC, et al. Macrophages and chronic renal allograft nephropathy. *Kidney Int Suppl* 1996; **57**: S42–49.

120. Andersen CB, Ladefoged SD, Larsen S. Acute kidney graft rejection. A morphological and immunohistological

study on "zero-hour" and follow-up biopsies with special emphasis on cellular infiltrates and adhesion molecules. *APMIS* 1994; **102**: 23–37.

121. Gallon L, Gagliardini E, Benigni A, Kaufman D, et al. Immunophenotypic analysis of cellular infiltrate of renal allograft biopsies in patients with acute rejection after induction with alemtuzumab (Campath-1H). *Clin J Am Soc Nephrol* 2006; **1**: 539–545.

122. Weir MR, Hall-Craggs M, Shen SY, Posner JN, et al. The prognostic value of the eosinophil in acute renal allograft rejection. *Transplantation* 1986; **41**: 709–712.

123. Kormendi F, Amend WJ, Jr. The importance of eosinophil cells in kidney allograft rejection. *Transplantation* 1988; **45**: 537–539.

124. Zand MS. B-cell activity of polyclonal antithymocyte globulins. *Transplantation* 2006; **82**: 1387–1395.

125. Lehnhardt A, Mengel M, Pape L, Ehrich JH, et al. Nodular B-cell aggregates associated with treatment refractory renal transplant rejection resolved by rituximab. *Am J Transplant* 2006; **6**: 847–851.

126. Hsu AC, Arbus GS, Noriega E, Huber J. Renal allograft biopsy: A satisfactory adjunct for predicting renal function after graft rejection. *Clin Nephrol* 1976; **5**: 260–265.

127. Schroeder TJ, Weiss MA, Smith RD, Stephens GW, et al. The efficacy of OKT3 in vascular rejection. *Transplantation* 1991; **51**: 312–315.

128. Macdonald FI, Ashraf S, Picton M, Dyer PA, et al. Banff criteria as predictors of outcome following acute renal allograft rejection. *Nephrol Dialysis Transplant* 1999; **14**: 1692–1697.

129. Gaber LW. Borderline changes in the Banff schema: rejection or no rejection? *Transplant Proc* 2004; **36**: 755–757.

130. Meehan SM, Siegel CT, Aronson AJ, Bartosh SM, et al. The relationship of untreated borderline infiltrates by the Banff criteria to acute rejection in renal allograft biopsies. *J Am Soc Nephrol* 1999; **10**: 1806–1814.

131. Schweitzer EJ, Drachenberg CB, Anderson L, Papadimetriou JC, et al. Significance of the Banff borderline biopsy. *Am J Kidney Dis* 1996; **28**: 585–588.

132. Zhang PL, Rothblum LI, Han WK, Blasick TM, et al. Kidney injury molecule-1 expression in transplant biopsies is a sensitive measure of cell injury. *Kidney Int* 2008; **73**: 608–614.

133. Gaber LW, Moore LW, Gaber AO, Tesi RJ, et al. Correlation of histology to clinical rejection reversal: a thymoglobulin multicenter trial report. *Kidney Int* 1999; **55**: 2415–2422.

134. Shimizu A, Yamada K, Sachs DH, Colvin RB. Persistent rejection of peritubular capillaries and tubules is associated with progressive interstitial fibrosis. *Kidney Int* 2002; **61**: 1867–1879.

135. Rush D, Nickerson P, Gough J, McKenna R, et al. Beneficial effects of treatment of early subclinical rejection: a randomized study. *J Am Soc Nephrol* 1998; **9**: 2129–2134.

136. Jurcic V, Jeruc J, Maric S, Ferluga D. Histomorphological assessment of phlebitis in renal allografts. *Croat Med J* 2007; **48**: 327–332.

137. Torbenson M, Randhawa P. Arcuate and interlobular phlebitis in renal allografts. *Hum Pathol* 2001; **32**: 1388–1391.

138. Stuht S, Gwinner W, Franz I, Schwarz A, et al. Lymphatic neoangiogenesis in human renal allografts: results from sequential protocol biopsies. *Am J Transplant* 2007; **7**: 377–384.

139. Lobo PI, Spencer CE, Isaacs RB, McCullough C. Hyperacute renal allograft rejection from anti-HLA class 1 antibody to B cells – antibody detection by two color FCXM was possible only after using pronase-digested donor lymphocytes. *Transplant Int* 1997; **10**: 69–73.

140. Dragun D, Muller DN, Brasen JH, Fritsche L, et al. Angiotensin II type 1-receptor activating antibodies in renal-allograft rejection. *N Engl J Med* 2005; **352**: 558–569.

141. Trpkov K, Campbell P, Pazderka F, Cockfield S, et al. Pathologic features of acute renal allograft rejection associated with donor-specific antibody. Analysis using the Banff grading schema. *Transplantation* 1996; **61**: 1586–1592.

142. Lobo PI, Spencer CE, Stevenson WC, Pruett TL. Evidence demonstrating poor kidney graft survival when acute rejections are associated with IgG donor-specific lymphocytotoxin. *Transplantation* 1995; **59**: 357–360.

143. Cosimi AB, Conti D, Delmonico FL, Preffer FI, et al. In vivo effects of monoclonal antibody to ICAM-1 (CD54) in nonhuman primates with renal allografts. *J Immunol* 1990; **144**: 4604–4612.

144. Sadahiro M, McDonald TO, Allen MD. Reduction in cellular and vascular rejection by blocking leukocyte adhesion molecule receptors. *Am J Pathol* 1993; **142**: 675–683.

145. Alpers CE, Gordon D, Gown AM. Immunophenotype of vascular rejection in renal transplants. *Modern Path* 1990; **3**: 198–203.

146. Saisu K, Morozumi K, Suzuki K, Fujita K. Significance of interstitial lesions as the early indicator for acute vascular rejection in human renal allografts. *Clin Transplant* 1999; **13 Suppl. 1**: 17–23.

147. Mauiyyedi S, Pelle PD, Saidman S, Collins AB, et al. Chronic humoral rejection: identification of antibody-mediated chronic renal allograft rejection by C4d deposits in peritubular capillaries. *J Am Soc Nephrol* 2001; **12**: 574–582.

148. Collins AB, Schneeberger EE, Pascual MA, Saidman SL, et al. Complement activation in acute humoral renal allograft rejection: diagnostic significance of C4d deposits in peritubular capillaries. *J Am Soc Nephrol* 1999; **10**: 2208–2214.

149. Russell PS, Chase CM, Colvin RB. Alloantibody- and T cell-mediated immunity in the pathogenesis of transplant arteriosclerosis: lack of progression to sclerotic lesions in B cell-deficient mice. *Transplantation* 1997; **64**: 1531–1536.

150. Delaney VB, Campbell WG, Jr., Nasr SA, McCue PA, et al. Efficacy of OKT3 monoclonal antibody therapy in steroid-resistant, predominantly vascular acute rejection. A report of three cases with morphologic and immunophenotypic evaluation. *Transplantation* 1988; **45**: 743–748.

151. Haas M, Kraus ES, Samaniego-Picota M, Racusen LC, et al. Acute renal allograft rejection with intimal arteritis: Histologic predictors of response to therapy and graft survival. *Kidney Int* 2002; **61**: 1516–1526.

152. Grimm PC, Nickerson P, Jeffery J, Savani RC, et al. Neointimal and tubulointerstitial infiltration by recipient mesenchymal cells in chronic renal-allograft rejection. *N Engl J Med* 2001; **345**: 93–97.

153. Nolan CR, Saenz KP, Thomas CA, 3rd, Murphy KD. Role of the eosinophil in chronic vascular rejection of renal allografts. *Am J Kidney Dis* 1995; **26**: 634–642.

154. Axelsen RA, Seymour AE, Mathew TH, Canny A, et al. Glomerular transplant rejection: a distinctive pattern of early graft damage. *Clin Nephrol* 1985; **23**: 1–11.

155. Habib R, Broyer M. Clinical significance of allograft glomerulopathy. *Kidney Int* 1993; **43**: S95–98.

156. Tuazon TV, Schneeberger EE, Bhan AK, McCluskey RT, et al. Mononuclear cells in acute allograft glomerulopathy. *Am J Pathol* 1987; **129**: 119–132.

157. Messias NC, Eustace JA, Zachary AA, Tucker PC, et al. Cohort study of the prognostic significance of acute transplant glomerulitis in acutely rejecting renal allografts. *Transplantation* 2001; **72**: 655–660.

158. Richardson WP, Colvin RB, Cheeseman SH, Tolkoff-Rubin NE, et al. Glomerulopathy associated with cytomegalovirus viremia in renal allografts. *N Engl J Med* 1981; **305**: 57–63.

159. Regele H, Bohmig GA, Habicht A, Gollowitzer D, et al. Capillary deposition of complement split product C4d in renal allografts is associated with basement membrane injury in peritubular and glomerular capillaries: a contribution of humoral immunity to chronic allograft rejection. *J Am Soc Nephrol* 2002; **13**: 2371–2380.

160. Tinckam KJ, Djurdjev O, Magil AB. Glomerular monocytes predict worse outcomes after acute renal allograft rejection independent of C4d status. *Kidney Int* 2005; **68**: 1866–1874.

161. Magil AB. Infiltrating cell types in transplant glomerulitis: relationship to peritubular capillary C4d deposition. *Am J Kidney Dis* 2005; **45**: 1084–1089.

162. Herrera GA, Alexander RW, Cooley CF, Luke RG, et al. Cytomegalovirus glomerulopathy: a controversial lesion. *Kidney Int* 1986; **29**: 725–733.

163. Olsen S, Spencer E, Cockfield S, Marcussen N, et al. Endocapillary glomerulitis in the renal allograft. *Transplantation* 1995; **59**: 1421–1425.

164. Ozdemir BH, Demirhan B, Gungen Y. The presence and prognostic importance of glomerular macrophage infiltration in renal allografts. *Nephron* 2002; **90**: 442–446.

165. Gloor JM, Sethi S, Stegall MD, Park WD, et al. Transplant glomerulopathy: subclinical incidence and association with alloantibody. *Am J Transplant* 2007; **7**: 2124–2132.

166. Maryniak RK, First MR, Weiss MA. Transplant glomerulopathy: evolution of morphologically distinct changes. *Kidney Int* 1985; **27**: 799–806.

167. Zollinger HU, Mihatsch MJ. *Renal Pathology in Biopsy*, 1st edn, vol. 1. Springer Verlag: Berlin, 1978.

168. Drachenberg CB, Steinberger E, Hoehn-Saric E, Heffes A, et al. Specificity of intertubular capillary changes: comparative ultrastructural studies in renal allografts and native kidneys. *Ultrastruct Pathol* 1997; **21**: 227–233.

169. Sijpkens YW, Joosten SA, Wong MC, Dekker FW, et al. Immunologic risk factors and glomerular C4d deposits in chronic transplant glomerulopathy. *Kidney Int* 2004; **65**: 2409–2418.

170. Smith RN, Kawai T, Boskovic S, Nadazdin O, et al. Chronic antibody mediated rejection of renal allografts: pathological, serological and immunologic features in non-human primates. *Am J Transplant* 2006; **6**: 1790–1798.

171. Zwirner J, Felber E, Burger R, Bitter-Suermann D, et al. Classical pathway of complement activation in mammalian kidneys. *Immunology* 1993; **80**: 162–167.

172. Zwirner J, Felber E, Herzog V, Riethmuller G, et al. Classical pathway of complement activation in normal and diseased human glomeruli. *Kidney Int* 1989; **36**: 1069–1077.

173. Feucht HE, Felber E, Gokel MJ, Hillebrand G, et al. Vascular deposition of complement-split products in kidney allografts with cell-mediated rejection. *Clin Exp Immunol* 1991; **86**: 464–470.

174. Feucht HE, Opelz G. The humoral immune response towards HLA class II determinants in renal transplantation. *Kidney Int* 1996; **50**: 1464–1475.

175. Kluth-Pepper B, Schneeberger H, Lederer SR, Albert E, et al. Impact of humoral alloreactivity on the survival of renal allografts. *Transplant Proc* 1998; **30**: 1772.

176. Lederer SR, Kluth-Pepper B, Schneeberger H, Albert E, et al. Impact of humoral alloreactivity early after transplantation on the long-term survival of renal allografts. *Kidney Int* 2001; **59**: 334–341.

177. Racusen LC, Colvin RB, Solez K, Mihatsch MJ, et al. Antibody-mediated rejection criteria—an addition to the Banff 97 classification of renal allograft rejection. *Am J Transplant* 2003; **3**: 708–714.

178. Thiel S, Vorup-Jensen T, Stover CM, Schwaeble W, et al. A second serine protease associated with mannan-binding lectin that activates complement. *Nature* 1997; **386**: 506–510.

179. Petersen SV, Thiel S, Jensen L, Steffensen R, et al. An assay for the mannan-binding lectin pathway of complement activation. *J Immunol Methods* 2001; **257**: 107–116.

180. Imai N, Nishi S, Alchi B, Ueno M, et al. Immunohistochemical evidence of activated lectin pathway in kidney allografts with peritubular capillary C4d deposition. *Nephrol Dial Transplant* 2006; **21**: 2589–2595.

181. Bohmig GA, Exner M, Habicht A, Schillinger M, et al. Capillary C4d deposition in kidney allografts: a specific marker of alloantibody-dependent graft injury. *J Am Soc Nephrol* 2002; **13**: 1091–1099.

182. Colvin RB. Pathology of renal allografts. In: Colvin RB, Bhan AK, McCluskey RT (eds). *Diagnostic Immunopathology*, 2nd edn. Raven Press: New York, 1995, pp. 329–366.

183. Colvin RB. General features of the allograft response. In: Colvin RB, Bhan AK, McCluskey RT (eds). *Diagnostic Immunopathology*, 2nd edn. Raven Press: New York, 1995, pp. 311–328.

184. Wahrmann M, Exner M, Schillinger M, Haidbauer B, et al. Pivotal role of complement-fixing HLA alloantibodies

in presensitized kidney allograft recipients. *Am J Transplant* 2006; **6**: 1033–1041.

185. Mengel M, Bogers J, Bosmans J-P, Serón D, et al. Incidence of C4d stain in protocol biopsies from renal allografts: Results from a multicenter trial. *Am J Transplant* 2005; **5(5)**: 1490–4.

186. Kato M, Morozumi K, Takeuchi O, Oikawa T, et al. Complement fragment C4d deposition in peritubular capillaries in acute humoral rejection after ABO blood group-incompatible human kidney transplantation. *Transplantation* 2003; **75**: 663–665.

187. Feucht HE. Complement C4d in graft capillaries – the missing link in the recognition of humoral alloreactivity. *Am J Transplant* 2003; **3**: 646–652.

188. Regele H, Exner M, Watschinger B, Wenter C, et al. Endothelial C4d deposition is associated with inferior kidney allograft outcome independently of cellular rejection. *Nephrol Dial Transplant* 2001; **16**: 2058–2066.

189. Seemayer CA, Gaspert A, Nickeleit V, Mihatsch MJ. C4d staining of renal allograft biopsies: a comparative analysis of different staining techniques. *Nephrol Dial Transplant* 2007; **22**: 568–576.

190. Magil AB, Tinckam K. Monocytes and peritubular capillary C4d deposition in acute renal allograft rejection. *Kidney Int* 2003; **63**: 1888–1893.

191. Demirci C, Sen S, Sezak M, Sarsik B, et al. Incidence and importance of c4d deposition in renal allograft dysfunction. *Transplant Proc* 2008; **40**: 174–177.

192. Haas M, Rahman MH, Racusen LC, Kraus ES, et al. C4d and C3d staining in biopsies of ABO- and HLA-incompatible renal allografts: correlation with histologic findings. *Am J Transplant* 2006; **6**: 1829–1840.

193. Merion RM, White DJ, Thiru S, Evans DB, et al. Cyclosporine: five years' experience in cadaveric renal transplantation. *N Engl J Med* 1984; **310**: 148–154.

194. Borel JF, Kis ZL. The discovery and development of cyclosporine (Sandimmune). *Transplant Proc* 1991; **23**: 1867–1874.

195. Danovitch GM. Cyclosporin or tacrolimus: which agent to choose? *Nephrol Dial Transplant* 1997; **12**: 1566–1568.

196. Randhawa PS, Shapiro R, Jordan ML, Starzl TE, et al. The histopathological changes associated with allograft rejection and drug toxicity in renal transplant recipients maintained on FK506. Clinical significance and comparison with cyclosporine. *Am J Surg Pathol* 1993; **17**: 60–68.

197. Japanese FK Study Group. Morphological characteristics of renal allografts showing renal dysfunction under FK 506 therapy: is graft biopsy available to reveal the morphological findings corresponding with FK 506 nephropathy? *Transplant Proc* 1993; **25**: 624–627.

198. Schmidt RJ, Venkat KK, Dumler F. Hemolytic-uremic syndrome in a renal transplant recipient on FK 506 immunosuppression. *Transplant Proc* 1991; **23**: 3156–3157.

199. Mihatsch MJ, Kyo M, Morozumi K, Yamaguchi Y, et al. The side-effects of ciclosporine-A and tacrolimus. *Clin Nephrol* 1998; **49**: 356–363.

200. Randhawa PS, Tsamandas AC, Magnone M, Jordan M, et al. Microvascular changes in renal allografts associated with FK506 (Tacrolimus) therapy. *Am J Surg Pathol* 1996; **20**: 306–312.

201. Fischer G, Wittmann-Liebold B, Lang K, Kiefhaber T, et al. Cyclophilin and peptidyl-prolyl cis-trans isomerase are probably identical proteins. *Nature* 1989; **337**: 476–478.

202. Takahashi N, Hayano T, Suzuki M. Peptidyl-prolyl cis-trans isomerase is the cyclosporin A-binding protein cyclophilin. *Nature* 1989; **337**: 473–475.

203. Borel JF, Baumann G, Chapman I, Donatsch P, et al. In vivo pharmacological effects of ciclosporin and some analogues. *Advance Pharmacol* 1996; **35**: 115–246.

204. Kapturczak MH, Meier-Kriesche HU, Kaplan B. Pharmacology of calcineurin antagonists. *Transplant Proc* 2004; **36**: 25S–32S.

205. Wiederrecht G, Hung S, Chan HK, Marcy A, et al. Characterization of high molecular weight FK-506 binding activities reveals a novel FK-506-binding protein as well as a protein complex. *J Biol Chem* 1992; **267**: 21753–21760.

206. Maki N, Sekiguchi F, Nishimaki J, Miwa K, et al. Complementary DNA encoding the human T-cell FK506-binding protein, a peptidylprolyl cis-trans isomerase distinct from cyclophilin. *Proc Natl Acad Sci USA* 1990; **87**: 5440–5443.

207. Keown P. Molecular and clinical therapeutics of cyclosporine in transplantation. In: Ginns I CA, Morris PJ, eds. (ed). *Transplantation*. Blackwell Science: Malden, MA, 1999.

208. Wong W, Venetz JP, Tolkoff-Rubin N, Pascual M. 2005 immunosuppressive strategies in kidney transplantation: which role for the calcineurin inhibitors? *Transplantation* 2005; **80**: 289–296.

209. Halloran PF. Immunosuppressive drugs for kidney transplantation. *N Engl J Med* 2004; **351**: 2715–2729.

210. First MR. Tacrolimus based immunosuppression. *J Nephrol* 2004; **17 Suppl. 8**: S25–S31.

211. Webster AC, Woodroffe RC, Taylor RS, Chapman JR, et al. Tacrolimus versus ciclosporin as primary immunosuppression for kidney transplant recipients: meta-analysis and meta-regression of randomised trial data. *BMJ* 2005; **331**: 810.

212. Kramer BK, Montagnino G, Del Castillo D, Margreiter R, et al. Efficacy and safety of tacrolimus compared with cyclosporin A microemulsion in renal transplantation: 2 year follow-up results. *Nephrol Dial Transplant* 2005; **20**: 968–973.

213. Bowman LJ, Brennan DC. The role of tacrolimus in renal transplantation. *Expert Opin Pharmacother* 2008; **9**: 635–643.

214. Kaplan B, Schold JD, Meier-Kriesche HU. Long-term graft survival with neoral and tacrolimus: a paired kidney analysis. *J Am Soc Nephrol* 2003; **14**: 2980–2984.

215. Meier-Kriesche HU, Kaplan B. Cyclosporine microemulsion and tacrolimus are associated with decreased chronic allograft failure and improved long-term graft survival as compared with sandimmune. *Am J Transplant* 2002; **2**: 100–104.

216. Nankivell BJ, Borrows RJ, Fung CL, O'Connell PJ, et al. Calcineurin inhibitor nephrotoxicity: longitudinal assessment by protocol histology. *Transplantation* 2004; **78**: 557–565.

217. Stratta P, Canavese C, Quaglia M, Balzola F, et al. Post-transplantation chronic renal damage in nonrenal transplant recipients. *Kidney Int* 2005; **68**: 1453–1463.

218. Mihatsch MJ, Theil G, Spichtin HP, Oberholzer M, et al. Morphological findings in kidney transplants after treatment with cyclosporine. *Transplantation Proc* 1983; **15 Suppl. 1**: 2821–2835.

219. Mihatsch MJ, Ryffel B, Gudat F. The differential diagnosis between rejection and cyclosporine toxicity. *Kidney International – Supplement* 1995; **52**: S63–69.

220. Mihatsch MJ, Morozumi K, Strom EH, Ryffel B, et al. Renal transplant morphology after long-term therapy with cyclosporine. *Transplant Proc* 1995; **27**: 39–42.

221. Mihatsch MJ, Gudat F, Ryffel B, Thiel G. Cyclosporine Nephropathy. In: Tisher CC, Brenner BM (eds). *Renal Pathology – With Clinical and Functional Correlations*, 2nd edn, vol. 2. J.B. Lippincott Company: Philadelphia, PA, 1994, pp. 1641–1681.

222. Ojo AO, Held PJ, Port FK, Wolfe RA, et al. Chronic renal failure after transplantation of a nonrenal organ. *N Engl J Med* 2003; **349**: 931–940.

223. English RF, Pophal SA, Bacanu SA, Fricker J, et al. Long-term comparison of tacrolimus- and cyclosporine-induced nephrotoxicity in pediatric heart-transplant recipients. *Am J Transplant* 2002; **2**: 769–773.

224. Mihatsch MJ, Thiel G, Basler V, Ryffel B, et al. Morphological patterns in cyclosporine-treated renal transplant recipients. *Transplant Proc* 1985; **17**: 101–116.

225. Hall BM, Tiller DJ, Duggin GG, Horvath JS, et al. Post-transplant acute renal failure in cadaver renal recipients treated with cyclosporine. *Kidney Int* 1985; **28**: 178–186.

226. Ryffel B, Siegel H, Thiel G, Mihatsch MJ. Experimental cyclosporine nephrotoxicity. In: J.F. Burdick LCR, G.M. Williams, K. Solez (ed). *Kidney Transplant Rejection: Diagnosis and Treatment*, 2nd edn. Marcel-Dekker: New York, 1992, pp. 601–627.

227. Mihatsch M, Thiel G, Ryffel B. Cyclosporine nephrotoxicity. *Advance Nephrol* 1988; **17**: 303–320.

228. Sacchi G, Benetti A, Falchetti M, Grigolato P, et al. Ultrastructural renal findings in allografted kidneys of patients treated with ciclosporin A. *Appl Pathol* 1987; **5**: 101–107.

229. Tsinalis D, Dickenmann M, Brunner F, Gurke L, et al. Acute renal failure in a renal allograft recipient treated with intravenous immunoglobulin. *Am J Kidney Dis* 2002; **40**: 667–670.

230. Haas M, Sonnenday CJ, Cicone JS, Rabb H, et al. Isometric tubular epithelial vacuolization in renal allograft biopsy specimens of patients receiving low-dose intravenous immunoglobulin for a positive crossmatch. *Transplantation* 2004; **78**: 549–556.

231. Moreau JF, Droz D, Sabto J, Jungers P, et al. Osmotic nephrosis induced by water-soluble triiodinated contrast media in man. A retrospective study of 47 cases. *Radiology* 1975; **115**: 329–336.

232. Yamaguchi Y, Teraoka S, Yagisawa T, Takahashi K, et al. Ultrastructural study of cyclosporine-associated arteriolopathy in renal allografts. *Transplant Proc* 1989; **21**: 1517–1522.

233. Bergstrand A, Bohmann SO, Farnsworth A, Gokel JM, et al. Renal histopathology in kidney transplant recipients immunosuppressed with cyclosporin A: results of an international workshop. *Clin Nephrol* 1985; **24**: 107–119.

234. Strom EH, Epper R, Mihatsch MJ. Ciclosporin-associated arteriolopathy: the renin producing vascular smooth muscle cells are more sensitive to ciclosporin toxicity. *Clin Nephrol* 1995; **43**: 226–231.

235. Strom EH, Thiel G, Mihatsch MJ. Prevalence of cyclosporine-associated arteriolopathy in renal transplant biopsies from 1981 to 1992. *Transplant Proc* 1994; **26**: 2585–2587.

236. Savoldi S, Scolari F, Sandrini S, Scaini P, et al. Cyclosporine chronic nephrotoxicity: Histologic follow up at 6 and 18 months after renal transplant. *Transplant Proc* 1988; **20**: 777–784.

237. Collins BS, Davis CL, Marsh CL, McVicar JP, et al. Reversible cyclosporine arteriolopathy. *Transplantation* 1992; **54**: 732–734.

238. Morozumi K, Thiel G, Albert FW, Banfi G, et al. Studies on morphological outcome of cyclosporine-associated arteriolopathy after discontinuation of cyclosporine in renal allografts. *Clin Nephrol* 1992; **38**: 1–8.

239. Franceschini N, Alpers CE, Bennett WM, Andoh TF. Cyclosporine arteriolopathy: effects of drug withdrawal. *Am J Kidney Dis* 1998; **32**: 247–253.

240. Bren A, Pajek J, Grego K, Buturovic J, et al. Follow-up of kidney graft recipients with cyclosporine-associated hemolytic-uremic syndrome and thrombotic microangiopathy. *Transplant Proc* 2005; **37**: 1889–1891.

241. Takeda A, Morozumi K, Uchida K, Yokoyama I, et al. Is cyclosporine-associated glomerulopathy a new glomerular lesion in renal allografts using CyA? *Transplant Proc* 1993; **25**: 515–517.

242. Nankivell BJ, Borrows RJ, Fung CL, O'Connell PJ, et al. Evolution and pathophysiology of renal-transplant glomerulosclerosis. *Transplantation* 2004; **78**: 461–468.

243. Rangel EB, Gonzalez AM, Linhares MM, Araujo SR, et al. Thrombotic microangiopathy after simultaneous pancreas-kidney transplantation. *Clin Transplant* 2007; **21**: 241–245.

244. Karthikeyan V, Parasuraman R, Shah V, Vera E, et al. Outcome of plasma exchange therapy in thrombotic microangiopathy after renal transplantation. *Am J Transplant* 2003; **3**: 1289–1294.

245. Hochstetler LA, Flanigan MJ, Lager DJ. Transplant-associated thrombotic microangiopathy: the role of IgG administration as initial therapy. *Am J Kidney Dis* 1994; **23**: 444–450.

246. Trimarchi HM, Truong LD, Brennan S, Gonzalez JM, et al. FK506-associated thrombotic microangiopathy: report of two cases and review of the literature. *Transplantation* 1999; **67**: 539–544.

247. Katafuchi R, Saito S, Ikeda K, Hirano T, et al. A case of late onset cyclosporine-induced hemolytic uremic syndrome resulting in renal graft loss. *Clin Transplant* 1999; **13 Suppl. 1**: 54–58.

248. Zarifian A, Meleg-Smith S, O'Donovan R, Tesi RJ, et al. Cyclosporine-associated thrombotic microangiopathy in renal allografts. *Kidney Int* 1999; **55**: 2457–2466.

249. Schwimmer J, Nadasdy TA, Spitalnik PF, Kaplan KL, et al. De novo thrombotic microangiopathy in renal transplant recipients: a comparison of hemolytic uremic syndrome with localized renal thrombotic microangiopathy. *Am J Kidney Dis* 2003; **41**: 471–479.

250. Sommer BG, Innes JT, Whitehurst RM, Sharma HM, et al. Cyclosporine-associated renal arteriopathy resulting in loss of allograft function. *Am J Surg* 1985; **149**: 756–764.

251. Candinas D, Keusch G, Schlumpf R, Burger HR, *et al.* Hemolytic-uremic syndrome following kidney transplantation: prognostic factors. *Schweizer Medizin Wochenschr J Suisse Med* 1994; **124**: 1789–1799.

252. Dominguez J, Kompatzki A, Norambuena R, Arenas J, et al. Benefits of early biopsy on the outcome of kidney transplantation. *Transplant Proc* 2005; **37**: 3361–3363.

253. Langer RM, Van Buren CT, Katz SM, Kahan BD. De novo hemolytic uremic syndrome after kidney transplantation in patients treated with cyclosporine-sirolimus combination. *Transplantation* 2002; **73**: 756–760.

254. Franco A, Hernandez D, Capdevilla L, Errasti P, et al. De novo hemolytic-uremic syndrome/thrombotic microangiopathy in renal transplant patients receiving calcineurin inhibitors: role of sirolimus. *Transplant Proc* 2003; **35**: 1764–1766.

255. Lewis RM, Verani RR, Vo C, Katz SM, et al. Evaluation of chronic renal disease in heart transplant recipients: importance of pretransplantation native kidney histologic evaluation. *J Heart Lung Transplant* 1994; **13**: 376–380.

256. Josephson MA, Chiu MY, Woodle ES, Thistlethwaite JR, et al. Drug-induced acute interstitial nephritis in renal allografts: histopathologic features and clinical course in six patients. *Am J Kidney Dis* 1999; **34**: 540–548.

257. Kormendi F, Amend W. The importance of eosinophil cells in kidney allograft rejection. *Transplantation* 1988; **45**: 537–539.

258. Hongwei W, Nanra RS, Stein A, Avis L, et al. Eosinophils in acute renal allograft rejection. *Transplant Immunol* 1994; **2**: 41–46.

259. Almirall J, Campistol JM, Sole M, Andreu J, et al. Blood and graft eosinophilia as a rejection index in kidney transplant. *Nephron* 1993; **65**: 304–309.

260. Hallgren R, Bohman SO, Fredens K. Activated eosinophil infiltration and deposits of eosinophil cationic protein in renal allograft rejection. *Nephron* 1991; **59**: 266–270.

261. Ten RM, Gleich GJ, Holley KE, Perkins JD, et al. Eosinophil granule major basic protein in acute renal allograft rejection. *Transplantation* 1989; **47**: 959–963.

262. Colvin RB, Fang LS-T. Interstitial nephritis. In: Tisher CC, Brenner BM (eds). *Renal Pathology*, 2nd edn. JB Lippincott: Philadelphia, PA, 1994, pp. 723–768.

263. Kirken RA, Wang YL. Molecular actions of sirolimus: sirolimus and mTor. *Transplant Proc* 2003; **35**: 227S–230S.

264. Bruns CJ, Koehl GE, Guba M, Yezhelyev M, et al. Rapamycin-induced endothelial cell death and tumor vessel thrombosis potentiate cytotoxic therapy against pancreatic cancer. *Clin Cancer Res* 2004; **10**: 2109–2119.

265. Guba M, Yezhelyev M, Eichhorn ME, Schmid G, et al. Rapamycin induces tumor-specific thrombosis via tissue factor in the presence of VEGF. *Blood* 2005; **105**: 4463–4469.

266. Guba M, von Breitenbuch P, Steinbauer M, Koehl G, et al. Rapamycin inhibits primary and metastatic tumor growth by antiangiogenesis: involvement of vascular endothelial growth factor. *Nat Med* 2002; **8**: 128–135.

267. Kahan BD. Sirolimus. In: Morris PJ (ed). *Kidney transplantation: principles and practice*, 5th edn. W.B. Saunders Company: Philadelphia, PA, 2001, pp. 279–288.

268. Fellstrom B. Cyclosporine nephrotoxicity. *Transplant Proc* 2004; **36**: 220S–223S.

269. Stallone G, Infante B, Schena A, Battaglia M, et al. Rapamycin for treatment of chronic allograft nephropathy in renal transplant patients. *J Am Soc Nephrol* 2005; **16**: 3755–3762.

270. Danovitch GM. Immunosuppressive medications and protocols for kidney transplantation. In: Danovitch GM (ed). *Handbook of kidney transplantation*, 3rd edn. Lippincott Williams and Wilkins: Philadelphia, PA, 2001, pp. 62–110.

271. Qi S, Xu D, Peng J, Vu MD, et al. Effect of tacrolimus (FK506) and sirolimus (rapamycin) mono- and combination therapy in prolongation of renal allograft survival in the monkey. *Transplantation* 2000; **69**: 1275–1283.

272. Podder H, Stepkowski SM, Napoli KL, Clark J, et al. Pharmacokinetic interactions augment toxicities of sirolimus/cyclosporine combinations. *J Am Soc Nephrol* 2001; **12**: 1059–1071.

273. Lo A, Egidi MF, Gaber LW, Shokouh-Amiri MH, et al. Observations regarding the use of sirolimus and tacrolimus in high-risk cadaveric renal transplantation. *Clin Transplant* 2004; **18**: 53–61.

274. Morelon E, Kreis H. Sirolimus therapy without calcineurin inhibitors: Necker Hospital 8-year experience. *Transplant Proc* 2003; **35**: 52S–57S.

275. Dean PG, Lund WJ, Larson TS, Prieto M, et al. Wound-healing complications after kidney transplantation: a prospective, randomized comparison of sirolimus and tacrolimus. *Transplantation* 2004; **77**: 1555–1561.

276. McTaggart RA, Tomlanovich S, Bostrom A, Roberts JP, et al. Comparison of outcomes after delayed graft function: sirolimus-based versus other calcineurin-inhibitor sparing induction immunosuppression regimens. *Transplantation* 2004; **78**: 475–480.

277. McTaggart RA, Gottlieb D, Brooks J, Bacchetti P, et al. Sirolimus prolongs recovery from delayed graft function after cadaveric renal transplantation. *Am J Transplant* 2003; **3**: 416–423.

278. Boratynska M, Banasik M, Patrzalek D, Szyber P, et al. Sirolimus delays recovery from posttransplant renal failure in kidney graft recipients. *Transplant Proc* 2005; **37**: 839–842.

279. Fervenza FC, Fitzpatrick PM, Mertz J, Erickson SB, et al. Acute rapamycin nephrotoxicity in native kidneys of patients with chronic glomerulopathies. *Nephrol Dial Transplant* 2004; **19**: 1288–1292.

280. Reynolds JC, Agodoa LY, Yuan CM, Abbott KC. Thrombotic microangiopathy after renal transplantation in the United States. *Am J Kidney Dis* 2003; **42**: 1058–1068.

281. Hardinger KL, Cornelius LA, Trulock EP, 3rd, Brennan DC. Sirolimus-induced leukocytoclastic vasculitis. *Transplantation* 2002; **74**: 739–743.

282. Pasqualotto AC, Bianco PD, Sukiennik TC, Furian R, et al. Sirolimus-induced leukocytoclastic vasculitis: the second case reported. *Am J Transplant* 2004; **4**: 1549–1551.

283. Sartelet H, Toupance O, Lorenzato M, Fadel F, et al. Sirolimus-induced thrombotic microangiopathy is associated with decreased expression of vascular endothelial growth factor in kidneys. *Am J Transplant* 2005; **5**: 2441–2447.

284. Novick AC, Hwei HH, Steinmuller D, Streem SB, et al. Detrimental effect of cyclosporine on initial function of cadaver renal allografts following extended preservation. Results of a randomized prospective study. *Transplantation* 1986; **42**: 154–158.

285. van den Akker JM, Wetzels JF, Hoitsma AJ. Proteinuria following conversion from azathioprine to sirolimus in renal transplant recipients. *Kidney Int* 2006; **70**: 1355–1357.

286. Letavernier E, Bruneval P, Mandet C, Van Huyen JP, et al. High sirolimus levels may induce focal segmental glomerulosclerosis de novo. *Clin J Am Soc Nephrol* 2007; **2**: 326–333.

287. Letavernier E, Pe'raldi MN, Pariente A, Morelon E, et al. Proteinuria following a switch from calcineurin inhibitors to sirolimus. *Transplantation* 2005; **80**: 1198–1203.

288. Merkel S, Mogilevskaja N, Mengel M, Haller H, et al. Side effects of sirolimus. *Transplant Proc* 2006; **38**: 714–715.

289. Mackenzie EF, Poulding JM, Harrison PR, Amer B. Human polyoma virus (HPV)—a significant pathogen in renal transplantation. *Proc Eur Dial Transplant Assoc* 1978; **15**: 352–360.

290. Binet I, Nickeleit V, Hirsch HH, Prince O, et al. Polyomavirus disease under new immunosuppressive drugs: a cause of renal graft dysfunction and graft loss. *Transplantation* 1999; **67**: 918–922.

291. Drachenberg CB, Beskow CO, Cangro CB, Bourquin PM, et al. Human polyoma virus in renal allograft biopsies: morphological findings and correlation with urine cytology. *Hum Pathol* 1999; **30**: 970–977.

292. Nickeleit V, Hirsch HH, Zeiler M, Gudat F, et al. BK-virus nephropathy in renal transplants-tubular necrosis, MHC-class II expression and rejection in a puzzling game. *Nephrol Dial Transplant* 2000; **15**: 324–332.

293. Randhawa PS, Finkelstein S, Scantlebury V, Shapiro R, et al. Human polyoma virus-associated interstitial nephritis in the allograft kidney. *Transplantation* 1999; **67**: 103–109.

294. Howell DN, Smith SR, Butterly DW, Klassen PS, et al. Diagnosis and management of BK polyomavirus interstitial nephritis in renal transplant recipients. *Transplantation* 1999; **68**: 1279–1288.

295. Cosio FG, Amer H, Grande JP, Larson TS, et al. Comparison of low versus high tacrolimus levels in kidney transplantation: assessment of efficacy by protocol biopsies. *Transplantation* 2007; **83**: 411–416.

296. Mengel M, Marwedel M, Radermacher J, Eden G, et al. Incidence of polyomavirus-nephropathy in renal allografts: influence of modern immunosuppressive drugs. *Nephrol Dial Transplant* 2003; **18**: 1190–1196.

297. Nickeleit V, Singh HK, Mihatsch MJ. Polyomavirus nephropathy: morphology, pathophysiology, and clinical management. *Curr Opin Nephrol Hypertens* 2003; **12**: 599–605.

298. Khamash HA, Wadei HM, Mahale AS, Larson TS, et al. Polyomavirus-associated nephropathy risk in kidney transplants: the influence of recipient age and donor gender. *Kidney Int* 2007; **71**: 1302–1309.

299. Ramos E, Drachenberg C, Hirsch HH, Munivenkatappa R, et al. BK polyomavirus allograft nephropathy (BKPVN): eight-fold decrease in graft loss with prospective screening and protocol biopsy. *Am J Transplant* **(Suppl.)** 2006; WTC 2006 congress abstracts: 121.

300. Gaber LW, Egidi MF, Stratta RJ, Lo A, et al. Clinical utility of histological features of polyomavirus allograft nephropathy. *Transplantation* 2006; **82**: 196–204.

301. Nickeleit V, Mihatsch MJ. Polyomavirus nephropathy in native kidneys and renal allografts: an update on an escalating threat. *Transplant Int* 2006; **19**: 960–973.

302. Sachdeva MS, Nada R, Jha V, Sakhuja V, et al. The high incidence of BK polyoma virus infection among renal transplant recipients in India. *Transplantation* 2004; **77**: 429–431.

303. Nada R, Sachdeva MU, Sud K, Jha V, et al. Co-infection by cytomegalovirus and BK polyoma virus in renal allograft, mimicking acute rejection. *Nephrol Dial Transplant* 2005; **20**: 994–996.

304. Mindlova M, Boucek P, Saudek F, Jedinakova T, et al. Kidney retransplantation following graft loss to polyoma virus-associated nephropathy: an effective treatment option in simultaneous pancreas and kidney transplant recipients. *Transplant Int* 2008; **21**: 353–356.

305. Polo C, Perez JL, Mielnichuck A, Fedele CG, et al. Prevalence and patterns of polyomavirus urinary excretion in immunocompetent adults and children. *Clin Microbiol Infect* 2004; **10**: 640–644.

306. Nickeleit V, Gordon J, Thompson D, Romeo C. Antibody titers and latent polyoma-BK-virus (BKV) loads in the general population: potential donor risk assessment for the development of BK-virus nephropathy (BKN) post transplantation. *J Am Soc Nephrol* (abstracts issue) 2004; **15**: 524A.

307. Hirsch HH, Knowles W, Dickenmann M, Passweg J, et al. Prospective study of polyomavirus type BK replication and nephropathy in renal-transplant recipients. *N Engl J Med* 2002; **347**: 488–496.

308. Nickeleit V, Hirsch HH, Binet IF, Gudat F, et al. Polyomavirus infection of renal allograft recipients: from latent infection to manifest disease. *J Am Soc Nephrol* 1999; **10**: 1080–1089.

309. Nickeleit V, Hirsch HH, Zeiler M, Gudat F, et al. BK-virus nephropathy in renal transplants-tubular necrosis, MHC-class II expression and rejection in a puzzling game. *Nephrol Dial Transplant* 2000; **15**: 324–332.

310. Nickeleit V, Klimkait T, Binet IF, Dalquen P, et al. Testing for polyomavirus type BK DNA in plasma to identify renal allograft recipients with viral nephropathy. *N Engl J Med* 2000; **342**: 1309–1315.

311. Nickeleit V, Steiger J, Mihatsch MJ. BK Virus Infection after Kidney Transplantation. *Graft* 2002; **5 (December Suppl.):** S46–S57.

312. Singh HK, Bubendorf L, Mihatsch MJ, Drachenberg CB, et al. Urine cytology findings of polyomavirus infections. In: Ahsan N (ed). *Polyomaviruses and Human Diseases*, 1st edn. Springer Science+Business Media, Landes Bioscience/Georgetown, TX, 2006, pp. 201–212.

313. Singh HK, Madden V, Shen YJ, Thompson D, et al. Negative staining electron microscopy of urine for the detection of polyomavirus infections. *Ultrastruct Pathol* 2006; **30(5):** 329–338.

314. Nickeleit V, Steiger J, MJ M. BK Virus Infection after Kidney Transplantation. *Graft* 2002; **5 (December Suppl.):** S46–S57.

315. Drachenberg CB, Papadimitriou JC, Hirsch HH, Wali R, et al. Histological patterns of polyomavirus nephropathy: correlation with graft outcome and viral load. *Am J Transplant* 2004; **4:** 2082–2092.

316. Drachenberg CB, Hirsch HH, Papadimitriou JC, Gosert R, et al. Polyomavirus BK versus JC replication and nephropathy in renal transplant recipients: a prospective evaluation. *Transplantation* 2007; **84:** 323–330.

317. Baksh FK, Finkelstein SD, Swalsky PA, Stoner GL, et al. Molecular genotyping of BK and JC viruses in human polyomavirus-associated interstitial nephritis after renal transplantation. *Am J Kidney Dis* 2001; **38:** 354–365.

318. Trofe J, Cavallo T, First MR, Weiskittel P, et al. Polyomavirus in kidney and kidney-pancreas transplantation: a defined protocol for immunosuppression reduction and histologic monitoring. *Transplant Proc* 2002; **34:** 1788–1789.

319. Kazory A, Ducloux D, Chalopin JM, Angonin R, et al. The first case of JC virus allograft nephropathy. *Transplantation* 2003; **76:** 1653–1655.

320. Milstone A, Vilchez RA, Geiger X, Fogo AB, et al. Polyomavirus simian virus 40 infection associated with nephropathy in a lung-transplant recipient. *Transplantation* 2004; **77:** 1019–1024.

321. Bruno B, Zager RA, Boeckh MJ, Gooley TA, et al. Adenovirus nephritis in hematopoietic stem-cell transplantation. *Transplantation* 2004; **77:** 1049–1057.

322. Nickeleit V, Hirsch HH, Binet IF, Gudat F, et al. Polyomavirus infection of renal allograft recipients: from latent infection to manifest disease. *J Am Soc Nephrol* 1999; **10:** 1080–1089.

323. Nickeleit V, Hirsch HH, Zeiler M, Gudat F, et al. BK-virus nephropathy in renal transplants-tubular necrosis, MHC-class II expression and rejection in a puzzling game. *Nephrol Dial Transplant* 2000; **15:** 324–332.

324. Celik B, Randhawa PS. Glomerular changes in BK virus nephropathy. *Hum Pathol* 2004; **35:** 367–370.

325. Nair R, Katz DA, Thomas CP. Diffuse glomerular crescents and peritubular immune deposits in a transplant kidney. *Am J Kidney Dis* 2006; **48:** 174–178.

326. Nickeleit V, Thompson B, Latour M, Chan G, et al. Tubulo-centric granulomatous interstitial nephritis in renal allograft recipients with polyomavirus nephropathy. *Lab Invest* 2007; **87 (Suppl. 1)** 274A (abstract).

327. Bracamonte ER, Furmanczyk PS, Smith KD, Nicosia RF, et al. Tubular basement membrane immune deposits associated with polyoma virus nephropathy in renal allografts. *Lab Invest* 2006; **86** 259A (abstract).

328. Singh D, Kiberd B, Gupta R, Alkhudair W, et al. Polyoma virus-induced hemorrhagic cystitis in renal transplantation patient with polyoma virus nephropathy. *Urology* 2006; **67:** 423 e411–423, e412.

329. Herawi M, Parwani AV, Chan T, Ali SZ, et al. Polyoma virus-associated cellular changes in the urine and bladder biopsy samples: a cytohistologic correlation. *Am J Surg Pathol* 2006; **30:** 345–350.

330. Weinreb DB, Desman GT, Burstein DE, Dikman SH, et al. Renal transplant patient with polyoma virus bladder infection and subsequent polyoma virus nephropathy. *Int J Urol* 2006; **13:** 439–441.

331. Nickeleit V, Mihatsch MJ. Polyomavirus nephropathy: pathogenesis, morphological and clinical aspects. In: Kreipe HH (ed). *Verh Dtsch Ges Pathol*, 88. Tagung. Urban & Fischer: Muenchen, Germany, 2004, pp. 6984.

332. Zambrano A, Villarreal LP. A monoclonal antibody specific for BK virus large T-antigen (clone BK.T-1) also binds the human Ku autoantigen. *Oncogene* 2002; **21:** 5725–5732.

333. Weinreb DB, Desman GT, Burstein DE, Kim DU, et al. Expression of p53 in virally infected tubular cells in renal transplant patients with polyomavirus nephropathy. *Hum Pathol* 2006; **37:** 684–688.

334. Randhawa PS, Vats A, Zygmunt D, Swalsky P, et al. Quantitation of viral DNA in renal allograft tissue from patients with BK virus nephropathy. *Transplantation* 2002; **74:** 485–488.

335. Schmid H, Burg M, Kretzler M, Banas B, et al. BK virus associated nephropathy in native kidneys of a heart allograft recipient. *Am J Transplant* 2005; **5:** 1562–1568.

336. Schmid H, Nitschko H, Gerth J, Kliem V, et al. Polyomavirus DNA and RNA detection in renal allograft biopsies: results from a European multicenter study. *Transplantation* 2005; **80:** 600–604.

337. Nickeleit V, Singh HK, Gilliland MGF, Thompson D, et al. Latent Polyomavirus Type BK Loads in Native Kidneys Analyzed by TaqMan PCR: What Can Be Learned To Better Understand BK Virus Nephropathy? (abstract). *J Am Soc Nep* 2003; **14:** 424A.

338. Boldorini R, Veggiani C, Barco D, Monga G. Kidney and urinary tract polyomavirus infection and distribution: molecular biology investigation of 10 consecutive autopsies. *Arch Pathol Lab Med* 2005; **129:** 69–73.

339. Randhawa P, Shapiro R, Vats A. Quantitation of DNA of polyomaviruses BK and JC in human kidneys. *J Infect Dis* 2005; **192:** 504–509.

340. Chesters PM, Heritage J, McCance DJ. Persistence of DNA sequences of BK virus and JC virus in normal human tissues and in diseased tissues. *J Infect Dis* 1983; **147:** 676–684.

341. Limaye AP, Smith KD, Cook L, Groom DA, et al. Polyomavirus nephropathy in native kidneys of non-renal transplant recipients. *Am J Transplant* 2005; **5:** 614–620.

342. Bracamonte E, Leca N, Smith KD, Nicosia RF, et al. Tubular basement membrane immune deposits in association with BK polyomavirus nephropathy. *Am J Transplant* 2007; **7(6):** 1552–60.

343. Binet I, Nickeleit V, Hirsch HH. Polyomavirus infections in transplant recipients. *Curr Opin Org Transplant* 2000; **5:** 210–216.

344. Nickeleit V, Mihatsch MJ. Polyomavirus allograft nephropathy and concurrent acute rejection: a diagnostic and therapeutic challenge. *Am J Transplant* 2004; **4:** 838–839.

345. Colvin RB, Nickeleit V. Renal transplant pathology. In: Jennette JC, Olson JL, Schwartz MM, Silva FG (eds). *Pathology of the Kidney*. 6th edn, vol. 2. Lippincott Williams & Wilkins: Philadelphia, PA, 2007, pp. 1347–1490.

346. Hirsch HH, Brennan DC, Drachenberg CB, Ginevri F, et al. Polyomavirus-associated nephropathy in renal transplantation: interdisciplinary analyses and recommendations. *Transplantation* 2005; **79:** 1277–1286.

347. Drachenberg RC, Drachenberg CB, Papadimitriou JC, Ramos E, et al. Morphological spectrum of polyoma virus disease in renal allografts: diagnostic accuracy of urine cytology. *Am J Transplant* 2001; **1:** 373–381.

348. van Gorder MA, Della Pelle P, Henson JW, Sachs DH, et al. Cynomolgus polyoma virus infection: a new member of the polyoma virus family causes interstitial nephritis, ureteritis, and enteritis in immunosuppressed cynomolgus monkeys. *Am J Pathol* 1999; **154:** 1273–1284.

349. Nickeleit V, Singh, HK, Mihatsch, MJ. Polyomavirus nephropathy: morphology, pathophysiology, and clinical management. *Curr Opin Nephrol Hypertension* 2003; **12:** 599–605.

350. Mayr M, Nickeleit V, Hirsch HH, Dickenmann M, et al. Polyomavirus BK nephropathy in a kidney transplant recipient: critical issues of diagnosis and management. *Am J Kidney Dis* 2001; **38:** E13.

351. Jeong HJ, Hong SW, Sung SH, Yim H, et al. Polyomavirus nephropathy in renal transplantation: a clinico-pathological study. *Transplant Int* 2003; **16:** 671–675.

352. Ahuja M, Cohen EP, Dayer AM, Kampalath B, et al. Polyoma virus infection after renal transplantation. Use of immunostaining as a guide to diagnosis. *Transplantation* 2001; **71:** 896–899.

353. Mannon RB, Hoffmann SC, Kampen RL, Cheng OC, et al. Molecular evaluation of BK polyomavirus nephropathy. *Am J Transplant* 2005; **5:** 2883–2893.

354. Mayr M, Nickeleit V, Hirsch HH, Dickenmann M, et al. Polyomavirus BK nephropathy in a kidney transplant recipient: critical issues of diagnosis and management. *Am J Kidney Dis* 2001; **38:** E13.

355. Buehrig CK, Lager DJ, Stegall MD, Kreps MA, et al. Influence of surveillance renal allograft biopsy on diagnosis and prognosis of polyomavirus-associated nephropathy. *Kidney Int* 2003; **64:** 665–673.

356. Nickeleit V, Klimkait T, Binet IF, Dalquen P, et al. Testing for polyomavirus type BK DNA in plasma to identify renal-allograft recipients with viral nephropathy. *N Engl J Med* 2000; **342:** 1309–1315.

357. Nickeleit V, Mihatsch MJ. Polyomavirus nephropathy in native kidneys and renal allografts: an update on an escalating threat. *Transplant Int* 2006; **19:** 960–973.

358. Hirsch HH, Drachenberg CB, Steiger J, Ramos E. Polyomavirus associated nephropathy in renal transplantation: critical issues of screening and management. In: Ahsan N (ed) *Polyomaviruses and Human Diseases*, 1st edn. Springer Science+Business Media, Landes Bioscience/Eurekah.com: New York, NY, 2006, pp. 160–173.

359. Drachenberg CB, Hirsch HH, Ramos E, Papadimitriou JC. Polyomavirus disease in renal transplantation: review of pathological findings and diagnostic methods. *Hum Pathol* 2005; **36:** 1245–1255.

360. Nickeleit V, Steiger J, Mihatsch MJ. Re: noninvasive diagnosis of BK virus nephritis by measurement of messenger RNA for BK virus VP1. *Transplantation* 2003; **75:** 2160–2161.

361. Tong CY, Hilton R, MacMahon EM, Brown L, et al. Monitoring the progress of BK virus associated nephropathy in renal transplant recipients. *Nephrol Dial Transplant* 2004; **19:** 2598–2605.

362. Singh S, Madden V, Detwiler R, Andreoni K, et al. Noninvasive diagnosis of polyomavirus allograft nephropathy by electron microscopy on voided urine samples. *Am Soc Nephrol* (in press).

363. Ramos E, Vincenti F, Lu WX, Shapiro R, et al. Retransplantation in patients with graft loss caused by polyoma virus nephropathy. *Transplantation* 2004; **77:** 131–133.

364. Hirsch HH, Ramos E. Retransplantation after polyomavirus-associated nephropathy: just do it? *Am J Transplant* 2006; **6:** 7–9.

365. Womer K, Meier-Krieschke HU, Patton P, Dibadj K, et al. Preemptive retransplantation for BK virus nephropathy: successful outcome despite active viremia. *Am J Transplant* 2006; **6:** 209–213.

366. Emovon OE, Chavin J, Rogers K, Self S. Adenovirus in kidney transplantation: an emerging pathogen? *Transplantation* 2004; **77:** 1474–1475.

367. Asim M, Chong-Lopez A, Nickeleit V. Adenovirus infection of a renal allograft. *Am J Kidney Dis* 2003; **41:** 696–701.

368. Nickeleit V. Critical commentary to: Acute adenoviral infection of a graft by serotype 35 following renal transplantation *Pathol Res Pract* 2003; **199:** 701–702.

369. Ito M, Hirabayashi N, Uno Y, Nakayama A, et al. Necrotizing tubulointerstitial nephritis associated with adenovirus infection. *Hum Pathol* 1991; **22:** 1225–1231.

370. Mazoyer E, Daugas E, Verine J, Pillebout E, et al. A case report of adenovirus-related acute interstitial nephritis in a patient with AIDS. *Am J Kidney Dis* 2008; **51:** 121–126.

371. Mathur SC, Squiers EC, Tatum AH, Szmalc FS, et al. Adenovirus infection of the renal allograft with sparing of pancreas graft function in the recipient of a combined kidney-pancreas transplant. *Transplantation* 1998; **65:** 138–141.

372. Friedrichs N, Eis-Hubinger AM, Heim A, Platen E, et al. Acute adenoviral infection of a graft by serotype 35 following renal transplantation. *Pathol Res Pract* 2003; **199:** 565–570.

373. Emovon OE, Lin A, Howell DN, Afzal F, et al. Refractory adenovirus infection after simultaneous kidney-pancreas transplantation: successful treatment with intravenous ribavirin and pooled human intravenous immunoglobulin. *Nephrol Dial Transplant* 2003; **18:** 2436–2438.

374. Lim AK, Parsons S, Ierino F. Adenovirus tubulointerstitial nephritis presenting as a renal allograft space occupying lesion. *Am J Transplant* 2005; **5:** 2062–2066.

375. Bilic M, Nickeleit V, Howell DN, Self S. Necrotizing granulomatous tubulointerstitial nephritis due to adenovirus infection in the renal allograft: a characteristic morphologic pattern with major clinical implications. *Lab Invest* 2006; **86 (Suppl. 1)** 259A (abstract).

376. Seidemann K, Heim A, Pfister ED, Koditz H, et al. Monitoring of adenovirus infection in pediatric transplant recipients by quantitative PCR: report of six cases and review of the literature. *Am J Transplant* 2004; **4:** 2102–2108.

377. Lion T, Baumgartinger R, Watzinger F, Matthes-Martin S, et al. Molecular monitoring of adenovirus in peripheral blood after allogeneic bone marrow transplantation permits early diagnosis of disseminated disease. *Blood* 2003; **102:** 1114–1120.

378. Myerowitz RL, Stalder H, Oxman MN, Levin MJ, et al. Fatal disseminated adenovirus infection in a renal transplant recipient. *Am J Med* 1975; **59:** 591–598.

379. Rubin RH, Colvin RB. Impact of cytomegalovirus infection on renal transplantation. In: L.C. R, Solez K, Burdick JF (eds). *Kidney Transplant Rejection: Diagnosis and Treatment*, 3rd edn. Marcel Dekker: New York, 1998, pp. 605–625.

380. Battegay EJ, Mihatsch MJ, Mazzucchelli L, Zollinger HU, et al. Cytomegalovirus and kidney. *Clin Nephrol* 1988; **30:** 239–247.

381. Joshi K, Nada R, Radotra BD, Jha V, et al. Pathological spectrum of cytomegalovirus infection of renal allograft recipients—an autopsy study from north India. *Ind J Pathol Microbiol* 2004; **47:** 327–332.

382. Sachdeva MS, Nada R, Jha V, Joshi K. Viral infections of renal allografts—an immunohistochemical and ultrastructural study. *Ind J Pathol Microbiol* 2004; **47:** 189–194.

383. Cozzutto C, Felici N. Unusual glomerular change in cytomegalic inclusion disease. *Virchows Arch A Pathol Anat Histol* 1974; **364:** 365–369.

384. Beneck D, Greco MA, Feiner HD. Glomerulonephritis in congenital cytomegalic inclusion disease. *Hum Pathol* 1986; **17:** 1054–1059.

385. Onuigbo M, Haririan A, Ramos E, Klassen D, et al. Cytomegalovirus-induced glomerular vasculopathy in renal allografts: a report of two cases. *Am J Transplant* 2002; **2:** 684–688.

386. Detwiler RK, Singh HK, Bolin P, Jr., Jennette JC. Cytomegalovirus-induced necrotizing and crescentic glomerulonephritis in a renal transplant patient. *Am J Kidney Dis* 1998; **32:** 820–824.

387. Kadereit S, Michelson S, Mougeno tB, Thibault P, et al. Polymerase chain reaction detection of cytomegalovirus genome in renal biopsies. *Kidney Int* 1992; **42:** 1012–1016.

388. Liapis H, Storch GA, Hill DA, Rueda J, et al. CMV infection of the renal allograft is much more common than the pathology indicates: a retrospective analysis of qualitative and quantitative buffy coat CMV-PCR, renal biopsy pathology and tissue CMV-PCR. *Nephrol Dial Transplant* 2003; **18:** 397–402.

389. Reinke P, Fietze E, Ode-Hakim S, Prosch S, et al. Late-acute renal allograft rejection and symptomless cytomegalovirus infection. *Lancet* 1994; **344:** 1737–1738.

390. Harris NL, Swerdlow SH, Frizzera G, Knowles DM. Post-transplant lymphoproliferative disorders. In: Jaffe ES, Harris NL, Stein H, Vardiman JW (eds). *Pathology and Genetics of Tumours of Haematopoietic and Lymphoid Tissues*. IARC Press: Lyon France, 2001, pp. 264–269.

391. Knowles DM, Cesarman E, Chadburn A, Frizzera G, et al. Correlative morphologic and molecular genetic analysis demonstrates three distinct categories of posttransplantation lymphoproliferatve disorders. *Blood* 1995; **85:** 552–565.

392. Wood A, Angus B, Kestevan P, Dark J, et al. Alpha interferon gene deletions in post-transplant lymphoma. *Bri J Haematol* 1997; **98:** 1002–1003.

393. Mueller-Hermelink HK, Ott G, Kneitz B, Ruediger T. The spectrum of lymphoproliferations and malignant lymphoma after organ transplantation. In: Kreipe HH (ed). *Verhandlungen der Deutschen Gesellschaft fuer Pathologie, 88. Tagung*, vol. 1. Urban & Fischer: Muenchen, Germany, 2004, pp. 63–68.

394. Caillard S, Dharnidharka V, Agodoa L, Bohen E, et al. Posttransplant lymphoproliferative disorders after renal transplantation in the United States in era of modern immunosuppression. *Transplantation* 2005; **80:** 1233–1243.

395. Shapiro R, Nalesnik M, McCauley J, Fedorek S, et al. Posttransplant lymphoproliferative disorders in adult and pediatric renal transplant patients receiving tacrolimus-based immunosuppression. *Transplantation* 1999; **68:** 1851–1854.

396. Saadat A, Einollahi B, Ahmadzad-Asl MA, Moradi M, et al. Posttransplantation lymphoproliferative disorders in renal transplant recipients: report of over 20 years of experience. *Transplant Proc* 2007; **39:** 1071–1073.

397. Frank D, Cesarman E, Liu Yf, Michler RE, et al. Posttransplantion lymphoproliferative disorders frequently contain type A and not type B Epstein-Barr virus. *Blood* 1995; **85:** 1396–1403.

398. Lager DJ, Burgart LJ, Slagel DD. Epstein-Barr virus detection in sequential biopsies from patients with a posttransplant lymphoproliferative disorder. *Mod Pathol* 1993; **6:** 42–47.

399. Kumar S, Kumar D, Kingma DW, Jaffe ES. Epstein-Barr virus-associated T-cell lymphoma in a renal transplant patient. *Am J Surg Path* 1993; **17:** 1046–1053.

400. Ferry JA, Harris NL. Pathology of posttransplant lymphoproliferative disorders. In: Solez K, Racussen LC, Billingham ME (eds). *Solid Organ Transplant Rejection*. Marcel Dekker: New York, 1996, pp. 277–298.

401. Penn I. The changing pattern of posttransplant malignancies. *Transplant Proc* 1991; **23:** 1101–1103.

402. Capello D, Rossi D, Gaidano G. Post-transplant lymphoproliferative disorders: molecular basis of disease histogenesis and pathogenesis. *Hematol Oncol* 2005; **23:** 61–67.

403. Weissman DJ, Ferry JA, Harris NL, Louis DN, et al. Posttransplant lymphoproliferative disorders in solid organ recipients are predominantly aggressive tumors of host origin. *Am J Clin Pathol* 1995; **103:** 748–755.

404. Renoult E, Aymard B, Gregoire MJ, Bellou A, et al. Epstein-Barr virus lymphoproliferative disease of donor origin after kidney transplantation: a case report. *Am J Kidney Dis* 1995; **26:** 84–87.

405. Nalesnik MA. Clinicopathologic characteristics of posttransplant lymphoproliferative disorders. *Recent Results Cancer Res* 2002; **159:** 9–18.

406. Bakker NA, van Imhoff GW, Verschuuren EA, van Son WJ, et al. Early onset post-transplant lymphoproliferative disease is associated with allograft localization. *Clin Transplant* 2005; **19**: 327–334.

407. Schmidtko J, Wang R, Wu CL, Mauiyyedi S, et al. Posttransplant lymphoproliferative disorder associated with an Epstein- Barr-related virus in cynomolgus monkeys. *Transplantation* 2002; **73**: 1431–1439.

408. Koike J, Yamaguchi Y, Hoshikawa M, Takahashi H, et al. Post-transplant lymphoproliferative disorders in kidney transplantation: histological and molecular genetic assessment. *Clin Transplant* 2002; **16 (Suppl. 8)** 12–17.

409. Randhawa PS, Magnone M, Jordan M, Shapiro R, et al. Renal allograft involvement by Epstein-Barr virus associated post-transplant lymphoproliferative disease. *Am J Surg Pathol* 1996; **20**: 563–571.

410. Senel MF, Van BCT, Riggs S, Clark Jr, et al. Post-transplantation lymphoproliferative disorder in the renal transplant ureter. *J Urol* 1996; **155**: 2025.

411. Delbello MW, Dick WH, Carter CB, Butler FO. Polyclonal B cell lymphoma of renal transplant ureter induced by cyclosporine: case report. *J Urol* 1991; **146**: 1613–1614.

412. Blaes AH, Peterson BA, Bartlett N, Dunn DL, et al. Rituximab therapy is effective for posttransplant lymphoproliferative disorders after solid organ transplantation: results of a phase II trial. *Cancer* 2005; **104**: 1661–1667.

413. Oertel SH, Verschuuren E, Reinke P, Zeidler K, et al. Effect of anti-CD 20 antibody rituximab in patients with post-transplant lymphoproliferative disorder (PTLD). *Am J Transplant* 2005; **5**: 2901–2906.

414. Radl J, Valentijn RM, Haaijman JJ, Paul LC. Monoclonal gammapathies in patients undergoing immunosuppressive treatment after renal transplantation. *Clin Immunol Immunopathol* 1985; **37**: 98–102.

415. Cockfield SM, Preiksaitis JK, Jewell LD, Parfrey NA. Post-transplant lymphoproliferative disorder in renal allograft recipients. Clinical experience and risk factor analysis in a single center. *Transplantation* 1993; **56**: 88–96.

416. Citterio F, Lauriola L, Nanni G, Vecchio FM, et al. Polyclonal lymphoma confined to renal allograft: case report. *Transplant Proc* 1987; **19**: 3732–3734.

417. Jones C, Bleau B, Buskard N, Magil A, et al. Simultaneous development of diffuse immunoblastic lymphoma in recipients of renal transplants from a single cadaver donor: transmission of Epstein-Barr virus and triggering by OKT3. *Am J Kidney Dis* 1994; **23**: 130–134.

418. Denning DW, Weiss LM, Martinez K, Flechner SM. Transmission of Epstein-Barr virus by a transplanted kidney, with activation by OKT3 antibody. *Transplantation* 1989; **48**: 141–144.

419. Nádasdy T, Park CS, Peiper SC, Wenzl JE, et al. Epstein-Barr virus infection-associated renal disease: diagnostic use of molecular hybridization technology in patients with negative serology. *J Am Soc Nephrol* 1992; **2**: 1734–1742.

420. Delecluse H-J, Kremmer E, Rouault J-P, Cour C, et al. The expression of Epstein-Barr virus latent proteins is related to the pathological features of post-transplant lymphoproliferative disorders. *Am J Pathol* 1995; **146**: 1113–1120.

421. Thomas JA, Hotchin NA, Allday MJ, Amolot P, et al. Immunohistology of Epstein-Barr virus-associated antigens in B cell disorders from immunocompromised individuals. *Transplantation* 1990; **49**: 944–533.

422. Hjelle B, Evans HM, Yen TS, Garovoy M, et al. A poorly differentiated lymphoma of donor origin in a renal allograft recipient. *Transplantation* 1989; **47**: 945–948.

423. Ulrich W, Chott A, Watschinger B, Reiter C, et al. Primary peripheral T cell lymphoma in a kidney transplant under immunosuppression with cyclosporine A. *Hum Pathol* 1989; **20**: 1027–1030.

424. Meduri G, Fromentin L, Vieillefond A, Fries D. Donor-related non-Hodgkin's lymphoma in a renal allograft recipient. *Transplant Proc* 1991; **23**: 2649–2650.

425. Colvin RB, Nickeleit V. Renal transplant pathology. In: Jennette JC, Olson JL, Schwartz MM, Silva FG (eds). *Pathology of the kidney*, 6 edn, vol. 2. Lippincott Williams & Wilkins: Philadelphia, PA, 2007, pp. 1347–1490.

CHAPTER 4

Histopathology of Liver Transplantation

Anthony J. Demetris, M.D.

Marida Minervini, M.D.

Michael Nalesnik, M.D.

Erin Ochoa, M.D.

Parmjeet Randhawa, M.D.

Eizaburo Sasatomi, M.D., Ph.D.

Tong Wu, M.D., Ph.D.

I. INTRODUCTION

It is becoming significantly more challenging to write a reasonably comprehensive chapter on liver allograft pathology because of the breadth and depth of such an undertaking. All of the various nuances of acute and chronic hepatitis, biliary diseases, and vascular complications, and how they are affected by immunosuppression, in addition to conditions unique to allografts, such as rejection, small-for-size syndrome, and preservation/reperfusion injury, should be covered. But one has to be somewhat selective and attempt to include only information that might be useful to practicing pathologists. The amount of literature on this subject is also overwhelming. Because the histopathology of liver allografts is so often based on clinicopathological correlations one should be aware of new immunosuppressive and antiviral drugs and treatment approaches. New therapies have the potential to influence histopathological findings. We recently contributed a similar chapter to a text on gastrointestinal pathology (1), which in turn, evolved from a previous chapter by our group on the same topic (2). The reader, therefore, will surely recognize some overlaps and similarities, which could not be avoided when covering exactly the same subject. This is particularly true in sections that are based primarily on consensus documents generated by the Banff Working Group. We have, however, made significant updates where needed.

i. Cadaveric Donor Biopsy Evaluation

Increased utilization of extended criteria donors (ECD) has prompted significantly more requests for frozen section evaluations of cadaveric donor organs. ECD have been defined, in recent reviews by Alkofer et al. (3) and Busuttil and Tanaka (4), as donors with increased age (more than sixty years), hypernatremia (>155 meq/l), macrovesicular steatosis (>40 percent), cold ischemia time exceeding twelve hours, partial-liver allografts, and donation after cardiac death (DCD). These factors adversely affect graft survival in several studies (3,4). Feng et al. (5), in a study of more than 20,000 transplants, identified ECD as old age (>60

years), black race, and short height, cerebrovascular cause of death, and DCD and split/partial grafts. Suboptimal donors have also been identified on the basis of hemodynamic instability, use of vasopressors, hypernatremia, hepatitis B virus (HBV) or hepatitis C virus (HCV) infection or anti-HBc antibody positivity, or presence of a liver mass, fibrosis, or other focal lesions, or history of cancer.

Most frequently, a frozen resection request is prompted by the gross appearance and/or "feel," or consistency of the donor liver, preexisting donor disease, the clinical history or circumstances surrounding donor death, or harvesting procedure. The tissue for frozen section evaluation should be obtained fresh and, preferably, in the presence of the pathologist who should also grossly inspect the donor liver. We routinely obtain three tissue samples if the gross appearance is uniform: two 1.0- to 2.0-cm needle cores, one each from the right and left lobes and one 1.0 cm^2 subcapsular wedge biopsy is also from the right lobe. Any areas of heterogeneity or obvious lesions are also sampled.

One should be aware of several pitfalls that can occur during preparation of the sample. First, the fresh liver tissue should be transported immediately to the frozen section room on a paper towel moistened with preservation solution or in a plastic specimen container. Prolonged storage in "physiological" saline, air drying, and placement of the tissue sample on an absorbent substrate all should be avoided. Extended storage in physiological saline can significantly distort hepatocyte morphology causing them to appear shrunken or necrotic. This can lead to an overestimation of ischemic injury. Avoidance of air drying is obvious. An absorbent substrate can blot fat out of the tissue. Consequently, the amount of fat in the biopsy is falsely underestimated in review of the frozen section. This can lead to transplantation of a fatty organ that otherwise should have been discarded.

If the pathologist finds it difficult to cut the frozen section then significant hepatic steatosis and/or necrosis should be suspected. It is not uncommon to detect hepatocytes in various stages of injury/necro-apoptosis because of ischemic damage. In such cases, reliable distinction between viable and damaged/nonviable hepatocytes can be enhanced by staining several sections for increasing lengths of time in eosin. This maneuver enhances contrast between viable and damaged/nonviable hepatocytes because of the latter are usually hypereosinophilic.

Following the histopathological examination, the findings should be correlated with the donor history and laboratory values before a diagnosis or opinion is given. It is not uncommon, however, to receive partial or a fragmented clinical history, which can be misleading in some cases. Therefore, if the biopsy findings do not correlate with the donor agonal history, the pathologist should requests additional information.

Donor organs are usually disqualified for transplantation if the donor is positive for certain serologically diagnosed infections (e.g., HIV); had a central nervous system malignancy subject to biopsy or other manipulation; had an extra-CNS malignancy, especially if it occurred within five years of donation; and sepsis. Biopsy findings that usually *disqualify* organs include diffuse necrosis involving more than 10 percent of all hepatocytes, severe macrovesicular steatosis involving 50 percent or more of hepatocytes, moderate or severe atherosclerosis of intrahepatic artery branches, and definite evidence of bridging fibrosis in donors with chronic hepatitis (6–9). We have found polarization microscopy to offer a quick, immediately available, and reasonably accurate estimate of liver fibrosis. It is helpful, therefore, if the frozen section microscope has polarizing capabilities.

Some factors that define ECD potentially have histopathological manifestations and justify biopsy evaluation (7,8,10). These include advanced age (>60 years), macrovesicular steatosis (>40 percent), DCD, HCV infection, and cardiovascular instability. Other factors that define ECD do not have reliable histopathological findings and do not justify biopsy evaluation. These include black race, short stature, cerebrovascular cause of death, hypernatremia (>155 meq/l), and cold ischemia time exceeding twelve hours, and partial-liver allografts.

DCD donors represent the most rapidly growing donor organ source. They currently represent about 4–5 percent of the total donor pool. DCD refers to donation only after the donor is removed from life support and allowed to undergo cardiac arrest/death. Consequently, the liver is exposed to a significant warm ischemic insult. This should be limited optimally to less than twenty minutes. Even under ideal circumstances, however, DCD donors are still more susceptible to ischemic damage, especially to the biliary tract. This often results in delayed biliary tract complications, such as biliary sludge, that develop several weeks to months after transplantation.

Each ECD factor independently contributes to the potential for graft dysfunction or failure after transplantation(5). A seventy-five-year-old donor on vasopressors prior to donation with a long cold ischemic time (more than fifteen hours) and hepatic artery atherosclerosis is very likely to evoke anxiety and disqualify the donor liver. In contrast, a seventy-year-old donor without any other ECD risk factors might be viewed more favorably. It should be remembered, however, that biopsy evaluation is only one laboratory test used in the evaluation of donor organs. The pathologist is unable to predict the adequacy of organ function after transplantation based on frozen section light microscopic evaluation prior to the operation in the absence of significant histopathological findings.

A grossly fatty appearance is the most common reason for requesting frozen section evaluation of a cadaveric donor liver. In our experience, the gross and microscopic correlation is good and an experienced donor surgeon is usually able to accurately estimate steatosis severity before biopsy evaluation. Livers with microvesicular steatosis, however, are an exception to this statement. Therefore, the pathologist needs to evaluate the liver for the presence of *macrovesicular* steatosis. Macrovesicular steatosis increases susceptibility to preservation/reperfusion injury, impairs regeneration and is increased with age [reviewed in (3,4)]. In contrast, *microvesicular* steatosis, is often found after a short period of warm ischemia or other insult, and usually does not adversely affect the clinical course after transplantation.

In our experience, the severity of steatosis can be roughly estimated on hematoxylin and eosin (H&E)–stained slides alone. Fat stains are not necessary. In general, steatotic donors are usually disqualified when the macrovesicular steatosis involves roughly 50–60 percent or more of the hepatocyte volume based on low-power microscopic examination. Livers with greater than 50 percent macrovesicular steatosis are at increased risk for dysfunction early after transplantation, and in general, the severity of post-transplant dysfunction is directly proportional to the macrovesicular steatosis. But graft failure in livers with less than 50 percent macrovesicular steatosis is uncommon (6–10). A majority of centers, therefore, agree that donor livers with more than 60 percent macrovesicular steatosis should not be used for transplantation. But recent studies from some centers suggest that even these severely steatotic donor livers can be used if other complications are absent (11,12). Therefore, the contraindication for use of livers with macrovesicular steatosis should not be considered absolute.

Some studies have applied an evenly distributed range for scoring macrovesicular steatosis (mild <30 percent, moderate 30–60 percent, and severe >60 percent) (13), but we and others (4,14) use a scale that more closely reflects the triage algorithm for ECD at our center. Our *algorithm* is as follows: mild donor macrovesicular steatosis (<10 percent) does not at all influence the decision making process. Livers with moderate macrovesicular steatosis (10–30 percent) are usually still used for transplantation, but other factors are also taken into consideration. Consequently, the macrovesicular steatosis impacts organ triage. For example, a liver with 25 percent macrovesicular steatosis, and two or three other ECD risk factors, might be discarded. Livers with more than 30 percent, or severe steatosis, are used only under special circumstances, such as when cold ischemic time is kept to a minimum (usually less than eight to nine hours) and there are very few or no other ECD risk factors, such as old age or cardiovascular instability. The outcome in such situations can be comparable to nonsteatotic donor livers (11,12).

Necrosis in donor biopsies can negatively impact outcome (10,13), but a reproducible method of quantifying the necrosis has not been reported. In our experience, the liver is usually disqualified if more than 10 percent (roughly estimated) of hepatocytes are necrotic and the necrosis diffusely involves both the wedge and needle cores, which more deeply sample the liver. It should be emphasized, however, that the assessment should be based on an overall evaluation of all three fragments and not on small areas of subcapsular necrosis. Correlation with the liver injury test profile can add additional useful information to determine if the biopsy observed necrosis is the result of a sampling problem.

Many centers utilize HCV+ donors because recurrent HCV infection after transplantation invariably occurs. But since some patients experience only a slow progression of fibrosis, liver replacement is justified. All HCV+ donors at our institution are subjected to frozen section biopsy analysis. Donor livers with nonbridging fibrosis (<3 by Ishak scale) are used after informed consent by the recipient; others are discarded. Studies evaluating the outcome of HCV+ donors show that the rates of recurrent hepatitis and serious disease after transplantation are not significantly affected by the donor HCV status (15). Mildly diseased HCV+ donor organs can be used, therefore, to prolong the life of a recipient with endstage HCV-induced liver failure. Properly selected HCV+ donors can result in graft and patient survival rates similar to HCV negative donors (16). Anti-HBc–positive donors can transmit HBV to naive and unvaccinated recipients (17). Donor biopsy evaluation is generally not helpful in this circumstance because the vast majority of biopsies do not show any specific features.

Unusual diseases and inadvertently transferred diseases such as amyloidosis, hepatocyte iron deposits, parasitic diseases (18), and small latent "histoplasmomas" (1) have been reported. Alternatively, a disease such as a familial amyloid polyneuropathy can be intentionally transferred with the donor organ in so-called "domino" transplants (19).

ii. Living Donor Biopsy Evaluation

Living donor liver transplant operations currently account for about 5 percent or less of the total number of liver transplants carried out in North America in Europe. The percentage of living donors is significantly higher in the Orient because cadaveric donors are less readily available (20). Because a major liver resection is a risky procedure with a mortality roughly estimated at about 2:700 (21), many centers routinely subject potential living donors to biopsy evaluation. This is done in an effort to further minimize the risk of donation (22–24).

The first step in the evaluation process is a thorough stepwise medical and surgical evaluation. This includes screening for any major medical diseases, obesity, previous major abdominal surgery, anatomic compatibility with between the donor and recipient, infectious diseases that could be transmitted to the recipient, psychosocial instability, and any liver function abnormality or disease that might put the donor at risk (21). Abnormalities detected during the workup can disqualify a potential donor, signal the need for a liver biopsy, or require further evaluation.

Several groups have reported the histopathological findings in potential living donors. The majority of biopsies are either entirely normal or show mild disease. However, 20–50 percent of potential living donor biopsies show abnormalities; the most common abnormalities are within the spectrum of mild nonalcoholic fatty liver disease (NAFLD). NAFLD is also the most common reason for donor disqualification (22–24). The rate of disqualification on biopsy findings alone varies from 3 to 21 percent (22–24).

Most programs try to limit the severity of macrovesicular steatosis in living donors to less than 30 percent. If the biopsy shows greater than 30 percent macrovesicular steatosis, diet modification and other treatments to reduce hepatic steatosis are advised. These potential donors are often subjected to a follow-up biopsy before donation is allowed to proceed. Other living donor biopsy findings include low-grade chronic hepatitis of undetermined etiology, granulomas, and a wide variety other unexpected findings. For example, we uncovered one case of primary biliary cirrhosis (PBC) in a middle-aged female with nearly normal liver injury tests (unpublished observation). We have found that mild (1+ on a scale of 0–4) hepatocellular iron deposits are present in about 10 percent of potential donors, and therefore, probably represent a "normal" finding.

II. DETERMINATION OF CAUSES OF GRAFT DYSFUNCTION AFTER TRANSPLANTATION

i. Understanding the Operation and Timing of Causes of Dysfunction

Accurate biopsy interpretation requires familiarity with the operation since many of the complications are directly or indirectly attributable to technical considerations. The most commonly utilized operative approach is an orthotopic liver transplant procedure where a whole cadaveric donor liver that replaces the native liver in an anatomically correct fashion. Usually, however, the donor gallbladder is resected prior to transplantation. End-to-end anastomoses connect the recipient and donor portal vein, hepatic artery, bile duct and vena cava (25). Donor and recipient are matched routinely for *size* and *ABO blood groups*. Numerous surgical variations, including live donors, split livers, alternate vena caval anastomoses, and etc., of the operation exist, but are beyond the scope of this chapter [for more details see (26)].

More complicated and technically demanding operative approaches are those that deviate from reconstruction of the normal anatomy. These alternative operative approaches also increase the risk of complications. Examples include increased risk of *hepatic artery thrombosis* in small caliber vessels from pediatric and/or living donors and recipients (26). Operative manipulation of the donor liver before transplantation such as occurs with "split" livers, reduced-size livers, and living donors, increase the risk of both vascular and biliary tract complications.

Accurate biopsy interpretation also requires understanding that the various causes of allograft dysfunction occur during characteristic time periods after transplantation (Table 4.1). Therefore, knowledge of the original disease and time after transplantation often provides enough information to generate a reasonably accurate differential diagnosis, even before looking at the biopsy slides. The primary diseases for which liver transplantation was carried out in the United States for 2006 are shown in Table 4.2. In addition, it is not uncommon for more than one cause of liver injury to be present. As previously mentioned, a thorough clinicopathological evaluation should be carried out before a final histopathological diagnosis is given.

ii. Post-transplant Allograft Needle Biopsies

Needle allograft biopsies are obtained after transplantation to 1) determine the cause of dysfunction, 2) examine the immunologic and/or architectural status, and 3) assess the effect of therapy and/or progression of disease. Triage of the tissue sample depends on the clinical differential diagnosis and time after transplantation.

Most diagnostically important histopathological studies can be completed on routinely processed, formalin-fixed, paraffin-embedded sections. A clinical differential that includes antibody mediated rejection optimally requires fresh frozen tissue for immunofluorescent staining for immunoglobulin and complement. Alternatively, formalin-fixed, paraffin-embedded samples can be used for C4d staining. For each biopsy we routinely review two H&E stained slides each containing two to four step sections. Most frequently utilized special stains, which are ordered only on indication after review of the H&E sections, include trichrome, iron, copper to detect chronic

cholestasis, and cytokeratin 7 or 19 to detect bile ducts in cases with equivocal ductopenia.

Information needed for interpretation of post-transplant allograft biopsies includes the original disease, time after transplantation, and type of transplant (i.e., standard whole organ cadaveric, donation after cardiac death livers, reduced-size cadaveric, living related). These variables greatly influence the susceptibility toward certain complications and consequently affect the histopathological differential diagnosis. It is also ideal to have a clinical differential diagnosis and the results of liver injury tests. This additional information, however, can bias the histopathological interpretation. In our opinion, it is best, therefore, to first review the slides, and then correlate the findings and differential diagnosis with the clinical history and laboratory results. Final interpretation should be based on a complete clinicopathological correlation.

During sign-out, we rely heavily on electronic medical records and our in-house transplant-specific information portal and software [EDIT (27)] for clinical and laboratory data. This information portal also contains outpatient notes, medical records, and outpatient laboratory results, which become increasingly important as the time after transplantation increases. Routinely comparing findings in previous biopsies with the current biopsy greatly assists with the overall interpretation and with assessment of therapeutic intervention and disease progression. Re-review of all liver allograft biopsies at a weekly clinicopathological conference provides viable feedback to the clinician and is a necessary quality assessment tool.

iii. Failed Allograft Evaluations

It is usually necessary to review previous biopsies and correlate the findings with the clinical course to determine the exact cause of allograft failure. The gross examination of failed allografts is the same as used for native hepatectomy specimens, described elsewhere (28). Special attention should be given to the dissection and inspection of hilar structures, especially the biliary and vascular anastomoses. This usually requires the assistance of the operative surgeon, who is more familiar with the anatomy, especially when the operative procedure is not standard. Tissue sampling for microscopy should follow the same protocol as used in the native livers; specific sampling of grossly obvious defects is intuitive.

The most common causes of allograft failure vary according to the time after transplantation. "Preservation/reperfusion" injury or primary nonfunction, vascular thrombosis, and patient death are the leading causes of *allograft failure within the first several weeks* after transplantation (29,30). Few allografts fail because of acute cellular or antibody-mediated rejection. Most episodes of acute cellular rejection are responsive to increased immunosuppression and liver allografts are naturally resistant to antibody mediated rejection (31). Recurrent

TABLE 4.1 Approximate Timing of Common Allograft Syndromes [adapted from (1) and (2)]

Syndrome	Clinical associations/observations	Peak time period
"Preservation" reperfusion injury	Older (>60 years), hemodynamically unstable, DCD, and hypernatremic donors, long cold (>12 hours) or warm (>120 minutes) ischemic time; reconstruction of vascular anastomoses; poor bile production; a prolonged cholestatic phase probably predisposed to biliary sludge syndrome	Recognized primarily in postreperfusion biopsies; changes can persist for several months depending on the severity of the injury
Antibody-mediated rejection	ABO-incompatible donor; high titer (>1:32) lymphocytotoxic cross-match; persistently low platelet counts and low complement levels after transplantation	Immediately after reperfusion persisting for several weeks to months; later onset less common
Acute cellular rejection	Younger, "healthier," female, and inadequately immunosuppressed recipients, long cold ischemic times, disorders of dysregulated immunity (e.g., PSC, AIH, PBC).	Three days to 6 weeks; later onset usually associated with inadequate immunosuppression
Chronic rejection	Moderate or severe or persistent episodes of acute rejection; noncompliant and inadequately immunosuppressed patients (e.g., infections, tumors, PTLD)	Bimodal distribution; early peak during first year and later increase in noncompliant and inadequately immunosuppressed patients
Hepatic artery thrombosis	Suboptimal anastomosis; pediatric/small caliber vessels; donor and/or recipient atherosclerosis; suboptimal or difficult arterial anastomosis; large difference in vessel caliber across anastomosis; hypercoagulopathy; suboptimal arterial flow	Bimodal distribution; early peak between 0 and 4 weeks and later peak between 18 and 36 months (see text)
Biliary tract obstruction or stricturing	Arterial insufficiency or thrombosis; long cold ischemia, DCD, difficult biliary anastomosis; antibody-mediated rejection; original disease of PSC	Variable
Venous outflow obstruction	Difficult "piggyback" hepatic vein reconstruction; cardiac failure	Usually during the first several weeks
"Opportunistic" viral and fungal infections (see text)	Seropositive donors to seronegative recipients (often pediatric); overimmunosuppression	0–8 weeks, much less common thereafter except for EBV-related PTLDs and other EBV-related tumors (see text)
Recurrent or new onset of viral hepatitis (e.g., HBV, HCV, HEV)	Original disease HBV, HCV, or acquired HEV-induced hepatitis	Usually first becomes apparent 4–6 weeks after transplantation and persists thereafter, but earlier onset (within 2 weeks) in aggressive cases
Recurrent AIH, PBC, and PSC	Original disease of AIH, PBC, or PSC. PBC: donor-recipient HLA-DR matching patients, immunosuppression weaning; living donor. PSC: intact colon with ulcerative colitis; male	Usually more than 6 months after transplantation; incidence of recurrence increases with time after transplantation
Alcohol abuse	High per day alcohol intake before transplantation; psychiatric comorbidity/social instability; noncompliance with treatment protocols; GGTP:ALP ratio >1.4	Usually >6 months
Nonalcoholic steatohepatitis	Original disease nonalcoholic steatohepatitis or cryptogenic cirrhosis; risk factors for NASH in general population	Usually >3–4 weeks and increases with time if risk factors persist

disease, delayed manifestations of technical complications, such as vascular thrombosis or biliary sludge syndrome, and patient death are most commonly responsible for *late graft failures* occurring more than one year after transplantation (29,32). Chronic rejection is relatively uncommon as a cause of graft failure and the incidence is decreasing (29,33), but recurrent HCV-induced cirrhosis is an emerging dilemma for organ allocation algorithms (34).

III. SPECIAL CONSIDERATIONS IN REDUCED-SIZE AND LIVING-RELATED LIVER ALLOGRAFTS

The shortage of cadaveric donor livers has forced surgeons to increasingly rely on alternative donor sources, such as reduced-size cadaveric liver allografts, where an adult liver is "split" for use in two recipients, and living donors. These procedures require considerable surgical skill and

TABLE 4.2 Indications for Liver Transplantation for Cadaveric Donors in the United States during the Calendar Year of 2006 [data obtained from the United Network for Organ Sharing (UNOS) Web site http://www.OPTN.org]

Diagnosis	Number	%
HCV cirrhosis*	1,914	29
Neoplasia	867	13
Biliary (PBC, PSC, BA, other)	792	12
Alcohol**	713	11
Cryptogenic cirrhosis	450	7
Fulminant hepatic failure	400	6
NAFLD	253	4
Metabolic disease	230	3
HBV cirrhosis	139	2
Autoimmune cirrhosis	162	2
Other	740	11
Total	6,650	100

* A minority of these patients also had coexistent HBV infection and/or alcohol use.

** Other patients with alcohol use were included with HCV group because of coexistent infection.

BA, biliary atresia; NALFD, nonalcoholic liver disease.

experience, however, the complication rate remains higher than in whole cadaveric liver transplantation (35). The histopathological manifestations of complications are similar to those seen for whole cadaveric organs, described later.

Adult-to-adult living donor liver transplantation requires the right lobe donation because there is a lower limit of the size of the allograft that can be safely transplanted. Adult left lobes, however, can often be used for adult-to-pediatric transplants because the adult donor is usually much larger than the pediatric recipient (36,37). In addition, normal liver structure and function is dependent on optimal portal venous and hepatic artery inflow and adequate venous outflow and biliary drainage. As expected, transplanting only a portion of the liver necessarily compromises at least one of these vascular or biliary conduits. This is especially true near the cut edge of the liver fragment. It is very important, therefore, to be aware of the technical details of the operation and the exact origin of the post-transplant biopsy, because sampling errors can be quite misleading in reduced size/living donor allografts.

For example, infarcted parenchyma and/or high-grade biliary or venous outflow obstruction changes can be seen in biopsies obtained near the cut surface of a reduced-size or living donor allograft in well recipients with near normal liver injury tests. This occurs because the histopathological changes are attributable to only localized defects of blood or bile flow and the biopsies are not representative of the entire liver. Thus, rendering a histopathological diagnosis of "infarcted liver" or "high-grade biliary obstruction" on a well patient can be avoided by inquiring about biopsy location and about the liver injury test profile. If the patient has more than one biliary anastomosis,

biopsy from one lobe might show obstructive cholangiopathy changes, whereas the other lobe might be normal, or show other histopathological changes.

Early after transplantation, reduced size/living donor allografts might be more susceptible to antibody-mediated rejection (38). Late after transplantation, low-grade ductular reactions and nodular regenerative hyperplasia changes are also fairly common in reduced-size and living donor liver allografts.

i. Preservation/Reperfusion Injury

1. Introduction

"Preservation/reperfusion" injury generally refers to the culmination of donor organ damage that occurs during the agonal phases in the donor, while being kept in preservation solution, and then when reperfused with blood in the recipient. Dysfunction usually occurs shortly after transplantation and it assumed that technical or vascular insults, such as arterial or venous thrombosis, alloimmunologic or adverse drug reactions, toxin exposure, and various infections have been reasonably excluded. Donor and recipient hypotension, warm ischemia, metabolic abnormalities, cold ischemia during organ preservation, and reperfusion injury all contribute to the syndrome of preservation/reperfusion injury.

2. Pathophysiology

Damage to the donor liver occurs during warm ischemia, cold ischemia, and rewarming/reperfusion injury. *Warm ischemia* refers to suboptimal perfusion with blood when the organ is at body temperature, which can occur before or during harvesting and during rewarming after implantation. Warm ischemic injury does not usually lead to clinical problems if limited to less than 120 minutes (39,40). DCD donors also suffer a warm ischemic insult, but instead of suboptimal perfusion, blood flow stops altogether. If, however, the time from pronouncement of cardiac death until infusion with preservation solution is limited to less than twenty minutes, post-transplant graft and patient survival rates are acceptable. Warm ischemia also preferentially targets hepatocytes and endothelial cells for injury [reviewed in (41–43)].

"Cold ischemia" refers to the damage that occurs when the donor organ is stored in preservation fluid and immersed in an ice bath; it preferentially damages sinusoidal endothelial cells (8, 44). In general, cold ischemic time should be less than twelve hours, if possible. Longer cold ischemic times can be tolerated, but at the expense of diminished outcome because of increased rates of dysfunction, post-transplant complications (especially biliary), and allograft failure (4,5).

Hypothermia lowers the metabolic rate and prolongs the time that anoxic cells can retain essential metabolic functions. But coexistent ischemic injury still depresses mitochondrial respiration, which in turn, causes ATP depletion [reviewed in (41–44)]. This results in deterioration of energy-dependent metabolic pathways and transport processes, activation of proteinases and metalloproteinases, and subsequent lifting of the sinusoidal endothelial cells from the underlying matrix. Loss of sinusoidal microvascular integrity and function and suboptimal microvascular blood flow after revascularization is the major determinant of subsequent graft viability and function [reviewed in (41–44)]. But ischemic/reperfusion damage to hepatocytes and biliary epithelial cells is receiving increasing attention as a cause of subsequent dysfunction [reviewed in (43)]. Significant steatosis in the donor liver also increases susceptibility to both warm and cold ischemic injury [reviewed in (41–44)].

Reperfusion of the liver with recipient blood is also an important cause of liver injury [reviewed in (41–44)]. Vascular congestion in the intestines during the anhepatic phase contributes to endotoxin leakage and tumor necrosis factor-α–induced activation of Kupffer's cells (44,45). Sequential hypoxia and re-oxygenation also activates complement factors. Activated Kupffer's cells, in turn, release reactive oxygen species and produce cytokines that potentiate granulocyte sludging within the sinusoids, which can undergo degranulation and cause further tissue damage. When severe, all of these processes contribute significantly to an imbalance of vasoconstrictors over vasodilators and microcirculatory failure after reperfusion [reviewed in (41–44)]. Vasodilators, therefore, such as endothelin antagonists, can mitigate reperfusion injury, whereas vasoconstrictors can make it worse (44).

The biliary tree is receiving increasing attention as a target of ischemia/reperfusion injury because suboptimally preserved and ECD organs frequently develop the "biliary sludge syndrome" (46–48). This complication is illustrative of the various pathophysiological mechanisms that contribute to preservation/reperfusion injury and wound healing in the biliary tree [reviewed in (46,47)]. Cold ischemic injury and/or sludging of whole blood in the plexus of a DCD donor damage the *microvasculature of the peribiliary plexus* which predisposes to microvascular thrombosis after reperfusion. This results in injury to the bile wall. Deep wounds cause inflammation and granulation tissue in the underlying stroma. The inflammation and bile contribute to poor wound healing, sludging of bile, and fibrosis, which leads to bile duct stricturing. Damage to the peribiliary plexus can be lessened by perfusing the hepatic artery with low viscosity preservation solutions, or thrombolytic agents before transplantation. This maneuver prevents microvascular thrombosis and promotes adequate reperfusion (49). Despite flushing the biliary tree with preservation solution, however, residual hydrophobic bile salts (43) often remain that directly damage hypoxic biliary epithelial cells, which are then shed into the bile after transplantation (50).

3. Clinical Presentation

Reliable early signs of *significant* preservation/reperfusion injury after complete revascularization include poor bile production and persistent elevation of serum lactate (51–53). This is usually associated with significant (>2500 IU/ml) increases of serum ALT and AST during the first few days after transplantation (8). Thereafter, the transaminases usually normalize rapidly during the first week (43,45). Typically, however, this is followed by a prolonged "cholestatic phase" of preservation/reperfusion injury characterized by persistent elevation of total bilirubin and γ-GTP. In cases that recover, there is slow gradual resolution of abnormal liver injury tests. Severely damaged allografts, however, are at risk for developing the biliary sludge syndrome.

Implantation and reperfusion of a donor liver with pre-existing macrovesicular steatosis often triggers intrahepatic coagulation and fibrinolysis. This results in wound site bleeding and difficulty in achieving hemostasis (6,13).

4. Histopathological Findings

Histopathological examination of the donor liver by light microscopy cannot reliably predict function after transplantation. Cold ischemia injury preferentially damages sinusoidal endothelial cells (8) and electron microscopy examination is needed to reliably assess the extent of injury (8).

Postreperfusion biopsies, or those obtained within several hours of complete revascularization, can reliably gauge the extent of preservation/reperfusion injury (8). In such biopsies, severe preservation injury is characterized by zonal or confluent coagulative necrosis, particularly if it is periportal or bridging, and severe neutrophilic inflammation. There is, however, considerable heterogeneity in biopsy findings because of uneven reperfusion and sampling errors should be kept in mind. For example, the subcapsular parenchyma is more vulnerable to injury, in general, and especially from manipulation. One should not mistake so-called surgical hepatitis characterized by sinusoidal neutrophilia in and around the central veins, as severe preservation/reperfusion injury.

Mild damage, which is present in many liver allografts, includes microvesicular steatosis, hepatocellular cytoaggregation, and hepatocellular swelling (8,28). The microvesicular steatosis is usually attributable to warm ischemia. Hepatocellular cytoaggregation refers to the detachment of individual hepatocytes from each other and "rounding up" of the cytoplasm. *Severe injury* is characterized by areas of confluent necrosis, which can show a zonal distribution. It can also be seen in cases with suboptimal regional perfusion. Significant necrosis is frequently accompanied by notable neutrophilic infiltration. Zones of bland hepatocyte dropout with residual intact reticulin architecture, but without hepatocytes, are usually attributable to previous damage that occurred in the donor.

Since normal hepatocytes require only four to six hours to undergo the entire apoptotic cycle, the presence of apoptotic hepatocytes or coagulative necrosis in a biopsy obtained more than several days after transplantation should arouse the suspicion of another, usually ischemic, insult. Such changes should not be passed off as residual preservation/reperfusion injury (43).

The liver initiates responses to repair the damage and regenerate hepatocytes and other cells lost during preservation/reperfusion injury. These responses are proportional to the insult and therefore can be used to gauge the severity of injury after the damaged cells have been removed. *Reparative responses* after mild injury are usually limited to hepatocellular mitosis, thickening of the plates, and nuclear enlargement. Mild centrilobular hepatocellular swelling and hepatocanalicular cholestasis are also common and can persist for several weeks. Severe centrilobular hepatocyte dropout usually triggers mitosis in neighboring nearby hepatocytes that rapidly proliferate to restore the normal architecture. Periportal and confluent bridging necrosis with collapse of the reticulin framework usually triggers *cholangiolar proliferation* (8,28) (Figure 4.1). This can link adjacent portal tracts and distort the architecture. Severe preservation/reperfusion injury is also usually accompanied by centrilobular hepatocellular swelling and hepatocanalicular and cholangiolar cholestasis (8,28) that often persist for one or two months. If the graft recovers, a normal architecture can be restored. But such patients are usually at risk for developing the biliary sludge syndrome and biliary strictures.

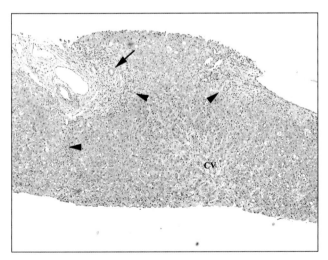

FIGURE 4.1:   *Severe preservation/reperfusion injury is usually seen during the first several weeks after transplantation and characterized by centrilobular hepatocellular swelling, cholangiolar proliferation (arrowhead), and mild, neutrophilic, or mixed portal inflammation without significant eosinophilia or blastic lymphocytes. Note the absence of edema around the true bile duct (arrow), which helps to distinguish severe preservation/ reperfusion injury from biliary tract obstruction/stricturing (PT = portal tract; CV = central vein).*

The histopathology is a bit more complicated if the donor liver had significant preexisting macrovesicular steatosis. Preservation/reperfusion injury of these livers causes death of some fat-containing hepatocytes and release of lipid droplets into the sinusoids. The extracellular lipid droplets coalesce into larger fat globules that trigger local fibrin deposition, neutrophilia, red blood cell congestion, and local obstruction of sinusoidal blood flow (6). Eventually, if the liver recovers, the large fat globules become surrounded by macrophages and eventually resolve over a period of several weeks.

5. Differential Diagnosis

Biliary obstruction/pancreatitis, sepsis, antibody-mediated rejection, and cholestatic hepatitis can produce histopathological changes that resemble preservation/reperfusion injury. The clinical context and history provide very important information when reviewing the slides. Detailed donor information, including age and type (e.g., ECD, DCD), cold and warm ischemic times, any operative difficulties, recipient clinical profile, and blood culture and cross-match results help to determine the likely source of injury and whether additional special stains such as C4d and/or immunofluorescent staining for immunoglobulin and complement might be warranted. In our experience, however, preservation/reperfusion injury and operative technical difficulties most often prove to be the cause of liver injury early after transplantation.

Examination of the "true" bile ducts contained within the portal tract connective tissue and cholangioles at the interface zone provide useful clues in distinguishing between preservation/reperfusion injury and biliary tract obstruction/stricturing and pancreatitis (Figure 4.1). Biliary obstruction and/or cholangitis usually cause at least some *periductal lamellar edema* surrounding the true bile ducts. An accompaniment by neutrophils within the lumen or infiltrating between biliary epithelial cells facilitates making the diagnosis of cholangiopathy. By comparison, preservation/reperfusion injury does not usually cause changes in and around the "true" bile ducts and neutrophils surround the cholangioles at the interface zone. Centrilobular hepatocanalicular changes, a prominent ductular reaction, cholangiolar cholestasis, and intralobular neutrophil clusters can be seen in both disorders. Discussion with the surgeon can also often help resolve this issue. The first several months after transplantation, the biliary tree is usually "stented" open by a T-tube stent. The long limb of the stent is brought to the skin surface and is used to monitor bile flow and to obtain cholangiograms. Therefore, the surgeons are usually aware of biliary tract obstructions during this time, unless a choledochoenteric biliary anastomosis was used.

It may be impossible to distinguish histopathologically between the histopathological changes associated with systemic *bacteremia* and preservation/reperfusion injury. And the development of sepsis in a recipient of an ECD organ with severe preservation/reperfusion injury is not uncommon. Fortunately, the clinical context and history can assist in this distinction.

A common problem is the recognition of *acute rejection* superimposed on preservation injury. The composition and severity of the portal and any perivenular inflammation is used to make this distinction. Significant rejection is usually accompanied by mild to moderate mixed portal inflammation containing blastic lymphocytes and eosinophils. In fact, significant portal eosinophilia early after transplantation is an excellent marker of an early emerging rejection reaction—in most circumstances. Moreover, the portal inflammation is usually associated with damage to true bile ducts and the cholangioles. Another reliable sign of rejection in this circumstance is the coalescence of a rejection-type infiltrate, similar to that seen in the portal tracts, around the central veins.

Distinction of preservation injury from antibody-mediated rejection is discussed under the section of antibody–mediated rejection.

Without the clinical context and history, it can be difficult to distinguish between preservation injury and *cholestatic hepatitis*. Cholestatic hepatitis, however, has only been reported in patients infected with HBV or HCV and is distinctly unusual before three to four weeks after transplantation. In addition, cholestatic hepatitis usually worsens with time unless the patient is specifically treated with decreased immunosuppression and/or antiviral therapy, where as the trend is toward gradual improvement with preservation/reperfusion injury.

ii. Portal Hyperperfusion or "Small-for-Size" Syndrome

1. Introduction and Pathophysiology
When a reduced size/living donor allograft is placed into the hyperdynamic and hypertensive portal circulation of a cirrhotic recipient, it might be unable to accommodate the significantly increased portal blood flow. This can result in injury to the portal venous and periportal sinusoids after reperfusion and a complication referred to as the "portal hyperperfusion" or "small-for-size graft syndrome (PHP/SFSS)."

The small-for-size syndrome occurs most commonly when the transplanted donor segment is less than 30 percent of the standard or expected liver volume of the recipient or less than 0.8 percent recipient body weight. But it can also occur occasionally following whole organ cadaveric transplantation and in reduced size allografts that are greater than 0.8 percent body weight. The ability to predict its occurrence on size matching alone before transplantation is suboptimal (54–56). Therefore, factors other than graft size must also be considered (57).

Regeneration of the reduced size/living donor allograft requires optimal and balanced portal venous and hepatic arterial blood inflow and adequate hepatic vein drainage (58). Afferent portal venous and hepatic artery hepatic blood flow inflow is reciprocally regulated by the arterial buffer response (59–61). This refers to the empirical observation that increased portal venous flow diminishes hepatic artery flow, whereas decreased portal venous flow increases arterial flow. Lautt (61) originally proposed that "adenosine washout" was responsible for this phenomenon.

Adenosine, a vasodilator substance, is constantly released among the hepatic arterioles and portal venules in the portal tracts. This maintains a physiologically balanced portal venous and hepatic artery inflow. Significantly increased portal flow *decreases* the local concentration of adenosine, which in turn, results in hepatic artery branch constriction and reduced arterial flow. This is exactly what occurs in liver allografts with PHP/SFSS (59–62). Low arterial flow, in turn, predisposes to *thrombosis* and *ischemic cholangitis*. Evidence supporting the importance of portal venous hyperperfusion is that this syndrome can be treated, in some cases effectively, by reducing portal blood flow using octreotide, splenic artery ligation, or mesocaval shunts (63–65). In addition to triggering the arterial buffer response, the high portal venous inflow directly causes mechanical damage to small periportal vein branches and vessels connecting portal veins and periportal sinusoids (57). This triggers a patho physiological cascade of events (57). At the most severe end of the spectrum, the PHP/SFSS manifests clinically as portal hypertension, ascites, coagulopathy, and hyperbilirubinemia (62,66–70). The underlying cause of the portal hypertension and ascites are self explanatory, based on the above description. Subsequent splanchnic venous stasis and perfusion of the liver with endotoxin-rich blood also probably contributes to the cholestasis (57).

All reduced size/living donor allograft that are required to grow after transplantation, however, likely experience the PHP/SFSS to some extent. In fact, it is probably an important physiological stimulus of liver regeneration (57). This contention is based on the observation that the rapidity and magnitude of hepatocyte regeneration is directly proportional to the increased portal blood flow (62). Therefore, failure of liver regeneration is not the major clinical problem associated with the PHP/SFSS. PHP/SFSS becomes pathological and clinically significant when the structural integrity of the hepatic vasculature is compromised. This can directly or indirectly, via the arterial buffer response, cause parenchymal or biliary ischemia and infarction.

2. Clinical Presentation
PHP/SFSS is classically defined as otherwise unexplained cholestasis, coagulopathy, and ascites that develops within the first week after a reduced size/living donor

transplantation (57). Frequently, the surgeon is aware of the potential for this complication because of portal hypertension and splanchnic congestion observed after complete revascularization. The clinical manifestations, however, are not entirely specific and can mimic other technical complications, such as portal vein thrombosis. Therefore, radiographic studies are often needed to exclude obvious mechanical or anastomotic complications. It is also often difficult to determine whether, and to what extent, the PHP/SFSS contributes to so-called "technical" complications encountered with reduced size/living donor allografts.

For example, a strong arterial buffer response can lead to significant arterial vasospasm. In such cases, hepatic arteriograms can show segmental narrowing, poor peripheral filling, at even reversal of flow (57). Diminished arterial flow, whatever the cause, predisposes to hepatic artery thrombosis and ischemic cholangitis. This is especially true when the blood vessels are smaller than normal size.

3. Histopathological Findings

Initial events in the PHP/SFSS are observed reliably in experimental animal models of PHP/SFSS (62,66,68,71), and occasionally in postreperfusion or early post-transplant allograft biopsies obtained within the first several days in humans (57). The most striking change and most severe form of injury is widespread portal venous and periportal sinusoidal *endothelial cell injury* (62,66,68, 71).

The vascular injury associated with the PHP/SFSS can be divided into early, intermediate, and late changes (57). The earliest changes include denudation of portal vein and periportal sinusoidal endothelium. This occurs as early as five minutes following transplantation in grafts of less than 30 percent expected liver volume (62). The microvascular connecting the portal veins and the sinusoids can rupture in severe cases. This results in hemorrhage into the portal and periportal connective tissue that can dissect into hepatic parenchyma, in extreme cases (69,72).

Reparative changes begin to occur if the allograft survives the initial crisis. These include endothelial cell hypertrophy, subendothelial edema accompanied by an in-growth of myofibroblasts and endothelial cells into the subendothelial space. Eventually, this leads to fibrointimal hyperplasia/intimal thickening and luminal obliteration or re-canalization of thrombi. Late sequelae of the early portal venous injury includes obliterative portal venopathy, which triggers nodular regenerative hyperplasia changes because of the same arterial buffer response, described above (57).

Venous findings typical, or nearly diagnostic, of PHP/SFSS are relatively uncommon in peripheral core needle biopsies. Instead, one often observes a constellation of nonspecific findings that usually include centrilobular hepatocanalicular cholestasis and centrilobular hepatocyte

steatosis and/or atrophy or necrosis. These are often combined with a low-grade ductular reaction at the interface zone. Review of the operative and radiographic reports and clinical history and discussion with the surgeon are useful in determining whether histopathological changes and graft dysfunction in peripheral needle biopsy can be attributed to PHP/SFSS.

Eventually, if the graft recovers, portal hypertension and ascites resolve over a period of several weeks. This is accompanied by restoration of the normal architecture, except that some grafts eventually develop significant nodular regenerative hyperplasia, as a result of portal venopathy (57).

Hilar sections of allografts that fail from PHP/SFSS frequently show changes of traumatic injury to larger portal vein endothelium, focal fibrointimal hyperplasia of the vein branches, evidence of arterial vasospasm, and in some cases, ischemic cholangitis, particularly if the hepatic artery has thrombosed (57).

4. Differential Diagnosis

The major histopathological differential for PHP/SFSS includes suboptimal arterial flow because of arterial thrombosis or stricturing not related to the SFSS, sepsis, hypotension, and biliary tract obstruction/structuring and ischemic cholangitis. Preservation injury might also be a differential diagnostic consideration, but living donor grafts are usually not affected significantly. Since portal hyperperfusion can lead to diminished arterial flow and thrombosis, it is also not surprising that more than one complication might be present. Biliary tract obstruction/stricturing alone, however, is usually not accompanied by either portal tract connective tissue hemorrhage or centrilobular hepatocyte ischemic changes, or significant nodular regenerative hyperplasia. Therefore, when these other changes are present, the PHP/SFSS should be considered.

Arterial vasospasm is usually detectable microscopically in failed allografts and typically only when it is severe. The vessels most commonly affected are medium-sized perihilar arteries.

iii. Vascular Complications

1. General Considerations

Complications involving the vascular anastomoses are the most frequent major technical issue that has the potential to cause serious allograft damage and/or failure. Most occur during the first several months after transplantation and are related to anastomotic imperfections, including preexisting atherosclerotic disease, manipulation of the vascular tree, metabolic or physiological abnormalities that predispose to thrombosis, or a combination of these factors. Anastomotic narrowing and other irregularities including intimal flaps, intimal and/or medial tears, and dramatic reductions in caliber across a suture line, and the creation of "kinks" or abnormal tortuosity are common mechanical/surgical problems. Potential problems can become real because of preexisting atherosclerotic disease and factors that increase the technical difficulty of the vascular anastomoses. Examples include small caliber vessels in pediatric recipients and reduced size/living donor grafts and/or abnormal anatomy, such as a piggyback venal caval anastomosis. Physiological or metabolic abnormalities that decrease hepatic blood flow and/or promote coagulation, such as cardiac failure, clotting abnormalities, rejection, and infections also increase the risk of complications, often at sites of abnormal anatomy, such as the anastomotic line.

Vascular interposition arterial grafts or small venous segments that link the donor and recipient arteries or veins, respectively, can be a convenient solution to make the donor and recipient anatomy compatible. This latter solution can also be a source of problems because of the number of anastomoses required for vascular reconstruction. In addition, vascular grafts are often cryopreserved or stored in preservation fluid for one to several days before implantation. Some, therefore, are marginally viable at the time of placement and can trigger thrombosis, stimulate atherogenesis, and/or serve as nidus for infection.

2. Hepatic Artery Thrombosis

a. Introduction and Pathophysiology The hepatic arterial tree is the most frequent and important site of vascular complications and a major cause of allograft damage and failure (51–53,73). Allografts are more susceptible to arterial ischemia than native livers because they are devoid of a collateral arterial circulation, at least early after transplantation.

The hepatic artery supplies primarily the extra- and intrahepatic bile ducts, hilar and portal tract connective tissue, and hilar lymph nodes. It is these structures, therefore, that are preferentially damaged by inadequate arterial flow or after arterial thrombosis. Ischemic damage to the biliary tree results in poor wound healing and subsequent biliary leaks because of poor anastomotic healing, biliary tract ulcers, and cholangitic abscesses. Ischemic biliary tract injury usually results in biliary tract strictures and the biliary sludge syndrome because of improper wound healing (46). The phrase "ischemic cholangitis" (28,74) or "ischemic cholangiopathy" (75) is often used to describe this sequence of events (Figures 4.2 and 4.3).

The initial and largest wave of arterial thromboses occur within the first several months after transplantation and these take place most frequently at or near the suture line. A second, smaller, wave of technically related arterial

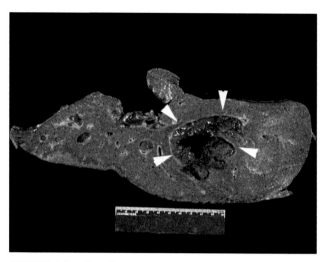

FIGURE 4.2: *Hepatic artery thrombosis frequently results in necrosis of the large bile ducts and formation of biliary sludge (surrounded by white arrowheads). This gross image illustrates why biopsies obtained from the periphery of the liver are not a good method to establish the diagnosis of hepatic artery thrombosis; they can show various changes, or even be misleading.*

thromboses occurs between one and three years after transplantation (76). *Suboptimal arterial anastomoses* can cause turbulent arterial flow immediately downstream from the suture line, which eventually leads to arterial fibrointimal hyperplasia, luminal narrowing, and thrombosis. Fibrointimal hyperplasia also often develops more quickly in arterial interposition grafts, predisposing them to thrombosis. Any physiological or metabolic abnormalities that decrease hepatic blood flow and/or promote coagulation, such as cardiac failure, PHP/SFSS, rejection, clotting abnormalities, and infections also predispose to thrombosis, particularly at the anastomosis site or other structural abnormality.

b. Clinical Presentation Most hepatic artery thromboses cause significant problems such as hepatic infarcts, ischemic cholangiopathy, and occasionally fulminant hepatic failure (51–53,73). Up to one third, however, can be asymptomatic. Symptoms, when present, are usually related to hepatic infarcts, abscesses, ischemic cholangiopathy and subsequent impaired bile flow. The major manifestations include right upper abdominal pain/discomfort, intermittent fever because of relapsing bacteremia/fungemia, biliary leaks and/or obstruction, bile peritonitis, and jaundice. Ultrasonography is usually used as a screening tool to inspect hepatic arterial blood flow, but angiography is the most reliable method of establishing the diagnosis with certainty.

Surgeons often attempt to salvage allografts with a thrombosed artery by thrombectomy. They are often encouraged by a grossly and microscopically "viable" appearance at the capsular surface. Unfortunately, there

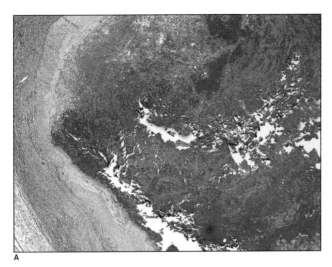
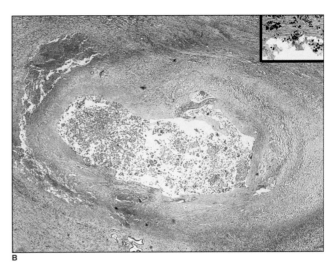

FIGURE 4.3: Sections through the hilum of a failed allograft with hepatic artery thrombosis (upper panel) shows necrosis of the large bile ducts with leakage of bile into the surrounding connective tissue (lower panel). This necrotic tissue frequently becomes seated with bacteria and fungi (right upper inset).

may still be development of bile duct necrosis and/or the biliary sludge syndrome because the biliary tree has already been ischemically damaged at the time of thrombectomy.

c. Histopathological Findings A diagnosis of hepatic artery thrombosis cannot be reliably made on needle biopsy evaluation (28,77). This is because needle biopsies sample the subcapsular parenchyma, which is variably affected. Sampling errors, therefore, are significant problem. Structures most commonly and reliably susceptible to ischemic injury, such as the perihilar tissue and large bile ducts, are not routinely sampled.

Findings in peripheral core needle biopsies of allografts with a thrombosed artery can therefore be quite variable. Frank coagulative necrosis or marked centrilobular hepatocyte swelling, cholangiolar proliferation with or without bile plugs, and acute cholangiolitis are all within the spectrum of the hepatic artery thrombosis. The biopsy might even be unremarkable, either because the patient has developed vascular collaterals and the thrombosis is inconsequential, or there has been necrosis of hilar bile ducts and changes secondary to biliary sludging have not yet developed in the periphery. More frequent findings include biliary tract obstruction or stricturing. Occasionally, hepatic artery thrombosis can present as spotty acidophilic necrosis of hepatocytes or so-called ischemic hepatitis and mimic acute viral hepatitis. Chronic suboptimal arterial flow can cause centrilobular hepatocellular atrophy and sinusoidal widening.

Examination of failed allografts with hepatic artery thrombosis illustrates the pathophysiological consequences of suboptimal arterial flow. Necrosis of hilar/perihilar bile ducts with leakage of bile into the surrounding connective tissue, biliary sludge, infarction of hepatic hilar lymph nodes, and patchy parenchymal infarction are common findings (Figure 4.3). Since the necrotic tissue can become seeded with bacteria and fungi, special stains for micro-organisms should be carried out routinely.

d. Differential Diagnosis The histopathological presentation and differential diagnosis for hepatic artery narrowing or thrombosis is broad and includes almost every syndrome associated with graft dysfunction. *Ischemic necrosis,* often centrilobular, is the finding that most reliably points toward arterial thrombosis. More often, however, are centrilobular hepatocyte swelling and/or biliary tract obstruction/cholangitis. The relationship between arterial thrombosis and biliary tract complications is so common that examination of hepatic arterial patency should be routinely considered when biliary tract complications are encountered. Chronic suboptimal arterial flow can cause biliary epithelial cell senescence changes that resemble chronic rejection. And ischemic hepatitis, presenting as spotty hepatocyte apoptosis, can be virtually indistinguishable from the lobular phase of viral hepatitis. Unless a high index of suspicion is maintained, these less common presentations of hepatic artery thrombosis are easily misdiagnosed.

3. Portal Vein Thrombosis

a. Introduction and Pathophysiology The portal vein is much less frequently the site of complications than the hepatic artery. The various portal venous complications include thrombosis, strictures, and poor flow because of persistent collateral circulation or hypotension (51–53,78,79) and their incidence is increased in reduced-size and living donor transplants and when cryopreserved venous interposition grafts are used (80). Long-surviving liver allografts recently as with cirrhosis are also are susceptible to portal vein thrombosis, as in any cirrhotic liver with portal hypertension. Significantly suboptimal flow and complete occlusion are usually clinically significant.

b. Clinical Presentation The clinical presentation of portal vein thrombosis in a cirrhotic allograft is the same as those in a native liver with cirrhosis: variceal hemorrhage, splenomegaly, and ascites. Portal vein thrombosis in a noncirrhotic allograft can cause widespread necrosis (Figure 4.4) and present with fulminant hepatic failure and portal hypertension with massive ascites and edema. If the thrombus is partial or only narrowing is present, or there is suboptimal flow, small infarcts can develop or the liver can become seeded by intestinal bacteria resulting in relapsing fever.

c. Histopathological Findings The histopathological findings depend on the severity of portal vein flow compromise, the time after transplantation, and the condition/structure of the allograft. Complete portal venous obstruction early after transplantation in a noncirrhotic allograft often causes *massive coagulative necrosis*. Suboptimal portal vein flow because of strictures, kinks or persistent collateral circulation can cause periportal and/or midzonal coagulative necrosis (Figure 4.5), hepatocyte atrophy, unexplained zonal or panlobular steatosis, or nodular

regenerative hyperplasia. Bacterial or fungal infection of a partial portal vein thrombus can result in miliary seeding of the liver with small abscesses.

d. Differential Diagnosis It can be quite difficult to distinguish suboptimal portal vein blood flow from suboptimal hepatic venous drainage. Red blood cell congestion within central veins and centrilobular sinusoids and obliterative central venopathy suggests that suboptimal hepatic venous drainage is the correct diagnosis. Otherwise unexplained linear zones of ischemic necrosis and/or hepatocellular atrophy should raise the possibility of compromised portal vein blood flow. Frequently, however, ultrasonography and/or angiography are needed to specifically characterize the cause of the vascular abnormality. Suboptimal portal venous blood flow can also present with massive hepatic steatosis and, therefore, has to be considered in the differential diagnosis of steatosis/hepatitis in allografts. In our experience, blood flow–associated allograft steatosis is usually associated with persistent venous collaterals that have failed to close, or reopened after transplantation.

4. Hepatic Vein and Vena Caval Complications

a. Introduction and Pathophysiology Complications involving the hepatic venous outflow, including the hepatic veins and vena cava are relatively uncommon. Risk factors include reduced-size/living donor allografts and difficulties reconstructing the venous outflow tract or alternative anastomoses such as the "piggyback" approach (26). Significant stenosis or thrombosis of the outflow tract is mostly always associated with either significant clinical or histopathological manifestations.

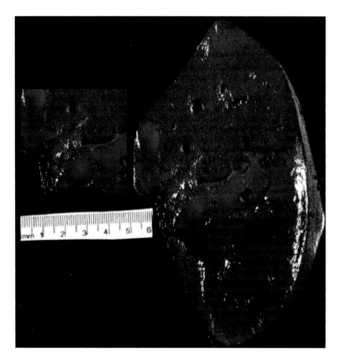

FIGURE 4.4: *Thrombosis of the large extrahepatic portion of the portal vein in a noncirrhotic allograft is relatively uncommon early after transplantation. When it does occur it frequently results large areas of necrosis and in zones of hepatocyte atrophy and/or necrosis represented by the mottled areas in this image.*

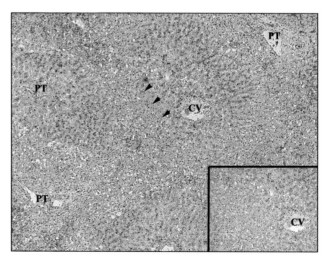

FIGURE 4.5: *Microscopic examination of a liver with portal vein thrombosis often shows linear zones of ischemic hepatocytes, which can manifest as hepatocyte atrophy or coagulative necrosis (outlined by arrowheads) that are often periportal or mid zonal in distribution (lower right inset).*

b. Clinical Presentation The clinical presentation depends on the severity of outflow tract compromise. Severe stenosis or thrombosis presents as the *Budd-Chiari syndrome* including hepatic enlargement, tenderness, and ascites and edema. Less severe stenosis might initially result only in histopathological manifestations or an increase in the portal vein/vena cava pressure gradient.

c. Histopathological Findings The most reliable *acute* findings include *centrilobular congestion and hemorrhage* involving the hepatic venules and surrounding perivenular sinusoids. Red blood cell stasis is usually observed within the lumen of at least some obstructed hepatic venules. Bland centrilobular hepatocyte necrosis and dropout are also usually present. *Chronic changes* can include nodular regenerative hyperplasia, perivenular fibrosis, and central vein occlusion, particularly if outflow obstruction is severe and/or of long duration, and venocentric cirrhosis. The chronic changes can also be accompanied by a prominent ductular reaction at the interface zone and perivenular areas, which can make it difficult to recognize architectural landmarks and to exclude biliary obstruction.

d. Differential Diagnosis The differential diagnosis for centrilobular or perivenular congestion, hemorrhage and hepatocyte necrosis is quite extensive. If these changes are *not* accompanied by any significant inflammation a mechanical/outflow obstruction cause should be suspected. If, however, the centrilobular changes are accompanied by significant lymphocytic, histiocytic and/or lymphoplasmacytic inflammation, an immunologically mediated cause of injury, such as acute and chronic rejection, adverse drug reactions, and viral and autoimmune hepatitis (AIH) should be suspected.

It is important to remember, however, that the inflammation can be transient even in some cases of "immune-mediated" centrilobular injury. These particular cases can present at a later stage when they are indistinguishable from mechanical causes of venous outflow obstruction (81). A review of the clinical history and previous biopsies can help to determine the underlying cause. Examination of venous outflow patency is warranted in cases where there is no, or minimal, associated inflammation.

iv. Bile Duct Complications

1. General Considerations and Pathophysiology

The biliary tree is often referred to as the "Achilles' heel" of liver transplantation and is frequently the site of both minor and major complications. Biliary tract reconstruction during transplantation varies considerably. The most common anastomoses are an end-to-end, duct-to-duct, or a donor biliary–recipient enteric communication. Most

biliary tract complications are ultimately attributable to ischemic and/or traumatic injury or a surgically-introduced abnormal anatomy that predispose to poor wound healing, inadequate drainage, or inordinate reflux. The terminal portion of the donor bile duct is particularly vulnerable to ischemic-injury since it it supplied by only one of the three terminal branchings of the hepatic artery (*the peribiliary plexus*) (82) and arterial flow originates more proximal to the resection margin of the donor extrahepatic bile duct. To ascertain adequate arterial flow and viability, therefore, the terminal end of the donor extrahepatic bile duct is "trimmed" backward toward the liver until bleeding occurs from the cut surface.

The is particularly vulnerable to preservation/reperfusion injury and damage during operative manipulation (83). For example, in DCD donors, sludging of blood, or use of the more viscous University of Wisconsin solution (84,85), can prevent adequate reperfusion of the peribiliary plexus in the recipient [reviewed in (46,47)]. This can be avoided by arterial, and consequently peribiliary plexus, perfusion by thrombolytic agents and/or less viscous preservation solutions (e.g., HTK) (84,85) before reperfusion in the recipient [reviewed in (46,47)].

There are several other causes of biliary tract ischemia because of arterial and/or peribiliary plexus injury. Included are: 1) small-for-size syndrome and severe arterial vasospasm (57); and 2) prolonged cold ischemia; and 3) preformed anti-donor antibodies (31). Biliary tract complications are also more common after reduced size liver transplants, such as living donors (86,87) and split liver transplant operations (88). Once this myriad of other causes of biliary tract complications have been reasonably excluded, recurrent primary sclerosing cholangitis (PSC) should be considered in patients who have the disease before transplantation.

Biliary tract complications, including anastomotic dehiscence, transmural necrosis, bile leakage, cholangitic abscesses, ascending cholangitis, bile casts, strictures, obstruction, ampullary dysfunction, and biliary-vascular fistulas [reviewed in (89–93)], occur in about 15 percent in whole cadaveric allografts and up to 30–40 percent of reduced-size/living donor allografts (35,89). By far, *strictures* are the most common complication. They are categorized according to time after transplantation and location; into those occurring early and late; and into anastomotic and nonanastomotic or intrahepatic [reviewed in (89–93)]. Intrahepatic strictures are further categorized into hilar versus peripheral.

Anastomotic strictures usually appear within the first several months after transplantation. They continue to appear, but at a reduced rate, for many years after transplantation [reviewed in (89,90)]. Risk factors for the development of anastomotic strictures include postoperative bile leaks, female donor–male recipient sex combination, and more recent year of transplantation (89,90).

Compared to nonanastomotic strictures, anastomotic strictures are generally more amenable to radiographically directed and/or surgical intervention and have less of a negative impact on long-term graft and patient survival (89,90).

Conversely, nonanastomotic strictures usually occur later after transplantation, are generally untreatable and progressive, and negatively impact graft and patient survival (89–93). Risk factors for nonanastomotic strictures include use of high viscosity preservation solution, PSC original disease, Roux-en-Y biliary anastomoses, and cytomegalovirus (CMV) infection (91–93).

Early (less than one year) nonanastomotic strictures are often associated with preservation-related injury (93,94) and usually located in perihilar bile ducts. As expected, risk factors include long cold and warm ischemic times, high viscosity preservation solution, older recipient age, a duct-to-duct biliary anastomosis, and bile leaks (93). Late (greater than one year) nonanastomotic strictures are usually peripheral and associated with immunologic risk factors, such as PSC as the original disease.

2. Clinical Presentation

Routine monitoring of liver injury tests showing selective elevation of γ-glutamyltranspeptidase and alkaline phosphatase is the usual method of detecting early and/or minor biliary tract complications, such as strictures and stones. Clinical signs and symptoms are infrequent unless the patient becomes jaundiced. Biliary tract problems are often first suspected on biopsy evaluation, but cholangiography [MRCP, ERCP (duct-to-duct) or percutaneous transhepatic cholangiography (PTC)] is needed to *confirm* the diagnosis and localize the defects (89,90). During the first several months after transplantation, T-tube stents provide ready access for cholangiograms, which are routinely performed before clamping and one week and again at the time of T-tube removal at three months.

More serious biliary tract complications, such as obstruction, cholangitic abscesses and ascending cholangitis usually present with fever, jaundice, upper right quadrant pain, and intermittent bacteremia. As mentioned above, complications occurring at or near the biliary anastomosis are generally more amenable to treatment than those occurring within the liver.

3. Histopathological Findings

Allograft biliary tract complications are histopathologically identical to those seen in native livers. Portal and periductal edema, predominantly neutrophilic portal inflammation, intraepithelial, and intraluminal neutrophils within true bile ducts, an interface ductular reaction of varying severity, centrilobular hepatocanalicular cholestasis, and small clusters of neutrophils throughout the

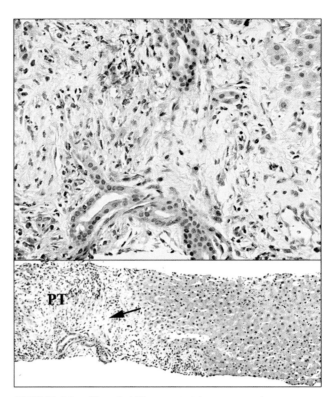

FIGURE 4.6: *Chronic biliary tract strictures can show predominantly mononuclear inflammation with interface activity resembling late-onset acute rejection and chronic hepatitis. In this particular biopsy, obtained from a recipient with chronic biliary strictures years years after transplantation showed mild predominantly lymphoplasmacytic portal inflammation with interface activity (arrowheads, right panel, and upper left inset). However, periductal edema surrounding the true bile ducts (arrow, right panel), periportal Mallory's hyalin (arrow, upper left panel), and deposition of copper in periportal hepatocytes (lower left panel) were the changes that pointed toward chronic biliary tract strictures.*

lobules are the typical findings of stricturing/obstructive cholangiopathy. Over time chronic biliary tract strictures, or intermittent obstruction, is often associated with mixed or predominantly chronic portal inflammation, biliary epithelial cell senescence changes, and low-grade ductopenia involving the small bile ducts (Figure 4.6). More than one year after transplantation, in addition to the classic features described above, biliary strictures are a relatively common cause of portal eosinophilia (Figure 4.7).

Biliary-vascular fistulas are recognized by red blood cells in lumina of bile ducts or bile concretions in blood vessels. Occasionally, inordinate elevations of the serum bilirubin, beyond normal pathophysiological ranges, can also be seen with a fistula. Prompt surgical intervention is usually required for these findings. In contrast, *periductal* hemorrhage surrounding small interlobular bile ducts is an inconsequential finding in asymptomatic patients when a biopsy is obtained within a day or so after transhepatic cholangiography (95).

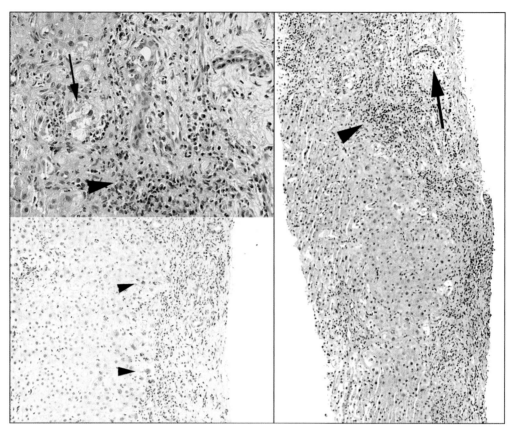

FIGURE 4.7: *This example of obstructive cholangiopathy was detected about fourteen months after liver transplantation. Features used to establish the diagnosis included the prominent portal edema surrounding the true bile ducts, ductular reaction, and predominantly acute portal inflammation. Note the significant portal eosinophilia (upper panel). In contrast to early after transplantation, late after transplantation, portal edema with eosinophilia should suggest obstructive cholangiopathy—especially in a patient with adequate immunosuppressive drug levels.*

4. Differential Diagnosis

The histopathological differential diagnosis for biliary tract complications is significantly influenced by the time after transplantation. Biliary obstruction/cholangitis can be difficult to distinguish from preservation/reperfusion injury and acute rejection within the first several weeks after transplantation. It can be made more difficult if the patient is treated with increased immunosuppression before the biopsy was obtained.

Features used to distinguish between preservation/reperfusion injury and biliary obstruction was discussed above in Preservation/Reperfusion Injury.

Features that favor biliary tract obstruction/stricturing over acute cellular rejection early after transplantation include neutrophilic-predominant portal infiltrate, periductal edema, and retention of the normal nuclear: cytoplasmic ratio and biliary epithelial cells, and an absence of perivenular mononuclear inflammation. In contrast, features that favor acute rejection include a mixed portal infiltrate comprised of blastic and small lymphocytes, plasma cells, and eosinophils; lymphocytic cholangitis, and increased nuclear-cytoplasmic ratio in biliary epithelial

cells, and perivenular inflammation. Portal eosinophilia in early acute rejection can be quite striking, especially in patients treated with "steroid-sparing" immunosuppressive regimens (96). But late after transplantation biliary stricturing is not an uncommon cause of portal eosinophilia. Checking blood immunosuppression levels is helpful in making the distinction.

Late-onset and/or chronic biliary tract complications can occasionally present with predominantly mononuclear portal inflammation and biliary epithelial cell senescence changes and low-grade ductopenia can develop (97). Such cases can mimic acute and chronic rejection, viral hepatitis, and recurrent autoimmune disorders (Figure 4.6). Portal fibrosis with stellate expansion and a ductular reaction at the interface zone, portal neutrophilic and/or eosinophilic inflammation, and centrilobular cholestasis are features that favor obstructive cholangiopathy. Usually, however, late-onset and/or chronic biliary tract complications present with the typical changes described under the "histopathological findings."

Clinicopathological correlation can also be quite helpful in distinguishing late-onset biliary tract complications from late-onset acute rejection. Adequate immunosuppressive drug levels with preferential elevation of the γGTP and alkaline phosphatase (98) favors obstructive cholangiopathy because late-onset acute rejection is unusual in this circumstance.

Chronic obstructive cholangiopathy can be difficult to distinguish from chronic viral hepatitis. Cholangitis favors a biliary tract complication, whereas cholangiolitis and lobular disarray favor chronic hepatitis. The cholestatic liver injury tests profile favors obstructive cholangiopathy, unless the patient has cholestatic variant of viral hepatitis. Therefore, review of HBV and/or HCV nucleic acid levels in the blood helps to distinguish between the two because cholestatic viral hepatitis is variably associated with high levels of viral replication. With long-standing biliary strictures, prominent deposits of *copper or copper-associated protein* in periportal hepatocytes favor obstructive cholangiopathy.

It is often very difficult to distinguish between chronic rejection and biliary strictures, especially recurrent PSC, in peripheral core needle biopsies. At-risk populations are similar; both can cause "cholestatic" elevation of liver injury tests and intrahepatic cholestasis, biliary epithelial cell senescence changes, and small bile duct loss. Careful examination of the clinical history, evaluation of serial biopsies, and histopathology are needed to distinguish with confidence between biliary strictures/recurrent PSC and chronic rejection (99). Features that *favor* biliary strictures/recurrent PSC over chronic rejection in a needle biopsy include a history of biliary tract complications and/or PSC original disease, periductal lamellar edema involving the true bile ducts, stellate portal expansion, portal neutrophilia, and a ductular reaction affecting at least some portal tracts, and deposition of copper or copper-associated protein in periportal hepatocytes. Features that favor acute and/or chronic rejection include a previous history of rejection and/or inadequate immunosuppression, lymphoplasmacytic portal inflammation, small portal tracts, absence of a ductular reaction, and active central perivenulitis and/or perivenular fibrosis.

Additional findings in *failed allografts* can also be used to distinguish between biliary strictures/recurrent PSC and chronic rejection. Chronically rejected livers are usually of normal or slightly increased weight, whereas those with obstructive cholangiopathy are usually significantly enlarged. In the hilar lymph nodes, obstructive cholangiopathy usually causes bile-pigmented sinus histiocytosis, whereas chronically rejected nodes are usually atrophic and/or fibrotic. The perihilar arteries are either normal or show mild and focal eccentric fibrointimal hyperplasia, whereas foam cell arteriopathy and significant concentric fibrointimal hyperplasia are typical of chronic rejection. In obstructive cholangiopathy, extrahepatic/large intrahepatic bile ducts often show focal ulceration, periductal lymphoplasmacytic inflammation,

and fibrosis, whereas in chronic rejection ulceration is unusual.

Angiography and cholangiography are also useful in making the distinction between obstructive cholangiopathy and chronic rejection. "Pruning" of the peripheral arterial and biliary trees and poor peripheral filling are seen in chronic rejection, whereas some intrahepatic duct dilation is observed with obstructive cholangiopathy and arterial changes are either not present or not significant.

In our opinion it is not yet possible to reliably distinguish recurrent PSC from other causes of biliary tract obstruction or stricturing of the bases of needle biopsy evaluation alone.

v. Rejection

1. *General Considerations*

Rejection is generally categorized into antibody-mediated, acute cellular, and chronic (100). Antibody-mediated rejection usually occurs within the first several weeks after transplantation in ABO-incompatible allografts and in recipients with a strongly positive lymphocytotoxic cross-match (101). Acute cellular rejection can occur at any time after transplantation, but is most common during the first month (102) and is mediated primarily by cell-mediated immunity. Chronic rejection usually develops directly from severe or persistent and unresolved acute rejection and is probably mediated by a combination of both antibodies and cellular immunity.

2. *Antibody-Mediated Rejection*

a. General Considerations In general, liver allografts are much *less susceptible* than other solid organ allografts to injury from antibody-mediated rejection because of preformed lymphocytotoxic and blood group antibodies [reviewed in (31)]. Lymphocytotoxic cross-match results, therefore, do not routinely influence organ triage/recipient selection at most centers. Crossing ABO blood group barriers, however, is avoided in most programs because it leads to a high incidence (~60 percent) of significant antibody-mediated rejection and/or graft failure [reviewed in (31)]. ABO-incompatible liver allografts are still utilized in some countries, such as Japan, where the donor pool is more limited. Vigorous anti-rejection therapy is needed to achieve reasonable results under these circumstances, and even so, the recipients are still at risk for late biliary tract complications, such as ischemic cholangitis (31). One case of late onset, combined antibody and cell-mediated, rejection has recently been reported (103). However, whether antibody-mediated rejection is reliably detectable late after transplantation and whether it adversely impacts long-term allograft survival requires further study.

Living donor liver allografts appear to be more susceptible to antibody-mediated rejection than whole liver cadaveric donors (104). This is probably related to several factors unique to reduced sized/living donor allografts such as small caliber blood vessels and mechanical microvascular injury and arterial vasospasm because of portal hyperperfusion (see considerations in reduced-size allografts).

b. Pathophysiology The consequences of anti-donor antibodies depend on the class, titer, timing of the antibody response, and the density and distribution of target antigens in the liver (31,105). High-titer preformed antibodies directed at antigens expressed on endothelial cells, such as the isoagglutinins and lymphocytotoxic (anti-MHC class I) antibodies are potentially the most dangerous. Antibody binding to the allograft endothelium precipitates complement fixation, endothelial damage, deposition of platelet-fibrin thrombi, and initiation of the clotting and fibrinolytic cascades. This, in turn, leads to microvascular thrombosis, arterial vasospasm, and coagulopathy that in concert act to impair blood flow and cause hemorrhagic necrosis. Hyperacute rejection can occur within the first several hours to days after transplantation and is usually associated with preformed, high titer, isoagglutinins, or anti-MHC lymphocytotoxic antibodies, but this is rare because liver allografts have a natural resistance to antibody mediated rejection [reviewed in (31)].

Resistance of liver allografts to antibody mediated rejection has been attributed to 1) secretion of soluble MHC class I antigens that bind to and neutralize the antibodies; 2) Kupffer's cell phagocytosis of subsequent immune complexes and activated platelet aggregates; 3) dual afferent hepatic blood supply; 4) unique hepatic sinusoidal microvasculature, which is devoid of a conventional basement membrane (reviewed in references) (31); and 5) possibly, a homologous source of complement (106).

Risk factors for antibody-mediated rejection include ABO-incompatible transplants and recipients with a strongly positive lymphocytotoxic cross-match, which is more frequently seen in female recipients because of pregnancies and recipients of previous organ transplants or blood transfusions. Risk factors for acute rejection include younger, "healthier" (e.g., Child-Pugh grade A, good renal function and muscle mass), black, female recipients, and patients with disorders of immune regulation before transplantation, such as PBC, PSC, AIH [reviewed in (107)], inadequate immunosuppression, and exposure to the same or similar alloantigens via blood transfusions or previous transplants or pregnancies. Since chronic rejection usually develops from acute rejection, risk factors for chronic rejection overlap with those for acute rejection.

In general, isoagglutinins cause more damage than lymphocytotoxic antibodies; lymphocytotoxic antibodies do not reliably cause clinically relevant allograft damage

unless present at a relatively high titer (>1:32). As in other organs, IgG usually cause more damage than IgM lymphocytotoxic antibodies [reviewed in (31,108)]. In our experience, positive lymphocytotoxic cross-match results are encountered in 8–12 percent, mostly female, recipients. Only 30 percent of recipients with a positive cross-match have titers high enough to cause clinically significant liver injury. Since the patient population at risk for severe antibody-mediated rejection is fairly small, antibody mediated rejection is often overlooked as a cause of dysfunction or failure. This occurs because 1) the incidence is relatively low, 2) many programs do not routinely conduct pretransplant cross-matching, and 3) even if cross-matches are performed, the titer and post-transplant monitoring are not routinely carried out.

c. Clinical Presentation The most severe and dramatic form of antibody mediated rejection, hyperacute, begins immediately after reperfusion in unconditioned ABO-incompatible recipients, but is rare (109–112). Liver hyperacute rejection allograft dysfunction usually becomes recognizable over a period of hours to days, rather than minutes to hours, as in other organs [reviewed in (31)]. In such cases, the first signs of dysfunction usually develop in the operating room after complete revascularization and recognized by uneven reperfusion, swelling, dusky appearance, and cessation of bile flow in a liver that initially produced adequate bile. These signs are often accompanied by coagulopathy manifested as difficulty in achieving hemostasis and an inordinate need for platelets and other blood component replacement therapy.

Precipitous allograft failure, however, is distinctly unusual. A more common scenario is a relentless rise in liver injury tests during the first several post-transplant days and other signs of impending hepatic failure. Hepatic angiograms, often obtained at this point to exclude an arterial thrombosis, usually show changes indicative of immunologically mediated arterial vasospasm (31). A persistent rise in serum bilirubin, refractory thrombocytopenia, and low complement activity during the first week after transplantation are signs of an ongoing antibody mediated reaction.

d. Histopathological Findings The histopathological manifestations of antibody mediated rejection depend on the timing of the biopsy and the class, titer, and specificity of the anti-donor antibodies [reviewed in (31)]. In general, ABO incompatibility causes more red blood cell congestion and necrosis than lymphocytotoxic antibodies (Figures 4.8–4.10). If isoagglutinins are present at high titer, prominent red blood cell, and focal neutrophil sludging in the sinusoids, platelet-fibrin thrombi in portal and central veins, and acidophilic hepatocyte necrosis biopsies can be seen within 2–6 hours after reperfusion. In such cases, confluent coagulative necrosis, prominent sinusoidal and

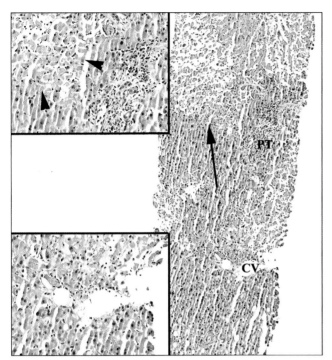

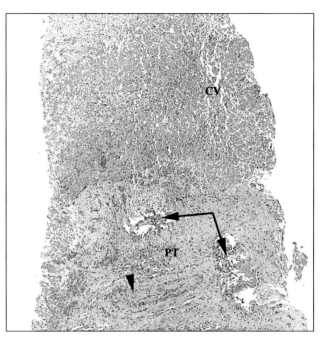

FIGURE 4.9: *Follow-up biopsy at fourteen days after liver transplantation of the same patient illustrated in Figure 4.8. The biopsy now shows widespread coagulative necrosis, flame-shaped portal vein thrombi (arrows), and focal fibrinoid necrosis of a hepatic artery branch (arrowhead).*

FIGURE 4.8: *Antibody-mediated rejection of an ABO-incompatible liver allograft usually causes significantly more damage than lymphocytotoxic antibodies. This biopsy was obtained eight days after transplantation of an ABO-incompatible liver. Note the mild, predominantly neutrophilic, portal inflammation (upper left inset) and patchy areas of coagulative necrosis (arrow), which is illustrated at higher magnification in the upper left inset. Note also the endothelial cell reactivity of the central vein illustrated at higher magnification in the lower left inset. (PT = portal tract; CV = central vein). Follow-up tissue samples from this particular patient are illustrated in Figures 4.9 and 4.10.*

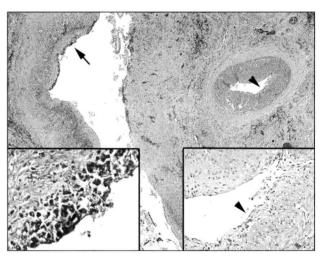

venous congestion, and hemorrhage into the portal tract connective tissue begin to appear within one or five days (Figure 4.8). Portal veins often show circumferential fibrin deposition (Figure 4.9). The most common arterial findings include endothelial cell hypertrophy and evidence of arterial vasospasm, such as mural myocyte vacuolization, wrinkling of the elastic lamina, and thickening of the wall with narrowing of the lumen. In severe cases, neutrophilic and/or necrotizing arteritis is seen (Figure 4.10). Portal neutrophilia, cholangiolar proliferation, and small areas of confluent hepatic necrosis usually began to appear at two–three days. If untreated, progressive hemorrhagic infarction of the organ can occur in ABO-incompatible organs over a relatively short period of time.

The gross exam of failed ABO-incompatible grafts shows findings similar to "hyperacute" rejection in other organs. They are usually quite enlarged, cyanotic and mottled with areas of necrosis. Capsular ruptures, hepatic artery or portal vein thrombosis are seen in severe cases. Microscopically, changes in the hilum/perihilar region can be particularly helpful in establishing a diagnosis of

FIGURE 4.10: *Follow-up failed allograft specimen from the patient whose biopsy specimens were illustrated in Figures 4.8 and 4.9, obtained at eighteen days after transplantation. This ABO-incompatible liver allograft showed findings typical of severe antibody-mediated rejection, such as fibrointimal hyperplasia of the peri-hilar hepatic artery branches (arrowhead). When viewed at higher magnification (lower right inset) significant neutrophilic and lymphocytic intimal inflammation was easily detectable. Note also that the large bile duct is totally necrotic and bile has leaked into the surrounding connective tissue, which is severely inflamed. This illustrates that antibody mediated rejection is an important cause of ischemic cholangitis. Note also the bacterial colonies in the necrotic bile duct wall (left lower inset).*

antibody-mediated rejection. Included are congestion and leukocyte margination in the peribiliary vascular plexus, partially organized thrombi in arterial branches, focal mural necrosis of large septal bile ducts, and inflammatory and/or necrotizing arteritis (Figure 4.10). Late sequelae of antibody-mediated rejection can include biliary sludge and stricturing with obstructive cholangiopathy, and obliterative arteriopathy and loss of small bile ducts, or chronic rejection.

A diagnosis of antibody-mediated rejection is more difficult to establish in patients harboring preformed lymphocytotoxic antibodies because the changes are generally less florid. Reperfusion biopsies from patients with high titer lymphocytotoxic antibodies contain platelet aggregates in the portal and or central veins more often than cross-match negative controls. Spotty acidophilic necrosis of hepatocytes and centrilobular hepatocellular swelling, accompanied by cholangiolar proliferation and hepatocanalicular cholestasis often appear during the first week after transplantation in those with high-titer (>1:32). Inflammatory or necrotizing arteritis is rarely present, but nearly diagnostic when found. More commonly, the histopathological changes closely resemble those seen in preservation/reperfusion injury and clinicopathological correlation and staining for immune deposits are needed to confirm the diagnosis (Figures 4.11 and 4.12).

Unfortunately, intrahepatic *immune deposits* are ephemeral in antibody-mediated rejection, even when using the more sensitive technique of immunofluorescence on frozen tissue. For example, immunofluorescent deposits are usually detectable only in post-reperfusion biopsies and biopsies obtained within a few days after transplantation in allografts known to be damaged by antibody-mediated rejection (e.g., ABO-incompatible). In severe cases, selective deposits of IgG and/or IgM, C3, and C4 are usually detectable diffusely along the sinusoids and in perihilar arteries, portal veins, and peribiliary plexus. Thereafter, immune deposits become patchy in distribution and may be difficult to distinguish from background staining, unless antibody titers are quite high. Usually, however, frozen tissue has not been saved for immunofluorescence testing, unless the surgeon/clinician is suspicious of a diagnosis of antibody mediated rejection.

Therefore, detection of immune reactants often depends on localization of *C4d deposits* in formalin-fixed, paraffin-embedded tissues (Figure 4.12). This stain has been a reliable marker of antibody-mediated rejection in kidney and heart allografts (113,114). In liver allografts, however, interpretation of C4d staining is more difficult (112,115–122). Bellamy recently reported a small series and reviewed the literature (112,115–122) concluding that the practical utility of C4d immunohistochemistry is limited. It may, however, identify a small subgroup of individuals in whom chronic humoral microvascular injury contributes to allograft dysfunction (115).

Endothelial cell C4d staining is most specific for antibody-mediated rejection and is also frequently seen

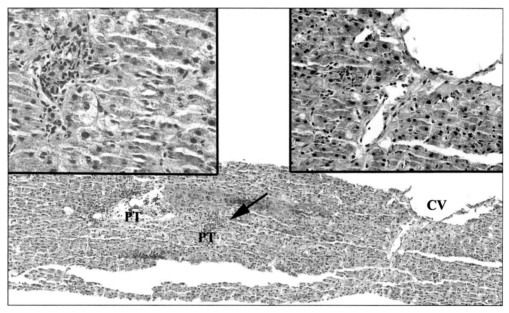

FIGURE 4.11: *Antibody-mediated rejection in a recipient with a strong (usually >1:32–64) lymphocytotoxic cross-match is usually detected within the first week after transplantation and closely resembles preservation/reperfusion injury. Features include mild, predominantly neutrophilic portal inflammation and mild cholangiolar proliferation (upper left inset), sinusoidal leukocytosis, and reactive appearing endothelial cells in the portal and/or central veins (upper right inset). These changes, however, can be subtle, are not entirely specific, and require clinical pathological correlation (see text) and demonstration of immunoglobulin and complement in the tissues (see Figure 4.3) (PT = portal tract; CV = central vein).*

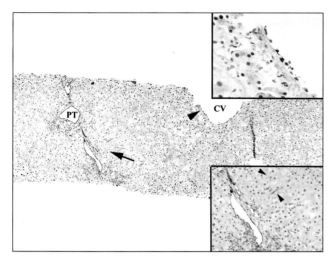

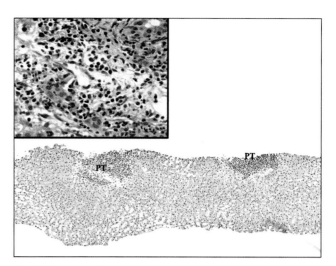

FIGURE 4.12: *C4d staining can be used to detect complement deposition in formalin-fixed, paraffin-embedded tissue samples. This biopsy is the same biopsy as illustrated in Figure 4.2, obtained from a recipient with a strongly positive lymphocytotoxic cross-match six days after liver transplantation. Note the strong staining in the portal vein (lower right inset), hepatic artery, sinusoidal (lower right inset, arrowheads), and central vein endothelium (upper right inset), which also shows minimal neutrophilic infiltration of the subendothelial space (PT = portal tract; CV = central vein).*

FIGURE 4.13: *This biopsy shows histopathological evidence of mild acute cellular rejection. Only the two portal tracts shown in this biopsy, which contains ten other portal tracts, were inflamed. The upper left inset shows the characteristic "rejection-type" portal infiltrate comprised of blastic and or lymphocytes and eosinophils and focal bile duct inflammation and damage.*

during acute cellular rejection. For example, C4d staining of portal capillary and venous and hepatic artery endothelium is detected in 10–80 percent of patients recipients with acute cellular rejection (112,115–122). C4d staining has been reported to be proportional to the Banff grades of acute cellular rejection being more widespread and intense with severe acute cellular rejection. Portal venous, arterial, and capillary endothelial C4d staining is also usually detected in cross-match positive recipients that develop severe antibody-mediated rejection (120) and in those who develop hyperacute rejection (122). Necrotic hepatocytes can also show C4d staining, but this type of staining is not specific for antibody mediated rejection. Normal liver allograft biopsies are usually C4d negative.

A minority of recipients with other causes of allograft dysfunction, such as biliary tract obstruction or stricturing (115), recurrent HBV (116), and HCV (118) show portal microvascular C4d deposition. But these deposits tend to be less widespread than in severe acute cellular or antibody-mediated rejection. In one study, diffuse sinusoidal C4d staining, in addition to portal vasculature positivity, distinguished moderate-to-severe rejection from other complications (121). In our experience, C4d staining can be helpful in suspected cases of antibody-mediated rejection and sinusoidal staining in nonnecrotic areas is a more specific but insensitive sign of antibody-mediated damage (Figure 4.13). C4d deposition has also been associated with macrophage and plasma cell infiltrates, similar to kidney and heart allografts (117).

e. Differential Diagnosis Precipitous allograft failure from severe antibody-mediated rejection can be difficult to distinguish from hemorrhagic liver necrosis caused by hypotension and poor perfusion, sepsis, or vascular thrombosis. Unless unequivocal evidence of antibody-mediated rejection are detected, such as inflammatory/necrotizing arteritis and/or diffuse immunoglobulin and complement deposition, the cause of allograft failure can be extremely difficult to determine with certainty. More commonly changes diagnostic of antibody mediated rejection are not present and the diagnosis requires a thorough clinico-pathological correlation, immunofluorescence, and/or immunoperoxidase staining for immunoglobulins and complement.

Knowing that the recipient harbors high titer lympho-cytotoxic antibodies or that the allograft is ABO-blood group incompatible often facilitates biopsy interpretation. This information heightens recognition of typical patterns of histopathological injury, described above, and correlation with clinical course and laboratory findings. Haga et al. suggested that portal stromal C4d deposition is a hallmark of antibody mediated rejection in ABO-incompatible allografts (112); we have also detected portal and sinusoidal microvascular endothelial cell staining in ABO-incompatible grafts.

Distinguishing antibody-mediated rejection from preservation/reperfusion injury can be quite difficult, but the pre-sensitization state and post-transplant clinical and laboratory profile provide discriminating information (see Clinical Presentation, above). For example, antibody mediated rejection should be suspected in a female liver allograft recipient with high-titer, donor-specific, lymphocytotoxic antibodies, who received a liver with a short cold ischemic time, but shows persistence of the antibodies after transplantation and develops graft dysfunction, refractory and otherwise unexplained thrombocytopenia, and circulating low complement levels after transplantation (108).

Antibody-mediated rejection should be favored over preservation/reperfusion injury when the following histopathological findings are detected: 1) neutrophils, macrophages, and to a lesser extent, lymphocytes, marginating on the luminal aspect and beneath the portal and central veins, along with diffuse endothelial cell reactivity and 2) blastic lymphocytes and eosinophils and other features of acute cellular rejection in the portal and/or perivenular areas. Immunoperoxidase staining for C4d can be confirmatory in moderate to severe cases, as described above.

3. Acute (Cellular) Rejection

a. General Considerations Acute (cellular) rejection has been defined as, "inflammation of the allograft, elicited by a genetic disparity between the donor and recipient, primarily affecting interlobular bile ducts and vascular endothelia, including portal and hepatic veins and occasionally the hepatic artery and its branches" (100). Most episodes occur within 30 days after transplantation because the reaction is precipitated by mass migration of donor cells into recipient lymphoid tissues (123,124). Early acute rejection episodes rarely lead to allograft failure or permanent allograft damage because they are, for the most part, easily controlled by increased immunosuppression (27).

b. Pathophysiology The pathophysiology of acute cellular and chronic rejection is beyond the scope of this chapter. A basic concept, however, is that mobile donor leukocytes transplanted with the donor organ traffic to recipient lymphoid tissues after revascularization into recipient. Conversely, recipient leukocytes enter the allograft. This leads to immunologic recognition of the allograft as foreign in both the allograft and the recipient lymphoid tissues. The mass migration of leukocytes triggers a cascade of events that changes both the recipient and the allograft. Recipient leukocytes sensitized in the lymphoid tissue traffic into the allograft within several days after transplantation, where they join recipient leukocytes sensitized in the allograft to cause rejection.

Secretion of cytokines and chemokines within the allograft alters the expression of MHC, adhesion, and costimulatory molecules on various cell populations within the liver. This causes retention of inflammatory cells within the graft, especially in the portal tracts and perivenular tissues. Early after transplantation the subsequent immune response preferentially targets the biliary epithelia of small bile ducts, endothelia of portal and central

veins and hepatic artery branches (in severe rejection), which leads to the characteristic histopathological appearance of acute and chronic rejection.

Immunologic effector mechanisms that contribute to graft injury during acute rejection include antibody and complement-mediated injury, cytolytic T-cell lympholysis (Fas FasL interactions), and effector molecules and cytokines release from various inflammatory cells (e.g., TNF, eosinophil cationic protein, reactive oxygen species). These various effector mechanisms injure parenchymal and endothelial cells, which, in turn, can interfere with blood flow and cause ischemic injury (125,126). The prevalence and severity of inflammation and damage are used to grade acute rejection histopathologically. Immunologically mediated microcirculatory damage and poor arterial flow or thrombosis has the potential to cause the most significant injury. Compared to other solid organ allografts, acute rejection uncommonly leads to graft fibrosis and chronic rejection (27).

c. Clinical Presentation Acute cellular rejection first presents clinically usually between five and thirty days after transplantation. Earlier presentations can be seen in presensitized patients or in those who receive less than optimal baseline immunosuppression. Later presentations can be seen in recipients treated with lymphocyte-depleting antibodies. Clinical findings are often absent early in the course when the tissue damage is mild. Later in the course or with severe acute rejection, fever and allograft enlargement, cyanosis, and tenderness frequently occur. The change in the quantity and/or quality of bile is also a gross, but reliable, marker of graft dysfunction. Decreased bile flow and thin and pale bile are commonly seen. Ascites can occasionally develop because of increased intrahepatic hydrostatic pressure that results in liver swelling and increased lymph production (127).

Biochemical evidence of liver dysfunction usually includes nonselective elevations of some or all of the standard liver injury tests [e.g., total bilirubin, alanine aminotransferase, aspartate aminotransferase, γ-glutamyl transpeptidase, and alkaline phosphatase (127)]. Leukocytosis and eosinophilia are also frequently present in peripheral blood counts. Elevations of various proteins in the peripheral blood have been associated with acute rejection. Included are various interleukin levels or their receptors, neopterin, amyloid A protein, and anti-donor class I MHC antibodies. Since many of these clinical and laboratory findings lack sensitivity or specificity, none is routinely used to monitor recipients. Instead, a diagnosis of acute cellular rejection is usually suspected on clinical grounds and confirmed by examination of a core needle biopsy specimen, which is considered the "gold standard" method of establishing the diagnosis.

Risk factors for developing early acute rejection depend on the immunosuppressive regimen. But most studies include young recipient age, "healthy" recipients (normal serum creatinine, Child-Pugh classification, etc.), donor/recipient human leukocyte antigen (HLA)-DR mismatch, patients with immune dysregulated syndromes (e.g., PSC, AIH, and PBC), long cold ischemic time, and increased donor age [reviewed in (107)]. Late-onset acute rejection occurring more than one year after transplantation can have a slightly different histopathological appearance, is often associated with inadequate immunosuppression, is more difficult to control with increased immunosuppression, and more frequently leads to allograft damage and failure [reviewed in (107)].

The decision to treat liver allograft recipients with increased immunosuppression is usually based on the clinicopathological correlation. The following is an algorithm that is generally followed at our institution. Patients with indeterminate or mild acute rejection according to the Banff schema who are without, or have only minor, liver function abnormalities are generally not treated with increased immunosuppression. Some are treated with a slight increase in baseline immunosuppressive agents. This approach usually does not lead to long-term complications (27,128,129). Patients with mild acute rejection who show significant liver function abnormalities are usually treated with increased baseline immunosuppression and/or additional corticosteroid therapy. Recipients who develop moderate or severe acute rejection are generally treated more aggressively than those with less significant rejection. Most commonly, the treatment includes increased baseline immunosuppression and/or corticosteroid recycles. If unsuccessful, this is usually followed by lymphocyte depleting antibodies. The use of more aggressive immunosuppressive therapy is justified because higher grades of acute rejection show a small, but definite, increased risk of persistent and/or recurrent acute rejection and development of chronic rejection and allograft failure (27,130).

d. Histopathological Findings and Grading
Acute rejection is characterized by 1) predominantly mononuclear but mixed portal inflammation containing blastic or activated lymphocytes, neutrophils, and eosinophils; 2) subendothelial inflammation of portal and/or terminal hepatic venules; and 3) bile duct inflammation and damage (127,131). Minimal diagnostic criteria needed to establish the diagnosis of acute rejection include at least two of the above histopathological findings. The diagnosis is strengthened if greater than 50 percent of the ducts or terminal hepatic veins are damaged or if unequivocal endotheliitis of portal or terminal hepatic vein branches can be identified. Histopathological evidence of *severe injury*, which is used for histopathological grading, includes perivenular inflammation, centrilobular necrosis, arteritis, and inflammatory, usually central-to-central, bridging inflammation/necrosis (27,127).

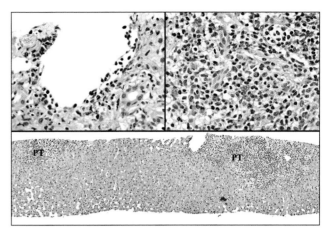

FIGURE 4.14: *In moderate acute cellular rejection, a rejection type infiltrate noticeably expands most or all of the portal tracts, as shown in this photomicrograph. The upper left inset illustrates classic "endothelialitis," or infiltration of inflammatory cells into the subendothelial space. The upper right inset nicely illustrates the pleomorphic, typical, "rejection-type" infiltrate comprising blastic and small lymphocytes eosinophils and neutrophils.*

Acute rejection-related infiltrates are most commonly encountered in the portal tracts (Figure 4.13) and around the central veins. The population is usually comprised of blastic and smaller lymphocytes, and eosinophils (Figure 4.14), which are more conspicuous in recipients treated with "steroid-sparing" and/or lymphocyte depleting immunosuppressive regimens. "Endotheliitis" or "endothelialitis" describes the localization of lymphocytes underneath the portal and central vein endothelium (Figure 4.14), which is characteristic of acute rejection, but it is also seen with other causes of allograft dysfunction (132). Therefore, endothelialitis should not be relied upon too heavily for a diagnosis of acute rejection, especially if it is only a focal finding.

The immunophenotypic profile of acute rejection infiltrates usually shows a predominance of T lymphocytes, as expected, and CD8+ cells often surround and invade damaged bile ducts (133,134). B cells usually comprise a minor fraction of the infiltrates. Macrophages and other leukocytes are also present and can predominate in severe acute rejection (133–135). In our experience, routine immunophenotypic analysis of graft infiltrating lymphocytes is not prognostically or clinically useful for establishing the diagnosis of acute rejection, except when attempting to distinguish acute rejection (T-cell predominant) from a post-transplant lymphoproliferative disorder (PTLD) (B-cell predominant; also see Differential Diagnosis).

Inflammatory bile duct damage is an important feature used to recognize acute rejection. Typically, small bile ducts less than 30 μm in diameter are preferentially affected and lymphocytes are found inside the ductal basement membrane. Histopathological evidence of biliary epithelial cell injury/response includes paranuclear vacuolization, increased nuclear: cytoplasmic ratio, mitoses, nucleoli, and occasional apoptotic bodies. Cytoplasmic eosinophilia and multinucleation usually signal chronic injury. Breaks in the basement membrane signify severe bile duct damage. Portal and/or peribiliary granulomas are not a feature of either acute or chronic rejection. When they are encountered a nonrejection-related cause of duct injury, such as recurrent PBC or a coexistent mycobacterial or fungal infection or sarcoidosis should be suspected.

Inflammatory and/or necrotizing *arteritis* can be an important feature of severe acute rejection, but this finding is uncommon and the vessels most commonly affected are located in the hilum and not sampled in needle biopsies. Furthermore, histopathological recognition of arteritis in peripheral needle biopsies is poorly reproducible (136). Inflammatory arteritis, therefore, is not generally included in grading schema unless it is unequivocally identified in an artery branch containing an internal elastic lamina. If unequivocal arteritis is identified, the biopsy is graded as severe acute cellular rejection.

The interface zone is usually unremarkable in typical early mild and moderate acute cellular rejection. In severe acute rejection, however, *spillover* of the inflammatory infiltrate into the periportal sinusoids is seen. Late-onset (>100 days) acute rejection show more interface activity and be more difficult to distinguish from chronic hepatitis (137). Acute rejection can also be associated with a slight increase of lymphocytes in the sinusoids.

A rejection-type infiltrate, similar to that seen in the portal tracts, can also be seen in the connective tissue and perivenular sinusoids surrounding the terminal hepatic veins. This has been referred to as "central perivenulitis" (137), and is present in up to 30 percent of acute rejection episodes. It is more frequent late (>100 days) after transplantation. Severe acute cellular rejection is diagnosed only when typical portal changes of acute rejection are accompanied by perivenular inflammation and zonal centrilobular congestion, hemorrhage, and hepatocyte necrosis and dropout (Figures 4.15 and 4.16).

Several well-known grading systems for acute rejection were melded into the Banff schema by the Banff Working Group that is comprised of recognized experts in liver transplant pathology, hepatology, and surgery from many of the major hepatic transplant centers in North America, Europe, and Asia (Table 4.3A,B) (131). It is widely utilized (138), simple and easy to apply, reproducible (139), scientifically correct, and shown to have prognostic significance in a prospective (27) and retrospective study (140).

The Banff schema includes descriptive grades of indeterminate, mild, moderate, and severe (Table 4.3A), and a semiquantitative *rejection activity index* (RAI) (Table 4.3B) (131). The RAI was included because it was part of the European grading system (130) and the conceptual equivalent of the hepatitis activity index (141). The RAI semiquantitatively scores the prevalence and severity of three separate histopathological features on a scale of

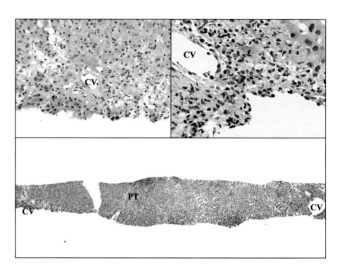

FIGURE 4.15: *This example, a moderate to severe acute cellular rejection, shows noticeable expansion of most or all of the portal tracts by a significant infiltrate. In addition, this biopsy shows a similar infiltrate in the perivenular regions (upper right inset) in some areas with congestion and hemorrhage (upper left inset) in other areas.*

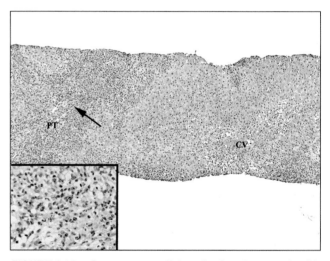

FIGURE 4.16: *Severe acute cellular rejection shows noticeable expansion of most or all portal tracts by a rejection-type infiltrate, as in moderate acute cellular rejection. Note is, however, that there is also prominent central perivenulitis is associated with perivenular hepatocyte necrosis and dropout. Biopsy showing only the perivenular changes, without the portal tract changes, should not be diagnosed as "severe" acute cellular rejection.*

0 to 3: portal inflammation, bile duct damage, and subendothelial inflammation. The individual components are then added together for a total RAI score.

In general, there is a direct correlation between the total RAI score and the descriptive rejection grade and an increased risk of persistent/recurrent acute rejection, chronic rejection, and graft failure (27). The *usual ranges of RAI scores* are indeterminate (1–2), mild (3–4), moderate (5–6), and severe acute rejection (>6). The maximum possible total RAI score is "9," but biopsies rarely achieve this

TABLE 4.3A Banff Grading of Acute Liver Allograft Rejection (349)

Global assessment	Criteria
Indeterminate	Portal inflammatory infiltrate that fails to meet the criteria for the diagnosis of acute reject (see text)
Mild	Rejection infiltrate in a minority of the triads, which is generally mild, and confined within the portal spaces
Moderate	Rejection infiltrate, expanding most or all of the triads
Severe	As above for moderate, with spillover into periportal areas and moderate to severe perivenular inflammation that extends into the hepatic parenchyma and is associated with perivenular hepatocyte necrosis

Note: Global assessment of rejection grade is made on review of the entire biopsy, and only after the diagnosis of rejection has been established. It is inappropriate to provide a "rejection grade" when the diagnosis of rejection is uncertain.

* Verbal description of mild, moderate, or severe acute rejection could also be labeled as grades I, II, and III respectively.

score (27). Instead, in our experience, most episodes of acute rejection are mild, have a total RAI less than 6, respond to increased immunosuppression, and do not lead to significant fibrosis, bile duct loss, or arteriopathy in subsequent or follow-up biopsies (27). Graft failure from acute rejection is unusual.

Additional immunosuppression given *before* a biopsy specimen is obtained can make the histopathological inter-pretation much more difficult because resolution of some characteristic findings, such as subendothelial infiltration of veins, can occur within twenty-four hours. Treatment before biopsy can also contribute to centrilobular hepatocyte swelling and hepatocanalicular cholestasis causing further confusion. In general, seven to ten days are usually required for rejection-related changes to completely resolve after therapy.

Considerable attention has recently been devoted to the histopathological appearance of *late acute rejection*, occurring more than several months after transplantation. Several studies show that it can show slightly different features than typical acute rejection seen early after transplantation [reviewed in (137)]. Late-onset acute rejection is usually characterized by fewer blastic lymphocytes, more necro-inflammatory type interface activity, less venous subendothelial inflammation, a higher incidence of perivenular inflammation, and slightly more lobular activity. This profile of late acute rejection causes the biopsies to more closely resemble chronic hepatitis [reviewed in (137)].

Late acute rejection can present as exclusively or predominantly perivenular inflammation and hepatocyte dropout with minimal or no portal tract changes—or *isolated* "central perivenulitis" (142–144). These cases can later evolve into typical chronic rejection with ductopenia and perivenular fibrosis. In such cases, subendothelial inflammation of portal or central veins is *not* a required finding. Perivenular fibrosis and a Budd-Chiari or a veno-occlusive-like clinical syndrome can develop as a consequence of the severe perivenular injury (81). Late acute rejection, however, is still most commonly characterized by findings seen in early acute cellular rejection, described above. Previously proposed Banff criteria (131) should be

TABLE 4.3B Acute RAI (349)

Category	Criteria	Score
Portal inflammation	Mostly lymphocytic inflammation involving, but not noticeably expanding, a minority of the triads	1
	Expansion of most or all of the triads, by a mixed infiltrate containing lymphocytes with occasional blasts, neutrophils, and eosinophils	2
	Marked expansion of most or all of the triads by a mixed infiltrate containing numerous blasts and eosinophils with inflammatory spillover into the periportal parenchyma	3
Bile duct inflammation damage	A minority of the ducts are cuffed and infiltrated by inflammatory cells and show only mild reactive changes such as increased nuclear: cytoplasmic ratio of the epithelial cells	1
	Most or all of the ducts infiltrated by inflammatory cells. More than an occasional duct shows degenerative changes such as nuclear pleomorphism, disordered polarity, and cytoplasmic vacuolization of the epithelium.	2
	As above for 2, with most or all of the ducts showing degenerative changes or focal luminal disruption	3
Venous endothelial inflammation	Subendothelial lymphocytic infiltration involving some but not a majority of the portal and/or hepatic venules	1
	Subendothelial infiltration involving most or all of the portal and/or hepatic venules.	2
	As above for 2, with moderate or severe perivenular inflammation that extends into the perivenular parenchyma and is associated with perivenular hepatocyte necrosis.	3

Note: Total RAI score = sum of all component scores for portal inflammation, bile duct inflammation/damage, and venous endothelial inflammation.

used for grading unless late acute rejection presents as isolated central perivenulitis. For these cases, the following descriptors are recommended (137).

Late Acute Rejection Descriptor	Findings
Minimal/Indeterminate	Perivenular inflammation involving a minority of terminal hepatic veins with patchy perivenular hepatocyte loss without confluent perivenular necrosis.
Mild	As above, but involving a majority of terminal hepatic veins.
Moderate	As above, with at least focal confluent perivenular hepatocyte dropout and mild moderate inflammation, but without bridging necrosis (Figure 4.17).
Severe	As above, with confluent perivenular hepatocyte dropout and inflammation involving a majority of hepatic venules with central-to-central bridging necrosis.

"Minimal" and "mild" cases, as described above, may resolve spontaneously (144). More severe perivenular changes probably warrant more aggressive treatment, but no prospective studies on the effect of therapy have been carried out.

e. Differential Diagnosis The differential diagnosis for acute rejection is significantly dependent on the *time* since transplantation. Acute rejection should be distinguished from preservation injury and obstructive cholangiopathy/cholangitis during the first several months after transplantation. These differentials were already discussed above in previous sections.

Distinguishing acute rejection from recurrent viral hepatitis B or C and AIH can be particularly difficult because both hepatitis and rejection show predominantly mononuclear portal inflammation, bile duct damage, and acidophilic necrosis of hepatocytes. The distinction, however, can be achieved by closely examining the severity and prevalence of the bile duct damage, interface activity, lobular changes, and perivenular inflammation and hepatocyte dropout (145). Features that favor acute rejection include inflammatory bile duct damage and perivenular inflammation involving a majority of the ducts and central veins, respectively; and low-grade or absent lobular and interface necro-inflammatory activity. In essence, inflammatory bile duct changes and perivenular necro-inflammatory activity predominate over interface and lobular necro-inflammatory activity (145). Conversely, recurrent and/or new-onset viral or AIH is favored when the interface and lobular necro-inflammatory activity predominate

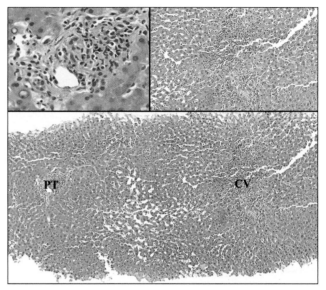

FIGURE 4.17: *Acute rejection can occasionally present as "isolated central perivenulitis" without, or with minimal, accompanying portal tract changes (PT = portal tract; shown at higher magnification in the upper left inset). Severe acute rejection should not be diagnosed in such cases. Similar changes can be seen with new-onset and recurrent AIH. In this case of "moderate" central perivenulitis, note the prominent perivenular inflammation and perivenular confluent necrosis (CV= central vein; shown at higher magnification in the upper right inset). The changes are less prominent in "mild," but "severe" central perivenulitis changes similar to those seen here, but with at least focal central-to-central bridging necrosis.*

over bile duct damage and perivenular changes. AIH resembles viral hepatitis in most respects, except AIH more often shows conspicuous plasma cells as a component of the infiltrate and more commonly shows aggressive interface activity. A subpopulation of patients with AIH can also show prominent central perivenulitis involving a majority of central veins. In such cases, severe interface activity, plasma cell predominance in the infiltrate, and relatively mild bile duct damage favor AIH over acute rejection.

Low-grade and/or chronic obstructive cholangiopathy can be associated with histopathological findings that are nearly indistinguishable from those of acute rejection. In such cases, it is helpful to remember that acute rejection occurring more than six months after transplantation is unusual in adequately immunosuppressed patients. Checking immunosuppression blood levels and the liver injury test profile often provides sufficient data to suggest a cholangiogram before increasing immunosuppressive therapy. More subtle histopathological features that favor chronic biliary strictures over acute rejection include a low-grade ductular reaction, sinusoidal neutrophil clusters, and periportal hepatocyte deposition of elemental copper, centrilobular hepatocanalicular cholestasis, and lamellar periduct edema involving true bile ducts. Central perivenulitis, as described above, is not seen with obstructive cholangiopathy.

4. Chronic Rejection

a. General Considerations Chronic rejection has been defined by a panel convened for the terminology of liver rejection and the Banff Working Group as an immunologic injury to the liver allograft, which usually evolves from severe or persistent acute rejection, and results in potentially irreversible damage to the bile ducts, arteries and veins [reviewed in (146)]. The term "chronic" technically implies a time parameter, but none is strictly intended (127). Chronic rejection often occurs within several months after transplantation and allograft failure can occur within the first year after transplantation [reviewed in (146)]. The incidence does not appear to increase with time after transplantation and has been decreasing in recent years—it currently affects about 3–5 percent liver allograft recipients by 5 years after transplantation. This represents a dramatic decrease since the 1980s when the incidence was 15–20 percent (146). Better recognition and control of acute rejection, reversibility of the early phases of chronic rejection, the unique immunologic properties of liver allografts, and the ability of the liver to regenerate without fibrosis after recovery from acute rejection probably all contribute to this decline.

Chronic rejection, however, has not been entirely eliminated and is still an important cause of late liver allograft dysfunction and failure. Chronic rejection is now most often seen in noncompliant patients, HCV+ recipients treated with an activating drugs such as alpha interferon (147,148), and recipients who have immunosuppression lowered because of medication adverse side effects, such as lymphoproliferative disorders (149).

Risk factors for chronic rejection have generally been divided into two general categories: 1) "Alloantigen-dependent," immunologic or rejection-related factors are the most important, especially the number and severity of acute rejection episodes [reviewed in (107,146)]. In cyclosporine-treated cohorts, late-onset acute rejection; younger recipient age; male-to-female sex mismatch; a primary diagnosis of AIH or biliary disease; baseline immunosuppression, interactions between HLA-DR3, TNF-2 status, and CMV infection (150), non-Caucasian recipient race [reviewed in (146)], and use of interferon alpha to treat recurrent HCV (147,148) were chronic rejection risk factors. The effects of histocompatibility differences and CMV infection are controversial. In a large tacrolimus-treated cohort, most matching factors described above for the cyclosporine-treated cohort were eliminated as significant risk factors, but the influence of the number and severity of acute rejection episodes remained (149). 2) Non-alloantigen–dependent or "non-immunologic" risk factors include donor age greater than forty years (149).

b. Pathophysiology Immunologic mechanisms of injury that contribute to allograft damage during acute rejection also likely contribute to the development of chronic rejection (146,151) because chronic rejection at higher risk when there is previous severe and/or persistent acute rejection episodes (27,149,152,153). *Bile duct damage and loss* in chronic rejection has been attributed to a combination of direct immunologic damage and indirect ischemic damage because of obliterative arteriopathy, small artery/arteriolar loss, and destruction of the peri-biliary capillary plexus (154,155). Cumulative damage enhances biliary epithelial cell senescence (97) detectable by nuclear p21 expression in biliary epithelial cells without coexistent Ki-67 labeling (97). These senescence related changes precede bile duct loss (146,152). Several studies have shown that the early phase of chronic rejection is potentially reversible (97,152,156,157), which in turn, depends on preservation of ductules and surrounding microvasculature (158).

c. Clinical Presentation Chronic rejection is usually suspected in a patient with a history of acute rejection, who develops progressive cholestasis and an increase in canalicular enzymes that is unresponsive to anti-rejection treatment (127). The three typical clinical settings include 1) the culmination of unresolved/persistent acute rejection, 2) the culmination of multiple episodes of acute rejection, and 3) an indolent presentation without preceding clinically recognizable episodes of acute rejection. The first two scenarios are the most common. These usually occur within the first year after transplantation in patients resistant to increased immunosuppressive therapy for acute rejection. An indolent presentation of chronic rejection is relatively uncommon and likely reflects inadequate monitoring, although it has been recently described in the setting of interferon treatment for recurrent HCV (148). Late-onset chronic rejection occurring more than one year after transplantation is typically seen in inadequately immunosuppressed patients, either as a result of noncompliance or because immunosuppression had to be lowered because of infectious, neoplastic or toxic complications of chronic immunosuppression (149).

Standard liver injury tests in a patient with chronic rejection usually show a cholestatic or "biliary" pattern manifest as preferential elevation of γ-glutamyl transpeptidase and alkaline phosphatase (98,127,159). Persistent elevation of alanine aminotransferase and total bilirubin usually marked the transition from acute to chronic rejection and can presage allograft failure (142,149,152). Clinical symptoms, if present, resemble those of acute rejection until dysfunction becomes significant enough to cause jaundice. Biliary sludging, biliary strictures, hepatic infarcts, and loss of hepatic

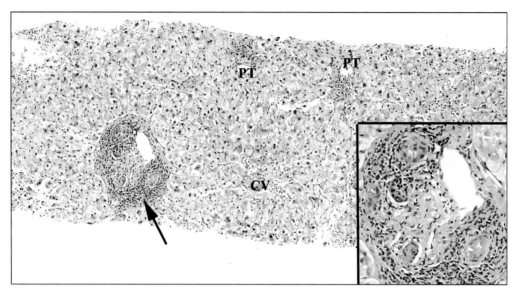

FIGURE 4.18: *Early chronic rejection is characterized by mild, predominantly mononuclear inflammation with variable bile duct loss and biliary epithelial senescence changes (lower right inset) involving a majority of bile ducts. The senescence changes include eosinophilic transformation of the cytoplasm, an increased nuclear: cytoplasmic ratio, uneven nuclear spacing, and multinucleation.*

synthetic function, manifest as coagulopathy and malnutrition, are other late findings that often occur immediately before allograft failure (127). Hepatic angiograms, in a typical case with obliterative arteriopathy, show pruning of the intrahepatic arteries with poor peripheral filling and segmental narrowing (127,160).

d. Histopathological Findings and Staging Chronic rejection primarily affects the portal tracts and perivenular regions and is divided into "early" (Figure 4.18) and "late" (Figure 4.19) stages according to the Banff Schema (Table 4.4) (146). *Early chronic rejection* in the portal tracts is characterized by mild lymphocytic cholangitis, biliary epithelial cell senescence changes involving a majority of small bile ducts, and variable small bile duct loss (Figure 4.18). The portal inflammation in chronic rejection is usually less severe and eosinophils are less common than in acute rejection; and the inflammatory infiltrate is comprised primarily of lymphocytes, plasma cells, and mast cells (161).

Recognition of *biliary epithelial cell senescence changes* is critical to the diagnosis of early chronic rejection (97). Include are eosinophilic transformation of the cytoplasm; uneven nuclear spacing; syncytia formation; nuclear enlargement and hyperchromasia resembling cytological dysplasia; ducts only partially lined by biliary epithelial cells (Figure 4.18); and positive staining for p21$^{WAF1/Cip1}$ (but not for Ki-67), which inhibits cell cycle progression and becomes upregulated in cells under severe stress or showing replicative senescence (97). *Late-stage chronic rejection* is characterized by bile duct loss in most or all the portal tracts, and in severe cases by arteriolar loss. Both of these features are recognized and quantified by careful morphometric analysis.

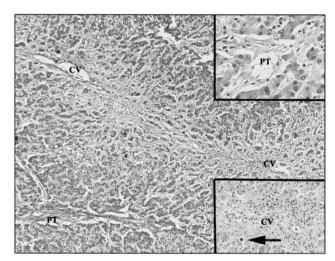

FIGURE 4.19: *The typical case of late chronic rejection is characterized by small bile duct loss involving a majority of the portal tracts and/or severe perivenular fibrosis with at least focal central to central bridging, as illustrated in this photomicrograph. Many cases of late chronic rejection show loss of both small bile ducts and hepatic artery branches in the portal tracts (upper right inset), such that it is difficult to distinguish between portal tracts and central veins. However, the cholestasis in late chronic rejection is centrilobular, which helped to identify the fibrotic central veins (lower right inset).*

Crawford et al. (162) defined a portal tract as "a focus within the parenchyma containing connective tissue (by Masson's trichrome stain) and at least two luminal structures embedded in the connective tissue mesenchyme, each with a continuous connective tissue circumference." Accordingly, bile ducts and hepatic artery branches are detectable in 93 $\pm$ 6 and 91 $\pm$ 7 percent of portal tracts, respectively, in a needle biopsy from a normal liver (162).

TABLE 4.4 Features of Early and Late Chronic Liver Allograft Rejection [Adapted from (146)]

Structure	Early CR	Late CR
Small bile ducts (<60 μm)	Bile duct loss in <50% of portal tracts Degenerative change involving a majority of ducts: eosinophilic transformation of the cytoplasm; nuclear hyperchromasia; uneven nuclear spacing; ducts only partially lined by biliary epithelial cells	Loss in ≥50% of portal tracts. Degenerative changes in remaining bile ducts.
Terminal hepatic venules and zone 3 hepatocytes	Intimal/luminal inflammation; lytic zone 3 necrosis and inflammation; mild perivenular fibrosis	Focal obliteration; variable inflammation; severe perivenular fibrosis, defined as central-to-central bridging fibrosis
Portal tract hepatic arterioles Other	Occasional loss involving <25% of portal tracts So-called transitional* hepatitis with spotty necrosis of hepatocytes	Loss involving >25% of portal tracts Sinusoidal foam cell accumulation; marked cholestasis
Large perihilar hepatic artery branches	Intimal inflammation, focal foam cell deposition without luminal compromise	Luminal narrowing by subintimal foam cells; fibrointimal proliferation
Large perihilar bile ducts	Inflammation damage and focal foam cell deposition	Mural fibrosis

* "Transitional" hepatitis: mild lobular disarray and spotty acidophilic necrosis of hepatocytes that can occur during evolution or transition from early to late stages of chronic rejection (163).

Lower figures were cited by others using larger tissue samples (154). Using two standard deviations from the normal as a cutoff, *bile duct loss* is considered present when less than 80 percent of the portal tracts contain bile ducts; *arterial loss* is considered present when less than 77 percent of the portal tracts contain hepatic artery branches.

Late chronic rejection, however, can cause both bile duct and arterial loss (154,155) (Figure 4.19). Recognizing portal tracts and conducting a morphometric analysis in such cases can be problematic. Portal tract recognition should be based primarily on the location of the structure—cholestasis in chronic rejection is centrilobular. Quantification of bile duct and arterial loss should be based on a count of the total number of portal tracts with and without bile ducts and arteries compared with expected values from normal livers, as above.

A ductular reaction at the interface zone is unusual in chronic rejection, unless the liver is recovering from chronic rejection. In such cases, several studies have reported the appearance of ductular reaction before and during the regrowth or re-emergence of bile ducts (152,156,157).

Early chronic rejection in the terminal hepatic venules and surrounding perivenular parenchyma is characterized by subendothelial and/or perivenular mononuclear inflammation (Figure 4.18). The perivenular infiltrate usually consists of lymphocytes, macrophages, and plasma cells (146,153) and is accompanied by perivenular hepatocyte dropout, an accumulation of pigment-laden macrophages, and mild perivenular fibrosis (146). Spotty acidophilic hepatocytes, or so-called transitional hepatitis can be seen during evolution from early to late chronic rejection (163).

Perivenular changes in late chronic rejection are characterized by severe (bridging) *perivenular fibrosis* with at least focal central-to-central or central-to-portal bridging and occasional obliteration of terminal hepatic venules (Figure 4.19) (146). Well-developed cirrhosis, primarily attributable to chronic rejection, is unusual until the very late stages when venous obliteration leads to areas of parenchyma extinction and veno-centric cirrhosis (151). True "regenerative" nodules are uncommon. Perhaps this is because a combination of venopathy and obliterative arteriopathy blunts any regenerative response (82). Perivenular hepatocyte ballooning and dropout; centrilobular hepatocanalicular cholestasis, nodular regenerative hyperplasia changes, and intra-sinusoidal foam cell clusters are other common findings in late chronic rejection (Figure 4.19).

A final diagnosis of chronic rejection should be based on a combination of the clinical, radiological, laboratory, and histopathological findings. In a biopsy specimen, minimal diagnostic criteria for chronic rejection are 1) senescent changes, affecting a majority of the bile ducts, with or without bile duct loss; 2) convincing foam cell obliterative arteriopathy; or 3) bile duct loss affecting greater than 50 percent of the portal tracts (146).

The diagnosis of chronic rejection is much easier to establish, with certainty, in an explanted failed allograft. This is because characteristic/diagnostic findings can be directly observed in the first-, second-, and third-order branches of the hepatic arterial tree in and around the liver hilum. In our experience, obliterative arteriopathy is usually seen in at least some of the perihilar arteries, except in cases characterized by bile duct loss and/or perivenular fibrosis alone. A progressive accumulation of the foamy macrophages usually first occurs in the intima. This, in turn, triggers proliferation of intimal, and migration of medial, donor-derived myofibroblasts, which eventually causes intimal thickening/luminal narrowing. This triggers thinning of media as the arteries attempt to dilate and compensate for the reduced arterial flow. But eventually, this compensation mechanism fails and the entire wall can be completely replaced by foam cells. The narrowing can predispose to arterial thrombosis, which in turn, causes necrosis of the large bile ducts and ischemic cholangiopathy.

Foamy macrophages can also be seen around bile ducts and veins in the connective tissue. Large perihilar bile ducts can also show focal sloughing of the epithelium, papillary hyperplasia, mural fibrosis, and acute and chronic inflammation.

Staging of chronic rejection assumes that the diagnosis has already been correctly established (146). *Early chronic rejection* implies that a significant potential for recovery exists if the source/cause of immunologic can be controlled or reversed. *Late chronic rejection*, in contrast, implies that the potential for recovery is limited and retransplantation should be considered, if otherwise clinically indicated. More study, however, is needed in this area. It is not well established that all patients proceed sequentially in an orderly fashion from the early to late chronic rejection. Some patients appear to persist in the acute/early stage for months or years, while others rapidly develop severe fibrosis and late changes within the first year after transplantation or within weeks or months after the first onset. Also, some cases show predominantly or exclusively either bile duct loss or arteriopathy alone, but usually both features occur together (146).

The important practical implication of chronic rejection staging is that the biopsy findings do not absolutely define a point of no return. Instead they provide information about the likelihood of reversal, which should be correlated with other clinical and laboratory parameters, such as persistently elevated serum bilirubin higher than 20 mg/dl, progressive decline in synthetic function, superimposed hepatic artery thrombosis, and bile duct necrosis or biliary sludging.

e. Differential Diagnosis In needle biopsy specimens, the diagnosis of chronic rejection is primarily based on damage and loss of small bile ducts and perivenular fibrosis; arteries with pathognomonic changes are rarely present in needle biopsy specimens (146). Duct injury and ductopenia can also occur because of nonrejection-related complications, such as obstructive cholangiopathy, hepatic artery stricturing or thrombosis, adverse drug reactions, and CMV infection. In addition, perivenular fibrosis can be caused by suboptimal hepatic venous drainage and other causes of perivenular injury. Therefore, a diagnosis of chronic rejection based on biliary epithelial senescence or loss or perivenular fibrosis alone should first exclude other nonrejection-related causes of ductal injury and loss or perivenular fibrosis.

The most difficult differential diagnosis is between chronic rejection and biliary tract obstruction or stricturing, including recurrent PSC [reviewed in (99)]. Features that favor obstructive cholangiopathy include 1) bile duct loss in some portal tracts accompanied by a ductular reaction in other portal tracts, 2) neutrophil clusters within the lobules, 3) bile infarcts, 4) deposition of copper and copper-associated protein in periportal hepatocytes, and 5) significant hepatocanalicular cholestasis, out of proportion to the prevalence of ductopenia (<50 percent). Features that favor chronic rejection include 1) bile duct changes combined with central perivenulitis and/or fibrosis and 2) an absence of changes typical of recurrent PSC, described above. Cholangiography and/or angiography may be required in some case to distinguish between chronic rejection and biliary obstruction. Such studies usually show "pruning" and poor peripheral filling in chronic rejection.

In other cases, isolated ductopenia involving less than 50 percent of the portal tracts can be seen without significant elevations of liver injury tests. Whether these uncommon cases are an early phase of chronic rejection is uncertain. Isolated perivenular fibrosis can be caused by mechanical outflow obstruction, adverse drug reactions and all of the nonrejection causes of veno-occlusive disease and Budd-Chiari syndrome in native livers.

The safest approach to the diagnosis of chronic rejection in any setting is to review prior biopsies and closely correlate the histopathological findings with the clinical course. The usual scenario is a history of severe or unresolved acute rejection preceding the development of histologic findings interpreted as chronic rejection.

vi. Bacterial and Fungal Infections

A high index of suspicion for infection should always be maintained when reviewing tissue specimens from liver allograft recipients. However, because of stress and tissue damage from the operation, combined with high immunosuppression needed to prevent acute rejection, most serious "opportunistic" fungal and viral infections generally occur within the first two months after transplantation. Infections occurring after six months are more often bacterial in origin. Fever, anastomotic or wound dehiscence, retransplantation, persistent abdominal pain, and vascular thrombosis are clinical situations, signs and symptoms that should further arouse suspicion of a serious infection.

Since many bacterial and fungal infections arise in nonviable tissue, most necrotic tissue should be routinely subjected to special stains for bacteria and fungi. Coexistent acute and chronic inflammation and granulomas are always good surrogate markers of infection but might not appear because of heavy immunosuppression. The histopathological manifestations of deep fungal and bacterial infections are familiar to most pathologists and beyond the intended scope of this chapter.

vii. "Opportunistic" Hepatitis Viruses

The term "opportunistic" is used for infections with CMV, Epstein-Barr virus (EBV), and herpes simplex virus (HSV) or varicella-zoster virus (VZV), and adenovirus because they usually do not usually cause clinically significant acute hepatitis in the general population. None causes chronic hepatitis in either liver allograft recipients or the general population. Most adult liver allograft recipients have already been infected; and the normal immune system adequately controls latent infection, which persists for life. In contrast, most pediatric recipients and a minority of adults are naive and have not been previously infected; these recipients are susceptible to primary infection with these viruses.

Immunosuppression needed to prevent rejection renders all liver allograft recipients vulnerable to acute hepatitis caused by these viruses. Those carrying latent infections develop "reactivation" infection/disease. "Naive" recipients develop primary infection/disease. In general, primary infection/diseases are significantly more severe than reactivation infection/disease. An important aspect of latent infection is that it results in periodic viral shedding into the peripheral circulation where it can be monitored by measuring viral antigens or nucleic acids. When viral levels surpass certain, empirically set, thresholds, preemptive lowering of immunosuppression and/or treatment with specific antiviral agents is used to prevent active disease (164). Monitoring and preemptive therapy has dramatically reduced the incidence of, but has not eliminated, diseases caused by these viruses. In our experience, therefore, a histopathological diagnosis of hepatitis because of one of these viruses is becoming uncommon.

1. CMV Hepatitis

a. Introduction and Pathophysiology Effective prophylactic and preemptive therapy have greatly lessened the incidence and impact of symptomatic disease CMV (165–167). Symptomatic infection/disease usually develops between three and eight weeks after transplantation often shortly after a cycle of increased immunosuppressive therapy used to treat acute rejection. Primary infections pose greater risk of significant disease than reactivation (168–171). Viral latency in granulocytes or endothelial cells (172) and monocytes might explain the early appearance of CMV antigens in the sinusoidal cells that precedes symptomatic disease (168). CMV infection has also been cited as a risk factor for hepatic artery thrombosis, especially in pediatric patients (173,174), chronic rejection [reviewed in (107)], biliary strictures (175), and fibrosis progression in recurrent HCV (176).

b. Clinical Presentation Any organ system can be involved depending on the extent of viral dissemination. But the most common signs and symptoms of active CMV infection/disease arise from gastrointestinal involvement and include fever, diarrhea and gastrointestinal ulcers, leukopenia, and low-grade hepatitis with modestly elevated liver injury tests [reviewed in (2)]. Respiratory insufficiency/pneumonia and retinitis are signs of severe disseminated disease. CMV can also occasionally cause a syndrome that mimics EBV-associated PTLD with lymphadenopathy, fever, and atypical lymphocytosis [reviewed in (2)].

c. Histopathological Findings CMV hepatitis has become an uncommon histopathological diagnosis because of serological monitoring for antigenemia and preemptive antiviral therapy (175). The usual case of CMV hepatitis is characterized by spotty lobular necrosis, Kupffer's cell hypertrophy, mild lobular disarray, and patchy lobular inflammation, described below. Infected hepatocytes occasionally contain diagnostic nuclear and/or cytoplasmic inclusions, but inclusions are now usually limited to patients who are over-immunosuppressed and not adequately monitored or treated. Any cell type can be infected. Diagnostic features include large eosinophilic intranuclear inclusions surrounded by a clear halo accompanied by small basophilic or amphophilic cytoplasmic inclusions (Figure 4.20). In severe cases, which are largely of historical significance, numerous cells containing CMV inclusions can be spread throughout the liver allograft. CMV alone does not cause submassive or massive necrosis [reviewed in (2)].

The infected cells are often surrounded by neutrophils, or microabscess, or clusters of macrophages and lymphocytes—microgranulomas. CMV hepatitis can also be associated with mild lymphoplasmacytic portal inflammation showing bile duct cell infiltration and damage that can superficially resemble acute or early chronic rejection. In fact, bile duct loss and chronic rejection have been associated with persistent allograft CMV infection (177,178).

Since characteristic inclusions are now uncommon, CMV hepatitis often presents as the parenchymal alterations, described above. Some of these cases can show "fragmented" nuclear CMV inclusions, which makes them difficult to recognize without immunoperoxidase staining to detect viral antigens or in situ hybridization to detect nucleic acids. Rapidly dividing tissues such as young granulation tissue, proliferating cholangioles, edges of infarcts, abscesses, or other intraparenchymal defects are fertile soil for CMV growth (28).

d. Differential Diagnosis CMV hepatitis can be difficult to distinguish from early HBV or HCV recurrence, and on occasion, EBV hepatitis, especially when no viral inclusions are detected and mononuclear portal inflammation is present. It is also difficult to distinguish CMV from HSV hepatitis because both can cause multinucleation and intra-nuclear eosinophilic inclusions surrounded by halos. CMV inclusion–containing cells, however, can also show small basophilic or amphophilic cytoplasmic inclusions, which distinguish them from HSV infected cells. Circumscribed foci of coagulative necrosis characteristic of HSV are not a feature of CMV hepatitis.

In cases without inclusions, subtle clues distinguishing CMV hepatitis from early acute HBV or HCV hepatitis include a lesser amount of lobular disarray and hepatocyte swelling in CMV. Microabscesses or microgranulomas are not generally seen in HBV or HCV. A definitive diagnosis of CMV hepatitis, however, often relies on demonstration of viral antigens or viral nucleic acids using immunostaining or in situ hybridization and correlation with the clinical and serological profile.

CMV hepatitis can superficially resemble EBV hepatitis because of the mild lymphoplasmacytic portal and lobular inflammation and both occasionally contain blastic and atypical lymphocytes. In such cases, EBV hepatitis usually causes more lymphoplasmacytic cytologic atypia, whereas CMV hepatitis usually causes more intralobular foci of inflammation (e.g., microgranulomas and microabscesses). Deeper sections, staining for EBV and CMV viral antigens and in situ hybridization for EBV nucleic acids are usually required to establish the final diagnosis with certainty.

CMV hepatitis most commonly develops in patients who have recently completed an augmented immunosuppressive regimen for rejection. In some cases, therefore, it is difficult to determine whether the liver inflammation/injury is attributable to residual CMV hepatitis or relapse of acute rejection or development of chronic rejection because of low immunosuppression levels used to treat the viral infection. O'Grady et al. and others described an association between CMV infection and chronic rejection (177,178) although others have not seen this relationship (179). We recommend that priority be given to the CMV inclusions or antigens, administration of anti-CMV therapy and follow-up biopsy after one–two weeks, if liver function abnormalities persist.

2. Herpes Simplex and Varicella-Zoster Viral Hepatitis

a. Introduction HSV (type I and II) or Varicella-Zoster (VZ) hepatitis can occur virtually any time after transplantation [reviewed in (2)] and often presents with fever, vesicular skin rashes, and fatigue and body pain, and elevated liver injury tests. Undetected HSV hepatitis can rapidly lead to submassive or massive hepatic necrosis, hypotension, disseminated intravascular coagulation, metabolic acidosis, and death (180). Fulminant cases occur more often as a result of a primary infection/disease in patients without evidence of prior immunity.

b. Histopathological Findings Recognition and prompt reporting of HSV and VZ hepatitis on needle biopsy evaluation is essential because effective pharmacologic therapy is available, and without treatment, they can be rapidly fatal. Two histopathological patterns of HSV hepatitis, localized and diffuse, have been described (180). Distinction between these two patterns, however, is probably related to swiftness in establishing the diagnosis and the level of immune competence. Both patterns cause characteristic circumscribed areas of coagulative-type necrosis showing no respect for the lobular architecture [reviewed in (2,180)]. The center of the necrotic zones is occupied by ghosts of hepatocytes, intermixed with neutrophils and nuclear debris, whereas more viable hepatocytes rimming the periphery usually contain recognizable HSV/VZ inclusions, if present. Infected cells are usually slightly enlarged and contain "smudgy," ground-glass nuclei or characteristic Cowdry type A eosinophilic inclusions. Multinucleate cells are occasionally present, but not infrequently, diagnostic inclusions of HSV or VZ will be absent on the H&E slides. In such cases, immunoperoxidase stains for HSV antigens can be confirmatory. In our experience, antibody preparations used to detect HSV subtypes can show cross reactivity making it difficult, in some cases, to separate HSV I from HSV II using immunohistochemistry. Monoclonal antibodies can be extremely helpful in distinguishing between HSV and VZ, which is not possible on H&E-stained sections.

c. Differential Diagnosis If a histopathological diagnosis of HSV or VZV hepatitis is considered on H&E sections, regardless if the diagnosis is confirmed, the clinical physicians should be immediately notified. This will prompt effective antiviral therapy that can be discontinued if the diagnosis is not confirmed using immunostains. Necrotic lesions of HSV/VZ hepatitis are distinguished from infarcts by examining viable or marginally viable cells at the edge of the necrotic lesions for characteristic viral inclusions. Frequently, however, only cells with a smudged nuclear chromatin are seen at this location. It is our policy to over diagnose HSV hepatitis on H&E sections followed by HSV/VZ immunostains to confirm or exclude the diagnosis.

The histopathological differential diagnosis of CMV and HSV hepatitis has been discussed above.

3. Epstein-Barr Virus

a. Introduction and Pathophysiology EBV infection "immortalizes" B lymphocytes, in vitro, and lies dormant in B lymphocytes and some epithelial cells, in vivo, because the immune system effectively controls viral replication following a primary infection (181,182). Potent immunosuppressive therapy after transplantation depresses T-cell immune surveillance that normally keeps EBV replication, and B-cell proliferation, in check. This enhances EBV replication and increases the risk of various EBV disease manifestations, discussed below. The reader is referred elsewhere for a more detailed discussion of EBV patho-physiology in this situation (181–183) (Chapter 10).

b. Clinical Presentation Up to 1–2 percent of all liver allograft recipients with preexisting anti-EBV immunity will develop reactivation disease (EBV) after transplantation; primary infection in patients without EBV immunity occurs more frequently. Pleomorphic disease manifestations (184) include hepatitis, gastroenteritis, post-transplant lymphoproliferative diseases [including B cell (185–188), Hodgkin's disease (189), T-cell lesions (190)], and smooth muscle stromal tumors (191). EBV-related syndromes often resemble classical infectious mononucleosis presenting with fever, lymphadenitis, pharyngitis, and jaundice (182,185–188). Atypical signs and symptoms include jaw pain, arthralgia, joint space effusions, diarrhea, encephalitis, pneumonitis, and mediastinal lymphadenopathy, and ascites (182,185–188). Laboratory tests usually show mildly elevated ALT and AST and circulating atypical lymphocytes; pancytopenia is noted on occasion (182,185–188).

PTLD are the result of unresolved and/or uncontrolled EBV replication and B-cell proliferation (182,192) that most frequently first manifest as lymph node enlargement and/or a mass lesion involving the hepatic allograft or gastrointestinal tract (182,192). Other organ/sites usually become commonly involved in disseminated disease. The first line of therapy, regardless of the clinical or histopathological manifestation or clonality, is withdrawal or dramatic reduction in immunosuppression to restore immune surveillance. This is usually combined with antiviral agents to inhibit viral replication (182,192). If unsuccessful, anti-CD20 antibodies or conventional chemotherapy are usually next considered (182,192).

Risk factors for the development of serious EBV-associated disease include primary infection, heavy immunosuppression, underlying Langerhans cell histiocytosis (182,185–188,193), and coexistent CMV disease (194). The risk of developing PTLD late after transplantation does not appear to be influenced by the type of immunosuppressive agents, but by the duration and intensity of immunosuppression (195).

As for CMV, peripheral blood monitoring for EBV nucleic acids is used follow viral replication. Monitoring of anti-EBV specific T cell responses using ELISPOT or tetramer staining is another emerging technology (181). If these tests are abnormal, the patient is examined for lymphadenopathy and other signs of EBV-related disease—preemptive reductions in immunosuppression are usually made before more serious EBV-related disease occurs [reviewed in (183)]. This treatment algorithm has decreased the incidence of severity of EBV-related disease.

c. Histopathological Findings The range of histopathological manifestations of EBV disease in liver allograft is broad. It ranges from EBV hepatitis characterized by mild nonspecific portal and sinusoidal lymphocytosis to PTLDs, resembling diffuse large B-cell lymphomas (182,185–188,196). In patients with enhanced EBV replication occasional EBV-containing cells can appear admixed among other inflammatory cells associated with rejection and other causes of allograft dysfunction (196).

So-called typical *EBV hepatitis* usually manifests as mild portal lymphoplasmacytic inflammation combined with sinusoidal lymphocytosis comprised of small or mildly atypical lymphocytes (Figure 4.21). "Lining-up" of lymphocytes in the sinusoids should suggest an EBV-related disorder, as in native livers. Lobular changes include focal hepatocellular swelling, mild acidophilic necrosis of hepatocytes, and mild lobular disarray/regenerative activity (185–187,196).

PTLDs represent a more severe manifestation of EBV disease and usually present with lymphoplasmacytic portal infiltrates that contain cells with cytologic atypia. In early or polymorphic lesions, atypical cells are usually intermixed with small and blastic lymphocytes, plasmacytoid lymphocytes, and plasma cells (185–187,196) (Figure 4.22). In late and/or monomorphic lesions atypical cells

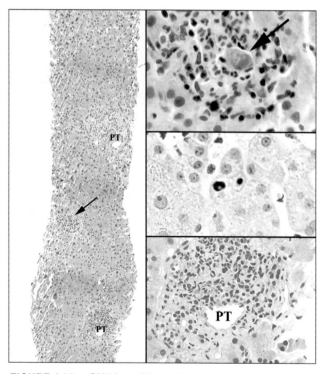

FIGURE 4.20: *CMV hepatitis has become an uncommon histopathological diagnosis because of peripheral blood monitoring and preemptive adjustments in immunosuppression and/or antiviral drug therapy. The typical case usually shows variable lymphoplasmacytic portal inflammation (lower right inset), minimal lobular disarray, and microgranulomas, or microabscesses (arrow, and upper right inset) scattered throughout the lobules. A CMV-infected cell is shown at higher magnification in the upper right inset (arrow). Immunostaining for CMV antigens is diagnostic when viral inclusions are not seen (right middle inset).*

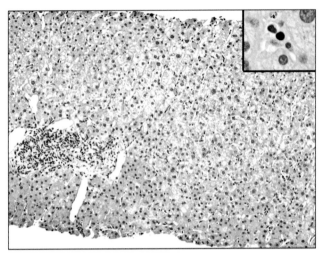

FIGURE 4.21: *EBV hepatitis is characterized by variable, but usually mild, mononuclear portal inflammation without bile duct damage, accompanied by mild sinusoidal lymphocytosis and low grade hepatocyte apoptosis. In situ hybridization for EBV RNA in occasional portal and/or sinusoidal lymphocytes is confirmatory (upper right inset).*

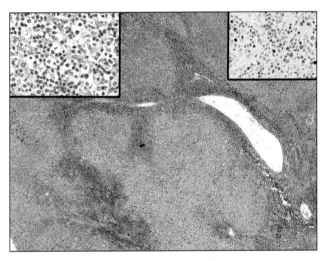

FIGURE 4.22 *Uncontrolled EBV replication results in the development of PTLDs. Characteristic features include a dense portal infiltrate comprised of a relatively monomorphic population of lymphocytes and plasmacytoid lymphocytes (upper left inset) that overrun the normal portal architecture or landmarks. In contrast to CMV, PTLDs can cause confluent or even larger, map-like areas of necrosis. Compare this infiltrate with that seen in acute rejection from Figure 4.14. In situ hybridization for EBV RNA (upper right inset) confirmed the diagnosis.*

predominate. This more severe form of hepatic involvement usually manifests as map-like enlargement of portal tracts because of sheets of atypical immunoblastic cells. The infiltrates obscure the normal portal architectural landmarks (185–187,196). Aggregates of similar cells can be seen in the sinusoids. Some cases are accompanied by significant hepatic necrosis. The cytologic features of the atypical cells resemble those of a diffuse immunoblastic

lymphoma. Hodgkin's-like lymphoma PTLDs with classical Reed-Sternberg cells can also occur and be associated with bile duct loss, as in native livers. Subendothelial localization of lymphocytes in portal and/or central veins can mimic acute rejection.

Diagnosis of any EBV-related disorder is confirmed by in situ hybridization for EBV RNA (EBER sequence). Our routine workup also includes immunohistochemical stains or in situ hybridization for kappa and lambda light chains, and CD20 to determine possible responsiveness to anti-CD20 antibodies (182). Occasionally, we also examine EBV antigen expression, and if enough fresh tissue is available, a portion is also submitted for flow cytometry and molecular analyses, which enable a more detailed phenotypic characterization and immunoglobulin gene rearrangements studies. A more detailed discussion of the extrahepatic manifestation of PTLD in lymph nodes and other tissues is present elsewhere (182,192).

d. Differential Diagnosis EBV hepatitis can be difficult to distinguish from nonspecific "reactive hepatitis" and acute HBV, HCV, or CMV hepatitis (185–187,196). HCV and EBV hepatitis can both show sinusoidal lymphocytosis, but EBV-related disorders usually contain at least occasional atypical cells. In contrast, lymphocytes associated with HCV hepatitis are usually small, round, and inactive appearing and form nodular aggregates in the portal tracts (185–187,196). The clinicopathological profile, including peripheral blood EBV levels, can also help making this distinction.

EBV hepatitis/PTLDs are most difficult to distinguish from *acute rejection* (Figure 4.14 versus 4.22). Features that favor acute rejection over EBV-related disorders include pleomorphic, "rejection-type" portal, and/or perivenular inflammatory infiltrates, including prominence of eosinophils; and severe and prevalent bile duct damage that are proportional to the severity of the inflammation. Features that favor EBV over acute rejection include: relatively monomorphic portal infiltrates, consisting primarily of activated and immunoblastic mononuclear cells, many of which show features of plasmacytic differentiation and some of which show atypical cytologic features; and patchy/mild inflammatory bile duct damage less than would be expected based on the severity of the portal infiltrate (185–187,196).

In most cases, however, the final diagnosis of EBV-related disorders is heavily dependent on in situ hybridization for EBV RNA (EBER probing) (185–187,196). But EBER probe results have to be interpreted with caution (197) because rare EBER+ cells are not uncommon in lymphoid tissues from the general population and such cells are found with slightly increased frequency in allograft recipients, the significance of which is open to debate (197). In our opinion, clustering of EBER+ cells into aggregates, or the presence of EBER positive cells in tissues showing other histopathological features of EBV-associated disease, is indicative of enhanced EBV replication. Such patients are at increased risk of developing EBV-related disease, including PTLD. Closer follow-up, including more frequent peripheral blood monitoring and cautious immunosuppression management are warranted. It should be remembered, however, that up to thirty one percent of PTLD fail to show evidence of EBV infection (198).

4. Adenoviral Hepatitis

a. Introduction and Pathophysiology Adenoviral hepatitis is largely restricted to those with primary infection most of whom are pediatric recipients (199,200) but occasional cases have been reported in adults (201). The disease usually manifests clinically between one and ten weeks after transplantation. Needle biopsy examination is needed to confirm the diagnosis. Symptoms include fever, respiratory distress, diarrhea, and liver dysfunction. During symptomatic disease, viral subtypes 1, 2, and 5 have been isolated from the lung, and gastrointestinal tract (199,200,202). Allograft hepatitis is most often caused by viral subtype 5, but in the general population, hepatitis has also been caused by subtypes 2, 11, and 16. Therefore, these subtypes might also be expected to infect and cause hepatitis in liver allografts (199,200).

b. Histopathological Findings Considerable experience is required to diagnose adenoviral hepatitis with certainty on H&E examination alone. This is because the disease is relatively uncommon and typical nuclear inclusions are difficult to recognize with certainty. The typical case shows "pox-like" granulomas, consisting almost entirely of macrophages, or macrophages intermixed with neutrophils that are spread randomly throughout the parenchyma (Figure 4.23). In some cases, the granulomas surround small map-like areas of necrosis (199–201). As with the other opportunistic viruses, typical/diagnostic adenoviral inclusions are usually found in the nuclei of viable hepatocytes near the edge of the necrotic zones and/or granulomas. The typical adenoviral inclusion shows crowding of chromatin towards the nuclear membrane, which makes the nucleus look like a "baked muffin" and immunohistochemical staining is usually required to confirm the diagnosis (Figure 4.23).

c. Differential Diagnosis Recognizing typical adenoviral inclusions is the most reliable method for distinguishing adenoviral hepatitis from other causes of focal hepatic necrosis and hepatic granulomas such as HSV/VZ, infarcts, and deep fungal or mycobacterial infections. In addition to immunostaining for adenoviral, HSV/VZ, and CMV viral antigens and/or nucleic acids, microbiological cultures of the biopsy and negative special stains for granuloma-causing organisms can assist establishing a diagnosis.

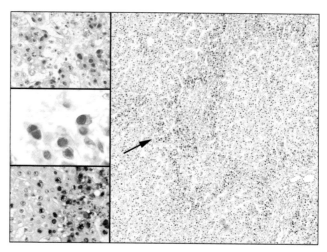

FIGURE 4.23: *Adenoviral hepatitis is characterized by map-like areas of necrosis, which are sometimes surrounded by macrophages and/or neutrophils. But in this case, the widespread necrosis is accompanied only by a few neutrophils. The area highlighted by the arrow is shown at higher magnification in the upper right inset; note the inclusion-containing cells located at the edge of the necrotic zone. The middle left inset shows characteristic adenoviral nuclear inclusions under oil immersion. Note the "baked-muffin" appearance of the nuclear inclusions and the smudgy appearance of infected cells. As with all other opportunistic viruses, immunostaining for viral antigens confirms the diagnosis (case courtesy of Dr. Ron Jaffe; Children's Hospital of Pittsburgh).*

Adenovirus can also cause changes similar to those seen with HSV/VZ and CMV hepatitis because of granulomatoid infiltrates and focal necrosis, respectively. Adenovirus generally usually causes less necrosis than either herpes simplex or VZ hepatitis. Granulomas associated with adenovirus usually consist almost solely of macrophages or mixtures of macrophages and neutrophils and are much larger than the "microgranulomas" typical of CMV hepatitis. Multinucleated giant cells are rare in adenoviral hepatitis. CMV hepatitis, in contrast, causes cytomegaly and produces eosinophilic intranuclear inclusions, surrounded by a clear halo, and basophilic or amphophilic small *cytoplasmic* inclusions. Adenovirus does not cause cytomegaly; the nucleus assumes a "smudgy" appearance and cytoplasmic inclusions are not seen.

Regardless, as with all other opportunistic virus infection, the diagnosis is first suspected on H&E sections and confirmed after immunohistochemical staining and/or in situ hybridization.

IV. CONSIDERATIONS INVOLVED IN THE EVALUATION OF LATE LIVER ALLOGRAFT DYSFUNCTION AND PROTOCOL BIOPSIES

Excellent short-term survival and a high incidence of recurrent original disease make liver allograft biopsy evaluation for late dysfunction an increasingly important aspect of liver transplant pathology. Interpretation of biopsies obtained more than six months after transplantation is significantly more difficult than early after transplantation. This is because a broader spectrum of insults can cause dysfunction and many of them show overlapping clinical, serological, and histopathological features. The Banff Working Group for liver allograft pathology, therefore, spent several years constructing a consensus document to help guide the evaluation and interpretation of such biopsies (137).

More than one year after liver transplantation, recipients are routinely monitored for liver allograft dysfunction using liver injury tests. In most programs, late biopsies are obtained when changes in liver injury tests represent a significant elevation from baseline values for that patient (137). Several studies [reviewed in (98)] described the structural integrity and listed the causes of dysfunction late liver allograft dysfunction in recipients one to nineteen years after transplantation. The results were remarkably similar among the various studies even though the recipient pool, immunosuppressive management policies and study designs differed significantly.

Leading causes of late liver allograft dysfunction include recurrence of the original disease and obstructive cholangiopathy. Dysfunction in only 4–38 percent of late biopsies was attributable to acute or chronic rejection. Knowledge of the original disease, changes in immunosuppression, findings in previous biopsies, the clinical and laboratory profile, and the result of any therapeutic or diagnostic tests or intervention should be incorporated into the interpretation and final diagnosis (98).

A minority of programs obtain *protocol* biopsies, except perhaps, in HCV+ recipients. For those with non-HCV–related disease, particularly pediatric recipients, obtaining protocol allograft biopsies in asymptomatic long-term survivors with normal or near normal liver tests is controversial. Considerations include morbidity and mortality, costs, inconvenience, resource utilization, and potential adverse impact of unexplained histopathological findings. These should be weighed against potential individual and/or societal benefits (98,203–208) such as 1) early detection of clinically unapparent disease (203,208), 2) identification of recipients that might be successfully weaned from immunosuppression (209), and 3) recognition of late-onset rapid HCV progression (205), and the impact of chronic low-grade injury and alcohol use (204) and long-term engraftment.

A majority (nearly 75 percent) of biopsies from recipients surviving more than one year with abnormal liver tests or symptoms will show histopathologically significant abnormalities (98,203–207). The abnormalities are usually attributable to recurrent disease or biliary tract strictures (98,203–207). In addition, nearly 25 percent of biopsies from long-surviving asymptomatic recipients with normal liver tests will show significant abnormalities if the original

disease is one that commonly recurs, such as HCV, PBC, and AIH (98,203–207). Minor histopathological abnormalities occur in about two-thirds of biopsies, even without recurrent disease in asymptomatic recipients with normal or near-normal liver tests (98,203–207). Common findings are portal venopathy and nodular regenerative hyperplasia; thickening and hyalinization of small hepatic artery branches (98,210), and "nonspecific" portal and lobular inflammation (98,206–208). The pathogenesis, significance, and long-term consequences of these otherwise unexplained long-term histopathological findings are in need of further study.

Many late post-transplant biopsies show portal-based mononuclear inflammation with variable necro-inflammatory-type interface activity (137). Subtle histopathological differences relied upon to distinguish among several possible specific causes of dysfunction are not always present or reliable. Rendering a definitive diagnosis may not be possible in the early stages of a disorder. In such case, using "features suggestive of early" emphasizes a tentative diagnosis (137).

Laboratory tests used to establish a diagnosis before transplantation may not have the same significance after transplantation. AMA and antinuclear antibodies (ANA) often persist after transplantation in patients with PBC or AIH, albeit at lower titers, even without histopathological evidence of recurrent disease. Patients without AIH before transplantation can develop auto-antibodies either as a complication of otherwise typical rejection (211–213) or in association with new-onset AIH (214–220). Conversely, the titer of autoantibodies might be influenced by chronic immunosuppression.

More than one insult can contribute to late post-transplant dysfunction. Biopsy analysis can help to determine the main component of injury but careful clinicopathological correlation is needed (137). Levels of immunosuppression can influence biopsy findings and the severity of recurrent viral hepatitis, AIH, and rejection. Late-onset acute rejection, for example, is often precipitated by inadequate immunosuppression and recipients with AIH and other autoimmune disorders are usually steroid dependent (137).

Criteria to determine the causes of late liver allograft dysfunction can be generalized to evaluate all the potential causes (137). First, the histopathological evidence of liver injury and liver injury tests should show patterns consistent with the diagnosis. Second, the diagnosis should be supported by positive serological, molecular biologic, immunologic, or radiographic evidence of pathogen or possible cause of injury. Third, other causes of similar histopathological changes and elevated liver tests should have been reasonably excluded. The typical histopathological findings, according to the Banff Working Group, of the various causes of late dysfunction are summarized in Table 4.5, important inclusionary and exclusionary criteria are shown in Table 4.6, and the approximate incidence, risk factors, and clinical observations in Table 4.7.

TABLE 4.5 Histopathological Features Most Commonly Detected with Various Causes of Late Liver Allograft Dysfunction*; Adapted from (137)

Histopathological features	Autoimmune hepatitis**	Acute rejection	Chronic rejection	Chronic viral hepatitis types B and C	PBC	PSC/BD strictures
Distribution, severity, and composition of portal inflammation	Usually diffuse predominantly mononuclear of varying intensity. Often prominent plasma cell component	Usually diffuse, variable intensity, mixed "rejection-type" (see text) infiltrate	Patchy, usually minimal or mild lymphoplasmacytic	Patchy, variable intensity; predominantly mononuclear; nodular aggregates	Noticeably patchy and variable intensity; predominantly mononuclear; nodular aggregates and granulomas	Usually patchy to diffuse depending on stage; mild neutrophilic, eosinophilic, or occasionally mononuclear predominant
Presence and type of interface activity	Usually prominent and defining feature: necro-inflammatory type; often plasma cell rich	Focally present and mild necro-inflammatory type	Minimal to absent	Variable, usually not prominent: necro-inflammatory and (ductular type)	Important feature later in disease development: ductular and necro-inflammatory type with copper deposition	Prominent and defining feature: ductular type with portal and peri-portal edema
Bile duct inflammation and damage	Variable; if present involves a minority of bile ducts	Present and usually involves a majority of bile ducts	Focal ongoing lymphocytic bile duct damage; inflammation wanes with duct loss	Variable; if present involves a minority of bile ducts	Granulomatous or focally severe lymphocytic cholangitis is diagnostic in proper setting	Periductal lamellar edema, "fibrous cholangitis," acute cholangitis, multiple intraportal ductal profiles
Biliary epithelial senescence changes and small bile loss	Absent or involves only a minority of ducts/portal tracts, but may be focally severe	Absent or involves only a minority of ducts	Senescence/atrophy/atypia involve a majority of remaining ducts (see text)	Absent or involves only a minority of ducts	Small bile duct loss associated with ductular reaction	Small bile duct loss associated with ductular reaction
Perivenular mononuclear inflammation and/or hepatocyte dropout	Variable, can involve a majority of perivenular regions, similar to rejection (see text); may be plasma cell rich	Variable, if defining feature should involve a majority of perivenular regions; may also show subendothelial inflammation of vein (see text)	Usually present, but variable	Variable, but generally mild, if present involves a minority of perivenular regions	Variable, but generally mild, if present involves a minority of perivenular regions	Absent
Lobular findings and necro-inflammatory activity	Variable severity; rosettes may be present and/or prominent	Variable, if present, concentrated in perivenular regions	Variable, if present, concentrated in perivenular regions	Disarray variable; variable severity, necro-inflammatory activity	Mild disarray, parenchymal granulomas; periportal copper deposition and cholatestasis are late features	Disarray unusual; neutrophils clusters; ±cholestasis
Pattern of fibrosis during progression toward cirrhosis	Usually macronodular, posthepatitic pattern	Rare	Uncommon, if present usually a venocentric pattern; may evolve to biliary pattern over time	Usually macronodular, hepatitic pattern; may be micronodular (see text)	Biliary pattern	Biliary pattern

* The histopathological findings in this table should be combined with clinical, serological, radiographic, and important exclusionary criteria listed in Table 4.2 to arrive at a final diagnosis.

** The same findings apply to recurrent and de novo autoimmune hepatitis.

TABLE 4.6 Inclusionary and Exclusionary Criteria for the Diagnosis of Recurrent and New-Onset Chronic Necro-inflammatory Diseases after Liver Transplantation and Timing of First Onset and Pattern of Liver Test Elevations* adapted from (137) and (1)

Diagnosis	Original disease	Serology/molecular testing**	Timing and liver injury test profile***	Important exclusionary criteria
Recurrent AIH	AIH	Autoantibodies** (ANA, ASMA, ALKM) usually in high titers (>1:80); raised serum IgG	>6 months, hepatocellular	Acute and chronic rejection, HBV, HCV infection, as determined by third-generation ELISA assay and/or by serum PCR
De novo AIH Recurrent HBV or HCV	Other than AIH HBV- or HCV-induced cirrhosis	Same as above HBV or HCV infection using standard, third-generation serological criteria and/or positive molecular testing for HBV or HCV nucleic acids	>6 months, hepatocellular Usually 6–8 weeks, but as early as 10 days. Usually hepatocellular; but may be cholestatic	Same as above Acute and chronic rejection, AIH
Recurrent PBC	PBC	Positive AMA, but little additional benefit because AMA remains elevated in the majority of patients after transplantation	>1 year, cholestatic	Biliary tract obstruction/strictures
Recurrent PSC	PSC	NA	Usually >1 year, cholestatic	HA thrombosis/stenosis, chronic (ductopenic) rejection, abnormal surgical anatomy, anastomotic strictures alone, nonanastomotic strictures occurring <90 days after OLTx, and ABO incompatibility
Acute rejection	NA (see text for risk factors)	NA	Any time; usually hepatocellular; may be mixed if superimposed on chronic rejection	Inadequate immunosuppression usually, but not always present (see text); important exclusions: biliary tract obstruction/strictures, HBV, HCV, AIH
Chronic rejection	NA (see text for risk factors)	NA	Any time, but usually <1 year, cholestatic; rarely hepatocellular in veno-occlusive variant (see text)	Inadequate immunosuppression usually, but not always present (see text); important exclusions: biliary tract obstruction/strictures, HBV, HCV, AIH
Idiopathic post-transplant hepatitis	Nonviral and non-AIH	Negative testing for HBV and HCV infection and autoantibodies	> 1 year; usually hepatocellular	Acute and chronic rejection, all other causes of chronic hepatitis, and biliary tract obstruction/strictures reasonably excluded. All attempts should be made to determine a cause

*   See Table 4.5 for compatible histopathological findings.

**   Timing, usual timing of first onset; ASMA, anti-smooth muscle antibodies; ALKM, anti-liver-kidney microsomal antibodies.

***   Sustained elevation for more than one month, hepatocellular, ALT and/or AST > ALP and/or GGTP; cholestatic = ALP and/or GGTP > AST and/or ALT.

TABLE 4.7 Incidence, Risk Factors, and Clinical Observations for Causes of Late Dysfunction [adapted from (1, 2, 137)]

Diagnosis	Incidence at 5 years of recurrent disease	Risk factors for disease recurrence and/or severe recurrent disease	Clinical/immunologic/radiological observations
Viral hepatitis			
HAV	<5%	Preexisting anti-HAV titers decline following OLTx, but recurrent or new-onset HAV is rare after OLTx	Not an important cause of post-transplant dysfunction (228,350,351)
Recurrent HBV	100% if HBV DNA positive; less frequent if HBV DNA is negative	Anti-HBc+ donor (17,239,352)—inadequate anti-HBV treatment; HBV mutants	Recurrent HBV disease not usually significant problem because of treatment with effective antiviral drugs (240,353–367)
Recurrent HCV	Nearly universal in those with HCV replication before transplantation	HCV RNA in blood helpful in differential diagnosis: >30,000,000 IU/l increased risk of cholestatic hepatitis; moderate or severe acute and chronic rejection usually occurs in association with relatively low HCV RNA levels <5,000,000 IU/l (145)	Greater viral burden (368–372) and more rapid progression of fibrosis than in general population (373–377); severity of hepatitis often worse with genotype 1 and 4 viruses (252,255, 257,368,369,378–383); variable disease progression (384, 385); subset of recipients with late-onset rapid progression (205)
HEV	Newly described cause of late liver allograft hepatitis/dysfunction (230)	Recurrent disease has not yet been described because HEV usually does not cause chronic infection in nonimmunosuppressed patients	Infection and persistent viremia after transplantation. Infection early after transplantation and leukopenia might be significant risk factors for chronic infection. More studies are needed on this topic to delineate the prevalence of infection in various populations (230)
Disorders of dysregulated immunity			
Recurrent AIH	~30%	Suboptimal immunosuppression (290,386–388); type I > type II disease (296); severe inflammation in native liver before transplantation (389); longer duration of follow-up (296). HLA-DR3 or -DR4 recipient status (214,390,391) might reflect more severe disease (392)	Usually need higher baseline immunosuppression and/or are steroid-dependent (see text); HLA-DR3 and/or -DR4 genotype often present
De novo AIH	<5%	May be more common in children (215, 217,393–395), but this assumption has been questioned recently (216)	Same as above
Recurrent PBC	20–30% increases with time (98,293,386, 396–400)	Tacrolimus as baseline immunosuppression (287,288); living-related donor (289); steroid and other immunosuppression withdrawal (290, 291,401); may recur as AIH (219,402)	Initial diagnosis often made by biopsy in asymptomatic recipient without increased liver tests (98,293,386, 396–399)
Recurrent PSC	20–30% increases with time (98,285,310,312,314, 315,317,403,404)	Male sex; donor-recipient gender mismatch; HLA-DRB1*08 (307); intact colon at time of transplantation (309, 405); patients at increased risk of rejection (314, 315, 403, 404)	Cholangiographically confirmed biliary strictures occurring >90 days after OLTx (403,404); mural irregularity, diverticulum-like outpouchings, and an overall appearance resembling PSC (316); patient and allograft survival not adversely affected upto 5 years (310,312,314,315,403,404); later outcome uncertain
Rejection/other			
Acute rejection	Variable, <30% of causes of late dysfunction	Inadequate immunosuppression (27,406–408); treatment with immune activating drugs (e.g., interferon); original disease of immune dysregulation (e.g., AIH, PBC, PSC)	Much less common than early after transplantation; may be more difficult to treat, perhaps related to delay in diagnosis (409)

(Continued)

TABLE 4.7 *Continued*

Diagnosis	Incidence at 5 years of recurrent disease	Risk factors for disease recurrence and/or severe recurrent disease	Clinical/immunologic/radiological observations
Chronic rejection	~3% (149,410,411)	Inadequate immunosuppression; treatment with immune-activating drugs (e.g., interferon); refractory acute rejection (146,149,151–154, 156,157,163,412–417); chronic rejection in a previous failed allograft	Important cause of late dysfunction (76,98,207,418–420); most cases occur within first year (149,152,156, 410, 412); does not appear to increase with time after transplantation, but more follow-up is needed
Idiopathic post-transplant hepatitis	5–60%, wide variation (98, 203,207,217,389,421)	Might be more common in pediatric recipients (see text)	Up to 50% of patients followed for a minimum of 10 years will develop bridging fibrosis (337) or cirrhosis (296); incidence varies widely among centers
Toxic/metabolic			
Alcoholic	13–50%	Rate of relapse difficult to document precisely. Severe relapse can lead to graft loss or patient death, but recurrent alcoholic liver disease is not a significant problem for the majority of alcoholics up to 6 years after transplantation (204, 321–323)	Recurrent disease difficult to distinguish from NASH, alone on basis of histopathology alone, elevated ratio of GGTP:ALP, clinical history often suggestive of relapse
NAFLD	25–100%*	Incidence depends on whether NASH or cryptogenic cirrhosis was the original diagnosis and whether protocol biopsies were obtained (333, 334, 422)	Usually asymptomatic with minimal elevation of liver injury tests; most commonly detected in protocol liver biopsies or in imaging studies
Malignancies			
HCC	See Risk Factors	Recurrence depends on size, less likely with single tumor <5 cm or 3 tumors each <3 cm, stage ≤T2, and histological grade (well differentiated), and absence of vascular invasion, and lymph node metastasis (423–429)	Multiparameter modeling systems used to predict recurrence after OLTx and thus, eligibility for OLTx; in some cases of late recurrence important to distinguish between donor and recipient origin of recurrent tumor
Bile duct/CC	See Risk Factors	Prognosis is generally poor, but patients with peripheral cholangiocarcinomas, and those early-stage hilar tumors (stage 0–II) without lymph node metastasis, and negative resection margins can show reasonable (~40%) 5-year survival (430–433)	Generally poor indication for liver transplantation because of very high recurrence rate

V. RECURRENT DISEASES AND DISEASES INDUCED BY TRANSPLANTATION

Recurrence of the original disease and the side effects of chronic immunosuppression are the most significant obstacles to long-term morbidity free survival for liver allograft recipients. The following native liver disease classification is helpful in understanding the impact of disease recurrence: 1) infectious (viral hepatitis A, B, C, D, E, etc.); 2) dysregulated immunity, including AIH, PBC, PSC, and overlap syndromes; 3) hepatocellular and cholangiocarcinomas; 4) toxic insults, such as alcohol abuse and adverse drug reactions; and 5) hepatic-based metabolic diseases such as α-1-antitrypsin deficiency and Wilson's disease and extrahepatic-based metabolic disorders, such as hemochromatosis, Gaucher's disease, and cystic fibrosis.

Hepatic transplantation for hepatocellular carcinoma is based on the stage of the disease at the time of transplantation (221–223). In general, small, early stage, hepatocellular carcinomas without vascular invasion are cured by liver transplantation. Microscopic vascular invasion is a powerful predictor of hepatocellular carcinoma recurrence, as are multiple liver tumors, and larger overall tumor burden. Bile duct and cholangiocarcinomas are usually a contraindication for liver transplantation and generally have a poor prognosis after liver replacement.

Other diseases of uncertain etiologies also can recur after liver transplantation. These include sarcoidosis (224), idiopathic granulomatous hepatitis (98), post-infantile giant cell hepatitis (225), and the Budd-Chiari syndrome (51–53).

i. Hepatitis Virus Infections (A, B, C, D, and E)

1. Introduction

Hepatitis A (HAV)-induced fulminant hepatic failure is a rare indication for liver replacement. HBV-induced cirrhosis is a leading indication in Asia (226,227), whereas HCV-induced cirrhosis is one of the most common indications throughout the world. Since HAV does not generally cause chronic infection, even in immunosuppressed hosts, it not as yet been identified as a cause of allograft dysfunction. However, Fagan et al. (228) showed hepatic persistence, or re-infection, of a liver allograft without dysfunction, presumably from extrahepatic viral reservoirs.

Like the opportunistic viruses, HBV and HCV remain in the circulation and/or infect extrahepatic tissues. If HBV or HCV are capable of replication they will *universally* re-infect the new liver. Effective screening of blood products and organ donors has largely eliminated acquisition of new infections during the transplant, but *newly acquired infections* after transplantation are not rare (229). Clinical and histopathological presentation and evolution of HBV and HCV in liver allograft recipients are nearly the same as those observed in the general population, with several important general exceptions: 1) viral replication is significantly enhanced because of the immunosuppression; 2) inflammation might be slightly less, but fibrosis progression definitely occurs more rapidly after, than before, transplantation; and 3) in a small percentage of cases, markedly enhanced viral replication results in atypical clinical and histopathological presentations, described in more detail below. Hepatitis E virus (HEV) has recently been identified as a cause of chronic hepatitis in liver allograft recipients (230).

2. Hepatitis B and Delta

a. Introduction The incidence of HBV-induced cirrhosis, and liver transplantation for this indication, is decreasing significantly in the Western World because of mandatory HBV vaccination but it is the leading indication for liver replacement in China (226,227). Active viral replication before transplantation, recognized by HBeAg seropositivity or detection of HBV DNA in the circulation, almost assures re-infection of the allograft. Re-infection and recurrent disease is less predictable in patients who had HBV-induced fulminant liver failure or in those with chronic liver disease who had become anti-HBe positive and serum HBV DNA and HBeAg negative prior to transplantation (231–237). Effective immunologic control of HBV infection and/or integration of nonreplicative HBV viral DNA into the genome probably account for the observation that 10–25 percent of these patients will not "re-infect" the new liver or develop HBV disease in the allograft.

Donor and blood product screening has largely limited HBV-induced allograft dysfunction to those infected before transplantation, except for a small cohort of naive recipients who acquire HBV infection during or after transplantation (229,238). Livers from anti-HBc positive donors is one possible source; they effectively transmit HBV to naive unvaccinated recipients (17,239).

In addition to vaccination, which prevents infection, pharmacological treatment of HBV in those already infected has significantly diminished the clinical and histopathological manifestations of HBV induced allograft dysfunction. Treatment modalities include polyclonal and monoclonal hepatitis B immune globulin, interferon-α (IFN-α), and antiviral drugs such as foscarnet, ganciclovir, famciclovir, and lamivudine (240). Although HBV re-infection of the allograft cannot be prevented reliably, these drugs effectively control viral replication and recurrent disease [reviewed in (240)]. In fact, effective anti-HBV therapy has significantly reduced the morbidity and mortality of recurrent HBV compared to the era when these treatments were not available (241,242). The high cost of indefinite drug therapy and emergence of viral mutants that escape pharmacologic control of the major drawbacks to this treatment approach (241,242).

b. Pathophysiology Liver damage in HBV infection is thought to be mediated primarily by immunologic injury in nonimmunosuppressed hosts because HBV is generally considered to be noncytopathic. Liver allograft damage is also probably attributable to primarily virally directed immunologic injury (243). In this scenario, HBV peptides are presented to recipient memory T helper cells by host antigen presenting cells that repopulate the allograft after transplantation (244,245). The viral antigens drive memory T helper cells activation and expansion of antigen-specific TH1-type CD4+ lymphocytes, which in turn, release IFN-γ, the most potent activator of monocytes/macrophages. Macrophage activation results in TNF-α expression, and together with IFN-γ theses cytokines contribute to allograft damage by 1) recruiting and activating nonspecific inflammatory cells; 2) upregulating TNFR expression, which makes hepatocytes more vulnerable to TNF-α; 3) exerting a direct cytotoxic effect on the HBsAg-expressing hepatocytes; and 4) inducing local mediators of tissue injury such as nitric oxide. These mechanisms are still operative with donor and recipient HLA mismatching and immunosuppression (243). Massive HBV replication occurring in a small minority of heavily, over-immunosuppressed, recipients can lead to a clinicopathological pattern of injury referred to as "fibrosing cholestatic hepatitis" (232–234). In this situation, the virus appears to be directly cytopathic because there is clinical, serological, and histopathological evidence of liver injury despite minimally increased hepatic inflammation, described in detail below.

c. Clinical Presentation HBV re-infection of the allograft occurs immediately after transplantation but HBV hepatitis usually first becomes clinically/serologically obvious about six to eight weeks as otherwise unexplained elevations of liver ALT and AST. More significant hepatitis, as in native livers, is accompanied by nausea, vomiting, jaundice, and, in rare cases, fulminant hepatic failure. The clinical presentation, therefore, is quite similar to HBV hepatitis seen in other immunosuppressed hosts and nonimmunosuppressed patients from the general population (231–234). In the liver transplant setting, however, recipients treated with too much immunosuppression can develop severe disease because of fibrosing cholestatic hepatitis. In contrast, rapid tapering and/or withdrawal of immunosuppression should also be avoided in HBV+ recipients with evidence of active viral replication. This maneuver can "re-arm" the immune system and cause severe immunologically mediated liver injury and fulminant hepatic failure.

d. Histopathological Findings The histopathological manifestations of HBV infection of hepatic allografts have been recently reviewed (246). The findings are similar to that seen in native livers. Effective antiviral pharmacological therapy, however, can effectively control HBV replication and has reduced the incidence and severity of recurrent acute and chronic HBV hepatitis. Consequently, the need to diagnose and monitor disease progression for HBV+ recipients has decreased significantly in recent years. It is important, however, to recognize the various HBV disease histopathological manifestations because they reliably appear in inadequately treated recipients and those harboring drug-resistant viral mutants.

As with all of the other viruses that cause chronic hepatic infection, the evolution of liver disease typically begins with *acute hepatitis*. This phase is usually first recognizable within four to six weeks after transplantation as expression of hepatitis core antigen in the cytoplasm of occasional hepatocytes (231,232). Expression of core antigen spreads to involve more hepatocytes, followed by surface antigen expression (231,232), and then by spotty hepatocyte apoptosis, lobular inflammation, Kupffer's cell hypertrophy, and lobular disarray. Portal inflammation is variable. A small percentage of HBV+ recipients will develop confluent/bridging, and even submassive necrosis, particularly if immunosuppression is lowered or withdrawn (231). Rare liver allograft recipients will show complete histopathological resolution of acute disease activity or will actually "clear" or immunologically "control" the virus. Most, however, evolve into the chronic phase and cirrhosis can develop rapidly within 12–18 months after transplantation (231–237).

Evolution into *chronic HBV* in untreated patients with active viral replication is characterized by lymphoplasmacytic portal inflammation with relative sparing of the bile ducts and portal and hepatic veins. The portal/periportal inflammation is associated with variable interface necroinflammatory activity (Figure 4.24). Lobular findings in the chronic phase are usually much less conspicuous

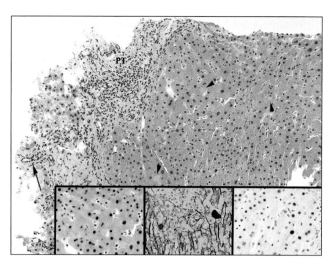

FIGURE 4.24: *Recurrent acute and chronic HBV hepatitis is becoming relatively uncommon because of vaccination and effective antiviral drugs, which inhibit HBV replication and prevent chronic liver inflammation. It is still seen occasionally, however, and the histopathological changes are usually typical of chronic hepatitis as seen in other settings, except perhaps, for enhanced viral replication. Note the abundant expression of hepatitis B core antigen (lower right inset), hepatitis B surface antigen (middle lower inset), and numerous ground-glass hepatocytes (arrowheads and lower left inset). Note also that the portal inflammation is not "bilio-centric"; instead, the bile ducts are intact (arrow).*

than during the acute phase and include ground glass hepatocytes or hepatocytes with sanded nuclei that stain positively for hepatitis B surface and core antigen, respectively, and mild disarray and low grade necroinflammatory activity.

Massive HBV replication because of the effects of (over) immunosuppression and MHC nonidentity between the liver and recipient can lead to the development of *fibrosing cholestatic hepatitis* (232,234,247,248). Other descriptive terms have been used to identify these cases (232–235,247,248). Fibrosing cholestatic hepatitis can also occur with the emergence of viral mutants. Typical histopathological findings include marked hepatocyte swelling, lobular disarray, and cholestasis combined with prominent ductular and fibrotic-type interface activity. These changes occur in the face of minimal or mild portal and lobular inflammation. The swollen and degenerating hepatocytes usually show massive hepatocellular expression of HB core and/or surface antigen, which have led several groups to suggest that HBV is directly cytopathic under these special circumstances (232–235,247,248). The prominent ductular and fibrotic type interface activity can lead to portal-to-portal bridging fibrosis over a period of weeks to months.

Delta agent coinfection of HBV+ recipients has resulted in reports of more severe and less severe HBV-related disease activity after transplantation compared to HBV+/delta recipients (237,249,250). There are also conflicting reports about the cytopathic effect of HDV and the relationship to HBV replication and allograft livers. David et al. (251) noted that HDV hepatitis associated with non-replicative HBV infection resulted in fibrosing cholestatic hepatitis, but without hepatic HBcAg expression. When active HBV replication was present, the HBV + HDV hepatitis produced necro-inflammatory activity similar to that seen in B and D viral hepatitis in patients from the general population (251).

e. Differential Diagnosis Acute HBV should be distinguished from other causes of acute hepatitis, such as CMV, HCV, and EBV and other causes of spotty hepatocyte apoptosis, such as a global ischemic insult or "ischemic" hepatitis and portal and so-called transitional hepatitis that accompanies the transition from acute to chronic rejection. The most reliable method of distinguishing acute HBV hepatitis from the other insults, listed above, is a review of the clinical, histopathological, and serological profile. Detection of viral antigens and/or nucleic acids in the blood or tissues combined with histological features of an active lobular hepatitis, and an absence of other causes, favor recurrent HBV.

Chronic HBV hepatitis should also be distinguished from other causes of chronic hepatitis such as HCV, AIH, and chronic adverse drug reactions. Detection of ground glass hepatocytes or viral antigens and/or nucleic acid in the blood or tissues, and an absence of other causes for chronic hepatitis favor chronic HBV. It should be remembered, however, that allograft HBV infection does not equate with HBV disease, or for that matter, exclude rejection or any other cause of allograft dysfunction (232). Detection of either core or surface antigen by immunohistochemistry may be seen in allografts that otherwise have all the features of acute or chronic rejection (232). Therefore, serological evidence of viral infection or detection of viral antigens or nucleic acid in the liver has to be *correlated* with the histological pattern of injury, which can include acute, chronic, or fibrosing cholestatic hepatitis.

Features used to distinguish between acute rejection and acute or chronic hepatitis have already been discussed (231,232) (see Acute Rejection – Differential Diagnosis).

3. Hepatitis C Virus

a. Introduction HCV-induced cirrhosis is the *leading* indication for liver replacement in the Western World; it currently accounts for about 25–30 percent of liver transplants. A significant percentage of HCV+ recipients also have a history of coexistent alcohol abuse and hepatocellular carcinoma. The allograft liver is almost immediately reinfected by HCV. Subsequent viremia is seen nearly all recipients within days after transplantation and HCV-induced hepatitis eventually develop in a majority, although the rate of fibrosis progression is quite variable.

The incidence of new-onset HCV infection after transplantation is usually low (<1 percent) in low prevalence areas (252,253), but as high as 10–20 percent in high prevalence regions (229,254).

As in the general population, recurrent chronic HCV disease evolves slowly after transplantation in the majority of recipients, but the progression of fibrosis is still significantly faster than in native livers. One small, but not insignificant, percentage of recipients develops very aggressive disease after transplantation. Another small percentage will show very slow fibrosis progression. But the majority develops an active chronic hepatitis and up to 20 percent are cirrhotic again by five years after transplantation. Therefore, liver transplantation for HCV-induced cirrhosis can significantly prolong survival, but recurrent disease is a very significant problem.

HCV disease progression after liver transplantation appears to be dependent on a variety of factors, some of which are influenced by local treatment policies. It is clear, however, that new and more effective anti-HCV therapy is needed. The hope is that HCV will become a chronic, but medically manageable, problem like that described for the evolution of HBV disease over the last two decades. Even if newer anti-HCV agents are employed, however, HCV-induced cirrhosis requiring liver transplantation will continue to be a major problem for the foreseeable future.

The *genotypes* of HCV seen after transplantation generally reflect those of recipient population. Type 1b is the most prevalent type in several European centers (255,256) and in a large North American site (257) accounting for 25–60 percent, of the patients, whereas in another American study, type 1a was predominant (257).

b. Pathophysiology Immunopathogenic mechanisms responsible for allograft liver injury in HCV-induced hepatitis are similar to those encountered in native livers [reviewed in (258) and (259)]. The important exception is that baseline immunosuppression and MHC mismatching greatly increase viral replication and interfere with viral clearance, respectively. These factors, in turn, drive more rapidly progressively fibrosis than is seen in native livers [reviewed in (259)].

HCV re-infection occurs almost immediately after transplantation and viral replication begins within days [reviewed in (259)]. HCV proteins interfere with 1) host innate immunity—by disrupting pathogen-associated pattern recognition pathways and subverting the activity of NK (natural killer) cells and 2) cellular immunoregulation via CD81 binding. Together, these impediments hinder development of the early antiviral response, diminish adaptive CD4+ and CD8+ T-cell responses needed for viral clearance, and therefore, promote viral persistence and chronic infection [reviewed in (258) and (259)].

An unending struggle between viral replication and mutational evasion of the antiviral immune response versus

TH1-mediated antiviral immunity continually damage the allograft liver. High levels of HCV replication also increase oxidative stress and trigger a liver-damaging, but ineffective, antiviral immune response (259). This response injures hepatocytes via the perforin/granzyme pathway and release of Fas ligand, inflammatory cytokines and other soluble effector molecules. Other "nonspecific" effector inflammatory cells are recruited to the site and damage nearby uninfected liver cells (bystander effect) [reviewed in (258) and (259)]. If viral replication persists, eventually, the continual struggle between the virus and the immune system causes liver fibrosis/cirrhosis [reviewed in (260)].

Charlton et al. (176) grouped factors associated with more aggressive HCV recurrence or diminished graft survival, or both, into the following four categories: viral, recipient, donor, and post-transplant. *Viral factors* include greater pre- and post-transplant viremia, viral genotypes 1 and 4, greater viral diversity (quasi-species), and lack of response to interferon therapy. *Donor factors* include increasing age, macrovesicular steatosis, and longer cold ischemic time. It is controversial whether living or reduced-size donor grafts are risk factors for more rapidly progressive HCV-induced fibrosis. *Recipient factors* include older age, black race, and MHC compatibility, presumably because anti-HCV memory T cells can cause more damage. *Factors operative after transplantation* include immunosuppression management, coexistent CMV, and acute rejection [reviewed in (176)].

Dramatic and rapid changes in immunosuppression and overimmunosuppression are associated with more rapidly progressive recurrent HCV (259). In our opinion, lymphocyte-depleting induction therapy followed by rapid "re-arming" of the immune system by rapid lowering of immunosuppression is a strategy to be avoided. This causes marked viral replication early after transplantation, and when the immunosuppression is rapidly lowered or withdrawn, the immune system significantly damages the allograft and causes more rapidly progressive fibrosis (261,262), as described above. Instead, one study reported that if immunosuppression is gradually tapered or withdrawn late (five years or more) after transplantation, fibrosis progression might be slowed or reversed (263).

Fibrosing cholestatic HCV, like cholestatic HBV, probably represents a direct viral cytopathic effect on hepatocytes because of massive HCV replication. This occurs in overimmunosuppressed recipients (259) most of whom typically show HCV RNA levels in the peripheral circulation of higher than 30 million IU/ml. The intrahepatic immune response in FCH HCV is typically TH2 like and infiltrating lymphocytes often lack HCV specificity (264).

c. Clinical Presentation
The clinical presentation of HCV hepatitis is not unlike that seen in the general population. *Acute hepatitis*, which develops in most recipients, is usually asymptomatic, and is recognized primarily by elevation of ALT and AST to four to eight times baseline levels. In most cases, this first becomes apparent between three and six weeks after transplantation in routinely monitored liver injury tests. An earlier onset within ten to fourteen days can be associated with more aggressive disease. Some cases also show significant elevations of the GGTP. Symptoms, when present, usually include fatigue and nausea. Jaundice at initial presentation is unusual unless the recipient is at risk for FCH. Fulminant liver failure is not seen outside of the setting of FCH. Needle biopsy evaluation is needed to confirm the diagnosis.

FCH HCV is clearly associated with "overimmunosuppression" and characterized clinically by malaise, jaundice, and marked and preferential elevations of bilirubin, alkaline phosphatase, and gamma glutamyltranspeptidase. The disease usually begins early after transplantation and evolves subacutely over a period of weeks to months. Later onset can also occur, most commonly when recurrent HCV is misdiagnosed as acute rejection and the patient is treated vigorously with increased immunosuppression. Early recognition of FCH HCV relies on a high index of suspicion, an understanding of the clinical circumstance surrounding its emergence, and markedly elevated HCV RNA levels.

d. Histopathological Findings
The evolution of HCV in liver allografts is quite similar to that seen in the general population, except in allografts the acute phase shows less inflammation and the chronic phase less often shows nodular aggregates of portal-based lymphocytes and there is more ductular-type interface activity (Figure 4.25).

Acute hepatitis usually first appears within three to six weeks, but can be detected as early as ten to fourteen days. It presents primarily as lobular hepatitis. Typical features include lobular disarray, Kupffer's cell hypertrophy, hepatocyte apoptosis, mild sinusoidal lymphocytosis; usually mild mononuclear portal inflammation, and macrovesicular steatosis involving periportal and midzonal hepatocytes. Focal mild lymphocytic cholangitis and reactive changes of the biliary epithelium can be seen focally, but is neither severe nor widespread. The acute/lobular phase is usually accompanied by an increase in HCV RNA levels in the peripheral blood.

The *transition* from acute to chronic hepatitis is marked by waning of the lobular changes and an increase in portal inflammation, formation of nodular portal-based lymphoid aggregates, and emergence of necro-inflammatory and ductular-type interface activity that begin to distort the architecture.

Chronic HCV usually begins between four and twelve months after transplantation and is usually dominated by portal and periportal changes. The predominant features are chronic portal inflammation, portal-based lymphoid aggregates, and necro-inflammatory and ductular-type interface activity of varying severity. Inflammatory bile

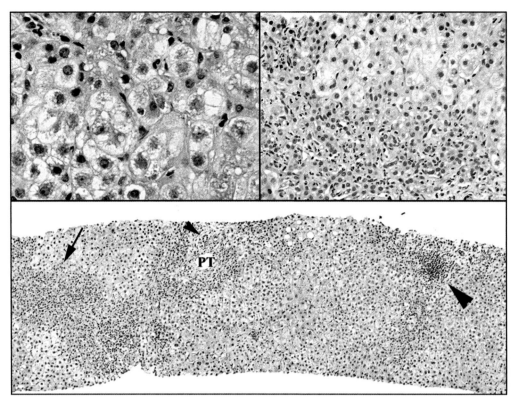

FIGURE 4.25: *Recurrent HCV appears histologically quite similar to that seen in native livers with predominantly mononuclear inflammation, portal-based nodular lymphoid aggregates (large arrowhead), and interface activity. However, in general, when compared to native livers, allografts usually show less inflammation and more often ductular-type interface activity is seen (arrow), which is shown at magnification, in the upper right inset. Note that the bile ducts are intact (small arrowhead). This particular case is bordering on FCH.*

duct damage can be seen, but it is usually not severe or widespread and there is usually no bile duct loss. Lobular changes are usually less conspicuous and include mild lobular disarray and necro-inflammatory activity. Inflammation in and around the connective tissue sheath of the central vein, known as "central perivenulitis," can also be seen in an occasional, or a minority, of central veins. But similar to the duct damage, it is neither severe nor widespread.

A *plasma cell–rich subtype* of recurrent HCV, "autoimmune-like," has recently been described by Khettry (265), which shows aggressive, plasma cell–rich, interface activity and some of these patients develop central perivenulitis (Figure 4.26). Many patients also develop auto-antibodies (ANA) and/or elevated serum gamma globulins (265) and are more prone to develop progressive fibrosis. Similar observations have been reported in native livers where features of clinical, serological, histopathological features of HCV and AIH overlap (266). If, however, central perivenulitis involves a majority of central veins, acute rejection has likely developed in the context of recurrent HCV. If the central perivenulitis is plasma cell–rich and involves a majority of central veins, then AIH, or autoimmune effector mechanism in the context of recurrent HCV, have developed. It is difficult to distinguish between rejection and AIH, but both are responsive to increased immunosuppression.

FCH HCV is characterized early by hepatocyte swelling and cholestasis, and only mild necro-inflammatory changes (267). Fully developed FCH HCV is characterized by extensive centrilobular hepatocyte swelling and degeneration, cholestasis, spotty acidophilic hepatocyte necrosis, and Kupffer's cell hypertrophy, combined with portal expansion because of prominent ductular-type and fibrotic-type interface activity, and mild mixed or even neutrophilic-predominant portal inflammation (268,269).

Some studies showed no correlation between viral genotype and/or levels and the severity of liver damage (270), while others showed that HCV RNA was higher during the acute/lobular phase of hepatitis and progression to chronic hepatitis was associated with significantly decreased liver HCV RNA, probably as a result of immune control of viral replication (discussed above). Other studies show that ballooning degeneration and cholestasis at initial presentation (271,272) correlate with more rapid development of allograft cirrhosis (271,272). One study showed no difference in the histopathological appearance or rate of progression of recurrent versus de novo HCV, whereas another showed that de novo infection caused more aggressive disease (268). HCV genotype 3 can present as hepatic steatosis, but exclusion of other causes of steatosis is required in this setting (273).

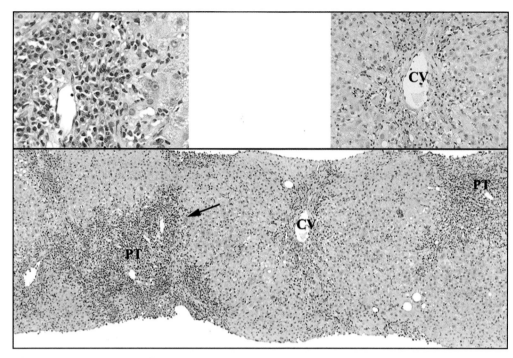

FIGURE 4.26: *Some cases of recurrent HCV show "autoimmune" features such as prominent plasmacytic inflammation (upper left inset), aggressive interface activity (arrow), and plasma cell-rich perivenular inflammation and hepatocyte dropout. This biopsy was obtained about twenty-six months after transplantation from a female recipient who was HCV RNA positive but also had serological evidence of coexistent autoimmunity. Bile duct damage was not a prominent feature, but a majority of the central veins showed central perivenulitis. It is difficult to distinguish between centrilobular-based rejection and autoimmune hepatitis in such cases. Both will respond to increased immunosuppression, but in HCV+ recipients, immunosuppressive therapy can hinder antiviral immunity.*

Acute and chronic rejection occurring in the context of recurrent HCV can be a difficult diagnosis to establish with certainty. If acute rejection is present it is important to determine whether recurrent HCV or rejection is the predominant process. In our prospective study, the following criteria reliably identified clinically significant acute rejection in the context of recurrent HCV: 1) portal inflammation with inflammatory bile duct damage involving 50 percent or more of the bile ducts or 2) mononuclear perivenular inflammation involving 50 percent or more of the terminal hepatic venules, associated with hepatocyte necrosis and/or dropout (145). Most such cases are graded as "moderate" acute cellular rejection according to the Banff criteria (145). In such cases, acute rejection should be listed as the predominant process, and more often than not, HCV RNA levels in the peripheral blood are relatively low (<5 million IU/ml).

Not unexpectedly, chronic rejection has been diagnosed with increased frequency in HCV+ recipients (274–276). A reduction in immunosuppression and/or treatment with an immune activating drug like alpha-interferon (277,278) can trigger rejection. An "inflammatory" microenvironment induced by HCV infection within the allograft can also upregulate adhesion, costimulatory and MHC antigens, and facilitate the rejection response. Partial donor-recipient MHC class I compatibility might also enable MHC-restricted T-cell–mediated antiviral immune responses to also target alloantigens (279).

Chronic HCV hepatitis does not change criteria needed to diagnose early and late chronic rejection, which have been already listed in previous sections.

Finally, two separate groups reported that routine immunostaining for *alpha smooth muscle protein* might provide important prognostic information. Prevalent and prominent staining of portal-based myofibroblasts at six months or one year after transplantation was predictive of rapid HCV disease progression (280,281) and likely illustrates mechanisms responsible for rapid development of cirrhosis in allografts [reviewed in (260)]. Livers from older donors also experience a faster rate of fibrosis progression (282).

e. Differential Diagnosis The differential diagnosis for acute and chronic HCV includes acute and chronic rejection, recurrent non-HCV viral hepatitis (e.g., HBV, CMV, EBV), and recurrent or new-onset AIH, PBC, and PSC, and biliary tract obstruction or stricturing. And as mentioned above, is important to recognize other causes of liver allograft dysfunction occurring in the background of recurrent HCV.

Acute and/or chronic rejection and recurrent HCV can occur together. Key features of acute rejection in this context are (137,145): 1) the prevalence and severity of mononuclear inflammatory bile duct damage and/or biliary epithelial senescence changes and 2) prevalence and severity of terminal hepatic vein inflammation and fibrosis. If either of these features involves a majority of bile ducts or terminal hepatic veins, then acute or chronic rejection, respectively, is present. Key features attributable to recurrent or new-onset HCV are the prevalence and severity of 1) lobular necro-inflammatory activity and 2) necro-inflammatory ductular type interface activity. These features are usually inconspicuous, or absent, in acute and chronic rejection. Prevalent and prominent ductular type interface activity strongly favors a nonrejection-related cause of allograft dysfunction.

The *timing* of the biopsy is also important. HCV is an uncommon cause of allograft dysfunction during the first several weeks after transplantation but occasional cases of acute HCV begin as early as ten to fourteen days. And most cases of recurrent hepatitis C begin between three and eight weeks after transplantation. Most acute rejection episodes, in contrast, occur within the first thirty days, with a median of eight days (102).

Trends in peripheral blood HCV RNA levels can be helpful in distinguishing recurrent HCV from acute rejection (145). In general, moderate or severe acute cellular and chronic rejection are associated with relatively low HCV RNA levels (<5 million IU/ml). Relatively high HCV RNA levels (>8 million IU/ml) are usually indicative of recurrent HCV (145).

It is important to remember that the most common mistake in published studies is the diagnosis of recurrent HCV as acute rejection [reviewed in (145)]. This leads to an inappropriate treatment of recurrent HCV with increased immunosuppression. Typically, liver injury tests transiently respond to the increased immunosuppression, but rapidly rebound to higher levels originally seen. Therefore, even though acute rejection and recurrent HCV can coexist, additional immunosuppression is usually given only when acute rejection is clearly the predominant process and of moderate severity according to the Banff criteria (145,283).

Distinguishing HCV from other causes of chronic hepatitis such as HBV, AIH, and drug-induced hepatitis is based on examination of the complete clinical, biochemical, and serological profile. A detailed histopathological examination can be extremely helpful in some cases. Viral antigen and/or nucleic acid detection, ground glass cells, or sanded nuclei distinguish HBV from HCV. In addition, confluent necrosis is more common in HBV, but is rarely, if ever seen in HCV, alone. Recurrent or de novo AIH and HCV are distinguished from each other on the basis of clinical, serological, and pathological profile used to diagnose AIH in the general population (284). Although there are no specific histopathological features that can reliably distinguish between AIH and HCV-induced hepatitis in an individual case, plasma cell–rich portal and perivenular inflammation with confluent perivenular necrosis favor AIH, whereas low-grade periportal and mid-zonal steatosis and portal lymphoid aggregates favor recurrent HCV.

FCH HCV can be difficult to distinguish from bile duct obstruction and hepatic artery thrombosis. Portal edema and portal, rather than periportal, neutrophilia is common in duct obstruction and/or acute cholangitis. In contrast, cholangiolar proliferation and acute cholangiolitis without portal edema is more characteristic of nonobstructive cholestatic hepatitis. In addition, lobular disarray and marked hepatocellular swelling is more usual for viral hepatitis in contrast to duct obstruction.

Exclusion of chronic HCV liver disease is based on negative RT-PCR results for HCV on liver tissue.

4. Hepatitis E Virus

a. Introduction, Pathophysiology, and Clinical Presentation The hepatotropic RNA virus, HEV, is an endemic cause of acute hepatitis in developing countries and appears to be an emerging disease in industrialized countries. It was recently identified as a cause of chronic hepatitis in immunosuppressed organ allograft recipients in France, including three liver transplant patients (230). HCV-induced chronic liver disease was discovered by screening all organ allograft recipients with short term, and otherwise unexplained, elevation of liver injury tests for HEV RNA and anti-HEV IgG. The prevalence of anti-HEV in their population was 10.4 percent in liver allograft recipients and three of eighty-six of these liver recipients (14/327 of all allograft recipients) developed acute infection. Seven of the fourteen acutely infected patients were asymptomatic, whereas the other seven developed fatigue, diffuse arthralgias, and myalgias over a period of one to two weeks; and one had marked weight loss.

Six of the patients showed complete resolution of liver injury tests abnormalities and cleared the HEV infection. The remaining eight patients developed chronic hepatitis characterized by continual elevation of liver injury tests and detection of HEV RNA in the serum and/or stool.

b. Histopathological Findings and Differential Diagnosis The acute and chronic phases of HEV hepatitis are similar to HBV and HCV as described above (230). The acute phase is predominantly lobular with inflammation but no ballooning, and spotty hepatocyte necrosis with acidophilic bodies. The portal tract show mild to moderate expansion by an inflammatory infiltrate composed mainly of lymphocytes. Mild "piecemeal necrosis" was observed in six patients (230).

Follow-up biopsies from patients with chronic infection showed features of typical chronic viral hepatitis, characterized by progressive fibrosis and portal hepatitis, with dense lymphocytic infiltrate and variable degrees of piecemeal necrosis. Lobular hepatitis was mild to moderate in all cases (230).

HEV adds yet another possible cause of chronic hepatitis in liver allograft recipients. Although we have not yet had experience with cases, from the histopathological descriptions, it is likely that the same criteria used to distinguish chronic HEV from acute and chronic rejection will use the same criteria as for HBV and HVC. It appears that serological and/or molecular biological studies for HEV RNA are needed to make a definitive diagnosis.

VI. DISORDERS OF DYSREGULATED IMMUNITY

i. Introduction

Immune dysregulation disorders including PBC, AIH, sclerosing cholangitis, and overlap syndromes commonly recur after liver transplantation. The approximate incidence is about 25 percent by five years after transplantation. The severity or rate of progression of recurrent disease, however, might be less than the same disease before transplantation [reviewed in (285) and (286)]. Long-term graft and patient survival for patients who underwent liver replacement for these indications have not yet been significantly influenced by recurrent disease although there appears to be a progressive increase in the incidence of recurrent disease with time. Thus, the diagnosis, management, and treatment of recurrent diseases of dysregulated immunity are likely to play an increasingly important role in the management of liver allograft recipients. It is also likely that recurrence of these diseases will begin to adversely impact long-term morbidity and mortality (286).

Establishing the diagnosis of recurrence can be especially problematic for this category of diseases. Even before transplantation the diagnosis is based, at least partially, on exclusionary criteria. Furthermore, various clinical, serological, histopathological, and radiographic findings compatible with recurrent disease also commonly occur with other causes of allograft dysfunction. For example, there are numerous other causes of intrahepatic biliary strictures besides recurrent PSC; and these complications can affect patients who underwent liver transplantation for this indication. Autoantibodies, such as ANA and AMA, used to establish the diagnosis of AIH or PBC before transplantation often persist after transplantation, albeit at lower titers, even in the absence of clinical or histopathological evidence of recurrent disease. A set of specific consensus criteria were recently proposed by the Banff Working Group to suggest a standardized approach to these uncertainties (137).

ii. Primary Biliary Cirrhosis

1. Introduction and Pathophysiology

The incidence of recurrent PBC varies considerably from 0 to 90 percent after one to nineteen years of follow-up; an average incidence of 20 percent at five years is typical [reviewed in (285) and (286)]. New-onset PBC has not been reported. The variation in the incidence of recurrent PBC is probably attributable to uncertainty about the pre- and post-transplant diagnosis, type of transplant, use of different immunosuppressive agents and management policies, monitoring by protocol biopsy, length of follow-up, operative techniques, and other factors that influence biliary tract physiology [reviewed in (285)]. *Risk factors* for recurrent disease include use of Tacrolimus versus Cyclosporine as baseline immunosuppression [(287,288) and unpublished observation], living-related liver transplantation (289), steroid withdrawal (290,291), and HLA-DR matching [Dvorchik, unpublished observation (286)].

2. Clinical Presentation

Recurrent PBC is usually first suspected because of a preferential increase in alkaline phosphatase and gamma glutamyl transpeptidase as part of routine serological monitoring. This usually occurs more than six months after transplantation and the diagnosis is confirmed on needle biopsy evaluation. Recurrent disease is usually first recognized histopathologically in the earliest stage and most affected recipients are asymptomatic. Discovering recurrent disease for the first time in protocol biopsies in recipients with normal, or near normal, liver injury tests is also not uncommon. In our experience, rare patients present with an acute febrile illness and increased liver injury tests (unpublished observation).

Left untreated recurrent PBC can progress after liver transplantation resulting in symptoms similar to those seen before transplantation such as jaundice, itching, hepatosplenomegaly and portal hypertension. Antimitochondrial antibodies are of little additional benefit in establishing the diagnosis of recurrent PBC because they remain elevated in the majority of patients after transplantation [reviewed in (285)], even in the absence of recurrent disease. The diagnosis is established on needle biopsies of the allograft. Ursodeoxycholic acid treatment of recurrent PBC after transplantation has not yet significantly impacted patient or allograft survival (292).

3. Histopathological Findings

Histopathological diagnosis of recurrent PBC is based on the same clinicopathological criteria as before transplantation. Diagnostic lesions include noninfectious,

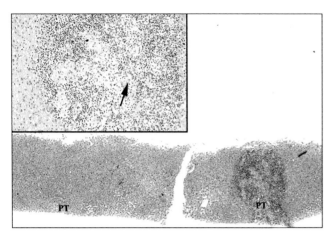

FIGURE 4.27: *Recurrent primary biliary cirrhosis is diagnosed using the same criteria as in native livers. Usually, there is significant mononuclear inflammation, but it only involves a minority of the portal tracts, at least in the early stages when recurrent disease is most often first discovered. The diagnosis is based on noninfectious, noncaseating, granulomatous duct destructive lesions, as shown in the upper left inset. The arrow highlights the damaged bile duct.*

noncaseating, granulomatous bile duct damage or severe lymphocytic cholangitis producing breaks in the ductal basement membranes (Figure 4.27). These findings are often referred to as "florid duct lesions." Diagnostic bile duct lesions, however, are not always present. Instead, cases often present with patchy mononuclear portal inflammation with focal lymphocytic cholangitis accompanied by portal lymphoid nodules and prominent ductular type interface activity resulting in a *"biliary" gestalt.* A biliary gestalt refers to a ductular reaction at the interface zone, periportal "clearing" or edema, cholestasis, accumulation of copper or copper associated pigment in periportal hepatocytes, and patchy small bile duct loss. Such cases are "strongly suggestive" of recurrent PBC if they occur in a proper context. The proper context includes an original disease of PBC with no other reasonable explanation for the biliary pathology; most patients also have preferential elevation of the γGTP and ALP.

The diagnosis of recurrent PBC is less certain in biopsies only with mild or without significant lymphocytic cholangitis or a biliary gestalt. For example, "possible" recurrent PBC might first present as unexplained chronic hepatitis (98,293) because a sampling problem may have missed the bile duct damage or the patient is presenting as an overlap syndrome with AIH (293) or as AIH, alone (219). In fact, plasma cell–rich periportal hepatitis early after transplantation might be an early marker of PBC recurrence (294).

Lobular findings in recurrent PBC are usually mild and nonspecific. Typical findings include mild spotty necrosis, slightly increased sinusoidal lymphocytes, mild nodular regenerative hyperplasia changes, and Kupffer's cell granulomas. More significant lobular findings usually signal another or coexistent insult. As in native livers, PBC pro-gression is characterized by development of "biliary-type" fibrosis, cholestasis, and deposition of copper and copper-associated proteins at the edge of the lobules, and portal-to-portal bridging fibrosis.

4. Differential Diagnosis

The differential diagnosis for recurrent PBC includes acute and chronic rejection, chronic obstructive cholangi-opathy, and chronic viral, AIH or idiopathic hepatitis, and adverse drug reactions. Some of these same disorders can also coexist with recurrent PBC. In cases with classic/diag-nostic biliary lesions, the diagnosis of recurrent PBC is relatively straightforward and based on identification of granulomatous duct destruction, or florid duct lesions, occurring in the proper context. Other causes of granu-lomatous cholangitis, such as fungal or acid-fast bacterial infections and HCV, should be reasonably excluded. Prominent focal lymphocytic cholangitis accompanied by portal lymphoid nodules containing germinal centers and a biliary gestalt in the portal/periportal areas is strongly suggestive of recurrent PBC.

The "biliary gestalt," described above, is one of the most helpful constellations of findings that can be used to distinguish biliary tract pathology from other, nonbili-ary, causes of liver allograft dysfunction. Neither acute nor chronic rejection shows a significant ductular reaction or lead to biliary fibrosis/cirrhosis. *Rejection-associated* portal inflammation and lymphocytic cholangitis usually involves a majority of portal tracts and preferentially involves small bile ducts (<20 μm in smallest diameter). *PBC-associated* portal inflammation and lymphocytic cholangitis, in con-trast, is typically patchy and preferentially involves medium-sized bile ducts (>40–50 μm in shortest diameter).

Patients that underwent liver transplant for PBC can develop "AIH" or an overlap syndrome after liver trans-plantation (219). This might represent "switching" of an autoimmune syndrome from PBC to AIH, new-onset AIH, or be an alternative form of rejection. The clinical, serological, and histopathological criteria used to establish the diagnosis of AIH and overlap syndrome before trans-plantation can also be used after transplantation. However, AMA and the titers of various other autoantibodies might not have the same significant after transplantation as they did before.

Recurrent PBC can be quite difficult to distinguish from obstructive cholangiopathy because both produce a biliary gestalt. Obviously, the clinical history and radio-graphic findings can be particularly helpful in making this distinction. For example, any history of biliary tract obstruction or stricturing, or any factors predisposing to one, should make one favor obstructive cholangiopathy because mechanical problems tend to persist. Histopatho-logical features that favor obstructive cholangiopathy over recurrent PBC include 1) edema and/or neutrophilic inflammation in and around the true bile ducts in the middle of the portal connective tissue, 2) centrilobular hepatocanalicular cholestasis, 3) bile infarcts, and 4) intralobular neutrophil clusters. In some cases, cholangiography may still be required to exclude a mechanical problem.

PBC can be difficult to distinguish from chronic viral and AIH since both can show chronic portal inflammation with necro-inflammatory-type interface activity. And some variant of recurrent HCV can show a prominent ductular reaction, mimicking a biliary gestalt, described above. The distinction in such cases is based on careful examination of the bile ducts for evidence of significant lymphocytic or granulomatous duct damage and small bile duct loss. In addition, most cases of chronic hepatitis do not produce the biliary gestalt. Portal granulomas have been reported with recurrent chronic HCV (295). In our experience, this observation is uncommon and the granulomas rarely cause significant ductal damage.

iii. Recurrent and New-Onset AIH

1. Introduction, Pathophysiology, and Clinical Presentation

In native livers, the diagnosis of AIH is based on a combination of clinical, pathologic, and serological findings, combined with the exclusion of other causes of chronic liver injury (284). A diagnosis of AIH is even more difficult to establish after transplantation because of significant overlapping pathophysiological mechanisms of injury and histopathological findings with rejection and other causes of late dysfunction (296,297). For example, recurrent HCV and rejection reactions, especially chronic rejection, can trigger "autoimmune" effector pathways (212,298–301) and "nonorgan-specific" autoantibodies have been detected in up to 71 percent of patients after liver transplantation (302), emphasizing the need for clinicopathological correlation (137). In addition, autoantibodies used to establish the diagnosis of AIH before transplantation often persist after transplantation, albeit usually at lower titers (303,304), even without histopathological evidence of recurrent hepatitis. The Banff Working Group, therefore, advocated relatively strict criteria (137) to establish the diagnosis of AIH after transplantation, but more study is needed in this area.

Risk factors for recurrent AIH include suboptimal immunosuppression; recipient HLA DR3 and DR4; type I AIH versus type II before transplantation; severe inflammation in the native liver; and longer follow-up [reviewed in (285) and (286)]. Acute rejection and steroid-dependence are risk factors for new-onset or de novo AIH in pediatric recipients (305).

Most patients with recurrent or new-onset AIH are first detected because of elevated liver injury tests, which are routinely monitored. This can occur when an attempt is made to routinely discontinue corticosteroids from the immunosuppression regimen, which in turn, results in elevations of liver injury tests. The diagnosis is established on needle biopsy combined with clinicopathological correlation.

2. Histopathology and Differential Diagnosis

AIH in native livers is histopathologically characterized primarily by aggressive, plasma cell–rich necro-inflammatory-type interface activity, variable perivenular inflammation and hepatocyte dropout, and rosetting/regeneration of hepatocytes with thickening of the plates. This constellation of features is a reasonably good, but not an infallible histopathological marker of autoimmunity (266,306). These are also reasonably good histopathological findings associated with AIH in liver allografts. Some patients will present with predominantly central perivenulitis, (as described under Acute Rejection) and in many of these cases, the perivenular infiltrate will also be plasma cell rich. In such cases, distinguishing between centrilobular-based acute rejection and AIH can be problematic. Coexistent and prevalent inflammatory bile duct damage favors rejection, whereas coexistent and prevalent interface activity and composition of plasma cells containing more than 30 percent of the infiltrate favor AIH.

But once a "chronic hepatitic" pattern of injury is considered or established histopathologically, examination of the clinicopathological and serological profiles are needed to 1) support an autoimmune etiology (e.g., ANA, ASMA, LKM, serum gamma globulins) and 2) reasonably exclude other causes of a chronic hepatitis pattern of injury, such as HBV, HCV, HEV, PBC, and obstructive cholangiopathy (284).

Distinguishing AIH from conventional acute and chronic rejection uses the same criteria as those used to distinguish acute and chronic rejection from viral hepatitis (see Hepatitis C Virus). Distinguishing chronic hepatitis from obstructive cholangiopathy and PBC has already been discussed in the sections on biliary tract complications and PBC, respectively.

iv. Recurrent PSC

1. Introduction, Pathophysiology, and Clinical Presentation

PSC is also a disease of dysregulated immunity, but of unknown etiology, that usually arises in patients with coexistent ulcerative colitis. The recurrence rate is roughly 20 percent by five years and appears to increase with time after transplantation more than other disorders of dysregulated immunity [reviewed in (285) and (286)]. Recurrent PSC can be quite difficult to diagnose with certainty. Many other insults, such as ischemic injury from prolonged preservation or non-heart–beating donors, imperfect biliary anastomoses, inadequate hepatic arterial flow, and antibody-mediated rejection, also cause nonanastomotic intrahepatic biliary strictures that mimic recurrent PSC.

The *early stage* of recurrent PSC usually first comes to clinical attention more than six to nine months after transplantation because of selective elevation of alkaline phosphatase and gamma glutamyl transpeptidase. These biochemical abnormalities are usually attributable to the development of nonanastomotic intrahepatic biliary strictures, typical of recurrent PSC. Occasionally, inadequately followed patients will first present with jaundice and/or signs and symptoms of ascending cholangitis. Nonanastomotic intrahepatic biliary strictures that develop *before* 90 days after transplantation are usually not attributable to recurrent disease, and therefore, other causes should be sought.

Risk factors for developing recurrent PSC include history of ACR and recipient HLA-DRB1*08(307), ulcerative colitis and steroid dependence after transplantation (308), male sex, and an intact colon before transplantation (309). Hilar bile duct cancer before transplantation significantly degrades survival after transplantation, as expected (310,311). Coexistent ulcerative colitis generally worsens after transplantation (312,313) and the risk of developing and dying from colon cancer is substantial (314). Patients with PSC are also at greater risk for acute and chronic and steroid-resistant rejection (311,315).

As in native livers, recurrent PSC progresses over a period of years and eventually results in biliary-type fibrosis/cirrhosis. But, up to five years after transplantation, patient and allograft survival are not adversely affected [reviewed in (285) and (286)]. Key cholangiographic findings that distinguish recurrent PSC from other causes of biliary strictures include mural irregularity, diverticulum-like outpouchings, and an overall appearance resembling PSC in native livers (316).

2. Histopathological Findings

The histopathological features of recurrent PSC are identical to those described for native livers. In our opinion, recurrent PSC cannot be reliably distinguished from other causes of biliary tract obstruction or stricturing in a needle biopsy. Findings typical of the *early stage* include mild non-specific acute and chronic "pericholangitis" and a variable, low-grade ductular reaction at the interface zone. A biliary gestalt appears as the disease becomes well developed. Included are irregular fibrous expansion of most portal tracts accompanied by variable portal edema, periductal lamellar edema, intraepithelial or intraluminal neutrophils within bile ducts, fibrous cholangitis, focal small bile duct loss, pigmented macrophages in the portal connective tissue, ductular-type interface activity surrounded by edema, and periportal deposition of golden pigment and copper and copper-associated protein. As is typical for biliary dis-

eases, the spatial relationship between the expanded portal tracts and the central veins remains intact until well-developed cirrhosis appears.

Lobular findings in early recurrent PSC include variable cholestasis, lobular neutrophil clusters, and mild nodular regenerative hyperplasia changes. Later stages are characterized by the development of biliary cirrhosis, cholestasis, intra-lobular foam cell clusters, marked deposition of copper and copper-associated protein, and Mallory's hyaline at the edge of the nodules.

3. Differential Diagnosis

Recognition of a biliary gestalt, described above, points toward a biliary etiology, as does preferential elevation of γ-glutamyl transpeptidase and alkaline phosphatase. Extensive clinicopathological and radiographic correlation are needed, however, to determine whether recurrent PSC or one of the many other causes of biliary tract pathology is responsible for the changes observed. In our opinion, this distinction is not possible on peripheral core needle biopsies. Instead, a diagnosis of recurrent PSC should be based on a complete analysis of clinical, histopathological and radiographic findings, including important exclusionary criteria. Harrison et al (317) suggested that classic "fibro-obliterative duct lesions" might be used to make the distinction, but we have seen similar lesions in patients with ischemic cholangitis and chronic reflux cholangiopathy.

VII. METABOLIC DISEASES AND TOXIC INSULTS

Jaffe (318) devised an algorithm/classification system to separate metabolic diseases into three categories for the purpose of understanding the impact of liver transplantation on the disease process and the possibility of recurrent disease (Table 4.8). The *classification system* is as follows: 1) the liver is the primary site of the defect and is associated with end-stage liver disease; 2) the liver is the primary site of the defect, but predominant adverse effects are systemic and not directly hepatotoxic; and 3) the defect is extrahepatic and effects on the liver are secondary.

Patients in the first group are prime candidates for liver transplantation because the cirrhotic liver is replaced by a genetically and structurally normal one that generally cures the disease. Examples include type 1 tyrosinemia, α-1-antitrypsin deficiency, Wilson's disease, neonatal hemochromatosis, and types 1, 3, and 4 glycogen storage disease (318). The liver is usually structurally normal or near normal in the second group. The goal of liver transplantation in this group of patients is to alleviate the systemic disease burden of the abnormal liver physiology. Examples of category two include familial amyloid polyneuropathy, type 1 oxalosis, urea cycle defects and hyperammonemia syndromes, familial hypercholesterolemia,

TABLE 4.8 Summary of Metabolic Disease Treated by Liver Transplantation Classified According the System of Jaffe et al. (318) (see text)

Liver is the site of the primary metabolic defect and liver is usually diseased (see text)	Liver is the site of primary metabolic defect, but liver is usually normal or near normal	Site of primary metabolic defect is probably extrahepatic and liver transplantation decreases morbidity and mortality associated with liver disease
α-1-antitrypsin deficiency (434,435)	Familial amyloid polyneuropathy (FAP) (436, 437). Mild liver abnormalities: amyloid deposits in portal tracts and nerve trunks; use of FAP-affected liver is controversial (19,438,439)	Hemochromatosis or (inadvertent transplantation of donor with hemochromatosis) reviewed in (440,441)
Wilson's disease (442–444)	Crigler-Najjar syndrome (445,446)	Niemann-Pick disease (318,447)
Tyrosinemia (448,449)	Type I hyperoxaluria (318,450,451)	Sea-blue histiocyte syndrome (452)
Type I and Ib glycogen storage disease (453,454)	Urea cycle enzyme deficiencies (318,450)	Erythropoietic protoporphyria (455–457)
Type III glycogen storage disease (454)	Protein C deficiency (458)	Cystinosis (318). Does not generally cause liver disease; one patient developed intrahepatic crystal deposits in liver with perivenular fibrosis and recurrent disease in the allograft (318).
Type IV glycogen storage disease (444,454)	Familial hypercholesterolemia (318,459)	Cystic fibrosis (460–462), cures liver disease, and if liver transplant is done early, lung function can improve
Inborn errors of bile acid synthesis (450)	Hemophilia A (463,464)	
	Hemophilia B (318,465)	

and hepatic clotting factor disorders (318). Some of the *resected native livers* from patients with familial amyloid polyneuropathy (FAP) are then transplanted in adult recipients with a different chronic liver disease in so-called domino transplants. Although these livers are structurally normal the FAP disease is also transferred. The reasoning is that the decades of survival are possible before FAP manifestations clinically in the recipient and the extended survival is worthwhile. The liver allograft is vulnerable to recurrent disease in the third group since the metabolic disorder persists after transplantation, but improved survival and/or quality of life issues rationalize liver replacement (318). Examples include lysosomal storage diseases such as Niemann-Pick, Gaucher's disease, cystinosis, and erythropoietic protoporphyria.

Toxic insults, other than alcohol, and adverse drug reactions do not generally recur after transplantation.

i. Recurrent Alcoholic Liver Disease

1. Introduction and Pathophysiology

End-stage alcoholic liver disease (ALD) is a leading indication for liver transplantation and is often combined with coexistent conditions such as HCV infection, hepatocellular carcinoma, and metabolic disorders, such as hemochromatosis and alpha one antitrypsin deficiency. The exact incidence of recurrent alcohol use/abuse after transplantation is difficult to determine with certainty, but reported

values range from 15 to 50 percent by five years after transplantation (204,319,320).

Recurrent alcohol abuse can directly damage the allograft, or indirectly contribute to allograft dysfunction because of rejection related to noncompliance with immunosuppression (321,322). The discussion of the pathophysiological mechanisms of alcoholic steatohepatitis is beyond the scope of this chapter.

2. Clinical Presentation

Problems with alcohol recidivism are usually detected because of elevation of liver injury tests that are routinely obtained in liver transplant populations (321), missed medical appointments (323), inappropriate social behavior (98), and noncompliance with immunosuppression (321,322). A high γ-glutamyl transpeptidase to alkaline phosphatase ratio might provide biochemical evidence of alcohol recurrence (98,321) but blood alcohol levels are more definitive proof of relapse. A small minority of patients experience a rapid downhill course after transplantation because of recidivism and recurrent alcoholic or nonalcoholic steatohepatitis (324–326), but in general, this course of events is rare.

Rigorous pretransplant screening programs attempt to identify patients who are likely to relapse after transplantation. *Risk factors* for alcoholic relapse include a duration of abstinence of less than six months before wait-listing, psychiatric comorbidities, or High-Risk Alcoholism Relapse Scale score greater than 3 (327); family

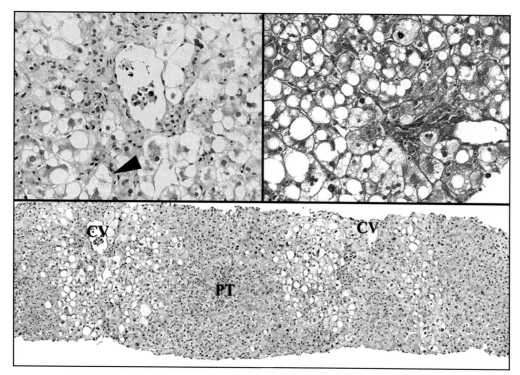

FIGURE 4.28: *Recurrent alcohol abuse is a relatively uncommon cause of significant allograft injury, although it is seen occasionally. In our experience, it is difficult to distinguish alcoholic from nonalcoholic fatty liver disease, but the strict perivenular distribution of mixed steatosis with so-called foamy degeneration of hepatocytes (upper left panel, arrowhead) is typical of recurrent alcohol use. Eventually, this can lead to subsinusoidal fibrosis (upper right inset).*

history of alcoholism (328); heavy daily ethanol consumption (321); and male sex, unstable social environment, and psychological instability (329).

Most alcoholics, however, do not relapse severely enough to cause noteworthy ALD in the allograft. Therefore, recurrent ALD minimally impacts long-term patient and allograft survival and is generally a good disease indication for liver replacement (204,321,330). Upper aerodigestive malignancies, attributable to a long history of alcohol, and often coexistent tobacco abuse are a significant source of morbidity and mortality in this patient population (321).

3. Histopathological Findings and Differential Diagnosis

The histopathological findings in alcoholic allograft liver disease are identical to those seen in native livers and will not be discussed in any detail. The most common histopathological presentation is mixed, but predominantly microvesicular steatosis, involving primarily the centrilobular hepatocytes. The zonal distribution pattern of the steatosis is usually distinctive (98,204,321,324) (Figure 4.28). More significant abuse can lead to so-called "foamy" degeneration of centrilobular hepatocytes (98), followed by fully developed "alcoholic hepatitis" with Mallory's hyaline, and ballooning degeneration of hepatocytes with associated lobular inflammation. Persistent abuse eventually causes

perivenular and subsinusoidal fibrosis. In our experience, relapse can also present with increased iron deposition in periportal hepatocytes and the reticular-endothelial cells and hepatocytes without significant steatosis (98). As in native livers, alcoholic steatohepatitis can co-exist with HCV and any other cause of allograft dysfunction and combined insults can lead to more rapid development of significant fibrosis (321,324).

For the differential diagnosis, please see the next section on nonalcoholic steatohepatitis.

ii. Recurrent Nonalcoholic Steatohepatitis

a. Introduction, Pathophysiology, and Clinical Presentation

NAFLD affects about 4–5 percent of recipients before transplantation, but the incidence is increasing. NAFLD recurs after liver transplantation because many risk factors, such as obesity, diabetes, metabolic syndrome/insulin resistance, and so forth persist, or are made worse after transplantation by the immunosuppression needed to prevent rejection (331). A significant proportion of patients who underwent liver transplantation for cryptogenic cirrhosis will also develop NAFLD after transplantation (332–335). Presumably, these patients also had undetected NAFLD before transplantation, but the histopathological features were not obvious in the explanted cirrhotic liver. In addition to the usual risk factors for NAFLD risk factors for recurrent NAFLD include cumulative steroid dose (333).

Recurrent NAFLD is usually first detected on protocol or indicated allograft biopsies in asymptomatic patients. Many of these patients have multiple risk factors for NAFLD such as obesity, diabetes, and hypertension. However, a minority of others are otherwise healthy and develop otherwise unexplained nonalcoholic liver disease after transplantation; in these patients, metabolic testing for insulin resistance and a search for more esoteric causes (see Differential Diagnosis) of NAFLD is warranted.

iii. Histopathology and Differential Diagnosis

A detailed description of the histopathology of hepatic steatosis and steatohepatitis are known to most pathologists and beyond the scope of this chapter. Readers are referred elsewhere for excellent reviews (336). The differential diagnosis for recurrent alcoholism and NAFLD includes all of the disorders known to cause steatohepatitis in the general population. ALD is very difficult to distinguish from nonalcoholic steatohepatitis. In nonallograft livers, steatosis and nuclear vacuoles appear more prevalent in the NAFLD group than in the ALD. In contrast, ballooning hepatocytes, lipogranuloma, focal necrosis, acidophilic bodies and fibrosis are more remarkable in ALD than in NAFLD and the severity of steatosis and lipogranulomata gradually decreases as the stage of liver fibrosis progresses.

The differential diagnosis for steatohepatitis in allografts is broader than in a native liver. Steatohepatitis is seen most commonly with morbid obesity, diabetes, insulin resistance, and alcohol abuse. However, it can also be associated with nutritional causes, such as protein calorie malnutrition, starvation, rapid weight loss, and various intestinal bypass or gastric stapling surgeries.

Hepatic steatosis and steatohepatitis can also be the result of medications, including amiodarone, perhexiline maleate, glucocorticoids, synthetic estrogens, calcium channel blockers, tamoxifen, methotrexate, valproic acid, cocaine, and antiviral agents (Zidovudine, Didanosine, and Fialuridine).

Metabolic disorders can also cause steatosis and steatohepatitis: hyperlipidemia, Wilson's disease, adult-onset citrullinemia (type II), lipodystrophy, dysbetalipoproteinemia, Weber-Christian disease, Wolman's disease, cholesterol ester storage disease, and fatty liver of pregnancy.

Other less common causes include inflammatory bowel disease, intestinal bacterial overgrowth, and exposure to environmental toxins, including phosphorous, petrochemicals, toxic mushrooms, and organic solvents. Hepatic blood flow abnormalities can also cause hepatic steatosis and steatohepatitis. Examples include pre-hepatic portal hypertension, portosystemic shunting, and patent ductus venosus.

A thorough clinicopathological correlation is needed to substantiate a suspicion of alcohol relapse or metabolic abnormalities leading to NAFLD. Awareness of the original diseases, detailed clinical history, including current alcohol use, blood alcohol levels, and the ratio of γ-glutamyl transpeptidase to alkaline phosphatase can be used to distinguish between these possibilities.

VIII. IDIOPATHIC POST-TRANSPLANT HEPATITIS

i. Introduction, Pathophysiology, and Clinical Presentation

Idiopathic post-transplant hepatitis is a diagnostic term coined by Hubscher (296) to describe patients that show chronic hepatitis changes on allograft biopsy (i.e., mononuclear portal inflammation with variable interface activity) but have no clinical or serological evidence of viral hepatitis infection, autoimmunity, or adverse drug reaction. According to the definition, features used to diagnose acute rejection, such as bile duct damage and venous endothelial inflammation, are neither severe nor widespread.

As with other "idiopathic" disease categories, the hope is that the diagnosis of "idiopathic post-transplant hepatitis" will become obsolete. As more information becomes available and causes of late liver allograft dysfunction can be determined more precisely, fewer patients should receive this diagnosis. For example, Hubscher originally included in this category a small subgroup of patients with inflammatory changes in zone 3 with foci of confluent necrosis (296). Currently, many centers would probably diagnose these changes as late-onset acute rejection if a majority of central veins were involved (142,143). Another small subgroup probably represents recurrent AIH, although strict criteria for AIH might not always be met (296). Both rejection and AIH should respond to increased immunosuppression (142,143,296). Yet another subgroup might represent chronic HEV infection as this has recently been described as a cause of chronic hepatitis in immunosuppressed patients (230). Currently, however, the underlying cause of the chronic hepatitis cannot be determined in most cases.

Most recipients with idiopathic post-transplant hepatitis are first detected after *protocol* allograft biopsy examination. As might be expected, these recipients are usually asymptomatic and have normal or near normal liver tests, although low-grade elevation of ALT and AST are not uncommon. The first study by the Birmingham group showed that approximately 5 percent of patients followed up for a minimum of ten years will develop progressive fibrosis/cirrhosis (296). A more recent follow-up study, however, showed that nearly 60 percent of pediatric recipients develop idiopathic post-transplant hepatitis by ten years after transplantation (337) and 15 percent of affected recipients had significant fibrosis/cirrhosis by ten years (337).

TABLE 4.9 Incidence of Idiopathic Post-transplant Hepatitis in Long-Term Biopsies from Various Centers; adapted from (338) and (1)

Study (no. of patients)	Length of follow-up	Incidence of unexplained inflammation in allograft	Conclusions/recommendations
Berenguer (203), adult (n = 248)	1–5 years	<10–30%	"Hepatitis" frequently seen in non-HCV recipients, but activity is mild. Therefore, protocol biopsies justified only in HCV+ patients. Non-HCV+ recipients with normal LFTs should not undergo protocol biopsies
Sebagh (206), adult (n = 143)	10 years	<10%	Chronic viral hepatitis and chronic rejection major causes of dysfunction. Protocol biopsies recommended because of frequent abnormalities when LFTs are normal
Pappo (98), adult (n = 65)	Mean survival 9.9 years	~35%	Recurrence of original disease and biliary tract complications were major problems. 6/17 patients with unexplained chronic hepatitis, but several of them had PBC as original disease. Protocol biopsies recommended
Slapak (207), adult (n = 116)	Mean 8.4 years	18–48%	13/27 patients had unexplained chronic hepatitis, but 8/13 had PBC as original disease. Protocol biopsies recommended
Heneghan (466), adult (n = 99)	>1 year	~15%	IPTH not mentioned as specific diagnosis or significant problem, but nonspecific inflammation seen in 15/99 patients transplanted for cryptogenic cirrhosis or alcohol
Contos, adult (n = 30)	Median follow-up of 3.5 years	Not mentioned	IPTH not mentioned as specific diagnosis or significant problem
Maor-Kendler (467), adult (n = 71)	Mean survival of ~4 years	~15%	IPTH not mentioned as specific diagnosis or significant problem, but listed as "nonspecific inflammation"
Burra (204), adult (n = 51)	>1 year	~25%, but difficult to determine timing of biopsy	IPTH not mentioned as specific diagnosis or significant problem, but alcoholic patients showed portal lymphocytic inflammation
Rosenthal (208), pediatric (n = 54)	1 year	~50%	IPTH not mentioned as significant problem, but "portal mononuclear inflammation" in nearly one half of recipients. Long-term follow-up not included. Argues against long-term protocol biopsies

There is considerable variation, however, in the *incidence* of idiopathic post-transplant hepatitis by center, and perhaps, by age [Table 4.9; reviewed in (338)]. A lack of protocol biopsies in low incidence centers; possible differences between pediatric and adult recipients; ambiguous criteria for distinguishing between "nonspecific portal and/or lobular inflammation" and "idiopathic post-transplant hepatitis"; different immunosuppressive management protocols/approach; undiscovered viruses such as HEV (230); and a combination of these reasons might explain the center variations (338). Clearly, more study is needed on this topic, particularly in pediatric allograft recipients. Liver injury tests are a relatively insensitive method of monitoring liver allograft pathology in long-term survivors. If a high percentage of recipients develop idiopathic post-transplant hepatitis, protocol biopsy evaluation might help guide therapy.

Current thinking suggests that many cases of idiopathic post-transplant hepatitis might represent a variant of late-onset acute rejection (337,338). Previous studies have already emphasized that histopathological features of late acute cellular rejection causes it to more closely resemble chronic hepatitis.

ii. Histopathology and Differential Diagnosis

As the name implies, the histopathology of idiopathic post-transplant hepatitis is that of chronic hepatitis with chronic portal inflammation, variable interface and lobular necro-inflammatory activity, but without prominent and prevalent bile duct damage and central perivenulitis. Obvious clinical, serological, and histopathological causes of chronic hepatitis, such as HBV, HCV, HEV, and AIH have been reasonably excluded. Therefore, these biopsies are unlikely to contain significant plasma cell inflammation comprising more than 30 percent of the infiltrates.

The differential diagnosis for idiopathic post-transplant hepatitis is the same as that for HBV or HCV infection or AIH, all of which have been previously described.

IX. CONSIDERATIONS IN IMMUNOSUPPRESSION MINIMIZATION PROTOCOLS

i. Introduction, Pathophysiology, and Clinical Presentation

Evaluation of allograft biopsies plays an important role in the *weaning* of liver allograft recipients from immunosuppression (261,263,290,291,339–342). This emerging field in transplantation pathology is being driven by the high cost and serious side effects of chronic immunosuppression. It is made possible because liver allografts are more "tolerogenic" than other solid organ allografts—liver allograft recipients can be more safely weaned from immunosuppression because they are less likely to experience rejection (261,263,290,291,339–342). If rejection does occur during or after weaning, it is usually rapidly reversible and the allografts heal without significant fibrosis or loss of function (27,290,291).

In the past several decades, occasional noncompliant patients and recipients deliberately removed from immunosuppression because of infectious or neoplastic complications occasionally did not develop rejection. This showed that early animal studies on hepatic tolerogenicity (343) also applied to humans. It was realized, therefore, that all long-term survivors might not need chronic immunosuppression (291) and studies were commenced to determine whether evaluation of these patients might provide insights into the immunologic mechanisms responsible for graft acceptance (261,263,290,291,339–342).

Discussion of the immunologic mechanisms responsible for allograft acceptance is beyond the scope of this chapter.

Studies to date have shown that roughly 15 percent of highly selected liver allograft recipients can be successfully weaned from immunosuppression [reviewed in (344)]. "Highly selected" refers to long-term survivors that have stable liver injury tests for several years, no technical complications, and are manageable with relatively low levels of immunosuppression. Currently, however, no reliable laboratory assay exists to prospectively identify patients that can be safely weaned from immunosuppression. Analysis of the peripheral blood has shown an increase in genes encoding for γδ T-cells (340,341) and NK receptors, and for proteins involved in cell proliferation arrest in tolerant recipients. "Tolerant" recipients also exhibit greater numbers of circulating, potentially regulatory, FoxP3+ T-cell subsets (CD4+ CD25+ T-cells), and Vδ1+ T cells than either nontolerant patients or healthy individuals (340,341).

Allograft dysfunction is usually first detected in patients being weaned from immunosuppression in the first several months after the process begins and manifests as increased liver injury tests. It should be noted, however, that not all elevations of liver tests that occur after weaning are related to rejection (290,291).

ii. Histopathology and Differential Diagnosis

Protocol biopsies are routinely obtained immediately before weaning. The purpose is to document any existing pathology and to exclude silent rejection and/or chronic hepatitis before drug withdrawal (209,263,290,291). Not unexpectedly, these protocol baseline biopsies show changes similar to those reported in long-term survivors maintained on immunosuppression, and discussed above. Common findings include recurrence of the original disease, such as viral hepatitis (261,263) and disorders of dysregulated immunity (290,291), biliary strictures (290,291), and nodular regenerative hyperplasia (290,291).

In some studies baseline biopsy findings proved to be associated with successful weaning. Included were less portal inflammation and less CD3+ and CD8+ lymphocytes within the lobules (209), more portal fibrosis in HCV+ recipients (263), and an increase of potentially regulatory FoxP3+ T cells (340) compared to recipients that required continual immunosuppression. Conversely, unsuccessful weaning was associated with significant chronic portal inflammation and lobular infiltration by CD8+ lymphocytes. These observations suggest that chronic portal inflammation and an increase in lobular CD8+ cells might represent a latent form of rejection, similar to idiopathic post-transplant hepatitis.

Most centers participating in these studies agree that protocol biopsies after minimization and/or withdrawal of immunosuppression are mandatory. Follow-up biopsies in the studies reveal some expected findings, such as acute rejection. Immunosuppression can also effectively inhibit immunologic allograft injury because of chronic viral hepatitis and disorders of dysregulated immunity, both of which can reappear and/or become more aggressive after weaning (290,291). It is difficult, however, to continue weaning when lowering of immunosuppression clearly correlates with elevation of liver tests. This is because most of the patients undergoing weaning were relatively stable before the process began. Clearly, more studies are needed in this area.

The Kyoto group also reported more portal fibrosis, ductular reactions, and decreased luminal diameter of bile ducts in recipients removed from immunosuppression compared to those maintained on immunosuppression (340,345). The suggestion was that the changes might represent a subtle variant of chronic rejection. However, the mean follow-up in their tolerant group was several years longer than in their control group. This raises some question about the etiology of these changes.

In our experience, acute rejection that occurs during or after weaning is still best recognized using standard criteria, discussed above (131,137,146). A histopathological diagnosis of "indeterminate" or "mild" acute cellular rejection, accompanied by a significant rise of liver injury tests above baseline levels, is usually a cause for greater concern in patients being weaned from immunosuppression than the same diagnoses early after transplantation. The fear is that the rejection will "get out of hand" in a long surviving recipient who already has experienced an otherwise excellent outcome—but with a need for low dose chronic immunosuppression. Consequently, weaning is commonly slowed, stopped altogether, or even reversed at this point. But whether the infiltrate will progress or resolve, as seen early after transplantation, has not been aggressively tested. It is also widely recognized that late-onset acute rejection more closely resembles chronic hepatitis than does early onset acute rejection and might present as central perivenulitis (137).

X. LONG-TERM CHANGES NOT READILY EXPLAINED BY RECURRENT DISEASE

Some histopathological changes in long-surviving allografts cannot be attributed to recurrence of a specific disease and might represent adverse side effects of medications and/or the effects of long-term engraftment and abnormal graft physiology. Included are portal venopathy and nodular regenerative hyperplasia; thickening and hyalinization of small hepatic artery branches (98,210), subsinusoidal fibrosis, and nonspecific portal and lobular inflammation (98,206–208). If NRH changes are detected early (less than four years) after transplantation progression to portal hypertension can occur (346).

XI. ADVERSE DRUG REACTIONS AND TOXIC INJURY

As a general rule, the morphologic manifestations associated with adverse drug reactions are the same in an allograft as in a native liver. An exception might be drugs that induce an immunologic response, or where altered self-antigens might precipitate or drive the reaction. These might be muted because of potent baseline immunosuppression. In the short term, Azathioprine use has been associated with centrilobular necrosis and central vein and subsinusoidal fibrosis (347), whereas nodular regenerative hyperplasia has been attributed to chronic toxicity (210).

Pseudo-ground-glass cells can be seen with increased frequency in liver allografts. Lefkowitch et al. (348) showed that they are composed of abnormal glycogen and closely resemble polyglucosan bodies. He speculated their appearance might be related to disturbed glycogen metabolism and polypharmacotherapy.

Acknowledgements: The editorial assistance and patience of Mrs. Linda Askren is gratefully acknowledged. Also, we apologize to the primary authors and readers for the reliance on reviews and the lack of primary literature citations: a limitation imposed on us by the editor.

REFERENCES

1. Demetris AJ, Crawford JM, Minvervini MI, Nalesnik M, Ochoa E, Randhawa P, et al. Transplantation pathology of the liver. In: Odze R, Goldblum J, Crawford JM, editors. Surgical Pathology of the GI Tract, Liver, Biliary Tract, and Pancreas. Philadelphia PA: Saunders Elsever; 2008.
2. Demetris AJ, Nalesnik M, Randhawa P, Wu T, Minervini M, Lai C, et al. Histologic patterns of rejection and other causes of liver dysfunction. In: Busuttil RW, Klintmalm GB, editors. Transplantation of the Liver. Philadelphia PA: Elsevier Saunders; 2005. pp. 1057–128.
3. Alkofer B, Samstein B, Guarrera JV, Kin C, Jan D, Bellemare S, et al. Extended-donor criteria liver allografts. Semin Liver Dis 2006;26(3):221–33.
4. Busuttil RW, Tanaka K. The utility of marginal donors in liver transplantation. Liver Transpl 2003;9(7):651–63.
5. Feng S, Goodrich NP, Bragg-Gresham JL, Dykstra DM, Punch JD, DebRoy MA, et al. Characteristics associated with liver graft failure: the concept of a donor risk index. Am J Transplant 2006;6(4):783–90.
6. Todo S, Demetris AJ, Makowka L, Teperman L, Podesta L, Shaver T, et al. Primary nonfunction of hepatic allografts with preexisting fatty infiltration. Transplantation 1989;47(5):903–5.
7. Kakizoe S, Yanaga K, Starzl TE, Demetris AJ. Frozen section of liver biopsy for the evaluation of liver allografts. Transplant Proc 1990;22(2):416–17.
8. Kakizoe S, Yanaga K, Starzl TE, Demetris AJ. Evaluation of protocol before transplantation and after reperfusion biopsies from human orthotopic liver allografts: considerations of preservation and early immunological injury. Hepatology 1990;11(6):932–41.
9. Zamboni F, Franchello A, David E, Rocca G, Ricchiuti A, Lavezzo B, et al. Effect of macrovescicular steatosis and other donor and recipient characteristics on the outcome of liver transplantation. Clin Transplant 2001;15(1):53–7.
10. Markin RS, Wisecarver JL, Radio SJ, Stratta RJ, Langnas AN, Hirst K, et al. Frozen section evaluation of donor livers before transplantation. Transplantation 1993;56(6):1403–9.
11. Angele MK, Rentsch M, Hartl WH, Wittmann B, Graeb C, Jauch KW, et al. Effect of graft steatosis on liver function and organ survival after liver transplantation. Am J Surg 2008;195(2):214–20.
12. McCormack L, Petrowsky H, Jochum W, Mullhaupt B, Weber M, Clavien PA. Use of severely steatotic grafts in liver transplantation: a matched case-control study. Ann Surg 2007;246(6):940–6; discussion 946–8.
13. D'Alessandro AM, Kalayoglu M, Sollinger HW, Hoffmann RM, Reed A, Knechtle SJ, et al. The predictive value of donor liver biopsies for the development of primary nonfunction after orthotopic liver transplantation. Transplantation 1991;51(1):157–63.
14. Fiorini RN, Kirtz J, Periyasamy B, Evans Z, Haines JK, Cheng G, et al. Development of an unbiased method for the estimation of liver steatosis. Clin Transplant 2004;18(6):700–6.
15. Testa G, Goldstein RM, Netto G, Abbasoglu O, Brooks BK, Levy MF, et al. Long-term outcome of patients transplanted with livers from hepatitis C- positive donors. Transplantation 1998;65(7):925–9.
16. Velidedeoglu E, Desai NM, Campos L, Olthoff KM, Shaked A, Nunes F, et al. The outcome of liver grafts procured from hepatitis C-positive donors. Transplantation 2002;73(4):582–7.
17. Dodson SF, Issa S, Araya V, Gayowski T, Pinna A, Eghtesad B, et al. Infectivity of hepatic allografts with

antibodies to hepatitis B virus. Transplantation 1997;64(11): 1582–4.

18. Pungpapong S, Krishna M, Abraham SC, Keaveny AP, Dickson RC, Nakhleh RE. Clinicopathologic findings and outcomes of liver transplantation using grafts from donors with unrecognized and unusual diseases. Liver Transpl 2006;12(2):310–5.

19. Nishizaki T, Kishikawa K, Yoshizumi T, Uchiyama H, Okano S, Ikegami T, et al. Domino liver transplantation from a living related donor. Transplantation 2000;70(8): 1236–9.

20. Tanaka K, Kiuchi T. Living-donor liver transplantation in the new decade: perspective from the twentieth to the twenty-first century. J Hepatobiliary Pancreat Surg 2002; 9(2):218–22.

21. Trotter JF, Wachs M, Everson GT, Kam I. Adult-to-adult transplantation of the right hepatic lobe from a living donor. N Engl J Med 2002;346(14):1074–82.

22. Nadalin S, Malago M, Valentin-Gamazo C, Testa G, Baba HA, Liu C, et al. Preoperative donor liver biopsy for adult living donor liver transplantation: risks and benefits. Liver Transpl 2005;11(8):980–6.

23. Tran TT, Changsri C, Shackleton CR, Poordad FF, Nissen NN, Colquhoun S, et al. Living donor liver transplantation: histological abnormalities found on liver biopsies of apparently healthy potential donors. J Gastroenterol Hepatol 2006;21(2):381–3.

24. Ryan CK, Johnson LA, Germin BI, Marcos A. One hundred consecutive hepatic biopsies in the workup of living donors for right lobe liver transplantation. Liver Transpl 2002;8(12):1114–22.

25. Starzl TE. History of liver and other splanchnic organ transplantation. In: Busuttil R, Klintmalm G, editors. Transplantation of the Liver. Philadelphia PA: W.B. Saunders Company; 1996. pp. 3–22.

26. Klintmalm G, Busuttil R. Transplantation of the Liver. Second ed. Philadelphia PA: Elsevier Saunders; 2005.

27. Demetris AJ, Ruppert K, Dvorchik I, Jain A, Minervini M, Nalesnik MA, et al. Real-time monitoring of acute liver-allograft rejection using the Banff schema. Transplantation 2002;74(9):1290–6.

28. Demetris AJ, Jaffe R, Starzl TE. A review of adult and pediatric post-transplant liver pathology. Pathol Annu 1987;22(Pt 2):347–86.

29. Jain A, Reyes J, Kashyap R, Dodson SF, Demetris AJ, Ruppert K, et al. Long-term survival after liver transplantation in 4,000 consecutive patients at a single center. Ann Surg 2000;232(4):490–500.

30. Sieders E, Peeters PM, TenVergert EM, de Jong KP, Porte RJ, Zwaveling JH, et al. Graft loss after pediatric liver transplantation. Ann Surg 2002;235(1): 125–32.

31. Demetris AJ, Murase N, Nakamura K, Iwaki Y, Yagihashi A, Valdivia L, et al. Immunopathology of antibodies as effectors of orthotopic liver allograft rejection. [Review]. Semin Liver Dis 1992;12(1):51–9.

32. Rabkin JM, de La Melena V, Orloff SL, Corless CL, Rosen HR, Olyaei AJ. Late mortality after orthotopic liver transplantation. Am J Surg 2001;181(5):475–9.

33. Jain A, Demetris AJ, Kashyap R, Blakomer K, Ruppert K, Khan A, et al. Does tacrolimus offer virtual freedom from chronic rejection after primary liver transplantation? Risk and prognostic factors in 1,048 liver transplantations with a mean follow-up of 6 years. Liver Transpl 2001;7(7): 623–30.

34. McCashland T, Watt K, Lyden E, Adams L, Charlton M, Smith AD, et al. Retransplantation for hepatitis C: Results of a U.S. multicenter retransplant study. Liver Transpl 2007;13(9):1246–1253.

35. Ghobrial RM, Busuttil RW. Challenges of adult living-donor liver transplantation. J Hepatobiliary Pancreat Surg 2006;13(2):139–45.

36. Marcos A, Fisher RA, Ham JM, Olzinski AT, Shiffman ML, Sanyal AJ, et al. Selection and outcome of living donors for adult to adult right lobe transplantation. Transplantation 2000;69(11):2410–5.

37. Shimada M, Shiotani S, Ninomiya M, Terashi T, Hiroshige S, Minagawa R, et al. Characteristics of liver grafts in living-donor adult liver transplantation: comparison between right- and left-lobe grafts. Arch Surg 2002;137(10):1174–9.

38. Astarcioglu I, Cursio R, Reynes M, Gugenheim J. Increased risk of antibody-mediated rejection of reduced-size liver allografts. J Surg Res 1999;87(2):258–62.

39. Takada Y, Taniguchi H, Fukunaga K, Yuzawa K, Otsuka M, Todoroki T, et al. Prolonged hepatic warm ischemia in non-heart-beating donors: protective effects of FK506 and a platelet activating factor antagonist in porcine liver transplantation. Surgery 1998;123(6):692–8.

40. Kootstra G, Kievit J, Nederstigt A. Organ donors: heartbeating and non-heartbeating. World J Surg 2002;26(2):181–4.

41. Selzner N, Rudiger H, Graf R, Clavien PA. Protective strategies against ischemic injury of the liver. Gastroenterology 2003;125(3):917–36.

42. Teoh NC, Farrell GC. Hepatic ischemia reperfusion injury: Pathogenic mechanisms and basis for hepatoprotection. J Gastroenterol Hepatol 2003;18(8):891–902.

43. Kukan M, Haddad PS. Role of hepatocytes and bile duct cells in preservation-reperfusion injury of liver grafts. Liver Transpl 2001;7(5):381–400.

44. Bilzer M, Gerbes AL. Preservation injury of the liver: mechanisms and novel therapeutic strategies. J Hepatol 2000;32(3):508–15.

45. Lichtman SN, Lemasters JJ. Role of cytokines and cytokine-producing cells in reperfusion injury to the liver. Semin Liver Dis 1999;19(2):171–87.

46. Demetris AJ, Fontes P, Lunz JG, 3rd, Specht S, Murase N, Marcos A. Wound healing in the biliary tree of liver allografts. Cell Transplant 2006;15 (Suppl. 1):S57–65.

47. Demetris AJ, Lunz JG, 3rd, Specht S, Nozaki I. Biliary wound healing, ductular reactions, and IL-6/gp130 signaling in the development of liver disease. World J Gastroenterol 2006;12(22):3512–22.

48. McDonald V, Matalon TA, Patel SK, Brunner MC, Sankary H, Foster P, et al. Biliary strictures in hepatic transplantation. J Vasc Interv Radiol 1991;2(4):533–8.

49. Pirenne J, Gunson B, Khaleef H, Hubscher S, Afford S, McMaster P, et al. Influence of ischemia-reperfusion injury

on rejection after liver transplantation. Transplant Proc 1997;29(1–2):366–7.

50. Carrasco L, Sanchez-Bueno F, Sola J, Ruiz JM, Ramirez P, Robles R, et al. Effects of cold ischemia time on the graft after orthotopic liver transplantation. A bile cytological study. Transplantation 1996;61(3):393–6.

51. Starzl TE, Demetris AJ. Liver transplantation: a 31-year perspective. Part I. Curr Probl Surg 1990;27(2):55–116.

52. Starzl TE, Demetris AJ. Liver transplantation: a 31-year perspective. Part II. [Review]. Curr Prob Surg 1990;27(3):117–78.

53. Starzl TE, Demetris AJ. Liver transplantation: a 31-year perspective. Part III. Curr Probl Surg 1990;27(4):187–240.

54. Lo CM, Fan ST, Chan JK, Wei W, Lo RJ, Lai CL. Minimum graft volume for successful adult-to-adult living donor liver transplantation for fulminant hepatic failure. Transplantation 1996;62(5):696–8.

55. Kiuchi T, Kasahara M, Uryuhara K, Inomata Y, Uemoto S, Asonuma K, et al. Impact of graft size mismatching on graft prognosis in liver transplantation from living donors. Transplantation 1999;67(2):321–7.

56. Nishizaki T, Ikegami T, Hiroshige S, Hashimoto K, Uchiyama H, Yoshizumi T, et al. Small graft for living donor liver transplantation. Ann Surg 2001;233(4):575–80.

57. Demetris AJ, Kelly DM, Eghtesad B, Fontes P, Wallis Marsh J, Tom K, et al. Pathophysiologic observations and histopathologic recognition of the portal hyperperfusion or small-for-size syndrome. Am J Surg Pathol 2006;30(8):986–993.

58. Marcos A, Orloff M, Mieles L, Olzinski AT, Renz JF, Sitzmann JV. Functional venous anatomy for right-lobe grafting and techniques to optimize outflow. Liver Transpl 2001;7(10):845–52.

59. Marcos A, Olzinski AT, Ham JM, Fisher RA, Posner MP. The interrelationship between portal and arterial blood flow after adult to adult living donor liver transplantation. Transplantation 2000;70(12):1697–703.

60. Smyrniotis V, Kostopanagiotou G, Kondi A, Gamaletsos E, Theodoraki K, Kehagias D, et al. Hemodynamic interaction between portal vein and hepatic artery flow in small-for-size split liver transplantation. Transpl Int 2002;15(7):355–60.

61. Lautt WW. Mechanism and role of intrinsic regulation of hepatic arterial blood flow: hepatic arterial buffer response. Am J Physiol 1985;249(5 Pt 1):G549–56.

62. Kelly DM, Demetris AJ, Fung JJ, Marcos A, Zhu Y, Subbotin V, et al. Porcine partial liver transplantation: a novel model of the "small-for-size" liver graft. Liver Transpl 2004;10(2):253–63.

63. Troisi R, Cammu G, Militerno G, De Baerdemaeker L, Decruyenaere J, Hoste E, et al. Modulation of portal graft inflow: a necessity in adult living-donor liver transplantation? Ann Surg 2003;237(3):429–36.

64. Ku Y, Fukumoto T, Nishida T, Tominaga M, Maeda I, Kitagawa T, et al. Evidence that portal vein decompression improves survival of canine quarter orthotopic liver transplantation. Transplantation 1995;59(10):1388–92.

65. Boillot O, Delafosse B, Mechet I, Boucaud C, Pouyet M. Small-for-size partial liver graft in an adult recipient; a new transplant technique. Lancet 2002;359(9304):406–7.

66. Man K, Lo CM, Ng IO, Wong YC, Qin LF, Fan ST, et al. Liver transplantation in rats using small-for-size grafts: a study of hemodynamic and morphological changes. Arch Surg 2001;136(3):280–5.

67. Liang TB, Man K, Kin-Wah Lee T, Hong-Teng Tsui S, Lo CM, Xu X, et al. Distinct intragraft response pattern in relation to graft size in liver transplantation. Transplantation 2003;75(5):673–8.

68. Asakura T, Ohkohchi N, Orii T, Koyamada N, Tsukamoto S, Sato M, et al. Portal vein pressure is the key for successful liver transplantation of an extremely small graft in the pig model. Transpl Int 2003;16(6):376–82.

69. Ayata G, Pomfret E, Pomposelli JJ, Gordon FD, Lewis WD, Jenkins RL, et al. Adult-to-adult live donor liver transplantation: a short-term clinicopathologic study. Hum Pathol 2001;32(8):814–22.

70. Shimamura T, Taniguchi M, Jin MB, Suzuki T, Matsushita M, Furukawa H, et al. Excessive portal venous inflow as a cause of allograft dysfunction in small-for-size living donor liver transplantation. Transplant Proc 2001;33(1–2):1331.

71. Man K, Fan ST, Lo CM, Liu CL, Fung PC, Liang TB, et al. Graft injury in relation to graft size in right lobe live donor liver transplantation: a study of hepatic sinusoidal injury in correlation with portal hemodynamics and intragraft gene expression. Ann Surg 2003;237(2):256–64.

72. Pantanowitz L, Pomfret EA, Pomposelli JJ, Lewis WD, Gordon FD, Jenkins RL, et al. Pathologic analysis of right-lobe graft failure in adult-to-adult live donor liver transplantation. Int J Surg Pathol 2003;11(4):283–94.

73. Lerut JP, Gordon RD, Tzakis AG, Stieber AC, Iwatsuki S, Starzl TE. The hepatic artery in orthotopic liver transplantation. Helv Chir Acta 1988;55(3):367–78.

74. Ludwig J, Batts KP, MacCarty RL. Ischemic cholangitis in hepatic allografts [see comments]. Mayo Clinic Proceedings 1992;67(6):519–26.

75. Cameron AM, Busuttil RW. Ischemic cholangiopathy after liver transplantation. Hepatobiliary Pancreat Dis Int 2005;4(4):495–501.

76. Backman L, Gibbs J, Levy M, McMillan R, Holman M, Husberg B, et al. Causes of late graft loss after liver transplantation. Transplantation 1993;55(5):1078–82.

77. Demetris AJ. The pathology of liver transplantation. Prog Liver Dis 1990;9:687–709.

78. Lerut J, Tzakis AG, Bron K, Gordon RD, Iwatsuki S, Esquivel CO, et al. Complications of venous reconstruction in human orthotopic liver transplantation. Ann Surg 1987;205(4):404–14.

79. Lerut J, Gordon RD, Iwatsuki S, Starzl TE. Surgical complications in human orthotopic liver transplantation. Acta Chirurgica Belgica 1987;87(3):193–204.

80. Kuang AA, Renz JF, Ferrell LD, Ring EJ, Rosenthal P, Lim RC, et al. Failure patterns of cryopreserved vein grafts in liver transplantation. Transplantation 1996;62(6):742–7.

81. Sebagh M, Debette M, Samuel D, Emile JF, Falissard B, Cailliez V, et al. "Silent" presentation of veno-occlusive disease after liver transplantation as part of the process of cellular rejection with endothelial predilection. Hepatology 1999;30(5):1144–50.

82. Wanless I. Physioanatomic considerations. In: Schiff ER, Sorrell MF, Maddrey WC, editors. Diseases of the Liver. 8th ed. Philadelphia PA: Lippincott Williams & Wilkins; 1999. pp. 3–37.

83. Demetris A, Crawford J, Nalesnik M, Randhawa P, Wu T, Minervini M. Transplantation pathology of the liver. In: Odze R, Goldblum J, Crawford JM, editors. Surgical Pathology of the GI Tract, Liver, Biliary Tract, and Pancreas. Philadelphia PA: WB Saunders; 2004. pp. 909–966.

84. Pirenne J, Van Gelder F, Coosemans W, Aerts R, Gunson B, Koshiba T, et al. Type of donor aortic preservation solution and not cold ischemia time is a major determinant of biliary strictures after liver transplantation. Liver Transpl 2001;7(6):540–5.

85. Minor T, Hachenberg A, Tolba R, Pauleit D, Akbar S. Fibrinolytic preflush upon liver retrieval from non-heart beating donors to enhance postpreservation viability and energetic recovery upon reperfusion. Transplantation 2001;71(12):1792–6.

86. Testa G, Malago M, Broelseh CE. Complications of biliary tract in liver transplantation. World J Surg 2001;25(10): 1296–9.

87. Cheng YF, Chen YS, Huang TL, Chen TY, de Villa V, Lee TY, et al. Biliary complications in living related liver transplantation. Chang Gung Med J 2001;24(3):174–80.

88. Amersi F, Farmer DG, Busuttil RW. Fifteen-year experience with adult and pediatric liver transplantation at the University of California, Los Angeles. Clin Transpl 1998:255–61.

89. Pascher A, Neuhaus P. Bile duct complications after liver transplantation. Transpl Int 2005;18(6):627–42.

90. Verdonk RC, Buis CI, Porte RJ, van der Jagt EJ, Limburg AJ, van den Berg AP, et al. Anastomotic biliary strictures after liver transplantation: causes and consequences. Liver Transpl 2006;12(5):726–35.

91. Verdonk RC, Buis CI, Porte RJ, Haagsma EB. Biliary complications after liver transplantation: a review. Scand J Gastroenterol Suppl 2006(243):89–101.

92. Verdonk RC, Buis CI, van der Jagt EJ, Gouw AS, Limburg AJ, Slooff MJ, et al. Nonanastomotic biliary strictures after liver transplantation, part 2: Management, outcome, and risk factors for disease progression. Liver Transpl 2007;13(5):725–732.

93. Buis CI, Verdonk RC, Van der Jagt EJ, van der Hilst CS, Slooff MJ, Haagsma EB, et al. Nonanastomotic biliary strictures after liver transplantation, part 1: radiological features and risk factors for early vs. late presentation. Liver Transpl 2007;13(5):708–718.

94. Foley DP, Fernandez LA, Leverson G, Chin LT, Krieger N, Cooper JT, et al. Donation after cardiac death: the University of Wisconsin experience with liver transplantation. Ann Surg 2005;242(5):724–31.

95. Hartshorne N, Hartman G, Markin RS, Demetris AJ, Ferrell L. Bile duct hemorrhage: a biopsy finding after cholangiography or biliary tree manipulation. Liver 1992;12(3):137–9.

96. Nagral A, Ben-Ari Z, Dhillon AP, Burroughs AK. Eosinophils in acute cellular rejection in liver allografts. Liver Transpl Surg 1998;4(5):355–62.

97. Lunz JG, 3rd, Contrucci S, Ruppert K, Murase N, Fung JJ, Starzl TE, et al. Replicative senescence of biliary epithelial cells precedes bile duct loss in chronic liver allograft rejection: increased expression of p21(WAF1/Cip1) as a disease marker and the influence of immunosuppressive drugs. Am J Pathol 2001;158(4):1379–90.

98. Pappo O, Ramos H, Starzl TE, Fung JJ, Demetris AJ. Structural integrity and identification of causes of liver allograft dysfunction occurring more than 5 years after transplantation. Am J Surg Pathol 1995;19(2):192–206.

99. Demetris AJ. Distinguishing between recurrent primary sclerosing cholangitis and chronic rejection. Liver Transpl 2006;12(11 Suppl. 2):S68–72.

100. Terminology of chronic hepatitis, hepatic allograft rejection, and nodular lesions of the liver: summary of recommendations developed by an international working party, supported by the World Congresses of Gastroenterology, Los Angeles, 1994. Am J Gastroenterol 1994;89(8 Suppl): S177–81.

101. Demetris AJ, Nakamura K, Yagihashi A, Iwaki Y, Takaya S, Hartman GG, et al. A clinicopathological study of human liver allograft recipients harboring preformed IgG lymphocytotoxic antibodies. Hepatology 1992;16(3): 671–81.

102. Wiesner RH, Demetris AJ, Belle SH, Seaberg EC, Lake JR, Zetterman RK, et al. Acute hepatic allograft rejection: incidence, risk factors, and impact on outcome. Hepatology 1998;28(3):638–45.

103. Wilson CH, Agarwal K, Carter V, Burt AD, Hubscher S, Talbot D, et al. Late humoral rejection in a compliant ABO-compatible liver transplant recipient. Transplantation 2006;82(7):988–9.

104. Takakura K, Kiuchi T, Kasahara M, Uryuhara K, Uemoto S, Inomata Y, et al. Clinical implications of flow cytometry crossmatch with T or B cells in living donor liver transplantation. Clin Transplant 2001;15(5):309–16.

105. Furuya T, Murase N, Nakamura K, Woo J, Todo S, Demetris AJ, et al. Preformed lymphocytotoxic antibodies: the effects of class, titer and specificity on liver vs. heart allografts. Hepatology 1992;16(6):1415–22.

106. Valdivia LA, Fung JJ, Demetris AJ, Celli S, Pan F, Tsugita M, et al. Donor species complement after liver xenotransplantation. The mechanism of protection from hyperacute rejection. Transplantation 1994;57(6):918–22.

107. Neuberger J. Incidence, timing, and risk factors for acute and chronic rejection. Liver Transpl Surg 1999;5(4 Suppl. 1): S30–6.

108. Manez R, Kelly RH, Kobayashi M, Takaya S, Bronsther O, Kramer D, et al. Immunoglobulin G lymphocytotoxic antibodies in clinical liver transplantation: studies toward further defining their significance. Hepatology 1995; 21(5):1345–52.

109. Demetris AJ, Jaffe R, Tzakis A, Ramsey G, Todo S, Belle S, et al. Antibody-mediated rejection of human orthotopic liver allografts. A study of liver transplantation across ABO blood group barriers. Am J Pathol 1988;132(3): 489–502.

110. Woodle ES, Perdrizet GA, Brunt EM, So SK, Jendrisak MD, McCullough CS, et al. FK 506: reversal of humorally mediated rejection following ABO-incompatible liver transplantation. Transplant Proc 1991;23(6):2992–3.

111. Gugenheim J, Samuel D, Reynes M, Bismuth H. Liver transplantation across ABO blood group barriers. Lancet 1990;336(8714):519–23.

112. Haga H, Egawa H, Fujimoto Y, Ueda M, Miyagawa-Hayashino A, Sakurai T, et al. Acute humoral rejection and C4d immunostaining in ABO blood type-incompatible liver transplantation. Liver Transpl 2006;12(3):457–64.

113. Tan CD, Baldwin WM, 3rd, Rodriguez ER. Update on cardiac transplantation pathology. Arch Pathol Lab Med 2007;131(8):1169–91.

114. Colvin RB. Antibody-mediated renal allograft rejection: diagnosis and pathogenesis. J Am Soc Nephrol 2007;18(4):1046–56.

115. Bellamy CO, Herriot MM, Harrison DJ, Bathgate AJ. C4d immunopositivity is uncommon in ABO-compatible liver allografts, but correlates partially with lymphocytotoxic antibody status. Histopathology 2007;50(6):739–49.

116. Bu X, Zheng Z, Yu Y, Zeng L, Jiang Y. Significance of C4d deposition in the diagnosis of rejection after liver transplantation. Transplant Proc 2006;38(5):1418–21.

117. Dankof A, Schmeding M, Morawietz L, Gunther R, Krukemeyer MG, Rudolph B, et al. Portal capillary C4d deposits and increased infiltration by macrophages indicate humorally mediated mechanisms in acute cellular liver allograft rejection. Virchows Arch 2005;447(1):87–93.

118. Jain A, Mohanka R, Orloff M, Abt P, Romano J, Bryan L, et al. Characterization of CD4, CD8, CD56 positive lymphocytes and C4d deposits to distinguish acute cellular rejection from recurrent hepatitis C in post-liver transplant biopsies. Clin Transplant 2006;20(5):624–33.

119. Krukemeyer MG, Moeller J, Morawietz L, Rudolph B, Neumann U, Theruvath T, et al. Description of B lymphocytes and plasma cells, complement, and chemokines/receptors in acute liver allograft rejection. Transplantation 2004;78(1):65–70.

120. Sakashita H, Haga H, Ashihara E, Wen MC, Tsuji H, Miyagawa-Hayashino A, et al. Significance of C4d staining in ABO-identical/compatible liver transplantation. Mod Pathol 2007;20(6):676–84.

121. Sawada T, Shimizu A, Kubota K, Fuchinoue S, Teraoka S. Lobular damage caused by cellular and humoral immunity in liver allograft rejection. Clin Transplant 2005;19(1):110–14.

122. Troxell ML, Higgins JP, Kambham N. Evaluation of C4d staining in liver and small intestine allografts. Arch Pathol Lab Med 2006;130(10):1489–96.

123. Demetris AJ, Qian S, Sun H, Fung JJ, Yagihasi A, Murase N, et al. Early events in liver allograft rejection: delineation of sites of simultaneous intragraft and recipient lymphoid tissue sensitization. Am J Pathol 1991;138:609–18.

124. Demetris AJ, Murase N, Fujisaki S, Fung JJ, Rao AS, Starzl TE. Hematolymphoid cell trafficking, microchimerism, and GVH reactions after liver, bone marrow, and heart transplantation. Transplantation Proceedings 1993;25(6):3337–44.

125. Nawaz S, Fennell RH. Apoptosis of bile duct epithelial cells in hepatic allograft rejection. Histopathology 1994;25(2):137–42.

126. Vierling JM. Immunology of acute and chronic hepatic allograft rejection. Liver Transpl Surg 1999;5(4 Suppl. 1):S1–S20.

127. Anonymous. Terminology for hepatic allograft rejection. International Working Party. [Review]. Hepatology 1995;22(2):648–54.

128. Seiler CA, Renner EL, Czerniak A, Didonna D, Buchler MW, Reichen J. Early acute cellular rejection: no effect on late hepatic allograft function in man. Transpl Int 1999;12(3):195–201.

129. Dousset B, Conti F, Cherruau B, Louvel A, Soubrane O, Houssin D, et al. Is acute rejection deleterious to long-term liver allograft function? J Hepatol 1998;29(4):660–8.

130. Hubscher S. Diagnosis and grading of liver allograft rejection: a European perspective. Transplant Proc 1996;28(1):504–7.

131. anonymous. Banff schema for grading liver allograft rejection: an international consensus document. Hepatology 1997;25(3):658–63.

132. Yeh MM, Larson AM, Tung BY, Swanson PE, Upton MP. Endotheliitis in chronic viral hepatitis: a comparison with acute cellular rejection and non-alcoholic steatohepatitis. Am J Surg Pathol 2006;30(6):727–33.

133. Demetris AJ, Lasky S, Thiel DHV, Starzl TE, Whiteside T. Induction of DR/IA antigens in human liver allografts: an immunocytochemical and clinicopathologic analysis of twenty failed grafts. Transplantation 1985;40:504–9.

134. McCaughan GW, Davies JS, Waugh JA, Bishop GA, Hall BM, Gallagher ND, et al. A quantitative analysis of T lymphocyte populations in human liver allografts undergoing rejection: the use of monoclonal antibodies and double immunolabeling. Hepatology 1990;12(6):1305–13.

135. Steinhoff G, Behrend M, Wonigeit K. Expression of adhesion molecules on lymphocytes/monocytes and hepatocytes in human liver grafts. Hum Immunol 1990;28(2):123–7.

136. Demetris AJ, Belle SH, Hart J, Lewin K, Ludwig J, Snover DC, et al. Intraobserver and interobserver variation in the histopathological assessment of liver allograft rejection. The Liver Transplantation Database (LTD) Investigators. Hepatology 1991;14(5):751–5.

137. Banff Working G, Demetris AJ, Adeyi O, Bellamy CO, Clouston A, Charlotte F, et al. Liver biopsy interpretation for causes of late liver allograft dysfunction. Hepatology 2006;44(2):489–501.

138. Cong WM, Zhang SY, Wang ZL, Xue L, Liu YS, Zhang SH. [Pathologic diagnosis of 1123 post-transplant liver biopsies from 665 liver transplant patients]. Zhonghua Bing Li Xue Za Zhi 2005;34(11):716–19.

139. Netto GJ, Watkins DL, Williams JW, Colby TV, dePetris G, Sharkey FE, et al. Interobserver agreement in hepatitis C grading and staging and in the Banff grading schema for acute cellular rejection: the "hepatitis C 3" multi-institutional trial experience. Arch Pathol Lab Med 2006;130(8):1157–62.

140. Demirhan B, Bilezikci B, Haberal AN, Sevmis S, Arat Z, Haberal M. Hepatic parenchymal changes and histologic eosinophilia as predictors of subsequent acute liver allograft rejection. Liver Transpl 2008;14(2):214–19.

141. Ishak K, Baptista A, Bianchi L, Callea F, De Groote J, Gudat F, et al. Histological grading and staging of chronic hepatitis. J Hepatol 1995;22(6):696–9.

142. Demetris AJ, Fung JJ, Todo S, McCauley J, Jain A, Takaya S, et al. Conversion of liver allograft recipients from

cyclosporine to FK506 immunosuppressive therapy—a clinicopathologic study of 96 patients. Transplantation 1992;53(5):1056–62.

143. Tsamandas AC, Jain AB, Felekouras ES, Fung JJ, Demetris AJ, Lee RG. Central venulitis in the allograft liver: a clinicopathologic study. Transplantation 1997;64(2):252–7.

144. Krasinskas AM, Ruchelli ED, Rand EB, Chittams JL, Furth EE. Central venulitis in pediatric liver allografts. Hepatology 2001;33(5):1141–7.

145. Demetris AJ, Eghtesad B, Marcos A, Ruppert K, Nalesnik MA, Randhawa P, et al. Recurrent hepatitis C in liver allografts: prospective assessment of diagnostic accuracy, identification of pitfalls, and observations about pathogenesis. Am J Surg Pathol 2004;28(5):658–69.

146. Demetris A, Adams D, Bellamy C, Blakolmer K, Clouston A, Dhillon AP, et al. Update of the International Banff Schema for Liver Allograft Rejection: working recommendations for the histopathologic staging and reporting of chronic rejection. An international panel. Hepatology 2000;31(3):792–9.

147. Walter T, Dumortier J, Guillaud O, Hervieu V, Paliard P, Scoazec JY, et al. Rejection under alpha interferon therapy in liver transplant recipients. Am J Transplant 2007;7(1):177–84.

148. Stanca CM, Fiel MI, Kontorinis N, Agarwal K, Emre S, Schiano TD. Chronic ductopenic rejection in patients with recurrent hepatitis C virus treated with pegylated interferon alfa-2a and ribavirin. Transplantation 2007;84(2):180–6.

149. Blakolmer K, Jain A, Ruppert K, Gray E, Duquesnoy R, Murase N, et al. Chronic liver allograft rejection in a population treated primarily with tacrolimus as baseline immunosuppression: long-term follow-up and evaluation of features for histopathological staging. Transplantation 2000;69(11):2330–6.

150. Evans PC, Smith S, Hirschfield G, Rigopoulou E, Wreghitt TG, Wight DG, et al. Recipient HLA-DR3, tumour necrosis factor-alpha promoter allele-2 (tumour necrosis factor-2) and cytomegalovirus infection are interrelated risk factors for chronic rejection of liver grafts. J Hepatol 2001;34(5):711–15.

151. Nakazawa Y, Jonsson JR, Walker NI, Kerlin P, Steadman C, Lynch SV, et al. Fibrous obliterative lesions of veins contribute to progressive fibrosis in chronic liver allograft rejection. Hepatology 2000;32(6):1240–7.

152. Blakolmer K, Seaberg EC, Batts K, Ferrell L, Markin R, Wiesner R, et al. Analysis of the reversibility of chronic liver allograft rejection implications for a staging schema. Am J Surg Pathol 1999;23(11):1328–39.

153. Neil DA, Hubscher SG. Histologic and biochemical changes during the evolution of chronic rejection of liver allografts. Hepatology 2002;35(3):639–51.

154. Oguma S, Belle S, Starzl TE, Demetris AJ. A histometric analysis of chronically rejected human liver allografts: insights into the mechanisms of bile duct loss: direct immunologic and ischemic factors. Hepatology 1989;9(2):204–9.

155. Matsumoto Y, McCaughan GW, Painter DM, Bishop GA. Evidence that portal tract microvascular destruction precedes bile duct loss in human liver allograft rejection. Transplantation 1993;56(1):69–75.

156. Freese DK, Snover DC, Sharp HL, Gross CR, Savick SK, Payne WD. Chronic rejection after liver transplantation: a

study of clinical, histopathological and immunological features. Hepatology 1991;13(5):882–91.

157. Hubscher SG, Buckels JA, Elias E, McMaster P, Neuberger J. Vanishing bile-duct syndrome following liver transplantation—is it reversible? Transplantation 1991;51(5):1004–10.

158. van den Heuvel MC, de Jong KP, Boot M, Slooff MJ, Poppema S, Gouw AS. Preservation of bile ductules mitigates bile duct loss. Am J Transplant 2006;6(11):2660–71.

159. Demetris AJ, Seaberg EC, Batts KP, Ferrell L, Lee RG, Markin R, et al. Chronic liver allograft rejection: a National Institute of Diabetes and Digestive and Kidney Diseases interinstitutional study analyzing the reliability of current criteria and proposal of an expanded definition. National Institute of Diabetes and Digestive and Kidney Diseases Liver Transplantation Database. Am J Surg Pathol 1998;22(1):28–39.

160. White RM, Zajko AB, Demetris AJ, Bron KM, Dekker A, Starzl TE. Liver transplant rejection: angiographic findings in 35 patients. AJR Am J Roentgenol 1987;148(6):1095–8.

161. O'Keeffe C, Baird AW, Nolan N, McCormick PA. Mast cell hyperplasia in chronic rejection after liver transplantation. Liver Transpl 2002;8(1):50–7.

162. Crawford AR, Lin XZ, Crawford JM. The normal adult human liver biopsy: a quantitative reference standard. Hepatology 1998;28(2):323–31.

163. Quaglia AF, Del Vecchio Blanco G, Greaves R, Burroughs AK, Dhillon AP. Development of ductopaenic liver allograft rejection includes a "hepatitic" phase prior to duct loss. J Hepatol 2000;33(5):773–80.

164. Bai X, Rogers BB, Harkins PC, Sommerauer J, Squires R, Rotondo K, et al. Predictive value of quantitative PCR-based viral burden analysis for eight human herpesviruses in pediatric solid organ transplant patients. J Mol Diagn 2000;2(4):191–201.

165. Badley AD, Seaberg EC, Porayko MK, Wiesner RH, Keating MR, Wilhelm MP, et al. Prophylaxis of cytomegalovirus infection in liver transplantation: a randomized trial comparing a combination of ganciclovir and acyclovir to acyclovir. NIDDK Liver Transplantation Database. Transplantation 1997;64(1):66–73.

166. Barkholt L, Lewensohn-Fuchs I, Ericzon BG, Tyden G, Andersson J. High-dose acyclovir prophylaxis reduces cytomegalovirus disease in liver transplant patients. Transpl Infect Dis 1999;1(2):89–97.

167. McGavin JK, Goa KL. Ganciclovir: an update of its use in the prevention of cytomegalovirus infection and disease in transplant recipients. Drugs 2001;61(8):1153–83.

168. Theise ND, Conn M, Thung SN. Localization of cytomegalovirus antigens in liver allografts over time. Hum Pathol 1993;24(1):103–8.

169. Bronsther O, Makowka L, Jaffe R, Demetris AJ, Breinig MK, Ho M, et al. Occurrence of cytomegalovirus hepatitis in liver transplant patients. J Med Virol 1988;24(4):423–34.

170. Snover DC, Hutton S, Balfour HH, Jr., Bloomer JR. Cytomegalovirus infection of the liver in transplant recipients. J Clin Gastroenterol 1987;9(6):659–65.

171. Wiesner RH, Marin E, Porayko MK, Steers JL, Krom RA, Paya CV. Advances in the diagnosis, treatment, and

prevention of cytomegalovirus infections after liver transplantation. Gastroenterol Clin North Am 1993;22(2):351–66.

172. Toorkey CB, Carrigan DR. Immunohistochemical detection of an immediate early antigen of human cytomegalovirus in normal tissues. J Infect Dis 1989;160(5):741–51.

173. Oh CK, Pelletier SJ, Sawyer RG, Dacus AR, McCullough CS, Pruett TL, et al. Uni- and multi-variate analysis of risk factors for early and late hepatic artery thrombosis after liver transplantation. Transplantation 2001;71(6):767–72.

174. Pastacaldi S, Teixeira R, Montalto P, Rolles K, Burroughs AK. Hepatic artery thrombosis after orthotopic liver transplantation: a review of nonsurgical causes. Liver Transpl 2001;7(2):75–81.

175. Lautenschlager I, Halme L, Hockerstedt K, Krogerus L, Taskinen E. Cytomegalovirus infection of the liver transplant: virological, histological, immunological, and clinical observations. Transpl Infect Dis 2006;8(1):21–30.

176. Charlton M, Wiesner R. Natural history and management of hepatitis C infection after liver transplantation. Semin Liver Dis 2004;24 (Suppl. 2):79–88.

177. O'Grady JG, Alexander GJ, Sutherland S, Donaldson PT, Harvey F, Portmann B, et al. Cytomegalovirus infection and donor/recipient HLA antigens: interdependent cofactors in pathogenesis of vanishing bile-duct syndrome after liver transplantation. Lancet 1988;2(8606):302–5.

178. Lautenschlager I, Hockerstedt K, Jalanko H, Loginov R, Salmela K, Taskinen E, et al. Persistent cytomegalovirus in liver allografts with chronic rejection. Hepatology 1997;25(1):190–4.

179. Paya CV, Wiesner RH, Hermans PE, Larson-Keller JJ, Ilstrup DM, Krom RA, et al. Lack of association between cytomegalovirus infection, HLA matching and the vanishing bile duct syndrome after liver transplantation. Hepatology 1992;16(1):66–70.

180. Kusne S, Schwartz M, Breinig MK, Dummer JS, Lee RE, Selby R, et al. Herpes simplex virus hepatitis after solid organ transplantation in adults. J Infect Dis 1991;163(5):1001–7.

181. Snow AL, Martinez OM. Epstein-Barr virus: evasive maneuvers in the development of PTLD. Am J Transplant 2007;7(2):271–7.

182. Nalesnik MA. Clinicopathologic characteristics of post-transplant lymphoproliferative disorders. Recent Results. Cancer Res 2002;159:9–18.

183. Bakker NA, van Imhoff GW, Verschuuren EA, van Son WJ. Presentation and early detection of post-transplant lymphoproliferative disorder after solid organ transplantation. Transpl Int 2007;20(3):207–18.

184. Koch DG, Christiansen L, Lazarchick J, Stuart R, Willner IR, Reuben A. Posttransplantation lymphoproliferative disorder—the great mimic in liver transplantation: appraisal of the clinicopathologic spectrum and the role of Epstein-Barr virus. Liver Transpl 2007;13(6):904–12.

185. Randhawa PS, Markin RS, Starzl TE, Demetris AJ. Epstein-Barr virus-associated syndromes in immunosuppressed liver transplant recipients. Clinical profile and recognition on routine allograft biopsy. Am J Surg Pathol 1990;14(6):538–47.

186. Randhawa PS, Jaffe R, Demetris AJ, Nalesnik M, Starzl TE, Chen YY, et al. The systemic distribution of Epstein-Barr virus genomes in fatal post-transplantation lymphoproliferative disorders. An in situ hybridization study. Am J Pathol 1991;138(4):1027–33.

187. Randhawa PS, Jaffe R, Demetris AJ, Nalesnik M, Starzl TE, Chen YY, et al. Expression of Epstein-Barr virus-encoded small RNA (by the EBER-1 gene) in liver specimens from transplant recipients with post-transplantation lymphoproliferative disease. N Engl J Med 1992;327(24):1710–14.

188. Nalesnik MA, Jaffe R, Starzl TE, Demetris AJ, Porter K, Burnham JA, et al. The pathology of posttransplant lymphoproliferative disorders occurring in the setting of cyclosporine A-prednisone immunosuppression. Am J Pathol 1988;133(1):173–92.

189. Bierman PJ, Vose JM, Langnas AN, Rifkin RM, Hauke RJ, Smir BN, et al. Hodgkin's disease following solid organ transplantation. Ann Oncol 1996;7(3):265–70.

190. Sivaraman P, Lye WC. Epstein-Barr virus-associated T-cell lymphoma in solid organ transplant recipients. Biomed Pharmacother 2001;55(7):366–8.

191. Lee ES, Locker J, Nalesnik M, Reyes J, Jaffe R, Alashari M, et al. The association of Epstein-Barr virus with smooth-muscle tumors occurring after organ transplantation. N Engl J Med 1995;332(1):19–25.

192. Nalesnik MA. The diverse pathology of post-transplant lymphoproliferative disorders: the importance of a standardized approach. Transpl Infect Dis 2001;3(2):88–96.

193. Newell KA, Alonso EM, Whitington PF, Bruce DS, Millis JM, Piper JB, et al. Posttransplant lymphoproliferative disease in pediatric liver transplantation. Interplay between primary Epstein-Barr virus infection and immunosuppression. Transplantation 1996;62(3):370–5.

194. Manez R, Breinig MC, Linden P, Wilson J, Torre-Cisneros J, Kusne S, et al. Posttransplant lymphoproliferative disease in primary Epstein-Barr virus infection after liver transplantation: the role of cytomegalovirus disease. J Infect Dis 1997;176(6):1462–7.

195. Cockfield SM. Identifying the patient at risk for post-transplant lymphoproliferative disorder. Transpl Infect Dis 2001;3(2):70–8.

196. Randhawa P, Blakolmer K, Kashyap R, Raikow R, Nalesnik M, Demetris AJ, et al. Allograft liver biopsy in patients with Epstein-Barr virus-associated posttransplant lymphoproliferative disease. Am J Surg Pathol 2001;25(3):324–30.

197. Hubscher SG, Williams A, Davison SM, Young LS, Niedobitek G. Epstein-Barr virus in inflammatory diseases of the liver and liver allografts: an in situ hybridization study. Hepatology 1994;20(4 Pt 1):899–907.

198. Muti G, Cantoni S, Oreste P, Klersy C, Gini G, Rossi V, et al. Post-transplant lymphoproliferative disorders: improved outcome after clinico-pathologically tailored treatment. Haematologica 2002;87(1):67–77.

199. Koneru B, Jaffe R, Esquivel CO, Kunz R, Todo S, Iwatsuki S, et al. Adenoviral infections in pediatric liver transplant recipients. JAMA 1987;258(4):489–92.

200. Michaels MG, Green M, Wald ER, Starzl TE. Adenovirus infection in pediatric liver transplant recipients. J Infect Dis 1992;165(1):170–4.

201. Saad RS, Demetris AJ, Lee RG, Kusne S, Randhawa PS. Adenovirus hepatitis in the adult allograft liver. Transplantation 1997;64(10):1483–5.

202. McGrath D, Falagas ME, Freeman R, Rohrer R, Fairchild R, Colbach C, et al. Adenovirus infection in adult orthotopic liver transplant recipients: incidence and clinical significance. J Infect Dis 1998;177(2):459–62.

203. Berenguer M, Rayon JM, Prieto M, Aguilera V, Nicolas D, Ortiz V, et al. Are posttransplantation protocol liver biopsies useful in the long term? Liver Transpl 2001;7(9):790–6.

204. Burra P, Mioni D, Cecchetto A, Cillo U, Zanus G, Fagiuoli S, et al. Histological features after liver transplantation in alcoholic cirrhotics. J Hepatol 2001;34(5):716–22.

205. Berenguer M, Aguilera V, Prieto M, Carrasco D, Rayon M, San Juan F, et al. Delayed onset of severe hepatitis C-related liver damage following liver transplantation: a matter of concern? Liver Transpl 2003;9(11):1152–8.

206. Sebagh M, Rifai K, Feray C, Yilmaz F, Falissard B, Roche B, et al. All liver recipients benefit from the protocol 10-year liver biopsies. Hepatology 2003;37(6):1293–301.

207. Slapak GI, Saxena R, Portmann B, Gane E, Devlin J, Calne R, et al. Graft and systemic disease in long-term survivors of liver transplantation. Hepatology 1997;25(1):195–202.

208. Rosenthal P, Emond JC, Heyman MB, Snyder J, Roberts J, Ascher N, et al. Pathological changes in yearly protocol liver biopsy specimens from healthy pediatric liver recipients. Liver Transpl Surg 1997;3(6):559–62.

209. Wong T, Nouri-Aria KT, Devlin J, Portmann B, Williams R. Tolerance and latent cellular rejection in long-term liver transplant recipients. Hepatology 1998;28(2):443–9.

210. Gane E, Portmann B, Saxena R, Wong P, Ramage J, Williams R. Nodular regenerative hyperplasia of the liver graft after liver transplantation. Hepatology 1994;20(1 Pt 1):88–94.

211. Dubel L, Farges O, Johanet C, Sebagh M, Bismuth H. High incidence of antitissue antibodies in patients experiencing chronic liver allograft rejection. Transplantation 1998;65(8):1072–5.

212. Duclos-Vallee JC, Johanet C, Bach JF, Yamamoto AM. Autoantibodies associated with acute rejection after liver transplantation for type-2 autoimmune hepatitis. J Hepatol 2000;33(1):163–6.

213. Shinkura N, Ikai I, Egawa H, Yamauchi A, Kawai Y, Inomata Y, et al. Presence of anti-FKBP12 autoantibodies in patients with liver allografts: its association with allograft rejection. Transplantation 1997;64(9):1336–42.

214. Salcedo M, Vaquero J, Banares R, Rodriguez-Mahou M, Alvarez E, Vicario JL, et al. Response to steroids in de novo autoimmune hepatitis after liver transplantation. Hepatology 2002;35(2):349–56.

215. Gupta P, Hart J, Millis JM, Cronin D, Brady L. De novo hepatitis with autoimmune antibodies and atypical histology: a rare cause of late graft dysfunction after pediatric liver transplantation. Transplantation 2001;71(5):664–8.

216. Heneghan MA, Portmann BC, Norris SM, Williams R, Muiesan P, Rela M, et al. Graft dysfunction mimicking autoimmune hepatitis following liver transplantation in adults. Hepatology 2001;34(3):464–70.

217. Hernandez HM, Kovarik P, Whitington PF, Alonso EM. Autoimmune hepatitis as a late complication of liver transplantation. J Pediatr Gastroenterol Nutr 2001;32(2):131–6.

218. Aguilera I, Wichmann I, Sousa JM, Bernardos A, Franco E, Garcia-Lozano JR, et al. Antibodies against glutathione S-transferase T1 (GSTT1) in patients with de novo immune hepatitis following liver transplantation. Clin Exp Immunol 2001;126(3):535–9.

219. Jones DE, James OF, Portmann B, Burt AD, Williams R, Hudson M. Development of autoimmune hepatitis following liver transplantation for primary biliary cirrhosis. Hepatology 1999;30(1):53–7.

220. Kerkar N, Hadzic N, Davies ET, Portmann B, Donaldson PT, Rela M, et al. De-novo autoimmune hepatitis after liver transplantation. Lancet 1998;351(9100):409–13.

221. Iwatsuki S, Gordon RD, Shaw BW, Jr., Starzl TE. Role of liver transplantation in cancer therapy. Ann Surg 1985;202(4):401–7.

222. Iwatsuki S, Starzl TE, Sheahan DG, Yokoyama I, Demetris AJ, Todo S, et al. Hepatic resection versus transplantation for hepatocellular carcinoma. Ann Surg 1991;214(3):221–8.

223. Iwatsuki S, Starzl TE. Role of liver transplantation in the treatment of hepatocellular carcinoma. Semin Surg Oncol 1993;9(4):337–40.

224. Hunt J, Gordon FD, Jenkins RL, Lewis WD, Khettry U. Sarcoidosis with selective involvement of a second liver allograft: report of a case and review of the literature. Mod Pathol 1999;12(3):325–8.

225. Pappo O, Yunis E, Jordan JA, Jaffe R, Mateo R, Fung J, et al. Recurrent and de novo giant cell hepatitis after orthotopic liver transplantation. Am J Surg Pathol 1994;18(8):804–13.

226. Huang J. Ethical and legislative perspectives on liver transplantation in the People's Republic of China. Liver Transpl 2007;13(2):193–6.

227. Zheng SS, Liang TB, Wang WL, Huang DS, Shen Y, Zhang M, et al. Clinical experience in liver transplantation from an organ transplantation center in China. Hepatobiliary Pancreat Dis Int 2002;1(4):487–91.

228. Fagan E, Yousef G, Brahm J, Garelick H, Mann G, Wolstenholme A, et al. Persistence of hepatitis A virus in fulminant hepatitis and after liver transplantation. J Med Virol 1990;30(2):131–6.

229. Cavallari A, De Raffele E, Bellusci R, Miniero R, Vivarelli M, Galli S, et al. De novo hepatitis B and C viral infection after liver transplantation. World J Surg 1997;21(1):78–84.

230. Kamar N, Selves J, Mansuy JM, Ouezzani L, Peron JM, Guitard J, et al. Hepatitis E virus and chronic hepatitis in organ-transplant recipients. N Engl J Med 2008;358(8):811–17.

231. Demetris AJ, Jaffe R, Sheahan DG, Burnham J, Spero J, Iwatsuki S, et al. Recurrent hepatitis B in liver allograft recipients. Differentiation between viral hepatitis B and rejection. Am J Pathol 1986;125(1):161–72.

232. Demetris AJ, Todo S, Van Thiel DH, Fung JJ, Iwaki Y, Sysyn G, et al. Evolution of hepatitis B virus liver disease after hepatic replacement. Practical and theoretical considerations. Am J Pathol 1990;137(3):667–76.

233. O'Grady JG, Smith HM, Davies SE, Daniels HM, Donaldson PT, Tan KC, et al. Hepatitis B virus reinfection after orthotopic liver transplantation. Serological and clinical implications. J Hepatol 1992;14(1):104–11.

234. Davies SE, Portmann BC, O'Grady JG, Aldis PM, Chaggar K, Alexander GJ, et al. Hepatic histological findings after transplantation for chronic hepatitis B virus infection, including a unique pattern of fibrosing cholestatic hepatitis. Hepatology 1991;13(1):150–7.

235. Mason AL, Wick M, White HM, Benner KG, Lee RG, Regenstein F, et al. Increased hepatocyte expression of hepatitis B virus transcription in patients with features of fibrosing cholestatic hepatitis. Gastroenterology 1993;105(1):237–44.

236. Todo S, Demetris AJ, Van Thiel D, Teperman L, Fung JJ, Starzl TE. Orthotopic liver transplantation for patients with hepatitis B virus- related liver disease. Hepatology 1991;13(4):619–26.

237. Samuel D, Bismuth H. Liver transplantation for hepatitis B. Gastroenterol Clin North Am 1993;22(2):271–83.

238. Prieto M, Gomez MD, Berenguer M, Cordoba J, Rayon JM, Pastor M, et al. De novo hepatitis B after liver transplantation from hepatitis B core antibody-positive donors in an area with high prevalence of anti-HBc positivity in the donor population. Liver Transpl 2001;7(1):51–8.

239. Uemoto S, Sugiyama K, Marusawa H, Inomata Y, Asonuma K, Egawa H, et al. Transmission of hepatitis B virus from hepatitis B core antibody-positive donors in living related liver transplants. Transplantation 1998;65(4):494–9.

240. Vargas HE, Dodson FS, Rakela J. A concise update on the status of liver transplantation for hepatitis B virus: the challenges in 2002. Liver Transpl 2002;8(1):2–9.

241. Marzano A, Angelucci E, Andreone P, Brunetto M, Bruno R, Burra P, et al. Prophylaxis and treatment of hepatitis B in immunocompromised patients. Dig Liver Dis 2007;39(5):397–408.

242. Eisenbach C, Sauer P, Mehrabi A, Stremmel W, Encke J. Prevention of hepatitis B virus recurrence after liver transplantation. Clin Transplant 2006;20 (Suppl. 17):111–16.

243. Marinos G, Rossol S, Carucci P, Wong PY, Donaldson P, Hussain MJ, et al. Immunopathogenesis of hepatitis B virus recurrence after liver transplantation. Transplantation 2000;69(4):559–68.

244. Porter KA. Pathology of liver transplantation. Transplant Rev 1969;2:129–70.

245. Gouw AS, Houthoff HJ, Huitema S, Beelen JM, Gips CH, Poppema S. Expression of major histocompatibility complex antigens and replacement of donor cells by recipient ones in human liver grafts. Transplantation 1987;43(2):291–6.

246. Thung SN. Histologic findings in recurrent HBV. Liver Transpl 2006;12(11 Suppl. 2):S50–3.

247. Phillips MJ, Cameron R, Flowers MA, Blendis LM, Greig PD, Wanless I, et al. Post-transplant recurrent hepatitis B viral liver disease. Viral-burden, steatoviral, and fibroviral hepatitis B. Am J Pathol 1992;140(6):1295–308.

248. Benner KG, Lee RG, Keeffe EB, Lopez RR, Sasaki AW, Pinson CW. Fibrosing cytolytic liver failure secondary to recurrent hepatitis B after liver transplantation. Gastroenterology 1992;103(4):1307–12.

249. Rizzetto M, Macagno S, Chiaberge E, Verme G, Negro F, Marinucci G, et al. Liver transplantation in hepatitis delta virus disease. Lancet 1987;2(8557):469–71.

250. Reynes M, Zignego L, Samuel D, Fabiani B, Gugenheim J, Tricottet V, et al. Graft hepatitis delta virus reinfection after orthotopic liver transplantation in HDV cirrhosis. Transplant Proc 1989;21(1 Pt 2):2424–5.

251. David E, Rahier J, Pucci A, Camby P, Scevens M, Salizzoni M, et al. Recurrence of hepatitis D (delta) in liver transplants: histopathological aspects. Gastroenterology 1993;104(4):1122–8.

252. Arnold JC, Kraus T, Otto G, Muller HM, Hofmann W, Gmelin K, et al. Recurrent hepatitis C virus infection after liver transplantation. Transplant Proc 1992;24(6):2646–7.

253. Mateo R, Demetris A, Sico E, Frye C, Wang LF, el-Sakhawi Y, et al. Early detection of de novo hepatitis C infection in patients after liver transplantation by reverse transcriptase polymerase chain reaction. Surgery 1993;114(2):442–8.

254. Marzano A, Smedile A, Abate M, Ottobrelli A, Brunetto M, Negro F, et al. Hepatitis type C after orthotopic liver transplantation: reinfection and disease recurrence. J Hepatol 1994;21(6):961–5.

255. Belli LS, Silini E, Alberti A, Bellati G, Vai C, Minola E, et al. Hepatitis C virus genotypes, hepatitis, and hepatitis C virus recurrence after liver transplantation. Liver Transpl Surg 1996;2(3):200–5.

256. Feray C, Samuel D, Gigou M, Paradis V, David MF, Lemonnier C, et al. An open trial of interferon alfa recombinant for hepatitis C after liver transplantation: antiviral effects and risk of rejection. Hepatology 1995;22(4 Pt 1):1084–9.

257. Gayowski T, Singh N, Marino IR, Vargas H, Wagener M, Wannstedt C, et al. Hepatitis C virus genotypes in liver transplant recipients: impact on posttransplant recurrence, infections, response to interferon-alpha therapy and outcome. Transplantation 1997;64(3):422–6.

258. Spengler U, Nattermann J. Immunopathogenesis in hepatitis C virus cirrhosis. Clin Sci (Lond) 2007;112(3):141–55.

259. McCaughan GW, Zekry A. Mechanisms of HCV reinfection and allograft damage after liver transplantation. J Hepatol 2004;40(3):368–74.

260. Demetris AJ, Lunz JG, 3rd. Early HCV-associated stellate cell activation in aggressive recurrent HCV: What can liver allografts teach about HCV pathogenesis? Liver Transpl 2005;11(10):1172–6.

261. Eghtesad B, Fung JJ, Demetris AJ, Murase N, Ness R, Bass DC, et al. Immunosuppression for liver transplantation in HCV-infected patients: Mechanism-based principles. Liver Transpl 2005;11(11):1343–52.

262. Berenguer M, Aguilera V, Prieto M, San Juan F, Rayon JM, Benlloch S, et al. Significant improvement in the outcome of HCV-infected transplant recipients by avoiding rapid steroid tapering and potent induction immunosuppression. J Hepatol 2006;44(4):717–22.

263. Tisone G, Orlando G, Cardillo A, Palmieri G, Manzia TM, Baiocchi L, et al. Complete weaning off immunosuppression in HCV liver transplant recipients is feasible and favourably impacts on the progression of disease recurrence. J Hepatol 2006;44(4):702–9.

264. Zekry A, Bishop GA, Bowen DG, Gleeson MM, Guney S, Painter DM, et al. Intrahepatic cytokine profiles associated with posttransplantation hepatitis C virus-related liver injury. Liver Transpl 2002;8(3):292–301.

265. Khettry U, Huang WY, Simpson MA, Pomfret EA, Pomposelli JJ, Lewis WD, et al. Patterns of recurrent hepatitis C after liver transplantation in a recent cohort of patients. Hum Pathol 2007;38(3):443–52.

266. Czaja AJ, Carpenter HA. Histological findings in chronic hepatitis C with autoimmune features. Hepatology 1997;26(2):459–66.

267. Dixon LR, Crawford JM. Early histologic changes in fibrosing cholestatic hepatitis C. Liver Transpl 2007;13(2):219–26.

268. Ferrell LD, Wright TL, Roberts J, Ascher N, Lake J. Hepatitis C viral infection in liver transplant recipients. Hepatology 1992;16(4):865–76.

269. Tsamandas AC, Furukawa H, Abu-Elmagd K, Todo S, Demetris AJ, Lee RG. Liver allograft pathology in liver/small bowel or multivisceral recipients. Mod Pathol 1996;9(7):767–73.

270. Asanza CG, Garcia-Monzon C, Clemente G, Salcedo M, Garcia-Buey L, Garcia-Iglesias C, et al. Immunohistochemical evidence of immunopathogenetic mechanisms in chronic hepatitis C recurrence after liver transplantation. Hepatology 1997;26(3):755–63.

271. Rosen HR, Martin P. Hepatitis C infection in patients undergoing liver retransplantation. Transplantation 1998;66(12):1612–16.

272. Rosen HR, Gretch DR, Oehlke M, Flora KD, Benner KG, Rabkin JM, et al. Timing and severity of initial hepatitis C recurrence as predictors of long-term liver allograft injury. Transplantation 1998;65(9):1178–82.

273. Gordon FD, Pomfret EA, Pomposelli JJ, Lewis WD, Jenkins RL, Khettry U. Severe steatosis as the initial histologic manifestation of recurrent hepatitis C genotype 3. Hum Pathol 2004;35(5):636–8.

274. Lumbreras C, Colina F, Loinaz C, Domingo MJ, Fuertes A, Dominguez P, et al. Clinical, virological, and histologic evolution of hepatitis C virus infection in liver transplant recipients. Clin Infect Dis 1998;26(1):48–55.

275. Charco R, Vargas V, Allende H, Edo A, Balsells J, Murio E, et al. Is hepatitis C virus recurrence a risk factor for chronic liver allograft rejection? Transpl Int 1996;9(Suppl. 1):S195–7.

276. Hoffmann RM, Gunther C, Diepolder HM, Zachoval R, Eissner HJ, Forst H, et al. Hepatitis C virus infection as a possible risk factor for ductopenic rejection (vanishing bile duct syndrome) after liver transplantation. Transplant International 1995;8(5):353–9.

277. Jain A, Demetris AJ, Manez R, Tsamanadas AC, Van Thiel D, Rakela J, et al. Incidence and severity of acute allograft rejection in liver transplant recipients treated with alfa interferon. Liver Transpl Surg 1998;4(3):197–203.

278. Dousset B, Conti F, Houssin D, Calmus Y. Acute vanishing bile duct syndrome after interferon therapy for recurrent HCV infection in liver-transplant recipients. N Engl J Med 1994;330(16):1160–1.

279. Ontanon J, Muro M, Garcia-Alonso AM, Minguela A, Torio A, Bermejo J, et al. Effect of partial HLA class I match on acute rejection in viral pre-infected human liver allograft recipients. Transplantation 1998;65(8):1047–53.

280. Russo MW, Firpi RJ, Nelson DR, Schoonhoven R, Shrestha R, Fried MW. Early hepatic stellate cell activation is associated with advanced fibrosis after liver transplantation in recipients with hepatitis C. Liver Transpl 2005;11(10):1235–41.

281. Gawrieh S, Papouchado BG, Burgart LJ, Kobayashi S, Charlton MR, Gores GJ. Early hepatic stellate cell activation predicts severe hepatitis C recurrence after liver transplantation. Liver Transpl 2005;11(10):1207–13.

282. Rayhill SC, Wu YM, Katz DA, Voigt MD, Labrecque DR, Kirby PA, et al. Older donor livers show early severe histological activity, fibrosis, and graft failure after liver transplantation for hepatitis C. Transplantation 2007;84(3):331–9.

283. Burton JR, Jr., Rosen HR. Acute rejection in HCV-infected liver transplant recipients: The great conundrum. Liver Transpl 2006;12(11 Suppl. 2):S38–47.

284. Alvarez F, Berg PA, Bianchi FB, Bianchi L, Burroughs AK, Cancado EL, et al. International Autoimmune Hepatitis Group Report: review of criteria for diagnosis of autoimmune hepatitis. J Hepatol 1999;31(5):929–38.

285. Faust TW. Recurrent primary biliary cirrhosis, primary sclerosing cholangitis, and autoimmune hepatitis after transplantation. Liver Transpl 2001;7(11 Suppl. 1):S99–108.

286. Gautam M, Cheruvattath R, Balan V. Recurrence of autoimmune liver disease after liver transplantation: a systematic review. Liver Transpl 2006;12(12):1813–24.

287. Dmitrewski J, Hubscher SG, Mayer AD, Neuberger JM. Recurrence of primary biliary cirrhosis in the liver allograft: the effect of immunosuppression. J Hepatol 1996;24(3):253–7.

288. Garcia RF, Garcia CE, McMaster P, Neuberger J. Transplantation for primary biliary cirrhosis: retrospective analysis of 400 patients in a single center. [In Process Citation]. Hepatology 2001;33(1):22–7.

289. Hashimoto E, Shimada M, Noguchi S, Taniai M, Tokushige K, Hayashi N, et al. Disease recurrence after living liver transplantation for primary biliary cirrhosis: a clinical and histological follow-up study. Liver Transpl 2001;7(7):588–95.

290. Mazariegos GV, Reyes J, Marino IR, Demetris AJ, Flynn B, Irish W, et al. Weaning of immunosuppression in liver transplant recipients. Transplantation 1997;63(2):243–9.

291. Ramos HC, Reyes J, Abu-Elmagd K, Zeevi A, Reinsmoen N, Tzakis A, et al. Weaning of immunosuppression in long-term liver transplant recipients. Transplantation 1995;59(2):212–17.

292. Charatcharoenwitthaya P, Pimentel S, Talwalkar JA, Enders FT, Lindor KD, Krom RA, et al. Long-term survival and impact of ursodeoxycholic acid treatment for recurrent primary biliary cirrhosis after liver transplantation. Liver Transpl 2007;13(9):1236–1245.

293. Hubscher SG, Elias E, Buckels JA, Mayer AD, McMaster P, Neuberger JM. Primary biliary cirrhosis. Histological evidence of disease recurrence after liver transplantation. J Hepatol 1993;18(2):173–84.

294. Sebagh M, Farges O, Dubel L, Samuel D, Bismuth H, Reynes M. Histological features predictive of recurrence

of primary biliary cirrhosis after liver transplantation. Transplantation 1998;65(10):1328–33.

295. Farges O, Bismuth H, Sebagh M, Reynes M. Granulomatous destruction of bile ducts after liver transplantation: primary biliary cirrhosis recurrence or hepatitis C virus infection? Hepatology 1995;21(6):1765–7.

296. Hubscher SG. Recurrent autoimmune hepatitis after liver transplantation: diagnostic criteria, risk factors, and outcome. Liver Transpl 2001;7(4):285–91.

297. Demetris AJ, Murase N, Delaney CP. Overlap between Allo- and Autoimmunity in the Rat and Human Evidence for Important Contribtuions for Dendritic and Regulatory Cells. Graft 2003;6:21–32.

298. Saadoun D, Landau DA, Calabrese LH, Cacoub PP. Hepatitis C-associated mixed cryoglobulinaemia: a crossroad between autoimmunity and lymphoproliferation. Rheumatology (Oxford) 2007;46(8):1234–42.

299. Fagiuoli S, Bruni F, Bravi M, Candusso M, Gaffuri G, Colledan M, et al. Cyclosporin in steroid-resistant autoimmune hepatitis and HCV-related liver diseases. Dig Liver Dis 2007;39 (Suppl. 3):S379–85.

300. Petersen-Benz C, Kasper HU, Dries V, Goeser T. Differential efficacy of corticosteroids and interferon in a patient with chronic hepatitis C-autoimmune hepatitis overlap syndrome. Clin Gastroenterol Hepatol 2004;2(5):440–3.

301. Lunel F, Cacoub P. Treatment of autoimmune and extrahepatic manifestations of hepatitis C virus infection. J Hepatol 1999;31 (Suppl. 1):210–16.

302. Salcedo M, Vaquero J, Banares R, al. e. Serum autoantibodies after liver transplantation. Prevalence and associated immunologic disorders. [Abstract]. J Hepatol 2003;34 (Suppl. 1):47.

303. Ratziu V, Samuel D, Sebagh M, Farges O, Saliba F, Ichai P, et al. Long-term follow-up after liver transplantation for autoimmune hepatitis: evidence of recurrence of primary disease. J Hepatol 1999;30(1):131–41.

304. Reich DJ, Fiel I, Guarrera JV, Emre S, Guy SR, Schwartz ME, et al. Liver transplantation for autoimmune hepatitis. Hepatology 2000;32(4 Pt 1):693–700.

305. Venick RS, McDiarmid SV, Farmer DG, Gornbein J, Martin MG, Vargas JH, et al. Rejection and steroid dependence: unique risk factors in the development of pediatric posttransplant de novo autoimmune hepatitis. Am J Transpl 2007;7(4):955–63.

306. Czaja AJ, Carpenter HA. Sensitivity, specificity, and predictability of biopsy interpretations in chronic hepatitis. Gastroenterology 1993;105(6):1824–32.

307. Alexander J, Lord JD, Yeh MM, Cuevas C, Bakthavatsalam R, Kowdley KV. Risk factors for recurrence of primary sclerosing cholangitis after liver transplantation. Liver Transpl 2008;14(2):245–51.

308. Cholongitas E, Shusang V, Papatheodoridis GV, Marelli L, Manousou P, Rolando N, et al. Risk factors for recurrence of primary sclerosing cholangitis after liver transplantation. Liver Transpl 2008;14(2):138–43.

309. Vera A, Moledina S, Gunson B, Hubscher S, Mirza D, Olliff S, et al. Risk factors for recurrence of primary sclerosing cholangitis of liver allograft. Lancet 2002;360(9349):1943–4.

310. Goss JA, Shackleton CR, Farmer DG, Arnaout WS, Seu P, Markowitz JS, et al. Orthotopic liver transplantation for primary sclerosing cholangitis. A 12-year single center experience. Ann Surg 1997;225(5):472–81.

311. Graziadei IW, Wiesner RH, Marotta PJ, Porayko MK, Hay JE, Charlton MR, et al. Long-term results of patients undergoing liver transplantation for primary sclerosing cholangitis. Hepatology 1999;30(5):1121–7.

312. Gow PJ, Chapman RW. Liver transplantation for primary sclerosing cholangitis. Liver 2000;20(2):97–103.

313. Dvorchik I, Subotin M, Demetris AJ, Fung JJ, Starzl TE, Wieand S, et al. Effect of liver transplantation on inflammatory bowel disease in patients with primary sclerosing cholangitis. Hepatology 2002;35(2):380–4.

314. Narumi S, Roberts JP, Emond JC, Lake J, Ascher NL. Liver transplantation for sclerosing cholangitis. Hepatology 1995;22(2):451–7.

315. Jeyarajah DR, Netto GJ, Lee SP, Testa G, Abbasoglu O, Husberg BS, et al. Recurrent primary sclerosing cholangitis after orthotopic liver transplantation: is chronic rejection part of the disease process? Transplantation 1998;66(10):1300–6.

316. Sheng R, Campbell WL, Zajko AB, Baron RL. Cholangiographic features of biliary strictures after liver transplantation for primary sclerosing cholangitis: evidence of recurrent disease. AJR Am J Roentgenol 1996;166(5):1109–13.

317. Harrison RF, Davies MH, Neuberger JM, Hubscher SG. Fibrous and obliterative cholangitis in liver allografts: evidence of recurrent primary sclerosing cholangitis? Hepatology 1994;20(2):356–61.

318. Jaffe R. Liver transplant pathology in pediatric metabolic disorders. Pediatr Dev Pathol 1998;1(2):102–17.

319. Osorio RW, Ascher NL, Avery M, Bacchetti P, Roberts JP, Lake JR. Predicting recidivism after orthotopic liver transplantation for alcoholic liver disease. Hepatology 1994;20(1 Pt 1):105–10.

320. Berlakovich GA, Steininger R, Herbst F, Barlan M, Mittlbock M, Muhlbacher F. Efficacy of liver transplantation for alcoholic cirrhosis with respect to recidivism and compliance. Transplantation 1994;58(5):560–5.

321. Bellamy CO, DiMartini AM, Ruppert K, Jain A, Dodson F, Torbenson M, et al. Liver transplantation for alcoholic cirrhosis: long term follow-up and impact of disease recurrence. Transplantation 2001;72(4):619–26.

322. Lucey MR, Carr K, Beresford TP, Fisher LR, Shieck V, Brown KA, et al. Alcohol use after liver transplantation in alcoholics: a clinical cohort follow-up study. Hepatology 1997;25(5):1223–7.

323. Abosh D, Rosser B, Kaita K, Bazylewski R, Minuk G. Outcomes following liver transplantation for patients with alcohol- versus nonalcohol-induced liver disease. Can J Gastroenterol 2000;14(10):851–5.

324. Conjeevaram HS, Hart J, Lissoos TW, Schiano TD, Dasgupta K, Befeler AS, et al. Rapidly progressive liver injury and fatal alcoholic hepatitis occurring after liver transplantation in alcoholic patients. Transplantation 1999;67(12):1562–8.

325. Molloy RM, Komorowski R, Varma RR. Recurrent nonalcoholic steatohepatitis and cirrhosis after liver transplantation. Liver Transpl Surg 1997;3(2):177–8.

326. Tang H, Boulton R, Gunson B, Hubscher S, Neuberger J. Patterns of alcohol consumption after liver transplantation. Gut 1998;43(1):140–5.

327. Haber PS, McCaughan GW. "I'll never touch it again, doctor!"—harmful drinking after liver transplantation. Hepatology 2007;46(4):1302–4.

328. Jauhar S, Talwalkar JA, Schneekloth T, Jowsey S, Wiesner RH, Menon KV. Analysis of factors that predict alcohol relapse following liver transplantation. Liver Transpl 2004;10(3):408–11.

329. Platz KP, Mueller AR, Spree E, Schumacher G, Nussler NC, Rayes N, et al. Liver transplantation for alcoholic cirrhosis. Transpl Int 2000;13 (Suppl. 1):S127–30.

330. Yusoff IF, House AK, De Boer WB, Ferguson J, Garas G, Heath D, et al. Disease recurrence after liver transplantation in Western Australia. J Gastroenterol Hepatol 2002;17(2):203–7.

331. Burke A, Lucey MR. Non-alcoholic fatty liver disease, non-alcoholic steatohepatitis and orthotopic liver transplantation. Am J Transplant 2004;4(5):686–93.

332. Ayata G, Gordon FD, Lewis WD, Pomfret E, Pomposelli JJ, Jenkins RL, et al. Cryptogenic cirrhosis: clinicopathologic findings at and after liver transplantation. Hum Pathol 2002;33(11):1098–104.

333. Contos MJ, Cales W, Sterling RK, Luketic VA, Shiffman ML, Mills AS, et al. Development of nonalcoholic fatty liver disease after orthotopic liver transplantation for cryptogenic cirrhosis. Liver Transpl 2001;7(4):363–73.

334. Kim WR, Poterucha JJ, Porayko MK, Dickson ER, Steers JL, Wiesner RH. Recurrence of nonalcoholic steatohepatitis following liver transplantation. Transplantation 1996;62(12):1802–5.

335. Ong J, Younossi ZM, Reddy V, Price LL, Gramlich T, Mayes J, et al. Cryptogenic cirrhosis and posttransplantation nonalcoholic fatty liver disease. Liver Transpl 2001;7(9):797–801.

336. Brunt EM. Nonalcoholic steatohepatitis: pathologic features and differential diagnosis. Semin Diagn Pathol 2005;22(4):330–8.

337. Evans HM, Kelly DA, McKiernan PJ, Hubscher S. Progressive histological damage in liver allografts following pediatric liver transplantation. Hepatology 2006;43(5):1109–17.

338. Shaikh OS, Demetris AJ. Idiopathic posttransplantation hepatitis? Liver Transpl 2007;13(7):943–6.

339. Sakaguchi S, Sakaguchi N, Shimizu J, Yamazaki S, Sakihama T, Itoh M, et al. Immunologic tolerance maintained by CD25+ CD4+ regulatory T cells: their common role in controlling autoimmunity, tumor immunity, and transplantation tolerance. Immunol Rev 2001;182:18–32.

340. Koshiba T, Li Y, Takemura M, Wu Y, Sakaguchi S, Minato N, et al. Clinical, immunological, and pathological aspects of operational tolerance after pediatric living-donor liver transplantation. Transpl Immunol 2007;17(2):94–7.

341. Martinez-Llordella M, Puig-Pey I, Orlando G, Ramoni M, Tisone G, Rimola A, et al. Multiparameter immune profiling of operational tolerance in liver transplantation. Am J Transplant 2007;7(2):309–19.

342. Reding R, Gras J, Bourdeaux C, Wieers G, Truong QD, Latinne D, et al. Stepwise minimization of the immunosuppressive therapy in pediatric liver transplantation. A conceptual approach towards operational tolerance. Acta Gastroenterol Belg 2005;68(3):320–2.

343. Calne RY, White HJO, Yoffa DE, Maginn RR, Binns RM, Samuel JR, et al. Observations of orthotopic liver transpantation in the pig. Br Med J 1967;2:478–80.

344. Lerut J, Sanchez-Fueyo A. An appraisal of tolerance in liver transplantation. Am J Transplant 2006;6(8):1774–80.

345. Yoshitomi M, Koshiba T, Sakashita H, Haga H, Tanaka K, Li Y, et al. Requirement of protocol biopsy before and after complete cessation of immunosuppression following living-donor liver transplantation. Am J Transpl 2006;6(Suppl. 2):173.

346. Devarbhavi H, Abraham S, Kamath PS. Significance of nodular regenerative hyperplasia occurring de novo following liver transplantation. Liver Transpl 2007;13(11):1552–6.

347. Sterneck M, Wiesner R, Ascher N, Roberts J, Ferrell L, Ludwig J, et al. Azathioprine hepatotoxicity after liver transplantation. Hepatology 1991;14(5):806–10.

348. Lefkowitch JH, Lobritto SJ, Brown RS, Jr., Emond JC, Schilsky ML, Rosenthal LA, et al. Ground-glass, polyglucosan-like hepatocellular inclusions: a "new" diagnostic entity. Gastroenterology 2006;131(3):713–8.

349. Harada K, Ozaki S, Gershwin ME, Nakanuma Y. Enhanced apoptosis relates to bile duct loss in primary biliary cirrhosis. Hepatology 1997;26(6):1399–405.

350. Gane E, Sallie R, Saleh M, Portmann B, Williams R. Clinical recurrence of hepatitis A following liver transplantation for acute liver failure. J Med Virol 1995;45(1):35–9.

351. McCaughan GW, Torzillo PJ. Hepatitis A, liver transplants and indigenous communities. Med J Aust 2000;172(1):6–7.

352. Douglas DD, Rakela J, Wright TL, Krom RA, Wiesner RH. The clinical course of transplantation-associated de novo hepatitis B infection in the liver transplant recipient. Liver Transpl Surg 1997;3(2):105–11.

353. Muller R, Gubernatis G, Farle M, Niehoff G, Klein H, Wittekind C, et al. Liver transplantation in HBs antigen (HBsAg) carriers. Prevention of hepatitis B virus (HBV) recurrence by passive immunization. J Hepatol 1991; 13(1):90–6.

354. Konig V, Hopf U, Neuhaus P, Bauditz J, Schmidt CA, Blumhardt G, et al. Long-term follow-up of hepatitis B virus-infected recipients after orthotopic liver transplantation. Transplantation 1994;58(5):553–9.

355. Tchervenkov JI, Tector AJ, Barkun JS, Sherker A, Forbes CD, Elias N, et al. Recurrence-free long-term survival after liver transplantation for hepatitis B using interferon-alpha pretransplant and hepatitis B immune globulin posttransplant. Ann Surg 1997;226(3):356–65.

356. Angus PW. Review: hepatitis B and liver transplantation. J Gastroenterol Hepatol 1997;12(3):217–23.

357. Roche B, Samuel D, Feray C, Majno P, Gigou M, Reynes M, et al. Retransplantation of the liver for recurrent hepatitis B virus infection: the Paul Brousse experience. Liver Transpl Surg 1999;5(3):166–74.

358. Cane PA, Mutimer D, Ratcliffe D, Cook P, Beards G, Elias E, et al. Analysis of hepatitis B virus quasispecies changes during emergence and reversion of lamivudine resistance in liver transplantation. Antivir Ther 1999;4(1):7–14.

359. Rayes N, Seehofer D, Bechstein WO, Muller AR, Berg T, Neuhaus R, et al. Long-term results of famciclovir for recurrent or de novo hepatitis B virus infection after liver transplantation. Clin Transplant 1999;13(6):447–52.
360. Mutimer D, Pillay D, Shields P, Cane P, Ratcliffe D, Martin B, et al. Outcome of lamivudine resistant hepatitis B virus infection in the liver transplant recipient. Gut 2000;46(1):107–13.
361. Seehofer D, Rayes N, Neuhaus R, Berg T, Muller AR, Bechstein WO, et al. Antiviral combination therapy for lamivudine-resistant hepatitis B reinfection after liver transplantation. Transpl Int 2000;13 (Suppl. 1):S359–62.
362. Gutfreund KS, Williams M, George R, Bain VG, Ma MM, Yoshida EM, et al. Genotypic succession of mutations of the hepatitis B virus polymerase associated with lamivudine resistance. J Hepatol 2000;33(3):469–75.
363. Seehofer D, Rayes N, Steinmuller T, Muller AR, Settmacher U, Neuhaus R, et al. Occurrence and clinical outcome of lamivudine-resistant hepatitis B infection after liver transplantation. Liver Transpl 2001;7(11):976–82.
364. Walsh KM, Woodall T, Lamy P, Wight DG, Bloor S, Alexander GJ. Successful treatment with adefovir dipivoxil in a patient with fibrosing cholestatic hepatitis and lamivudine resistant hepatitis B virus. Gut 2001;49(3):436–40.
365. Castells L, Esteban R. Hepatitis B vaccination in liver transplant candidates. Eur J Gastroenterol Hepatol 2001;13(4):359–61.
366. Ben-Ari Z, Mor E, Shapira Z, Tur-Kaspa R. Long-term experience with lamivudine therapy for hepatitis B virus infection after liver transplantation. Liver Transpl 2001;7(2):113–17.
367. Bock CT, Tillmann HL, Torresi J, Klempnauer J, Locarnini S, Manns MP, et al. Selection of hepatitis B virus polymerase mutants with enhanced replication by lamivudine treatment after liver transplantation. Gastroenterology 2002;122(2):264–73.
368. Gane EJ, Naoumov NV, Qian KP, Mondelli MU, Maertens G, Portmann BC, et al. A longitudinal analysis of hepatitis C virus replication following liver transplantation. Gastroenterology 1996;110(1):167–77.
369. Gane EJ, Portmann BC, Naoumov NV, Smith HM, Underhill JA, Donaldson PT, et al. Long-term outcome of hepatitis C infection after liver transplantation. N Engl J Med 1996;334(13):815–20.
370. Chazouilleres O, Kim M, Combs C, Ferrell L, Bacchetti P, Roberts J, et al. Quantitation of hepatitis C virus RNA in liver transplant recipients. Gastroenterology 1994;106(4):994–9.
371. McCaughan GW, Zekry A. Impact of immunosuppression on immunopathogenesis of liver damage in hepatitis C virus-infected recipients following liver transplantation. Liver Transpl 2003;9(11):S21–7.
372. Rosen HR. Hepatitis C virus in the human liver transplantation model. Clin Liver Dis 2003;7(1):107–25.
373. Sanchez-Fueyo A, Restrepo JC, Quinto L, Bruguera M, Grande L, Sanchez-Tapias JM, et al. Impact of the recurrence of hepatitis C virus infection after liver transplantation on the long-term viability of the graft. Transplantation 2002;73(1):56–63.
374. Bernard PH, Le Bail B, Rullier A, Trimoulet P, Neau-Cransac M, Balabaud C, et al. Recurrence and accelerated progression of hepatitis C following liver transplantation. Semin Liver Dis 2000;20(4):533–8.
375. Charlton M. Natural history of hepatitis C and outcomes following liver transplantation. Clin Liver Dis 2003;7(3):585–602.
376. Charlton M. Liver biopsy, viral kinetics, and the impact of viremia on severity of hepatitis C virus recurrence. Liver Transpl 2003;9(11):S58–62.
377. Wiesner RH, Sorrell M, Villamil F. Report of the first International Liver Transplantation Society expert panel consensus conference on liver transplantation and hepatitis C. Liver Transpl 2003;9(11):S1–9.
378. Feray C, Gigou M, Samuel D, Paradis V, Mishiro S, Maertens G, et al. Influence of the genotypes of hepatitis C virus on the severity of recurrent liver disease after liver transplantation. Gastroenterology 1995;108(4):1088–96.
379. Caccamo L, Gridelli B, Sampietro M, Melada E, Doglia M, Lunghi G, et al. Hepatitis C virus genotypes and reinfection of the graft during long- term follow-up in 35 liver transplant recipients. Transpl Int 1996;9 (Suppl. 1):S204–9.
380. Gordon FD, Poterucha JJ, Germer J, Zein NN, Batts KP, Gross JB, Jr., et al. Relationship between hepatitis C genotype and severity of recurrent hepatitis C after liver transplantation. Transplantation 1997;63(10):1419–23.
381. Gigou M, Roque-Afonso AM, Falissard B, Penin F, Dussaix E, Feray C. Genetic clustering of hepatitis C virus strains and severity of recurrent hepatitis after liver transplantation. J Virol 2001;75(23):11292–7.
382. Charlton M, Seaberg E, Wiesner R, Everhart J, Zetterman R, Lake J, et al. Predictors of patient and graft survival following liver transplantation for hepatitis C. Hepatology 1998;28(3):823–30.
383. Zhou S, Terrault NA, Ferrell L, Hahn JA, Lau JY, Simmonds P, et al. Severity of liver disease in liver transplantation recipients with hepatitis C virus infection: relationship to genotype and level of viremia. Hepatology 1996;24(5):1041–6.
384. Guido M, Fagiuoli S, Tessari G, Burra P, Leandro G, Boccagni P, et al. Histology predicts cirrhotic evolution of post transplant hepatitis C. Gut 2002;50(5):697–700.
385. Berenguer M, Crippin J, Gish R, Bass N, Bostrom A, Netto G, et al. A model to predict severe HCV-related disease following liver transplantation. Hepatology 2003;38(1):34–41.
386. Neuberger J, Portmann B, Calne R, Williams R. Recurrence of autoimmune chronic active hepatitis following orthotopic liver grafting. Transplantation 1984;37(4):363–5.
387. Sempoux C, Horsmans Y, Lerut J, Rahier J, Geubel A. Acute lobular hepatitis as the first manifestation of recurrent autoimmune hepatitis after orthotopic liver transplantation. Liver 1997;17(6):311–15.
388. Prados E, Cuervas-Mons V, de la Mata M, Fraga E, Rimola A, Prieto M, et al. Outcome of autoimmune hepatitis after liver transplantation. Transplantation 1998;66(12):1645–50.
389. Ayata G, Gordon FD, Lewis WD, Pomfret E, Pomposelli JJ, Jenkins RL, et al. Liver transplantation for autoimmune hepatitis: a long-term pathologic study. Hepatology 2000;32(2):185–92.

390. Gonzalez-Koch A, Czaja AJ, Carpenter HA, Roberts SK, Charlton MR, Porayko MK, et al. Recurrent autoimmune hepatitis after orthotopic liver transplantation. Liver Transpl 2001;7(4):302–10.

391. Wright HL, Bou-Abboud CF, Hassanein T, Block GD, Demetris AJ, Starzl TE, et al. Disease recurrence and rejection following liver transplantation for autoimmune chronic active liver disease. Transplantation 1992;53(1):136–9.

392. Czaja AJ, Strettell MD, Thomson LJ, Santrach PJ, Moore SB, Donaldson PT, et al. Associations between alleles of the major histocompatibility complex and type 1 autoimmune hepatitis. Hepatology 1997;25(2):317–23.

393. Birnbaum AH, Benkov KJ, Pittman NS, McFarlane-Ferreira Y, Rosh JR, LeLeiko NS. Recurrence of autoimmune hepatitis in children after liver transplantation. J Pediatr Gastroenterol Nutr 1997;25(1):20–5.

394. Faust TW. Recurrent primary biliary cirrhosis, primary sclerosing cholangitis, and autoimmune hepatitis after transplantation. Semin Liver Dis 2000;20(4):481–95.

395. McDiarmid SV. Liver transplantation. The pediatric challenge. Clin Liver Dis 2000;4(4):879–927.

396. Neuberger J, Portmann B, MacDougall BR, Calne RY, Williams R. Recurrence of primary biliary cirrhosis after transplantation. N Engl J Med 1982;306:1–4.

397. Balan V, Batts KP, Porayko MK, Krom RA, Ludwig J, Wiesner RH. Histological evidence for recurrence of primary biliary cirrhosis after liver transplantation [see comments]. Hepatology 1993;18(6):1392–8.

398. Polson RJ, Portmann B, Neuberger J, Calne RY, Williams R. Evidence for disease recurrence after liver transplantation for primary biliary cirrhosis. Clinical and histologic follow-up studies. Gastroenterology 1989;97(3):715–25.

399. Esquivel CO, Van Thiel DH, Demetris AJ, Bernardos A, Iwatsuki S, Markus B, et al. Transplantation for primary biliary cirrhosis. Gastroenterology 1988;94(5 Pt 1):1207–16.

400. Neuberger J. Liver transplantation for primary biliary cirrhosis. Autoimmun Rev 2003;2(1):1–7.

401. Jaeckel E, Tillmann HL, Manns MP. Liver transplantation and autoimmunity. Acta Gastroenterol Belg 1999;62(3):323–9.

402. Tan CK, Sian Ho JM. Concurrent de novo autoimmune hepatitis and recurrence of primary biliary cirrhosis post-liver transplantation. Liver Transpl 2001;7(5):461–5.

403. Graziadei IW, Wiesner RH, Batts KP, Marotta PJ, LaRusso NF, Porayko MK, et al. Recurrence of primary sclerosing cholangitis following liver transplantation. Hepatology 1999;29(4):1050–6.

404. Graziadei IW. Recurrence of primary sclerosing cholangitis after liver transplantation. Liver Transpl 2002;8(7):575–81.

405. Khettry U, Keaveny A, Goldar-Najafi A, Lewis WD, Pomfret EA, Pomposelli JJ, et al. Liver transplantation for primary sclerosing cholangitis: a long-term clinicopathologic study. Hum Pathol 2003;34(11):1127–36.

406. Anand AC, Hubscher SG, Gunson BK, McMaster P, Neuberger JM. Timing, significance, and prognosis of late acute liver allograft rejection. Transplantation 1995;60(10):1098–103.

407. Yoshida EM, Shackleton CR, Erb SR, Scudamore CH, Mori LM, Ford JA, et al. Late acute rejection occurring in liver allograft recipients. Can J Gastroenterol 1996;10(6):376–80.

408. D'Antiga L, Dhawan A, Portmann B, Francavilla R, Rela M, Heaton N, et al. Late cellular rejection in paediatric liver transplantation: aetiology and outcome. Transplantation 2002;73(1):80–4.

409. Neil DA, Hubscher SG. Delay in diagnosis: a factor in the poor outcome of late acute rejection of liver allografts. Transplant Proc 2001;33(1–2):1525–6.

410. Lowes JR, Hubscher SG, Neuberger JM. Chronic rejection of the liver allograft. Gastroenterol Clin North Am 1993;22(2):401–20.

411. Hoek BV, Wiesner R, Krom R, Ludwig J, Moore S. Severe ductopenic rejection following liver transplantation: incidence, time of onset, risk factors, treatment and outcome. Semin Liver Dis 1992;12:41–50.

412. Ludwig J, Wiesner RH, Batts KP, Perkins JD, Krom RA. The acute vanishing bile duct syndrome (acute irreversible rejection) after orthotopic liver transplantation. Hepatology 1987;7(3):476–83.

413. Fennell RH, Jr. Ductular damage in liver transplant rejection: its similarity to that of primary biliary cirrhosis and graft-versus-host disease. Pathol Annu 1981;16(Pt):289–94.

414. Grond J, Gouw ASH, Poppema S, Sloof MJH, Gips CH. Chronic rejection in liver transplants: a histopathologic analysis of failed grafts and antecedent serial biopsies. Transpl Proc 1986;16(5):128–35.

415. Vierling JM, Fennell RH, Jr. Histopathology of early and late human hepatic allograft rejection: evidence of progressive destruction of interlobular bile ducts. Hepatology 1985;5(6):1076–82.

416. Portmann B, Neuberger J, Williams R. Intrahepatic bile duct lesions. In: Calne R, editor. Liver Transplantation: The Cambridge-Kings College Hospital Experience. New York: Grune & Stratton; 1983. p. 279–87.

417. Wight DA. Chronic liver transplant rejection: definition and diagnosis. Transpl Proc 1996;28(1):465–7.

418. Quiroga J, Colina I, Demetris AJ, Starzl TE, Van Thiel DH. Cause and timing of first allograft failure in orthotopic liver transplantation: a study of 177 consecutive patients. Hepatology 1991;14(6):1054–62.

419. Starzl TE, Marchioro TL, Porter KA. Experimental and clinical observations after homotransplantation of the whole liver. Rev Int Hepatol 1965;15(8):1447–80.

420. Porte RJ, Ploeg RJ, Hansen B, van Bockel JH, Thorogood J, Persijn GG, et al. Long-term graft survival after liver transplantation in the UW era: late effects of cold ischemia and primary dysfunction. European Multicentre Study Group. Transpl Int 1998;11 (Suppl. 1):S164–7.

421. Nakhleh RE, Schwarzenberg SJ, Bloomer J, Payne W, Snover DC. The pathology of liver allografts surviving longer than one year [see comments]. Hepatology 1990;11(3):465–70.

422. Charlton M, Kasparova P, Weston S, Lindor K, Maor-Kendler Y, Wiesner RH, et al. Frequency of nonalcoholic steatohepatitis as a cause of advanced liver disease. Liver Transpl 2001;7(7):608–14.

423. Wong LL. Current status of liver transplantation for hepatocellular cancer. Am J Surg 2002;183(3):309–16.

424. Figueras J, Ibanez L, Ramos E, Jaurrieta E, Ortiz-de-Urbina J, Pardo F, et al. Selection criteria for liver transplantation in early-stage hepatocellular carcinoma with cirrhosis: results of a multicenter study. Liver Transpl 2001;7(10):877–83.

425. Frilling A, Malago M, Broelsch CE. Current status of liver transplantation for treatment of hepatocellular carcinoma. Dig Dis 2001;19(4):333–7.

426. Iwatsuki S, Dvorchik I, Marsh JW, Madariaga JR, Carr B, Fung JJ, et al. Liver transplantation for hepatocellular carcinoma: a proposal of a prognostic scoring system. J Am Coll Surg 2000;191(4):389–94.

427. Klintmalm GB. Liver transplantation for hepatocellular carcinoma: a registry report of the impact of tumor characteristics on outcome. Ann Surg 1998;228(4):479–90.

428. Marsh JW, Dvorchik I, Subotin M, Balan V, Rakela J, Popechitelev EP, et al. The prediction of risk of recurrence and time to recurrence of hepatocellular carcinoma after orthotopic liver transplantation: a pilot study [see comments]. Hepatology 1997;26(2):444–50.

429. Tamura S, Kato T, Berho M, Misiakos EP, O'Brien C, Reddy KR, et al. Impact of histological grade of hepatocellular carcinoma on the outcome of liver transplantation. Arch Surg 2001;136(1):25–30.

430. Casavilla FA, Marsh JW, Iwatsuki S, Todo S, Lee RG, Madariaga JR, et al. Hepatic resection and transplantation for peripheral cholangiocarcinoma. J Am Coll Surg 1997; 185(5):429–36.

431. Iwatsuki S, Todo S, Marsh JW, Madariaga JR, Lee RG, Dvorchik I, et al. Treatment of hilar cholangiocarcinoma (Klatskin tumors) with hepatic resection or transplantation. J Am Coll Surg 1998;187(4):358–64.

432. Meyer CG, Penn I, James L. Liver transplantation for cholangiocarcinoma: results in 207 patients. Transplantation 2000;69(8):1633–7.

433. Weimann A, Varnholt H, Schlitt HJ, Lang H, Flemming P, Hustedt C, et al. Retrospective analysis of prognostic factors after liver resection and transplantation for cholangiocellular carcinoma. Br J Surg 2000;87(9):1182–7.

434. Starzl T. Surgery for metabolic liver disease. In: WV M, editor. Surgery of the Liver. Boston MA: Blackwell Scientific Publications; 1986. pp. 127–136.

435. Putnam CW, Porter KA, Peters RL, Ashcavai M, Redeker AG, Starzl TE. Liver replacement for alpha1-antitrypsin deficiency. Surgery 1977;81(3):258–61.

436. de Carvalho M, Conceicao I, Bentes C, Luis ML. Long-term quantitative evaluation of liver transplantation in familial amyloid polyneuropathy (Portuguese V30M). Amyloid 2002;9(2):126–33.

437. Suhr OB, Ericzon BG, Friman S. Long-term follow-up of survival of liver transplant recipients with familial amyloid polyneuropathy (Portuguese type). Liver Transpl 2002;8(9):787–94.

438. Figueras J, Pares D, Munar-Ques M, Torras J, Fabregat J, Rafecas A, et al. Experience with domino or sequential liver transplantation in familial patients with amyloid polyneuropathy. Transplant Proc 2002;34(1):307–8.

439. Shaz BH, Lewis WD, Skinner M, Khettry U. Livers from patients with apolipoprotein A-I amyloidosis are not suitable as "domino" donors. Mod Pathol 2001;14(6):577–80.

440. Brandhagen DJ. Liver transplantation for hereditary hemochromatosis. Liver Transpl 2001;7(8):663–72.

441. Brandhagen DJ, Alvarez W, Therneau TM, Kruckeberg KE, Thibodeau SN, Ludwig J, et al. Iron overload in cirrhosis-HFE genotypes and outcome after liver transplantation. Hepatology 2000;31(2):456–60.

442. DuBois RS, Rodgerson DO, Martineau G, Shroter G, Giles G, Lilly J, et al. Orthotopic liver transplantation for Wilson's disease. Lancet 1971;1(7698):505–8.

443. Groth CG, Dubois RS, Corman J, Gustafsson A, Iwatsuki S, Rodgerson DO, et al. Metabolic effects of hepatic replacement in Wilson's disease. Transpl Proc 1973;5(1):829–33.

444. Zitelli BJ, Malatack JJ, Gartner JC, Shaw BW, Iwatsuki S, TE S. Orthotopic liver transplantation in children with hepatic-based metabolic disease. Transpl Proc 1983;15: 1284–1287.

445. Wolff H, Otto G, Giest H. Liver transplantation in Crigler-Najjar syndrome. A case report. Transplantation 1986; 42(1):84.

446. Kaufman SS, Wood RP, Shaw BW, Jr., Markin RS, Rosenthal P, Gridelli B, et al. Orthotopic liver transplantation for type I Crigler-Najjar syndrome. Hepatology 1986;6(6):1259–62.

447. Daloze P, Delvin EE, Glorieux FH, Corman JL, Bettez P, Toussi T. Replacement therapy for inherited enzyme deficiency: liver orthotopic transplantation in Niemann-Pick disease type A. Am J Med Genet 1977;1(2):229–39.

448. Fisch RO, McCabe ER, Doeden D, Koep LJ, Kohlhoff JG, Silverman A, et al. Homotransplantation of the liver in a patient with hepatoma and hereditary tyrosinemia. J Pediatr 1978;93(4):592–6.

449. Starzl TE, Zitelli BJ, Shaw BW, Jr., Iwatsuki S, Gartner JC, Gordon RD, et al. Changing concepts: liver replacement for hereditary tyrosinemia and hepatoma. J Pediatr 1985;106(4): 604–6.

450. Kayler LK, Merion RM, Lee S, Sung RS, Punch JD, Rudich SM, et al. Long-term survival after liver transplantation in children with metabolic disorders. Pediatr Transplant 2002;6(4):295–300.

451. Shneider BL. Pediatric liver transplantation in metabolic disease: clinical decision making. Pediatr Transplant 2002;6(1):25–9.

452. Gartner JC, Jr., Bergman I, Malatack JJ, Zitelli BJ, Jaffe R, Watkins JB, et al. Progression of neurovisceral storage disease with supranuclear ophthalmoplegia following orthotopic liver transplantation. Pediatrics 1986;77(1):104–6.

453. Malatack JJ, Finegold DN, Iwatsuki S, Shaw BW, Jr., Gartner JC, Zitelli BJ, et al. Liver transplantation for type I glycogen storage disease. Lancet 1983;1(8333):1073–5.

454. Matern D, Starzl TE, Arnaout W, Barnard J, Bynon JS, Dhawan A, et al. Liver transplantation for glycogen storage disease types I, III, and IV. Eur J Pediatr 1999;158 (Suppl. 2):S43–8.

455. Samuel D, Boboc B, Bernuau J, Bismuth H, Benhamou JP. Liver transplantation for protoporphyria. Evidence for the predominant role of the erythropoietic tissue in protoporphyrin overproduction. Gastroenterology 1988;95(3):816–19.

456. de Torres I, Demetris AJ, Randhawa PS. Recurrent hepatic allograft injury in erythropoietic protoporphyria [see comments]. Transplantation 1996;61(9):1412–13.

457. Dellon ES, Szczepiorkowski ZM, Dzik WH, Graeme-Cook F, Ades A, Bloomer JR, et al. Treatment of recurrent allograft dysfunction with intravenous hematin after liver transplantation for erythropoietic protoporphyria. Transplantation 2002;73(6):911–15.

458. Casella JF, Lewis JH, Bontempo FA, Zitelli BJ, Markel H, Starzl TE. Successful treatment of homozygous protein C deficiency by hepatic transplantation. Lancet 1988;1(8583): 435–8.

459. Starzl TE, Bilheimer DW, Bahnson HT, Shaw BW, Jr., Hardesty RL, Griffith BP, et al. Heart-liver transplantation in a patient with familial hypercholesterolaemia. Lancet 1984;1(8391):1382–3.

460. Cox KL, Ward RE, Furgiuele TL, Cannon RA, Sanders KD, Kurland G. Orthotopic liver transplantation in patients with cystic fibrosis. Pediatrics 1987;80(4):571–4.

461. Mieles LA, Orenstein D, Teperman L, Podesta L, Koneru B, Starzl TE. Liver transplantation in cystic fibrosis. Lancet 1989;1(8646):1073.

462. Milkiewicz P, Skiba G, Kelly D, Weller P, Bonser R, Gur U, et al. Transplantation for cystic fibrosis: outcome following early liver transplantation. J Gastroenterol Hepatol 2002;17(2):208–13.

463. Lewis JH, Bontempo FA, Spero JA, Ragni MV, Starzl TE. Liver transplantation in a hemophiliac. N Engl J Med 1985;312(18):1189–90.

464. Bontempo FA, Lewis JH, Gorenc TJ, Spero JA, Ragni MV, Scott JP, et al. Liver transplantation in hemophilia A. Blood 1987;69(6):1721–4.

465. Merion RM, Delius RE, Campbell DA, Jr., Turcotte JG. Orthotopic liver transplantation totally corrects factor IX deficiency in hemophilia B. Surgery 1988;104(5): 929–31.

466. Heneghan MA, Zolfino T, Muiesan P, Portmann BC, Rela M, Heaton ND, et al. An evaluation of long-term outcomes after liver transplantation for cryptogenic cirrhosis. Liver Transpl 2003;9(9):921–8.

467. Maor-Kendler Y, Batts KP, Burgart LJ, Wiesner RH, Krom RA, Rosen CB, et al. Comparative allograft histology after liver transplantation for cryptogenic cirrhosis, alcohol, hepatitis C, and cholestatic liver diseases. Transplantation 2000;70(2):292–7.

CHAPTER 5

Pathology of Cardiac Transplantation

Chi K. Lai, M.D., F.R.C.P.C.

Hui-Min Yang, M.D.

Seong Ra, M.D.

Michael C. Fishbein, M.D.

I. INTRODUCTION

Heart transplantation has evolved rapidly from experimental models to clinical practice for the treatment of end-stage heart disease. Over the past four decades, much has been learned about the immunologic responses to the allograft heart. In 1972, the Stanford group first used the endomyocardial biopsy (EMB) to diagnose rejection and institute therapy (1). Based on work done about a decade earlier by Sakakibara and Konno in Japan, Caves developed a cardiac bioptome to obtain right ventricular endomyocardium for histological evaluation (2,3). Implementation of the EMB immediately reduced the mortality rate after transplantation by 50 percent. Remarkably, in spite of many attempts to develop less invasive methods of monitoring for rejection, the EMB remains the gold standard. This chapter will focus on the pathology of cardiac transplantation with major emphasis on the use of the EMB to diagnose and guide therapy for patients after heart transplantation.

II. INDICATIONS

Cardiac transplantation is the treatment of choice for many patients with end-stage heart disease. These patients may have severe heart failure unresponsive to medical therapy or intractable, life-threatening cardiac arrhythmias. The goals of transplantation are to improve survival and the quality of life. It is estimated that in the United States each year, 4,000 patients could benefit from heart transplantation; however, only 2,000 donor hearts are available. Patients who qualify for transplantation have a variety of cardiac diseases. In most transplant centers, the most common diseases are coronary artery disease and cardiomyopathy. According to the 2007 International Society of Heart and Lung Transplantation (ISHLT) Registry report (4), adult patients underwent cardiac transplantation for the following heart diseases between 2004 and 2006: cardiomyopathy (45.2 percent), coronary artery disease (41.0 percent), valvular heart disease (2.6 percent), congenital heart disease (3.2 percent), retransplant (2.8 percent), and miscellaneous other causes (2.3 percent). The exact percentages obviously vary depending on the institution and the patient population. For example, there was a recent report published on the heart transplant experience from Padua, Italy, on patients transplanted from 1985 to 2004 (5). There were 600 heart transplants in 496 men, 104 women, and 42 children less than eighteen years old. In this series, 52 percent of patients were transplanted for cardiomyopathy, 37 percent for coronary artery disease, 6 percent for valvular disease, 27 percent for congenital heart disease, 1 percent for chronic rejection, 1 percent for "graft dysfunction," and 1 percent for other reasons. Among the 311 patients with cardiomyopathy, there were 83 percent with dilated cardiomyopathy, 6.5 percent with restrictive cardiomyopathy, 4.5 percent with arrhythmogenic right ventricular cardiomyopathy, 4 percent with hypertrophic cardiomyopathy, 4 percent with myocarditis, and 1 patient with amyloidosis. Moreover, in 10 percent of cases, there was discordance between the pretransplantation clinical diagnoses and the pathological diagnoses of the explanted heart. Some institutions exclude patients with certain cardiac illnesses, such as amyloidosis, HIV positivity, or cardiac sarcomas; however, these restrictions are not applied consistently.

III. ISCHEMIA/REPERFUSION INJURY

When myocardial blood flow and oxygenation is perturbed, such that oxygen demand exceeds oxygen supply, a state of ischemia exists. If the ischemia is of sufficient severity and duration, irreversible myocardial injury or necrosis occurs. If the ischemia is short lived and/or mild and if blood flow is restored, the myocardium returns to normal. In either case, reperfusion of blood seems to accentuate and amplify the myocardial injury after a period of ischemia.

Whether or not necrosis occurs after reperfusion, contractile function is impaired, sometimes for days. Morphological changes may range from mild edema to marked disruption of cellular organelles. ATP production is reduced, and if necrosis has occurred, myocardial proteins such as troponin and myoglobin leak into the blood. Better techniques of organ preservation are evolving to protect the donor organ from ischemia during harvesting and implantation. In addition to keeping the organ cold, additional measures are being tested to prevent ischemic injury to the graft. A cold ischemic time of more than four hours is a significant contributor to early death after transplantation (6). Early oxidative stress results in generation of reactive oxygen species and stimulates the production of cytokines. There is subsequent activation of the adhesion molecule cascade and increased inflammation in the graft (7). Acutely, if the ischemic/reperfusion injury is severe, it can result in early graft dysfunction and failure (8). In a study by Opelz and Wujciak (9), an ischemic time of six hours was associated with 25 percent greater graft loss than when ischemic time was less than two hours.

In the long term, ischemic/reperfusion injury can cause late graft failure. There is a strong relationship between an extended initial period of ischemia, development of cardiac allograft vasculopathy (CAV), and late graft failure. It is now recognized that allo-independent as well as allo-dependent mechanisms contribute to accelerated CAV. The consensus of opinion is that the tissue damage and resulting inflammatory changes associated with ischemic

injury increase exposure of donor antigens and upregulate the recipient immune system resulting in accelerated injury to the graft coronary arteries (10). Indeed, in the presence of allo-dependent mechanisms, ischemic/reperfusion injury potentiates CAV development.

The earliest and reversible changes of ischemic-reperfusion are best seen with the electron microscope. In routine light microscopic sections, if cell death has occurred, one may observe the classical changes of coagulation necrosis (Figure 5.1A). The associated tissue reaction will depend on the time interval between the transplant procedure and the EMB (Figure 5.1B) (11). In one study by Panizo et al. (12) in the first week after transplantation, coagulation necrosis was observed in twelve of thirty patients (40 percent). If one performs immunofluorescence (IF) studies in EMBs early after transplantation, necrotic fibers nonspecifically stain with immunoglobulins (Igs) and complement components (Figure 5.1C).

Once the cell membranes of the necrotic cells are compromised, there will be nonspecific uptake of these plasma proteins. It is unclear how early focal necrosis of myocardium affects long-term graft function (12).

IV. ACUTE CELLULAR REJECTION

Despite advances in immunosuppression and close surveillance, acute cellular rejection (ACR) remains an important concern. In our experience at UCLA medical center, 21–25 percent of EMBs showed ACR. Most were low-grade ACRs that do not require therapeutic intervention (Figure 5.2A, B). This is considerably lower than the incidence reported from other institutions at the ISHLT Registry (4). The incidence of ACR is highest during the first few months after transplantation.

In 2007, the ISHLT Registry reported that approximately 35–45 percent of the patients were treated for rejection during the first year after transplantation (4). In the patients transplanted between 1992 and 2006, acute rejection accounted for 6.4 percent of deaths in the first thirty days, 12.4 percent from thirty-one days to one year, 10.3 percent from one to three years, 4.4 percent from three to five years, 1.7 percent from five to ten years, and 1.2 percent at more than ten years. Notably, the long-term survival has increased due to improved maintenance immunosuppressive therapy and in the diagnosis and treatment of acute rejection (13). Nonetheless, acute rejection continues to be a significant clinical problem.

As with other solid organ transplants, ACR in the heart allograft is mediated by host cytotoxic and helper T cells targeting donor graft antigens (described in a previous chapter). Highly polymorphic donor major histocompatibility complex (MHC) or HLA antigens play a major role in cardiac ACR, while minor HLA antigens are less involved. Alloantigens in the donor heart graft are presented to naive T cells in two different ways: direct and

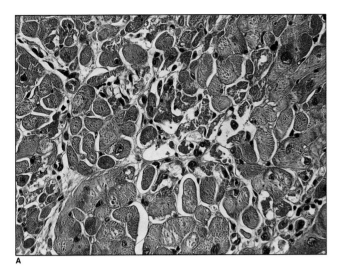

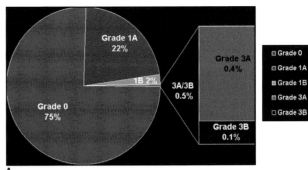

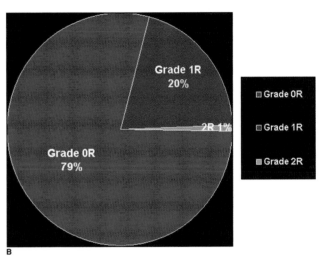

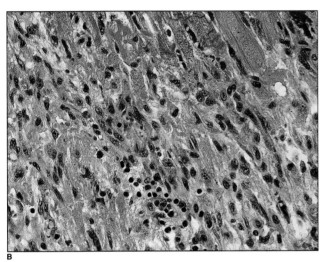

FIGURE 5.2: Incidence of rejection grades. (A) Distribution of rejection grade diagnoses in 2,240 surveillance endomyocardial biopsies obtained at UCLA Medical Center between 2004 and 2005 based on the 1990 ISHLT rejection grading system. (B) Distribution of rejection grade diagnoses in 1,321 surveillance endomyocardial biopsies obtained at UCLA Medical Center between 2006 and 2007 based on the new ISHLT rejection grading system.

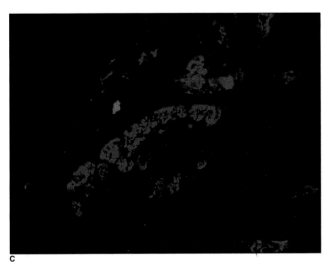

FIGURE 5.1: Ischemic/reperfusion injury. (A) In early stages, there is coagulation necrosis of myocytes, characterized by hypereosinophilia and loss of nuclei, with little or no inflammatory infiltrate (H&E; original magnification, 400×). (B) In later stages, granulation tissue with variable collagen deposition and mixed polymorphous inflammation are present (H&E; original magnification, 400×). (C) Necrotic fibers can nonspecifically stain with immunoglobulins or complement on IF studies (original magnification, 400×).

indirect allorecognition (14,15) (see Chapter 1). Direct allorecognition occurs when donor antigen-presenting cells (APCs) in the heart, such as dendritic cells, that express both the allogeneic MHC molecule and costimulatory molecules (e.g., B7-1, B7-2, and CD40), migrate to a regional lymph node to present donor peptide and activate recipient T cells. These cells then produce cytokines to initiate a delayed-type hypersensitivity response that results in graft injury. Sun et al. used a murine model of aortic transplantation to demonstrate that concurrent blockade against the CD28/B7 and CD40/CD40L costimulatory pathways can prolong graft survival (16). In indirect allorecognition, the recipient APCs take up allogeneic peptides from the graft, then process, and present them with self-MHC molecules to the recipient T cells. The allogeneic peptides presented include peptides from the foreign donor MHC molecules as well as the minor histocompatibility antigens (14,15). Although the immunologic mechanisms and relative contribution of CD8 T cells, CD4 T cells, and other inflammatory cells to myocyte injury has not been fully elucidated, Wagoner et al. found via a murine cardiac rejection model that only a small component of myocyte injury is mediated by cytotoxic CD8 T cells and that cell types involved in a delayed-type hypersensitivity response such as CD4 T cells, macrophages, and neutrophils may play a significant, if not more important, role in causing myocyte injury (17).

The *histopathological pattern* of ACR is characterized by a mononuclear infiltrate and its eventual damage to the myocardium and the vasculature (18). The inflammatory infiltrate consists predominantly of lymphocytes and macrophages, with occasional eosinophils (19). The lymphocytes appear "activated" or enlarged, with oval or reniform nuclei (20). The presence of eosinophils is usually associated with more severe ACR; however, they can occasionally be seen in lower grades of rejection. In the highest grade of rejection, the infiltrate is more polymorphous, consisting of neutrophils and eosinophils as well as lymphocytes and macrophages. *Immunohistochemical studies* performed by Michaels et al. demonstrated that identifying the type of infiltrating cell aids in the diagnosis of ACR (21). In ACR, more than 50 percent of the infiltrating cells are actually CD68-positive macrophages, whereas, T lymphocytes comprise less than 50 percent of the total inflammatory infiltrate. Only a small percentage of infiltrating cells are B lymphocytes.

Myocyte damage, sometimes termed "myocyte necrosis," is a crucial finding in ACR that is often difficult to recognize. Myocyte damage is often characterized by myocytolysis rather than actual coagulation necrosis. Features of myocytolysis include nuclear enlargement with occasional prominent nucleoli and clearing of the sarcoplasm and nuclei, which results in tinctorial changes (Figure 5.3A) (22). The injured myocyte is often surrounded by encroaching inflammatory cells, resulting in irregular, "scalloped" myocyte borders and architectural distortion (Figure 5.3B). The injured myocyte can be partially replaced

by the inflammatory infiltrate and the lymphocytes may appear to lie within the myocyte. Cell necrosis may be more widespread and apparent in more severe forms of ACR. Although myocytolysis is an important finding in ACR, it can also be seen in antibody-mediated rejection (AMR), Quilty effect (QE), and ischemic/reperfusion injury (20).

When the standard 7 or 9 French bioptome is used, the ISHLT recommends four fragments of endomyocardium for evaluation of acute rejection; however, three fragments may be adequate. If a smaller bioptome is used, some pathologists recommend that six pieces be obtained. Each piece should have at minimum 50 percent endomyocardium that is not a prior biopsy site or a scar. Multiple sections should be obtained from at least three levels through the tissue because findings of ACR may only be focally present. In most cases, routine hematoxylin and eosin (H&E) staining is sufficient for the diagnosis and grading of rejection. Special stains such as elastic and trichrome stains can be used to identify endocardium, and to highlight fibrosis or myocyte damage. Additional special stains for microorganisms may be used if there are clinical or histological findings suspicious for infection, which is extremely rare in the transplanted heart (20,23). In certain situations when AMR is suspected, fresh tissue may be processed for IF studies. In our experience, Zeus fixative results in excessive nonspecific fluorescence and is not recommended as a preservative for cardiac tissue for IF studies.

In the early days of cardiac transplantation, several grading schemes were used at different transplant centers with no consensus system. In 1990, the ISHLT established a standardized grading system for diagnosing rejection in EMBs (24). This grading scale has contributed to the overall improved communication in clinical and research settings. However, over the course of its usage, several issues have emerged. The main points of contention included the

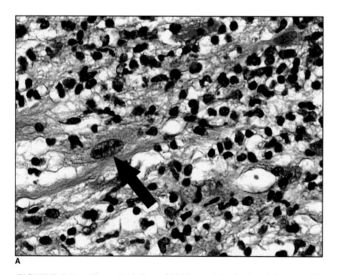
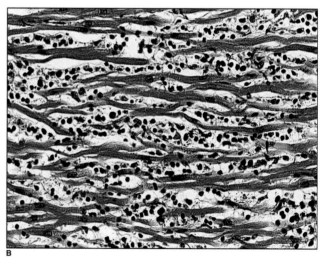

A   B

FIGURE 5.3: Myocyte injury. (A) Myocytolysis involving cardiac myocyte (arrow) is characterized by clearing of the sarcoplasm and nuclear enlargement with prominent nucleoli. Note that the inflammatory infiltrate encroaches upon and appears to lie within the injured myocyte (H&E; original magnification, 400×). (B) Significant myocyte damage with architectural distortion and considerable myocyte atrophy due to prominent inflammatory infiltrate (H&E; original magnification, 200×).

TABLE 5.1 Comparison of 1990 and 2004 ISHLT ACR Schemes (22)

1990	2004
Grade 0	Grade 0R
Grades 1A, 1B, and 2	Grade 1R
Grade 3A	Grade 2R
Grades 3B and 4	Grade 3R

poor interobserver reproducibility of the grading system, the diagnosis and treatment of grade 2 rejection, and the diagnosis of AMR (22). In particular, the existence of grade 2 rejection was questioned as most EMBs diagnosed as grade 2 rejection were shown to actually represent, on serial deeper sections, tangentially sectioned QE extending into the underlying myocardium, and therefore, not ACR (25). Further complicating the grade 2 rejection diagnosis is that some clinicians treated this grade of rejection, whereas others did not (26). In 2004, the ISHLT task forces made further modifications to the grading scale in an effort to resolve these issues (Table 5.1). For ACR, the 1990 ISHLT grading scale was simplified such that prior grades 1A, 1B, and 2 would be combined into the revised 2004 grade 1R, prior grade 3A would become grade 2R, and prior grades 3B and 4 would become grade 3R (22). The accuracy and reproducibility of the diagnosis was expected to be greatly improved with only three grades of rejection (26).

i. Histological Grading

The histological grade of ACR is based on the most severe findings present in the EMB (20,22,23).

Grade 0R (no ACR) remains the same as former grade 0 in the 1990 grading scale and is diagnosed in the absence of inflammatory infiltrate or myocyte injury (Figure 5.4A). The presence of *rare* interstitial lymphocytes is still regarded as grade 0R.

Grade 1R (mild ACR) encompasses former grades 1A, 1B, and 2 and includes lesions spanning the spectrum from focal perivascular infiltrates (Figure 5.4B) and/or diffuse sparse interstitial infiltrate (Figure 5.4C) with no accompanying myocyte injury to one discrete focus of mononuclear cells with associated myocyte damage (Figure 5.4D). Marboe et al. found that the concordance for the diagnosis of the 1990 ISHLT grade 2 rejection to be poor due to confusion with QE (27).

Grade 2R (moderate ACR) is the former grade 3A and is defined by *two or more foci* of lymphocytes and macrophages, with or without eosinophils, with associated myocyte damage. These infiltrates may involve one or more endomyocardial fragments; however, there are still intervening areas of uninvolved myocardium (Figure 5.4E). If two adjoining foci of inflammatory infiltrate with associated myocyte damage are present, deeper sectioning would most likely reveal one single focus (grade 1R). If the foci are more

widely separated by normal myocardium, they are most likely separate foci and should be regarded as grade 2R rejection. The presence of eosinophils may suggest a higher grade lesion; however, they may also be seen in QE.

Grade 3R (severe ACR) incorporates prior grades 3B and 4, and is characterized by a diffuse inflammatory process that may be predominantly mononuclear or polymorphous, consisting of large lymphocytes, eosinophils, and neutrophils, associated with myocyte damage (Figure 5.4F, G). Usually, most biopsy fragments are involved. Note that interstitial edema, hemorrhage, and vasculitis may be present in both severe ACR and AMR. When a diffuse interstitial infiltrate is present, the *intensity* of the infiltrate and its association with myocyte injury may be used to differentiate grade 3R from grade 1R rejection. Examination of multiple serial sections and the changes present in other fragments will usually help distinguish grade 3R from grade 1R. Diagnostic difficulty can also be encountered in deciding between 2R and 3R rejection. Stewart et al. suggested that the presence of a diffuse infiltrate with associated myocyte injury, even an intermittently sparse one, be regarded as grade 3R, whereas ample uninvolved areas between foci of myocyte damage is most likely grade 2R rejection. In practice, both grades 2R and 3R are treated.

As mentioned earlier, *myocyte damage* is a crucial finding in determining the severity of ACR. The spectrum of myocyte damage ranges from a single focus (grade 1R) to multiple foci (grade 2R) and a diffuse inflammatory infiltrate in association with myocyte damage (grade 3R) (20). However, preliminary results from an interobserver variability study have shown that grade 1R (in particular, 1990 ISHLT grade 1B) and grade 2R to have poor interobserver reproducibility, most likely due to difficulty in recognizing myocyte damage (28). The recognition of myocyte injury remains an area of difficulty in the current grading scheme. Occasionally, immunohistochemical staining for vimentin and actin can be used to determine the presence of myocyte damage. In our experience, these markers are fairly specific but not sensitive. Thus, better immunohistochemical markers are needed to reliably detect myocyte damage and help increase interobserver agreement.

Inflammatory infiltrates and/or myocyte injury in the cardiac allograft are present in several processes that must be distinguished from ACR (22).

ii. Lesions That May Resemble ACR

Perioperative ischemic injury resulting in myocardial necrosis can be the result of vasopressor therapy during acute care, donor trauma with catecholamine excess, prolonged warm and cold ischemia, or ischemia/reperfusion injury. In early ischemic injury that typically occurs up to six weeks after transplantation, there is usually a greater degree of myocyte necrosis that is out of proportion to the cellular infiltrate compared to that seen in ACR (22). More

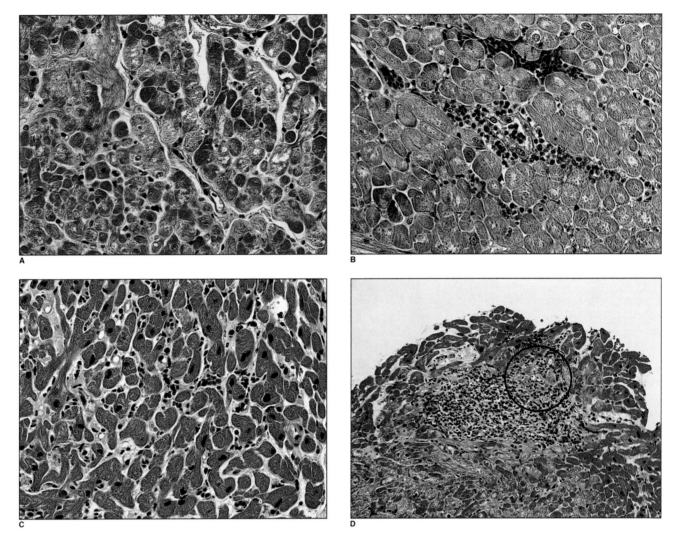

FIGURE 5.4:   ACR. (A) Grade 0R: normal myocardium contains few scattered lymphocytes and other interstitial cells (H&E, original magnification, 400×). (B) Grade 1R: focal perivascular lymphocytic infiltrate without myocyte injury (H&E; original magnification, 400×). (C) Grade 1R: diffuse sparse interstitial lymphocytic infiltrate without myocyte injury. (D) Grade 1R: single aggressive focus of lymphocytic infiltrate that extends into the adjacent myocardium and is associated with myocyte injury (circled area) (H&E; original magnification, 200×). (E) Grade 2R: multifocal aggressive lymphocytic infiltrates with associated myocyte injury (not apparent at this magnification). Note that there are still intervening areas of uninvolved myocardium (H&E; original magnification, 100×). (F) Grade 3R: diffuse predominantly mononuclear interstitial infiltrate with moderate architecture distortion and myocyte injury (H&E; original magnification, 400×). (G) Grade 3R: polymorphous inflammatory infiltrate with marked architectural distortion and myocyte injury (H&E; original magnification, 400×). (H) Although there are numerous CD3+ T lymphocytes, they usually comprise less than 50 percent of the inflammatory infiltrate (original magnification, 200×). (I) In ACR, CD68+ macrophages usually comprise more than 50 percent of the infiltrating cells (original magnification, 200×). (J) Scattered CD20+ B lymphocytes may be present in ACR (original magnification, 200×).

importantly, the necrosis present is coagulation necrosis, not myocytolysis as seen in rejection. The infiltrate and connective tissue present will vary depending on the time interval between the onset of ischemic injury and the EMB (11). Note that contraction bands are a common artifact in EMBs and should not be construed as contraction band necrosis indicative of ischemic injury (23).

Previous biopsy sites are common histological findings in EMBs that can potentially result in an erroneous diagnosis of ACR. Observed in only 16 percent of EMBs in the immediate postoperative period, they are more frequently seen in patients who have undergone repeated

biopsies (29). In one study, changes of a previous biopsy site were evident in nearly 70 percent of EMBs (30). Due to anatomical considerations and the fact that the bioptome is not easily maneuverable within the right ventricle, only a limited portion of the interventricular septum is sampled. A variety of histopathological findings can be seen depending on the stage of wound healing (30–32). Recent biopsy sites exhibit granulation tissue, surface thrombus, interstitial hemorrhage, coagulative necrosis of myocytes, mixed mononuclear and polymorphonuclear infiltrate, and karyorrhectic debris (Figure 5.5A). Later biopsy site changes include variable fibrosis,

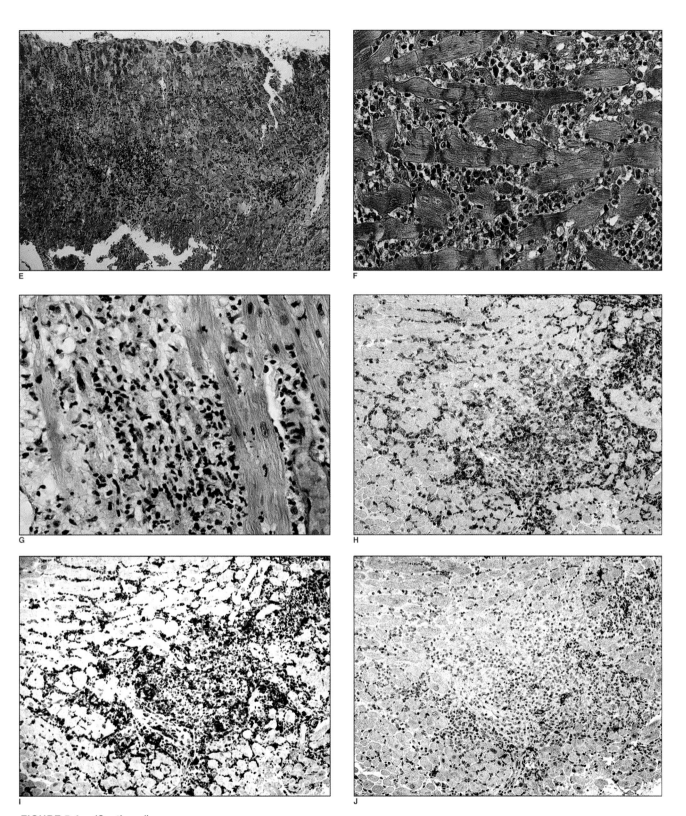

FIGURE 5.4: (Continued)

mononuclear cell infiltrate, hemosiderin-laden macrophages, and entrapped haphazardly arranged myocytes (Figure 5.5B). Old biopsy sites demonstrate endocardial and subendocardial dense fibrous scar tissue with scant

mononuclear cell infiltrate (Figure 5.5C). Confusion with ACR occurs when there is a prominent mononuclear cell infiltrate in association with myocyte damage (Figure 5.5D). However, ACR usually exhibits myocytolysis rather than coagulative necrosis of myocytes. Useful clues for a previous biopsy site include the endocardial location, the "punched-out" configuration, and the presence of fibrin, which is generally not seen in ACR.

QE is an inflammatory infiltrate that may be confined to the endocardium (Quilty A, QA) or infiltrate the myocardium (Quilty B, QB) and consists of varying proportions of T and B lymphocytes, macrophages, plasma cells, and occasional eosinophils. Characteristically, many small blood vessels are also present. QE can be mistaken for ACR when it extends into the myocardium and does not exhibit an obvious connection to the overlying endocardium due to tangential sectioning. This endocardial connection, however, can be demonstrated by obtaining serial deeper sections. In problematic cases, immunohistochemistry can be used to distinguish ACR from QE (21,33). In ACR, the majority of the infiltrating cells are CD3+ T lymphocytes (usually less than 50 percent) (Figure 5.4H) and CD68+ macrophages (usually more than 50 percent) (Figure 5.4I). Only a minor proportion of the inflammatory infiltrate consists of CD20+ B lymphocytes (Figure 5.4J). In contrast, QE consists of a significant proportion of CD3+ T lymphocytes (usually greater than 50 percent) and CD20+ B lymphocytes. Only scattered CD68+ macrophages (usually less than 50 percent) are present.

Post-transplant infections, notably cytomegalovirus (CMV) and toxoplasmosis, can produce a predominantly lymphocytic infiltrate in the myocardium (20,22). CMV can be distinguished from ACR by the characteristic viral inclusions in the myocytes and the presence of a significant neutrophilic component to the inflammatory infiltrate. The histological diagnosis of toxoplasmosis can be made when a toxoplasma cyst is visualized within the cardiomyocyte. Other infections, including Chagas disease, have also been reported.

Post-transplant lymphoproliferative disorders (PTLDs) can be distinguished from ACR by the presence of an intense inflammatory infiltrate consisting of large, atypical lymphocytes. In addition, there is usually little associated myocyte damage (20). Immunohistochemistry demonstrating sheets of CD20+ B cells or CD138+ plasmacytoid cells is also highly suggestive of PTLD. In addition, Epstein-Barr virus (EBV) genome can often be detected in the atypical lymphocytes using in situ hybridization. Molecular studies for Ig gene rearrangements can be performed on EMB material in difficult cases.

The majority of ACR cases are diagnosed by surveillance EMBs when the patients are asymptomatic. The *symptoms*, when present, are often vague and nonspecific and may include myalgia, low-grade fever, and flu-like symptoms. Some patients may present with symptoms of left ventricular dysfunction, such as orthopnea, dyspnea on exertion or at rest, paroxysmal nocturnal dyspnea, palpitations, near-syncope, or syncope. Less commonly, ACR manifests as atrial arrhythmias, including atrial premature depolarization, atrial flutter, or atrial fibrillation (34,35).

Gastrointestinal symptoms, likely secondary to hepatic congestion from the increase in central venous pressure, can occasionally occur, confound, and delay the diagnosis of rejection. Echocardiography may confirm left ventricular dysfunction by revealing an acute decline in systolic function or newly developed diastolic dysfunction.

Given the costs and possible complications arising from EMBs, many noninvasive methods to detect or monitor for ACR have been examined. However, despite extensive research and innovation in this field, the EMB remains the most sensitive, specific, and clinically useful method of rejection surveillance currently available (36). Noninvasive ancillary studies fall into two main categories: those that monitor changes in myocardial structure and function and those that assess immunologic or intragraft events. The former techniques include nuclear magnetic resonance imaging (37), magnetic resonance spectroscopy (38), Doppler echocardiography (39–43), hemodynamic monitoring electrocardiography (44), and intramyocardial electrograms (45–50). Intragraft and immunologic assessments include measurement of cardiac troponin T (51,52), coagulation markers (53), B-type natriuretic peptide (54), leukocyte membrane and complement activation markers (55,56), prostaglandin (57), markers of nitric oxide generation (58), annexin-V imaging (59), radiolabeled lymphocytes (60), anti-myosin antibody (61), soluble interleukin 2 (IL-2) receptor levels in serum (62), and gene expression profiling (GEP) of peripheral blood lymphocytes (63–65).

Since January 2005, GEP has been used clinically in several cardiac transplant programs to help exclude allograft rejection and assess risk for moderate/severe rejection. GEP has been shown to discriminate between quiescence (grade 0) and moderate/severe ACR (2004 revised ISHLT grade ≥2R) in the large, multicenter Cardiac Allograft Rejection Gene Expression Observational (CARGO) study (64). The test uses real-time polymerase chain reaction (PCR) technology to measure the expression of twenty genes in peripheral blood mononuclear cells (63–65). A multigene algorithm generates a score ranging from 0 to 40, with lower scores being associated with a very low likelihood of moderate/severe ACR (63). Beyond one year post-transplant, patients with a low score were very unlikely to have grade 2R or 3R rejection, obviating the need for biopsy in certain settings (64). However, transcriptome or gene expression studies are known to have poor replicability (66). To further validate the GEP method, long-term follow-up and independent confirmation of the above findings may be necessary.

Over the years, the immunosuppressive regimens have evolved from azathioprine, high-dose corticosteroids, and antithymocyte globulin used in the late 1960s to calcineurin inhibitors in the 1980s and 1990s (67,68). With the introduction of cyclosporine, a calcineurin inhibitor, there have been dramatic improvements in patient survival

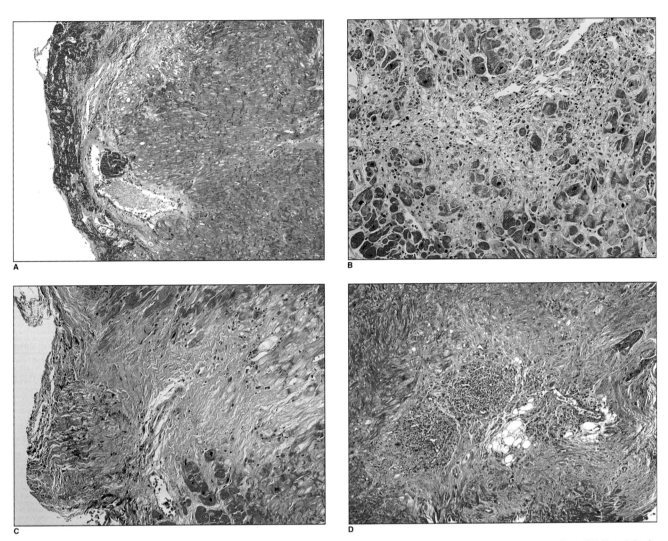

FIGURE 5.5: *Previous biopsy site. (A) Very recent biopsy site exhibiting fresh thrombus on the endocardial surface (H&E; original magnification, 100×). (B) Less recent biopsy site demonstrating granulation tissue with variable collagen deposition, myocyte injury, hemosiderin-laden macrophages, and a scattered mononuclear inflammatory infiltrate (H&E; original magnification, 200×). (C) Old biopsy site showing dense fibrous tissue with little or no inflammation. Note the punched out configuration (H&E; original magnification, 200×). (D) Old biopsy site with prominent mononuclear inflammatory infiltrate. Note the presence of hemosiderin-laden macrophages and the haphazardly arranged myocytes (H&E; original magnification, 100×).*

and decreased rejection (68); however, the use of cyclosporine is fraught with side effects, many that are severe (69). Tacrolimus, another calcineurin inhibitor, achieves comparable survival rates with somewhat fewer effects to other organ systems (70). Proliferation signal inhibitors such as sirolimus and everolimus are currently under study as complementary immunosuppressive therapy to calcineurin inhibitors. These proliferation signal inhibitors have been shown to prevent ACR and reduce the development of CAV (71). However, they are also associated with worsened renal function and impaired wound healing (72,73). Mycophenolate mofetil (MMF) has largely replaced azathioprine as patients treated with MMF had significant reduction in mortality at one year and decreased need for rejection treatment (74). Induction therapy with OKT3, IL-2 antagonists, and antithymocyte

globulins is used in approximately 40 percent of heart transplant patients to reduce rejection in the early post-transplant period (75).

The choice of therapy for ACR depends on the histological grade, presence of symptoms, signs of hemodynamic compromise, and the particular treatment protocol used at individual transplant centers. In general, low rejection grades (grades 1R) in the absence of hemodynamic dysfunction or worrisome symptoms are not treated since these patients are at low risk for progression into higher grade rejection, may resolve without treatment, and do not show significant resolution in response to treatment (76,77). The EMB may be repeated at an earlier time or blood levels of immunosuppressive agents may be measured. When there is concomitant hemodynamic compromise with the histological diagnosis of mild or focal moderate ACR, high-dose corticosteroids or antilymphocyte therapy such as antithymocyte globulin or OKT3 may be used. Grade 2R rejection without hemodynamic compromise warrants a transient increase in dose or an oral/intravenous pulse of corticosteroids (78,79). The patient usually undergoes weekly EMB for two weeks to ensure histological resolution after completion of treatment.

In cases of severe ACR, defined as grade 3R rejection, grade 2R rejection with hemodynamic compromise, or rejection refractory to corticosteroids, patients may be treated preferentially with antithymocyte globulin or OKT3. In cases of refractory or recurrent rejection, photopheresis has been a successful treatment modality by several reports (80–82).

V. ANTIBODY-MEDIATED REJECTION

AMR in cardiac transplantation is an underrecognized form of allograft dysfunction that was first described by Hammond et al. (83). Unlike ACR that involves better characterized cell-mediated immune mechanisms, graft injury results from deposition of antibody within the microvasculature of the cardiac allograft and subsequent complement activation via the classical pathway, that is, the humoral arm of the immune system. Also known as vascular (or microvascular) humoral rejection, this form of rejection typically targets the vasculature of the cardiac allograft, most notably the capillaries. Only recently has the ISHLT recognized AMR as a real and distinct clinicopathological entity (22,84).

The reported incidence of AMR is highly variable ranging from 2.7 to 59 percent (83,85–90). In one study, only 5 of 165 patients (3 percent) met the criteria of concurrent clinical and immunopathological evidence of AMR. This low rate was attributed to lack of allosensitization in most of the patients and fewer left ventricular assist device (LVAD) implantations prior to transplantation (90). In contrast, higher rates of AMR were observed in medical centers where antilymphocyte therapy such as OKT3 was frequently used (89,91,92). There are a variety of predisposing factors that have been identified for the development of AMR in cardiac transplant recipients, including female gender (89,93–95), CMV seropositivity (96–98), allosensitization as indicated by elevated panel reactive antibodies or a positive cross-match (99–101), and OKT3 therapy (89,91,92,102). Risk factors for allosensitization include pregnancy (103,104), multiple blood transfusions (104,105), prior organ transplantation (106), and LVAD implantation (107–111), possibly related to associated blood transfusions.

Typically, AMR is seen early after transplantation, most commonly within the first month (83,89,94). In patients presensitized to donor HLA antigens, it may occur as early as two to seven days after transplantation (112). Less commonly, AMR may develop months to years after transplantation. Clinically, patients with AMR may be asymptomatic or manifest evidence of mild to severe allograft dysfunction (83,86,89,94). A study by Michaels et al. showed that hemodynamic dysfunction, which consisted of shock, hypotension, decreased cardiac output/index, and/or a rise in capillary wedge or pulmonary artery pressure, was seen in 47 percent of patients at the time of AMR diagnosis (94). In addition, 68 percent of early AMR patients (less than one month) had graft dysfunction as compared to only 13 percent of late AMR patients (between one month and two years). Moreover, Michaels et al. observed that females with AMR were more likely to exhibit hemodynamic dysfunction than males (59 versus 33 percent).

The underlying pathogenesis of AMR is the deposition of alloantibodies and subsequent complement activation in the microvasculature of the cardiac allograft. For most patients with AMR, donor reactive antibodies develop de novo after transplantation and are generally absent pretransplant (113). It is well documented that most cardiac transplant patients develop alloantibodies within six months after transplantation (114). It appears that the allograft provides a powerful stimulus to alloantibody production that may possibly be related to antigen release subsequent to mechanical or immunological injury of the allograft (115,116). These alloantibodies are usually directed against MHC class I or II determinants, which are both constitutively expressed on capillary endothelium (116–118). However, other non-HLA antigens such as major histocompatibility class I–related chain A (MICA) (119), vimentin (120), skeletal muscle (121), and cardiac myosin (121) may also be targeted. The presence of anti-HLA antibodies is strongly correlated with AMR, decreased allograft survival, and increased mortality in cardiac transplant recipients (102,117,122,123).

The major target of circulating anti-HLA antibodies is the capillary endothelium of the cardiac allograft (113,124). Antibody binding to allograft endothelium triggers complement activation and formation of the terminal complement components, C5b-C9 (membrane attack complex), resulting in endothelial cell death (necrosis or apoptosis). This leads to detachment of the endothelial cells from the underlying matrix with resultant loss of vascular integrity and disruption of endothelial function. Moreover, complement fixation activates endothelial cells resulting in enhanced expression of surface leukocyte adhesion molecules, production and secretion of cytokines, and activation of the clotting and fibrinolytic systems. The consequences of endothelial cell death and activation include microvascular thrombosis, interstitial hemorrhage and edema, inflammatory cell infiltration, and myocardial and vascular necrosis, leading to cardiac allograft dysfunction and graft failure in occasional cases. Production of proliferative and fibrogenic growth factors by activated endothelial cells may play an important role in the pathogenesis of CAV (125).

In recent years, significant advances in the ability to detect circulating alloantibodies as well as better immunohistochemical techniques to detect complement-split products such as C3d and C4d have improved our ability to accurately diagnose AMR (84,126). This is further facilitated by the recent inclusion of diagnostic criteria for AMR in the revised ISHLT grading scheme for cardiac allograft rejection (Tables 5.2 and 5.3) (22,84). In this schema, every EMB specimen is subjected to a critical evaluation for the histological features of AMR. If such features are absent, the EMB should be designated negative for AMR (AMR 0). If features of AMR are present, confirmation using either IF on frozen tissue or immunoperoxidase (IP) staining on paraffinized tissue and testing for donor-specific HLA class I and II antibodies and non-HLA antibodies should be performed. A positive diagnosis of AMR (AMR 1) is rendered when these ancillary studies are positive. Moreover, patients with several episodes of documented acute AMR should subsequently be followed on future biopsies utilizing one of the immunohistochemical methods and monitored for production of donor-specific antibodies.

TABLE 5.2 ISHLT Recommendations for AMR (84)

AMR 0	Negative for AMR
	No histological evidence of AMR
AMR 1	Positive for AMR
	Histological features of AMR
	Positive IF for AMR
	Positive immunoperoxidase staining for AMR

TABLE 5.3 Diagnostic Criteria for AMR (84)

Clinical Evidence of Graft Dysfunction

Histological evidence of tissue injury (a and b required for diagnosis)
    Capillary endothelial changes: swelling or denudation
    Intravascular macrophages
    Intravascular neutrophils
    Interstitial edema, congestion, and/or hemorrhage

Immunopathological evidence for antibody-mediated injury
    Ig (G, M, and/or A) + C3d and/or C4d or C1q (equivalent staining in capillaries, 2+ to 3+) by IF studies on frozen tissue
    CD68+ macrophages within capillaries (identified using CD31 or CD34), and/or C4d capillary staining (2+ to 3+) by immunoperoxidase staining on paraffinized tissue
    Fibrin in vessels (optional; if present, process is reported as more severe)

Serological evidence of anti-HLA class I and/or class II antibodies or other anti-donor antibody at time of endomyocardial biopsy

Macroscopically, the heart is heavy and swollen with diffuse hemorrhagic discoloration of the myocardium and focal areas of coagulation necrosis (Figure 5.6A). *Histological* features of AMR include capillary congestion, "endothelial cell swelling," interstitial edema and hemorrhage (Figure 5.6B), neutrophil infiltration (Figure 5.6C), and intravascular thrombi (83,89). There is also a prominent intravascular accumulation of macrophages that often distends the capillaries (Figure 5.6D). The term, endothelial cell swelling, applies to the morphological appearance of injured endothelial cells, which is characterized by cytoplasmic swelling and nuclear enlargement. Although some swollen endothelial cells are present, most of the intravascular cells have been shown to be macrophages by IP staining for CD68 (Figure 5.6E) (94). The intravascular location can be confirmed by performing a CD34 (or CD31) immunostain (Figure 5.6F). Not infrequently, histological features of concurrent ACR may be present (83,89). The combination of AMR and ACR has been termed "mixed rejection." In one study, approximately half of AMR biopsies had mild ACR (89). Furthermore, five of thirty-three (15 percent) AMR biopsies with associated abnormal hemodynamics had moderate to severe ACR.

Although the revised ISHLT grading scheme for cardiac allograft rejection recommends a critical histological evaluation for AMR (22,84), a recent study by Hammond et al. showed that histological parameters of endothelial cell changes and intravascular accumulation of macrophages lacked sufficient sensitivity to serve as screening tools for further investigation of AMR (127). Examining their own experience with these histological parameters, they constructed ROC curves of the relationship of endothelial cell changes and intravascular accumulation of macrophages to AMR. They found that these histological features were poor predictors of AMR. In their study, only 30 percent of biopsies negative for ACR showed significant endothelial cell changes. Even when considering only positive endothelial activation, the sensitivity remained low at 63 percent. Thus, using this histological feature alone to screen for AMR would have resulted in more than 33 percent of AMR-positive biopsies that would not have been subjected to IP confirmation. For the histological feature of intravascular macrophage accumulation, they found that 92 percent of biopsies with this finding were positive for AMR by IF. However, this finding only occurred in 29 percent of AMR-positive biopsies. Consequently, intravascular macrophage accumulation was highly specific for AMR but lacked sufficient sensitivity to serve as a screening tool for AMR. If their results are validated by others, the authors believe that screening recommendations should be modified to include more sensitive IP screening methods for patients at high risk for AMR. Obviously, the ability to demonstrate the histopathology of AMR by light microscopy is highly dependent on the quality of the histological sections. This in turn is

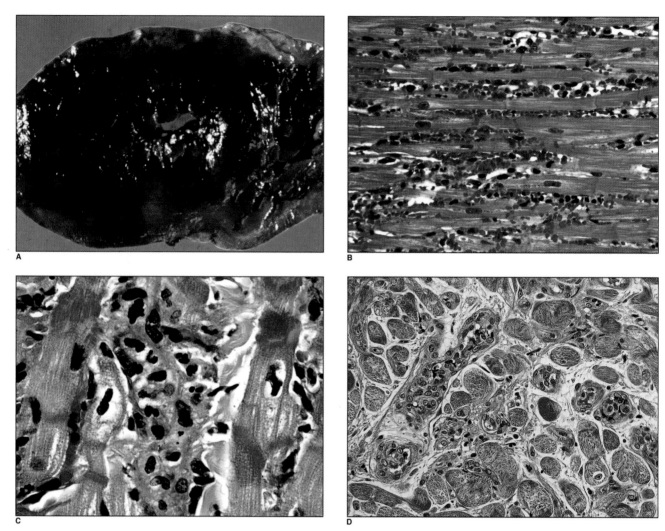

FIGURE 5.6: *AMR. (A) Grossly, the heart is swollen and heavy with a diffusely hemorrhagic myocardium. (B) Histological sections confirm the presence of prominent interstitial hemorrhage (H&E; original magnification, 400×). (C) A neutrophilic infiltrate may be present within the capillaries (H&E; original magnification, 400×). (D) The characteristic feature is intravascular accumulation of macrophages that distend the capillaries (H&E; original magnification, 400×). (E) Immunohistochemical staining for CD68 demonstrates that the majority of the intravascular inflammatory cells are indeed macrophages (original magnification, 400×). (F) The intravascular location of these macrophages can be confirmed by performing immunoperoxidase stains for CD34 (original magnification, 400×). (G) IF staining for C4d demonstrates strong and diffuse (3+) linear capillary staining (original magnification, 400×). (H) Immunoperoxidase staining for C4d also exhibits strong and diffuse (3+) linear capillary staining (original magnification, 400×).*

dependent on a number of factors including optimal fixation and processing of the tissue.

When the diagnosis of AMR is suspected histologically, it can be confirmed by performing IF microscopy on frozen tissue. Diffuse, linear staining (2+ to 3+) in capillaries for immunoglobulin (IgG, IgM, and/or IgA) and complement (C3d and/or C4d or C1q) is considered diagnostic of AMR (Figure 5.6G) (83,89). Moreover, some studies have shown that the accumulation of interstitial fibrin on IF denotes a more severe process (92,128). If frozen tissue is not available, IP staining can be performed on paraffinized tissue to demonstrate macrophages (CD68) within capillaries (CD31 or CD34) (94) and/or C4d deposition in capillaries (Figure 5.6H) (86,90,128). Only multifocal (2+)

or diffuse (3+) capillary staining is considered positive. C4d deposition can be evaluated using either IF or IP technique. A study comparing these two methods showed good sensitivity and specificity for the IP method, with the IF method being considered the gold standard (129).

C4d is the final split product derived from C4 during activation of the classical complement pathway (126,130). Due to a reactive thioester group, it is capable of forming a strong covalent bond with nearby structures such as the endothelium and can persist for several days to weeks. Its longer half-life allows it to serve as a good marker of complement activation and thus can be a useful indicator of AMR in cardiac transplant recipients (86,90,128). Microvascular deposition of C4d in cardiac allografts has been

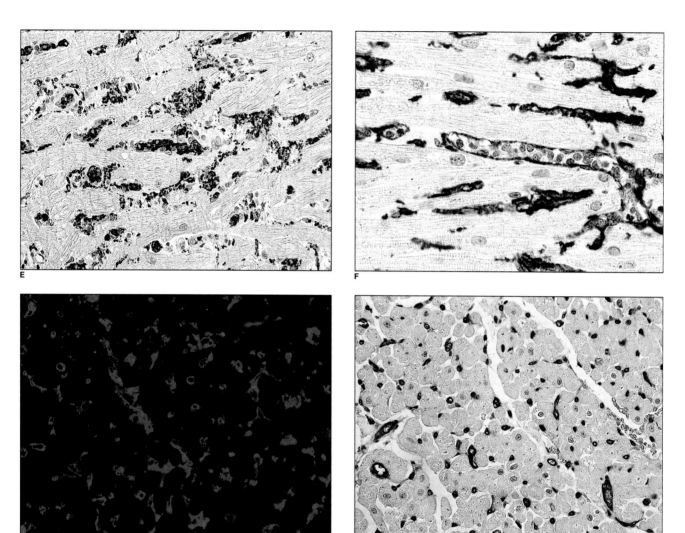

FIGURE 5.6: *(Continued)*

demonstrated to correlate with increased graft loss and development of CAV at one year after transplantation (128,131). It also correlated well with anti-donor serum alloantibodies with a sensitivity of 84 percent and a specificity of 89 percent (132). In another study, an association was found between C4d positivity and ischemic injury in early cardiac transplant biopsies (133). However, this association was not confirmed by others (129,134). Less commonly, C4d deposition may occur in the absence of clinical and/or histological evidence of AMR. One possible explanation is that these cardiac allografts have achieved a state of accommodation. Accommodation may result from abrogation or regulation of complement fixation by complement regulatory proteins such that tissue injury does not occur (135). Endothelial cells from "accommodated" allografts have shown increased expression of complement regulatory proteins such as CD59 as well as protective, anti-apoptotic molecules including A20, heme oxygenase-1 (HO-1), bcl-2, and bcl-xL (136–138). Consequently, C4d deposition by itself should *not* be equated with AMR.

The clearance of C4d from allografts has anecdotally been reported to occur within weeks (139). This is confounded by several factors including incomplete removal of circulating antibodies by plasmapheresis or other treatments, redistribution of antibodies from interstitial compartments, and continued antibody production. To overcome these confounding factors, Minami et al. (140) utilized a rat model of heart transplantation in which DA rat hearts were transplanted into Lewis rat recipients after pre-sensitization to DA rats via blood transfusions. When DA rat heart allografts from Lewis rat recipients were retransplanted back into isogeneic DA rat recipients, C4d deposits were decreased to minimal levels within five days. One possible explanation for this rapid clearance is that sublytic quantities of MAC (C5b-C9) cause exocytosis and endocytosis of portions of the cell membrane containing C4d.

Recently, Lepin et al. showed that phosphorylated S6 ribosomal protein (p-S6RP) is a potentially useful biomarker for the diagnosis of AMR (141). Using IP techniques to detect the level of S6RP in EMBs from heart transplant recipients, and correlating the results with histopathological diagnosis of rejection, C4d staining, production of post-transplant anti-HLA antibodies, and clinical outcome, the authors demonstrated a strong association between the diagnosis of AMR and the presence of p-S6RP in the graft capillary endothelium. The authors also found that C4d staining was positively associated with both AMR and p-S6RP. Moreover, post-transplant anti-HLA class II antibody production was significantly associated with a positive p-S6RP in cardiac biopsies.

AMR responds poorly to conventional therapy, which mainly targets cell-mediated immune function responsible for ACR. Behr et al. showed that immunosuppressive regimens that consisted of glucocorticosteroids, azathioprine, and either cyclosporine or FK506 were not capable of preventing AMR (142). Although both cyclosporine and FK506 prevent T-lymphocyte activation by inhibiting IL-2 synthesis (143,144), they do not suppress the B-cell–driven processes of AMR. Currently, AMR has been successfully treated with some combination of plasmapheresis, intravenous immune globulin, cyclophosphamide, anti-CD20 monoclonal antibody, or immunoadsorption (145–152).

VI. HYPERACUTE REJECTION

Hyperacute rejection (HAR) is a form of AMR that typically occurs within minutes to hours of implantation and results in extremely rapid destruction of the cardiac allograft. It is an extremely rare complication due to preformed antibodies to ABO, HLA, or donor vascular endothelial cell antigens. Classic HAR has been arbitrarily defined as developing within twenty-four hours following transplantation. The term, delayed HAR, is used when the onset occurs after twenty-four hours following transplantation. Classically, the pathogenesis of HAR is believed to result from antibody-mediated complement fixation and activation leading to destruction of capillary endothelial cells with associated secondary hemorrhage, thrombosis, and necrosis of the allograft. However, morphological studies in discordant xenografts indicate that antibody-mediated damage occurs primarily in the cardiac venules resulting in microvascular venular thrombosis (153–156). The morphological findings of HAR have been well described in discordant xenografts and human cardiac allografts and are similar to those of the previously described AMR (157,158).

VII. QUILTY EFFECT

The QE lesion is a nodular endocardial infiltrate that is frequently encountered in post-transplant EMBs. It consists of a chronic inflammatory cell infiltrate within the endocardium (QA) that can extend into the underlying myocardium (QB). QE is present in 10–20 percent of post-transplant EMBs (159,160) and is seen in 50–60 percent of post-cardiac transplant patients with a higher incidence in younger patients (161–163). QE is typically seen in EMBs within the first year after transplantation and in subsequent biopsies (163).

The etiology of QE is unknown. Most importantly, it has not been definitively shown to be a manifestation of ACR, chronic rejection, or to be associated with graft dysfunction (160,163). For this reason, QE is not treated with increased immunosuppression. A number of theories for its pathogenesis have been proposed since it was first described by Dr. Margaret Billingham in patients undergoing immunosuppressive regimens with cyclosporine. The original theory was that these endocardial inflammatory infiltrates were an idiosyncratic or toxic reaction to cyclosporine (159,164), or due to locally reduced cyclosporine levels in the endocardium (165). However, QE has been shown to occur with other immunosuppressive regimens such as FK506 (166). The pathogenesis of QE has also been associated with localized EBV infection (167) and early PTLD (168), but other studies have shown no definitive link (162–164,167).

QE is typically thought of as distinct from rejection, but a controversial link with ACR (169,170) and chronic rejection (161,171) has persisted. Some recent studies have analyzed the molecular pathways underlying QE and its possible links to rejection. A recent immunopathological study highlighted a similar molecular pathway (CXCL13-led B-cell recruitment) shared between QE and recurrent ACR episodes (172). The significance of this finding is unknown. Yamani et al. showed that increased expression of vitronectin receptor (integrin alphavbeta3) is present in ACR and chronic rejection (171,173). Another study demonstrated a link between low IL-10 production genotype and QE (174). It was suggested that this genotype may support the theory that QE represents abortive stages of ACR. Currently, a definitive explanation for the pathogenesis of QE has remained elusive.

QE can be unifocal or multifocal. Histologically, QE is a nodular collection of mononuclear cells in a background of abundant small blood vessels. Immunohistochemical evaluation demonstrates that the mononuclear cells are primarily T lymphocytes with admixed B lymphocytes, plasma cells, and scattered macrophages. QE has historically been divided into two subtypes: QA, which is confined to the endocardium (Figure 5.7A), and QB, in which the endocardial inflammatory infiltrate extends into the underlying myocardium (Figure 5.7B) where it can be associated with myocyte damage (Figure 5.7C). Less commonly, QE is encountered in the epicardium and deep within the myocardium (175). One case of QE within a coronary artery has recently been reported (176).

Because there was no clinical significance between QA and QB, the "A" and "B" designations were dropped in the most recent ISHLT classification (22). Although clinically insignificant, the nomenclature is still useful for practicing pathologists as QB can histologically mimic

ACR. Several studies have demonstrated the difficulties in distinguishing QB from 1990 ISHLT grade 2 or 3A ACR (27,177). The distinction between these two entities is important as a diagnosis of ACR may lead to unnecessary augmentation of immunosuppression and its accompanying comorbidities.

QE is ordinarily not difficult to differentiate from ACR when the lymphocytic infiltrate is confined to or connects with the endocardium. Difficulties in distinguishing these two lesions may arise due to tangential sectioning of the trabeculated endocardial surface. In these cases, there can be a myocardial lymphocytic infiltrate associated with myocyte damage with no obvious connection to the endocardium (Figure 5.7D) (25).

QB can be distinguished from ACR on H&E stains by the density of the infiltrate, presence of plasma cells, background fibrosis, and prominent vascularity (22). The use of deeper sections to demonstrate that the lymphocytic infiltrate is contiguous with the endocardium has been shown to help distinguish between QB and grade 2 rejection. One report using this methodology showed that 91 percent (thirty-two of thirty-five) of grade 2 rejections were actually QB calling into question the existence of grade 2 rejection (25). Moreover, IP studies can aid in distinguishing QB from ACR. The latter is characterized by greater than 50 percent macrophages in the inflammatory infiltrate, whereas the former exhibits scattered macrophages (Figure 5.7E) and greater than 50 percent T lymphocytes in the inflammatory infiltrate (Figure 5.7F) (21). B lymphocytes can be present in both ACR and QB, although they are usually more abundant in QB (Figure 5.7G) (33). A recent study showed that twenty-four of thirty-two QBs and twenty-three of twenty-four QBs larger than 0.3 mm contained a follicular dendritic cell network that can be highlighted by CD21 to help differentiate them from ACR (178).

In the latest ISHLT heart rejection scale, grade 2 rejection was grouped along with grade 1A and 1B rejection as mild ACR (grade 1R) (22). In this classification, neither QB nor grade 2 rejections are treated, so that any histological confusion between the two lesions is not clinically significant. Although the revised ISHLT heart rejection scale helped alleviate the burden on pathologists of differentiating QB from grade 2 rejection, there can still be confusion with higher grades of ACR (28).

Other lesions that may simulate QE are PTLDs and post-transplant myocardial infections. QE contains a mixed population of cells, whereas most cases of PTLDs are composed primarily of CD20+ B cells or CD138+ plasmacytoid cells that may be polyclonal or monoclonal. Ancillary studies such as in situ hybridization for the EBV genome and molecular studies for Ig gene rearrangements may be helpful in difficult cases. QE is normally easily distinguished from post-transplant myocardial infections. Infectious processes usually contain a more polymorphous inflammatory infiltrate with neutrophils or granulomas and may be associated with more myocyte coagulation necrosis. A search for microorganisms in these cases is warranted to potentially identify the cause of the inflammatory infiltrate.

VIII. POST-TRANSPLANT INFECTIONS

Infections are a common cause of morbidity and mortality after cardiac transplantation. Cardiac transplant patients are at an increased risk for bacterial, fungal, viral, and protozoal infections due to their immunosuppressed status. Infections are the most common cause of late deaths (more than thirty days) accounting for approximately 35 percent of mortalities and is a frequent cause of early deaths (less than thirty days) accounting for 18–44 percent of mortalities (179–181).

Although infections are still common after cardiac transplantation, the frequency of infectious episodes decreased from 2.83 episodes per patient in the 1970s (182) to 1.73 per patient between 1980 and 1996 (181). In comparison to a prior study by Hofflin et al. in the 1980s (183), a more recent study showed an increase in median onset (in days) after transplantation (MOT) for all infections (181). The decreased number of infections and increased MOT was attributed to improved immunosuppression, specifically the introduction of cyclosporine and new antimicrobial prophylaxis regimens. These regimens include gancyclovir against CMV infection, trimethoprim-sulfamethoxazole primarily against *Pneumocystis jiroveci*, and inhaled amphotericin B against fungal infections. The increased MOT of CMV from forty-four days (183) to seventy-one days (181) is significant as CMV infection has been postulated to worsen the net state of immunosuppression in patients after organ transplantation. It is postulated that CMV encodes proteins that affect the host immune environment by modulating molecules involved in immune recognition and inflammation leading to increased infections (184).

Several large series reveal variations in the incidence and types of infections that afflict patient populations of different institutions, primarily due to differences in the type, duration, and intensity of the immunosuppressive regimens (179–181,185,186). Augmentation of immunosuppression and steroid-containing immunosuppressive regimens have been associated with increased infections in cardiac transplant recipients (179). In addition, different antimicrobial prophylaxis regimens as well as geographical variations in the prevalence of microorganisms may influence the incidence and types of infections.

Bacterial and viral infections are the most common post-cardiac transplant infections accounting for approximately 80–90 percent of all infections (179–181,185,186). Fungal infections are less common accounting for approximately 5–15 percent of all infections but are associated with the highest mortality (23–36 percent)

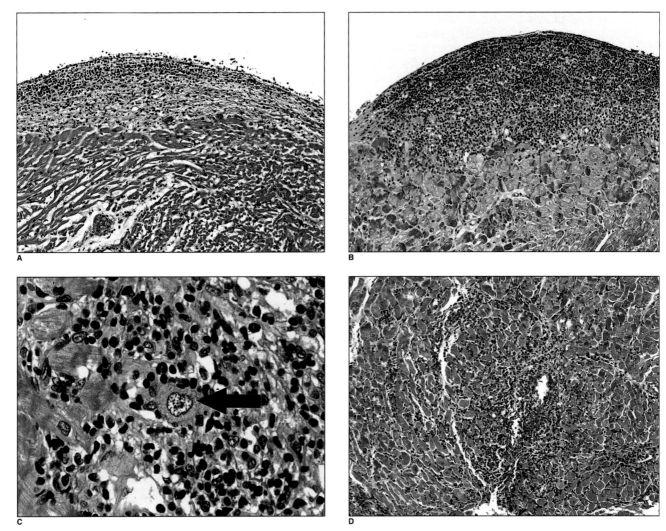

FIGURE 5.7: QE. (A) Quilty A lesion exhibiting nodular chronic inflammatory infiltrate involving the endocardium without significant infiltration of the subjacent myocardium (H&E; original magnification, 100×). (B) In contrast, Quilty B lesion infiltrates into the underlying myocardium (H&E; original magnification, 100×). (C) Occasionally, myocyte injury (arrow) may be observed in Quilty B lesions (H&E; original magnification, 400×). (D) Tangentially sectioned QE can be difficult to distinguish from ACR (H&E; original magnification, 200×). (E) CD68 immunostain shows only scattered macrophages in the inflammatory infiltrate (original magnification, 200×). (F) Most of the inflammatory infiltrate consists of CD3+ T lymphocytes (original magnification, 200×). (G) Both ACR and QE have CD20+ B lymphocytes; however, they are generally more numerous in QE as in this case (original magnification, 200×).

(179,181,185,186). Protozoal infections are the least common, accounting for less than 4 percent of all infections (179–181,185,186). The most common sites of infection are the lungs (179,181,185) and blood (180,186). Other common sites of infection include the oral cavity, urinary tract, skin, gastrointestinal tract, and surgical wound site (179–181,185,186). The heart is rarely the site of infection.

Most bacterial infections are caused by both gram-positive and gram-negative bacteria. Less common bacterial infections include *Nocardia asteroides*, mixed anaerobes, and *Mycoplasma pneumonia* (179,181). *Staphylococcus* species account for most of the gram-positive bacterial infections (36–52 percent of all infections), many of which are methicillin resistant (180,181,185). Other common gram-positive bacterial infections are due to *Enterococcus* and *Streptococcus*

species (181). *Escherichia coli* and *Pseudomonas aeruginosa* account for the majority of gram-negative bacterial infections (180,181,185). Other common gram-negative bacterial infections are due to *Klebsiella pneumoniae* (180) and *Legionella pneumophilia* (179,181).

Before the introduction of gancyclovir prophylaxis, CMV was the most common viral infection accounting for 23–26 percent of total infections (179,185,186). Two recent studies show that CMV is still a common post-cardiac transplant viral infection accounting for 4.7 percent (180) and 14.1 percent (181) of infections, but herpes simplex virus and varicella zoster virus are now more common (180,181).

The most common causes of fungal infections are *Candida* and *Aspergillus* species accounting for 83 percent of

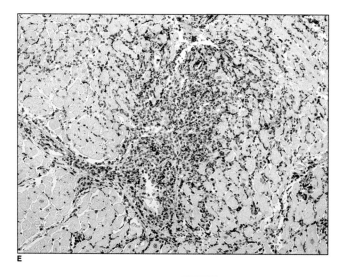

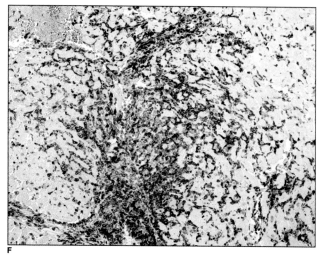

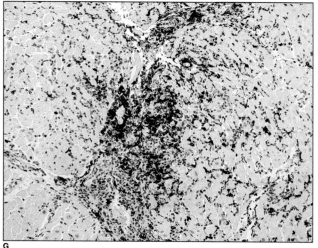

FIGURE 5.7: *(Continued)*

total fungal infections in one recent study (181). Infections due to *Aspergillus* (Figure 5.8A) are associated with high mortality rates (up to 60 percent) (181). *Toxoplasma* infections account for the majority of protozoal infections and are also associated with high mortality rates (up to 100 percent) (179,181,185). Other protozoal infections are due to vaginal trichomoniasis and intestinal giardiasis (181,185).

The incidence of some infections varies geographically with the patient population studied. *Mycobacterium tuberculosis* is an uncommon infection in post-cardiac transplant patients from the United States, accounting for less than 1 percent of infections (181,185). Hsu et al. demonstrated higher rates of *M. tuberculosis* infection in their series (3.6 percent), which the authors attributed to the endemic nature of this infection in Taiwan (180). The same study also showed less than 1 percent infection with *P. jiroveci* and a 4.7 percent infection rate with CMV, while several other studies showed higher rates of *Pneumocystis* infection (3–6.9 percent) (179,181,185) and CMV infection (15–25 percent) (179,181,185,186).

Rarely, some infections can disseminate from host organs to involve the allograft heart. The most commonly diagnosed microorganisms on EMBs are *Toxoplasma* and CMV. These infections can be primary or due to reactivation of the disease. Histologically, these infections can be associated with little to no inflammation, or alternatively, there can be a marked inflammatory infiltrate with neutrophils and eosinophils. When there is marked inflammation and myocyte damage, there may be confusion with ACR.

CMV infections are rarely diagnosed histologically. Myocardial involvement by CMV only occurs with primary infection (187). The characteristic enlarged cells with large, basophilic intranuclear inclusions and smaller intracytoplasmic inclusions (Figure 5.8B) are typically not seen on biopsy. Immunohistochemistry may be helpful in identifying CMV, but serology is more sensitive for diagnosing CMV infections.

Toxoplasma infections caused by the protozoan *Toxoplasma gondii* are more readily diagnosed on histology.

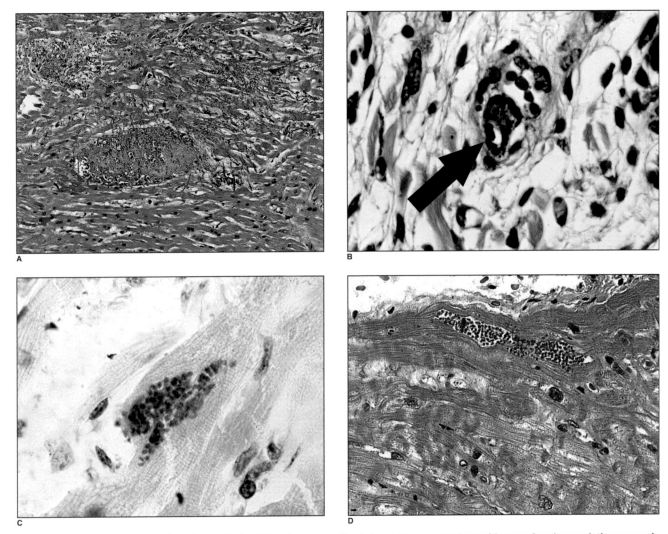

FIGURE 5.8:   *Post-transplant infections. (A) Angioinvasive aspergillosis involving myocardium with associated coagulation necrosis of myocytes (H&E; original magnification, 200×). (B) CMV infection involving the heart shows a characteristic cytomegalic endothelial cell (arrow) with intranuclear and cytoplasmic inclusions. Actual myocyte involvement is extremely rare and usually occurs with primary infection (H&E stain; original magnification, 400×). (C) Toxoplasma organisms within a cardiac myocyte with no significant associated inflammatory response (H&E stain; original magnification, 400×). (D) Trypanosoma organisms within a cardiac myocyte. Note the absence of surrounding inflammation (H&E; original magnification, 400×).*

These infections are characterized by tissue cysts and tachyzoites (Figure 5.8C), which can be identified on H&E stain. The Giemsa stain can help highlight these organisms. PCR studies are more sensitive and specific in detecting *Toxoplasma* infections and are important in diagnosing these infections.

Rare infections encountered in EMBs include Chagas disease due to infection by *Trypanosoma cruzi*. Two cases of Chagas disease in cardiac transplant recipients have been reported by the Center for Disease Control (188). At UCLA Medical Center, two cardiac transplant patients had evidence of *T. cruzi* infection in their EMBs. Review of donor and recipient demographics, one case was presumed to have originated from the donor and the second case was presumed to be reactivation of prior disease in the recipient. Histologically, rare cardiac myocytes from both

EMBs contained amastigotes with little to no surrounding inflammation (Figure 5.8D). Other portions of these biopsies showed a mixed inflammatory infiltrate consisting of lymphocytes, plasma cells, and scattered eosinophils. In a patient with suspected exposure to *T. cruzi*, a blood smear should be performed to look for trypomastigotes and tissue culture should be obtained to confirm the diagnosis. A high index of suspicion should be kept in areas where a large portion of the organ and blood donors have emigrated from countries where Chagas disease is endemic.

IX. POST-TRANSPLANT MALIGNANCY

De novo malignancy after solid organ transplantation is a well-established complication of chronic immunosuppression. Organ transplant recipients have a 100-fold greater risk of developing malignancy than the general population with an average incidence of 6 percent (range of 3–9 percent) (189). Post-transplant malignancies tend to affect a relatively younger population, the average age at the time of diagnosis being forty-seven years. Moreover, cancers that develop in the post-transplant setting are frequently more aggressive than those that occur in patients who have not undergone transplantation. In cardiac transplantation, malignancy is one of the leading causes of death three years or more after transplantation, accounting for approximately 23 percent of deaths (4). The one-, five-, and ten-year cumulative prevalence in survivors for all types of malignancy in adult heart transplant patients is 2.9, 15.1, and 31.9 percent, respectively. When compared to renal transplant recipients, there is a higher incidence of malignancy in cardiac transplant recipients, which may be a reflection of higher levels of immunosuppression to achieve rejection-free grafts (190).

Skin and lip cancers (36.8 percent) and lymphomas (16.8 percent) comprise the majority of de novo post-transplant malignancies (189). Commonly occurring cancers in the general population such as carcinomas of the lung, colon, breast, prostate, and uterine cervix are not significantly increased in transplant recipients. Other tumors that are seen in transplant patients but are uncommon in the general population include Kaposi's sarcoma, carcinomas of the kidney, carcinomas of the vulva and perineum, hepatobiliary tumors, and sarcomas (excluding Kaposi's sarcoma).

Cutaneous malignancies are the most commonly encountered type of malignancy after transplantation (189). Most of these are squamous cell carcinomas (50.1 percent), basal cell carcinomas (28.0 percent), or both (14.7 percent). In adult heart transplantation, they account for 46.1, 67.4, and 60.8 percent of malignancies at one, five, and ten years after transplantation (4). In one study, a high first-year rejection score after cardiac transplantation was independently associated with an increased risk of squamous cell carcinoma and may be related to the higher level of immunosuppression in heart transplant recipients (191). As compared to renal transplant recipients, there is a higher incidence, greater risk, and earlier development of squamous cell carcinoma (192–194).

PTLDs comprise 16.8 percent of de novo malignancies in organ allograft recipients (see chapter 10) (189). As compared to the general population, there is a greater proportion of PTLDs that are non-Hodgkin's lymphomas (93.5 versus 65 percent) and fewer Hodgkin's lymphomas and plasma cell neoplasms (2.7 versus 14 percent and 3.8 versus 21 percent, respectively). Of the non-Hodgkin's lymphomas studied immunologically, 87 percent were derived from B cells, 13 percent were derived from T cells, and less than 1 percent were of null-cell origin.

PTLDs have been reported to occur in 1.2–9 percent of cardiac transplant recipients, more frequently within the

first year after transplantation (195). In adult heart transplantation, they comprise 23.2, 9.1, and 6.4 percent of all malignancies at one, five, and ten years after transplantation, respectively (4). The risk of PTLDs is significantly greater in cardiac transplant recipients than their renal counterparts (196,197). This is likely due to differences in immunosuppressive protocols between these two transplant populations. PTLDs in cardiac transplant recipients carry a poor prognosis with Kaplan-Meier survival after PTLD diagnosis being 45, 33, 30, and 13 percent at one, three, five, and ten years, respectively (198).

EBV is a herpesvirus that has been implicated in the development of PTLD (199,200). Infection with EBV results in polyclonal activation and proliferation of B lymphocytes, which, under normal circumstances, are controlled by EBV-specific cytotoxic T lymphocytes. In the post-transplant setting, however, immunosuppressive drugs used to prevent allograft rejection suppress the activity of these cytotoxic T lymphocytes, allowing for persistence of EBV-infected B cells. Occasionally, uncontrolled proliferation of EBV-transformed B lymphocytes occurs, resulting in PTLD.

The WHO classification of tumors of hematopoietic and lymphoid tissues categorizes PTLDs into early lesions, polymorphic PTLD, monomorphic PTLD, and Hodgkin lymphoma and Hodgkin lymphoma–like PTLD (201) (see chapter 10). Early lesions consist of reactive plasma cell hyperplasia and infectious mononucleosis-like lesion. The former is characterized by the presence of abundant plasma cells and rare immunoblasts, whereas the latter has similar morphological features of infectious mononucleosis including paracortical expansion and numerous immunoblasts in a background of T cells and plasma cells. Both of these entities, however, are characterized by architectural preservation of the involved tissue. In contrast to early lesions, polymorphic PTLDs are characterized by destructive lesions that efface the lymph nodal architecture or form destructive extranodal masses. Unlike typical lymphomas, polymorphic PTLDs demonstrate the full gamut of B-cell maturation, from immunoblasts to plasma cells, with small and intermediate-sized lymphocytes and centrocyte-like cells (Figure 5.9A–C). Both B- and T-cell monomorphic PTLDs have sufficient architectural and cytological atypia to be recognized as neoplastic (Figure 5.9D, E). These should be classified according to their respective classification of B- and T-cell neoplasms. Hodgkin lymphomas should be diagnosed using both classical morphological and immunophenotypic features as polymorphic PTLDs may also have Reed-Sternberg–like cells.

Clinically, PTLDs may present as localized masses or as widely disseminated disease. In decreasing order of frequency, PTLDs may involve lymph nodes, lung, gastrointestinal tract, liver, central nervous system, spleen, and the heart (198). Involvement of the cardiac allograft by

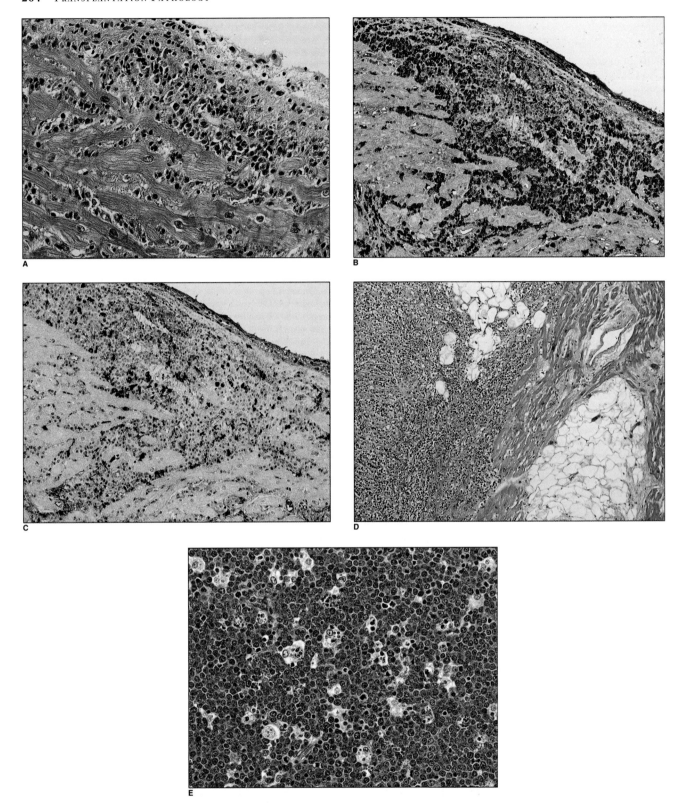

FIGURE 5.9: *PTLD. (A) Polymorphic PTLD exhibits the full range of B-cell maturation, from immunoblasts to plasma cells. The latter is prominent in this photomicrograph. Immunostains for kappa and lambda light chains demonstrate light chain restriction for kappa light chains (H&E; original magnification, 400×). (B) Immunostain for kappa light chains (original magnification, 200×). (C) Immunostain for lambda light chains (original magnification, 200×). (D) Monomorphic PTLDs should be classified according to their respective classification of B- and T-cell neoplasms. In this particular example, a Burkitt-type PTLD involves the epicardium with extension into the underlying myocardium. (E) Sheets of monomorphic, medium-sized lymphocytes with scant cytoplasm, round nuclei, and multiple nucleoli. Note the "starry-sky" appearance due to many tingible-body macrophages (H&E; original magnification, 400×).*

PTLD can be diagnosed utilizing the EMB (202). The main differential diagnostic considerations of PTLD on EMBs are ACR and QE. Distinguishing the former from PTLD is important as early diagnosis and subsequent reduction of immunosuppression may lead to regression in some cases (203). Ancillary studies to confirm the diagnosis can be performed on the EMB material including immunophenotyping, Ig gene rearrangement, and in situ hybridization or PCR detection of the EBV genome (204–208). A high index of suspicion should always be maintained for PTLDs given their potential for being aggressive and poor prognosis.

X. CARDIAC ALLOGRAFT VASCULOPATHY

CAV is a diffuse form of arteriosclerosis characterized by concentric fibromuscular proliferation of the intima that progressively obliterates the coronary vasculature. Despite advances in the therapy of acute rejection, CAV remains a major limiting factor in the long-term success of cardiac allografts. It is a major indication for retransplantation and is one of the leading causes of death after one year following transplantation. According to the ISHLT Registry, the cumulative prevalence of CAV in survivors was 7.1, 32.5, and 52.7 percent at one, five, and ten years after transplantation, respectively (4). In angiographic studies, the incidence of CAV has been reported to occur in 42 percent of all patients by the end of five years after heart transplantation (209). Using more sensitive techniques such as intravascular ultrasonography (IVUS), CAV has been detected in 75 percent of patients at one year (210).

The pathological features of CAV differ significantly from those of native coronary artery atherosclerosis (211–214). Typically, CAV diffusely involves the larger epicardial as well as the smaller epicardial and intramyocardial coronary vessels (215). Although both coronary arteries and veins can be involved in this process, the morphological changes in the veins are generally not as severe. The vascular lesions consist of relatively uniform, concentric intimal proliferation of modified smooth muscle cells within an extracellular matrix comprising collagen, lipid, and proteoglycans (Figure 5.10A) (216–223). Not infrequently, lipid-laden macrophages (also known as foam cells) can be quite prominent. These foam cells initially cluster near the internal elastic lamina (Figure 5.10B), but later on, they may be distributed throughout the intima. In addition, there may be changes of active or healed vasculitis including a variably dense inflammatory infiltrate comprised of lymphocytes and macrophages within the vessel wall, endothelialitis (Figure 5.10C), and medial fibrosis. Unlike native coronary artery atherosclerosis, early proliferative lesions of CAV lack necrosis, calcification, and cholesterol clefts. The internal elastic lamina is generally intact and the media is more or less of normal thickness (Figure 5.10B). Advanced CAV lesions, especially in

allografts greater than five years, or lesions in patients with risk factors for atherosclerosis, may exhibit superimposed changes of coronary artery atherosclerosis. In contrast to classical CAV, the atheromatous lesions of coronary artery atherosclerosis are typically focal, eccentric, and often associated with necrosis, calcification, and cholesterol clefts. Veins and intramyocardial vessels are usually not involved. There is often disruption of the internal elastic lamina as well as thinning of the media. Occasionally, a ruptured plaque with hemorrhage and associated occlusive thrombosis may be present.

The distal myocardium supplied by the narrowed epicardial and intramyocardial coronary arteries may exhibit changes of *ischemic injury* (224). One particular myocardial ischemic lesion, which is sublethal and potentially reversible, is subendocardial myocyte vacuolization (or myocytolysis) (Figure 5.10D). The other lesions reflect changes of myocardial infarction at different stages of evolution including multifocal to regional coagulation necrosis, granulation tissue, and healed scar (Figure 5.10E). Although more commonly present in the left ventricle, such myocardial ischemic lesions are also seen in the right ventricle, and thus, can be detected in EMBs. The latter typically do not allow for direct evaluation of CAV since sufficiently large vessels are rarely biopsied. However, one study showed that the specificity and sensitivity of myocardial ischemic pathology in biopsy specimens for diagnosing CAV is 98 and 17 percent, respectively, with a positive predictive value of 92 percent and a negative predictive value of 52 percent (225). Thus, the presence of ischemic myocardial pathology on an EMB indicates that there is a high likelihood of CAV; however, the absence of such changes does not exclude it.

CAV may represent a diagnostic challenge as many heart transplant patients do not experience angina due to cardiac denervation at the time of transplantation (226,227). Consequently, these patients often present late in the course of their disease with congestive heart failure, silent myocardial infarction, cardiac arrhythmias, or sudden death. Increasingly, more patients with CAV are presenting with chest pain; radionuclide and physiological studies indicate that re-innervation of the allograft is occurring in these patients. In the past, the gold standard for the detection of CAV was coronary angiography (228). Since this diagnostic modality measures luminal diameter rather than the vessel wall thickness, it may underestimate or even underdiagnose CAV. This has been attributed to vascular remodeling as well as the concentric and diffuse nature of CAV. IVUS has been shown to be a more sensitive technique in diagnosing CAV than coronary angiography, particularly in early lesions (43,229,230). Since IVUS is able to characterize the vessel wall morphology, it can determine the degree of intimal thickening and allows for assessment of vascular remodeling. However, the major disadvantage of IVUS is that it can only assess the larger epicardial coronary arteries due to the physical limitation of catheter size. Consequently, the

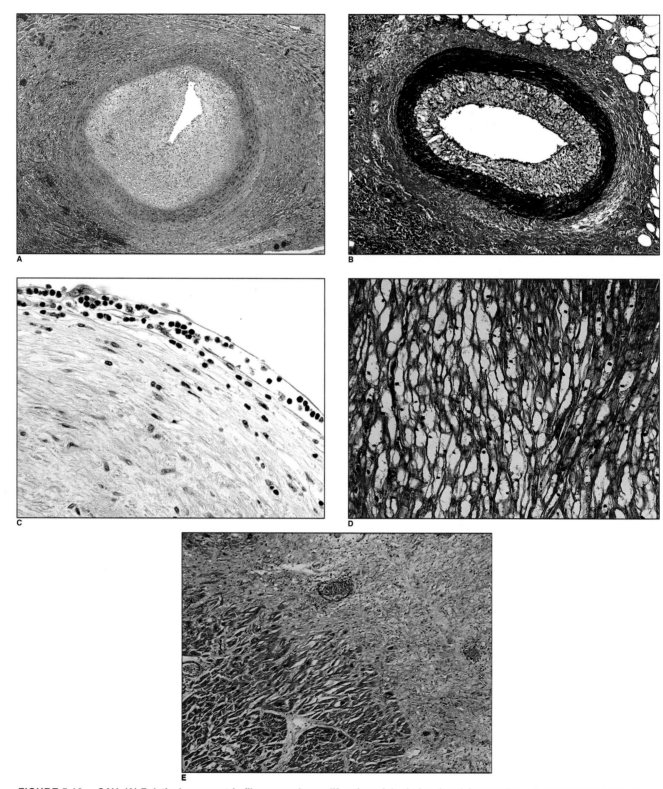

FIGURE 5.10: *CAV. (A) Relatively concentric fibromuscular proliferation of the intima involving medium-sized epicardial coronary artery. Notably absent are necrosis, calcification, and cholesterol clefts which are typical changes seen in native coronary artery atherosclerosis (H&E; original magnification, 40×). (B) Lipid-laden macrophages (or foam cells) are sometimes prominent and typically cluster near the internal elastic lamina in early lesions. Note that the internal elastic lamina is intact and the media is of normal thickness (trichrome-EVG; original magnification, 100×). (C) Endothelialitis, in which mononuclear inflammatory cells infiltrate the endothelium, is a fairly common finding in CAV (H&E; original magnification, 400×). (D) Myocytolysis of cardiac myocytes indicates sublethal, potentially reversible ischemic injury (H&E; original magnification, 200×). (E) Area of healed myocardial infarct adjacent to viable myocardium in cardiac allograft with severe CAV (H&E; original magnification, 100×).*

entire arterial tree cannot be evaluated for CAV. Dobutamine stress echocardiography has been reported to be the most sensitive noninvasive test for detecting CAV with a sensitivity of 79 percent and a specificity of 83 percent (231). Other possible future modalities, which may eventually replace the more invasive techniques such as coronary angiography and IVUS as screening tools, include pulse-wave tissue Doppler imaging (40), electron beam computed tomography (232), and magnetic resonance imaging looking at myocardial perfusion reserve after an adenosine infusion (233).

The pathogenetic mechanisms involved in the development of CAV have not been fully elucidated. Both immunologic and nonimmunologic risk factors have been identified for the development and progression of CAV (227,234–237). The importance of immunologic mechanisms has been suggested by the preferential involvement of the allograft vasculature by CAV with sparing of the host's native vessels. Although the relationship between ACR and CAV remains controversial, some studies have shown that the risk of developing CAV correlates with the number of HLA mismatches as well as the severity and frequency of rejection episodes (238–244). In particular, patients who experienced two or more rejection episodes had a 40 percent incidence of CAV (versus 23 percent incidence in patients with no rejection) (243). Moreover, the rate of CAV progression correlates with the severity of rejection (242).

The humoral (or antibody mediated) immune response has more recently been recognized as an important factor in the pathogenesis of CAV. Several studies have demonstrated an association between antibody production after heart transplantation and CAV (115–117,122,123,245,246). These studies indicate that both circulating anti-HLA and anti-endothelial antibodies are associated with CAV and poor survival. In addition, AMR has been shown to correlate with development of CAV (94,247). In particular, Hammond et al. found a significant difference in the time to the CAV development based on the pattern of rejection (247). They showed that patients with pure vascular and mixed (vascular and cellular) rejections developed CAV earlier than those with cellular rejection alone.

Various nonimmunologic risk factors that have been shown to be associated with the development and progression of CAV include donor- or recipient-related characteristics (age, gender) (209), donor-transmitted coronary atherosclerosis (248,249), ischemic/reperfusion injury (250,251), CMV infection (96,252–256), dyslipidemia (229,257–261), deficient fibrinolysis (262,263), and insulin resistance (258,259,264).

Overall, CAV appears to be initiated and propagated by both immune- and nonimmune-mediated mechanisms (227,234,235). The initiating event in CAV pathogenesis is most likely endothelial cell injury that results in a complex cascade of immunologic processes characterized by the release of inflammatory cytokines and growth factors as well as upregulation of cell surface adhesion molecules with subsequent binding of circulating leukocytes. This leads to induction of vascular smooth muscle cells, which proliferate and migrate from the media to the intima and produce various components of the extracellular matrix, resulting in the formation of a neointima. Further vascular narrowing occurs via constrictive remodeling (265–267).

XI. RECURRENT DISEASE IN THE CARDIAC ALLOGRAFT

The major problem that affects the transplanted heart is acute and/or chronic rejection. However, there are other potential problems including recurrence of the original heart disease in the allograft. Diseases such as amyloidosis, Chagas disease, Fabry's disease, giant cell myocarditis, and sarcoidosis have been reported to recur in the allograft heart (18). Recurrence has been reported as early as eight weeks for Fabry's disease, and up to sixty months after transplantation for amyloid heart disease (268,269). Biopsy of the recipient's native heart prior to transplantation may be helpful in documenting such conditions either to exclude the patient as a transplant candidate or for future monitoring of recurrent disease. In addition, the explanted heart should be examined carefully for any of the above disease entities and the clinicians alerted of the findings because their recurrence in the allograft heart may lead to allograft dysfunction (270,271). In the Padua experience (5), in 10 percent of cases, the pretransplantation clinical diagnosis was wrong, as pathological examination of the explanted native heart harbored unexpected pathology.

Recurrence of giant cell myocarditis is associated with arrhythmia but tends to respond favorably to therapy; therefore, giant cell myocarditis is not considered to be a contraindication for transplantation (268,272). Transplantation for amyloid heart disease is said to be contraindicated, due to concern for progression of systemic amyloidosis and recurrent amyloid deposition in the cardiac allograft. It has been shown that the long-term survival for patients transplanted for cardiac amyloidosis is reduced compared to patients transplanted for other indications (269,273). In spite of the known risks, patients with amyloidosis are still transplanted under special circumstances. Cardiac sarcoidosis is a diagnosis that may first be made at the time the explanted native heart is examined by the pathologist. Rare cases of recurrent sarcoidosis have been reported in the cardiac allograft (271,274). However, long-term consequences of recurrent sarcoidosis have yet to be elucidated. *Trypanosoma cruzi* infection, endemic in South America, is now of increased concern in the United States as more Latin American immigrants contribute to the U.S. blood supply and donate organs for human transplantation. Chagas disease in the transplanted heart may be from the donor or recipient, if either one has the disease but is undiagnosed. PCR has been reported to be a sensitive method for early diagnosis of reactivation of Chagas' disease after cardiac transplantation (275).

XII. CONCLUSIONS

Despite the success of cardiac transplantation in the past several decades, there are still several major limitations. One such limitation is the tremendous shortage of organs available for transplantation. Although an estimated 4,000 patients each year in the United States could benefit from heart transplantation, only 2,000 donor hearts are available. In addition, cardiac transplantation is an expensive therapy and consumes multiple resources. The EMB, for example, is a costly and invasive procedure for monitoring of cardiac allograft rejection. However, ongoing research in noninvasive techniques as well as proteomic and genomic markers to monitor for allograft rejection shows some promise. Finally, long-term complications such as infections, malignancy, and CAV continue to limit the life expectancy of cardiac allograft recipients. In spite of these limitations, the remarkable progress in basic science and clinical research has made cardiac transplantation a reasonable therapeutic option for patients with end-stage heart disease. A better understanding of the pathogenesis of acute and chronic rejection should continue to contribute to progress in this field.

REFERENCES

1. Heimansohn DA, Robison RJ, Paris JM 3rd, Matheny RG, Bogdon J, Shaar CJ. Routine surveillance endomyocardial biopsy: late rejection after heart transplantation. *Ann Thorac Surg*. 1997;64:1231–6.

2. Billingham ME. Dilemma of variety of histopathologic grading systems for acute cardiac allograft rejection by endomyocardial biopsy. *J Heart Transplant*. 1990;9:272–6.

3. Melvin KR, Mason JW. Endomyocardial biopsy: its history, techniques and current indications. *Can Med Assoc J*. 1982;126:1381–6.

4. Taylor DO, Edwards LB, Boucek MM, et al. Registry of the International Society for Heart and Lung Transplantation: twenty-fourth official adult heart transplantation report – 2007. *J Heart Lung Transplant*. 2007;26:769–781.

5. Valente M, Angelini A, Calabrese F, Thiene G. Heart and lung transplantation pathology: the Padua experience. *Transplant Proc*. 2006;38:1163–6.

6. Bourge RC, Naftel DC, Costanzo-Nordin MR, et al. Pretransplantation risk factors for death after heart transplantation: a multiinstitutional study. The Transplant Cardiologists Research Database Group. *J Heart Lung Transplant*. 1993;12:549–62.

7. Murata S, Miniati DN, Kown MH, et al. Superoxide dismutase mimetic m40401 reduces ischemia-reperfusion injury and graft coronary artery disease in rodent cardiac allografts. *Transplantation*. 2004;78:1166–71.

8. Koch A, Bingold TM, Oberlander J, et al. Capillary endothelia and cardiomyocytes differ in vulnerability to ische-

mia/reperfusion during clinical heart transplantation. *Eur J Cardiothorac Surg*. 2001;20:996–1001.

9. Opelz G, Wujciak T. The influence of HLA compatibility on graft survival after heart transplantation. The Collaborative Transplant Study. *N Engl J Med*. 1994;330:816–9.

10. Wang CY, Aronson I, Takuma S, et al. cAMP pulse during preservation inhibits the late development of cardiac isograft and allograft vasculopathy. *Circ Res*. 2000; 86:982–8.

11. Fishbein MC, Maclean D, Maroko PR. The histopathologic evolution of myocardial infarction. *Chest*. 1978;73:843–9.

12. Panizo A, Pardo FJ, Lozano MD, de Alava E, Sola I, Idoate MA. Ischemic injury in posttransplant endomyocardial biopsies: immunohistochemical study of fibronectin. *Transplant Proc*. 1999;31:2550–1.

13. John R, Rajasinghe HA, Chen JM, et al. Long-term outcomes after cardiac transplantation: an experience based on different eras of immunosuppressive therapy. *Ann Thorac Surg*. 2001;72:440–9.

14. Abbas AK. Disorders of the immune system. In: Kumar V, Fausto N, Abbas AK, editors. *Robbins & Cotran Pathologic Basis of Disease*. 7th ed. Philadelphia PA: Elsevier Saunders; 2005. pp. 218–222.

15. Janeway CA, Travers P, Walport M, Shlomchik MJ. Autoimmunity and transplantation. In: *Immunobiology: the Immune System in Health and Disease*. 6th ed. New York: Garland Science; 2005. pp. 569–603.

16. Sun H, Subbotin V, Chen C, et al. Prevention of chronic rejection in mouse aortic allografts by combined treatment with CTLA4-Ig and anti-CD40 ligand monoclonal antibody. *Transplantation*. 1997;64:1838–43.

17. Wagoner LE, Zhao L, Bishop DK, Chan S, Xu S, Barry WH. Lysis of adult ventricular myocytes by cells infiltrating rejecting murine cardiac allografts. *Circulation*. 1996;93: 111–19.

18. Winters GL, Schoen FJ. Pathology of cardiac transplantation. In: Silver MD, Gotlieb AI, Schoen FJ, editors. *Cardiovascular Pathology*. 3rd ed. New York: Churchill Livingstone; 2001. p. 725–62.

19. Marboe CC, Schierman SW, Rose E, Reemtsma K, Fenoglio JJ Jr. Characterization of mononuclear cell infiltrates in human cardiac allografts. *Transplant Proc*. 1984;16:1598–9.

20. Stewart S, Cary NRB, Goddard MJ, Billingham ME. Endomyocardial biopsies for heart and heart-lung transplant recipients based on International Society for Heart Lung Transplantation (ISHLT) Grading System. In: *Atlas of Biopsy Pathology for Heart and Lung Transplantation*. London: Arnold; 2001. pp. 2–52.

21. Michaels PJ, Kobashigawa J, Laks H, et al. Differential expression of RANTES chemokine, TGF-beta, and leukocyte phenotype in acute cellular rejection and Quilty B lesions. *J Heart Lung Transplant*. 2001;20:407–16.

22. Stewart S, Winters GL, Fishbein MC, et al. Revision of the 1990 working formulation for the standardization of nomenclature in the diagnosis of heart rejection. *J Heart Lung Transplant*. 2005;24:1710–20.

23. Marboe CC, Alobeid B. Pathology and the transplant patient. In: Edwards NM, Chen JM, Mazzeo PA, editors. *Cardiac Transplantation. The Columbia University Medical*

Center/New York-Presbyterian Hospital Manual. New Jersey: Humana Press; 2004. pp. 98–102.

24. Billingham ME, Cary NR, Hammond ME, et al. A working formulation for the standardization of nomenclature in the diagnosis of heart and lung rejection: Heart Rejection Study Group. The International Society for Heart Transplantation. *J Heart Transplant.* 1990;9:587–93.

25. Fishbein MC, Bell G, Lones MA, et al. Grade 2 cellular heart rejection: does it exist? *J Heart Lung Transplant.* 1994; 13:1051–7.

26. Billingham M, Kobashigawa JA. The revised ISHLT heart biopsy grading scale. *J Heart Lung Transplant.* 2005;24:1709.

27. Marboe CC, Billingham M, Eisen H, et al. Nodular endocardial infiltrates (Quilty lesions) cause significant variability in diagnosis of ISHLT grade 2 and 3A rejection in cardiac allograft recipients. *J Heart Lung Transplant.* 2005;24:S219–26.

28. Yang H, Lai C, Baruch-Oren T, et al. Has the 2004 revision of the International Society of Heart and Lung Transplantation (ISHLT) grading system improved the reproducibility of the diagnosis and grading of cardiac transplant rejection? *Cardiovasc Pathol.* 2008 Jul 10 [E-pub].

29. Zerbe TR, Arena V. Diagnostic reliability of endomyocardial biopsy for assessment of cardiac allograft rejection. *Hum Pathol.* 1988;19:1307–14.

30. Sibley RK, Olivari MT, Ring WS, Bolman RM, et al. Endomyocardial biopsy in the cardiac allograft recipient. A review of 570 biopsies. *Ann Surg.* 1986;203:177–87.

31. Novitzky D, Rose AG, Cooper DK, Reichart B, et al. Interpretation of endomyocardial biopsy after heart transplantation. Potentially confusing factors. *S Afr Med J.* 1986;70:789–92.

32. Rose AG, Novitzky D, Cooper DK, Reichart B. Endomyocardial biopsy site morphology. An experimental study in baboons. *Arch Pathol Lab Med.* 1986;110:622–5.

33. Radio SJ, McManus BM, Winters GL, et al. Preferential endocardial residence of B-cells in the "Quilty effect" of human heart allografts: immunohistochemical distinction from rejection. *Mod Pathol.* 1991;4:654–60.

34. Cui G, Tung T, Kobashigawa J, Laks H, Sen L. Increased incidence of atrial flutter associated with the rejection of heart transplantation. *Am J Cardiol.* 2001;88:280–4.

35. Scott CD, Dark JH, McComb JM. Arrhythmias after cardiac transplantation. *Am J Cardiol.* 1992;70:1061–3.

36. Mehra MR, Uber PA, Uber WE, Park MH, Scott RL. Anything but a biopsy: noninvasive monitoring for cardiac allograft rejection. *Curr Opin Cardiol.* 2002;17:131–6.

37. Walpoth BH, Lazeyras F, Tschopp A, et al. Assessment of cardiac rejection and immunosuppression by magnetic resonance imaging and spectroscopy. *Transplant Proc.* 1995; 27:2088–91.

38. Buchthal SD, Noureuil TO, den Hollander JA, et al. 31P-magnetic resonance spectroscopy studies of cardiac transplant patients at rest. *J Cardiovasc Magn Reson.* 2000;2:51–6.

39. Moidl R, Chevtchik O, Simon P, et al. Noninvasive monitoring of peak filling rate with acoustic quantification echocardiography accurately detects acute cardiac allograft rejection. *J Heart Lung Transplant.* 1999;18:194–201.

40. Dandel M, Hummel M, Muller J, et al. Reliability of tissue Doppler wall motion monitoring after heart transplantation for replacement of invasive routine screenings by optimally timed cardiac biopsies and catheterizations. *Circulation.* 2001;104:I184–91.

41. Mankad S, Murali S, Kormos RL, Mandarino WA, Gorcsan J 3rd. Evaluation of the potential role of color-coded tissue Doppler echocardiography in the detection of allograft rejection in heart transplant recipients. *Am Heart J.* 1999;138:721–30.

42. Valantine HA, Yeoh TK, Gibbons R, et al. Sensitivity and specificity of diastolic indexes for rejection surveillance: temporal correlation with endomyocardial biopsy. *J Heart Lung Transplant.* 1991;10:757–65.

43. St Goar FG, Pinto FJ, Alderman EL, et al. Intracoronary ultrasound in cardiac transplant recipients. In vivo evidence of "angiographically silent" intimal thickening. *Circulation.* 1992;85:979–87.

44. Graceffo MA, O'Rourke RA. Cardiac transplant rejection is associated with a decrease in the high-frequency components of the high-resolution, signal-averaged electrocardiogram. *Am Heart J.* 1996;132:820–6.

45. Hetzer R, Potapov EV, Muller J, et al. Daily noninvasive rejection monitoring improves long-term survival in pediatric heart transplantation. *Ann Thorac Surg.* 1998;66:1343–9.

46. Grasser B, Iberer F, Schreier G, et al. Intramyocardial electrogram variability in the monitoring of graft rejection after heart transplantation. *Pacing Clin Electrophysiol.* 1998; 21:2345–9.

47. Bourge R, Eisen H, Hershberger R, et al. Noninvasive rejection monitoring of cardiac transplants using high resolution intramyocardial electrograms: initial US multicenter experience. *Pacing Clin Electrophysiol.* 1998;21:2338–44.

48. Bainbridge AD, Cave M, Newell S, et al. The utility of pacemaker evoked T wave amplitude for the noninvasive diagnosis of cardiac allograft rejection. *Pacing Clin Electrophysiol.* 1999;22:942–6.

49. Ali A, Mehra MR, Malik FS, Uber PA, Ventura HO. Insights into ventricular repolarization abnormalities in cardiac allograft vasculopathy. *Am J Cardiol.* 2001;87:367–8, A10.

50. Frey AW, Uberfuhr P, Achakri H, Fuchs A, Reichart B, Theisen K. Detecting acute graft rejection in patients after orthotopic heart transplantation: analysis of heart rate variability in the frequency domain. *J Heart Lung Transplant.* 1998;17:578–85.

51. Dengler TJ, Zimmermann R, Braun K, et al. Elevated serum concentrations of cardiac troponin T in acute allograft rejection after human heart transplantation. *J Am Coll Cardiol.* 1998;32:405–12.

52. Vijay P, Scavo VA, Morelock RJ, Sharp TG, Brown JW. Donor cardiac troponin T: a marker to predict heart transplant rejection. *Ann Thorac Surg.* 1998;66:1934–9.

53. Segal JB, Kasper EK, Rohde C, et al. Coagulation markers predicting cardiac transplant rejection. *Transplantation.* 2001;72:233–7.

54. Masters RG, Davies RA, Veinot JP, Hendry PJ, Smith SJ, de Bold AJ. Discoordinate modulation of natriuretic peptides during acute cardiac allograft rejection in humans. *Circulation.* 1999;100:287–91.

55. Schowengerdt KO, Fricker FJ, Bahjat KS, Kuntz ST. Increased expression of the lymphocyte early activation

marker CD69 in peripheral blood correlates with histologic evidence of cardiac allograft rejection. *Transplantation*. 2000;69:2102–7.

56. Vallhonrat H, Williams WW, Dec GW, et al. Complement activation products in plasma after heart transplantation in humans. *Transplantation*. 2001;71:1308–11.

57. Zhao Y, Katz NM, Lefrak EA, Foegh ML. Urinary thromboxane B2 in cardiac transplant patients as a screening method of rejection. *Prostaglandins*. 1997;54:881–9.

58. Benvenuti C, Bories PN, Loisance D. Increased serum nitrate concentration in cardiac transplant patients. A marker for acute allograft cellular rejection. *Transplantation*. 1996;61:745–9.

59. Narula J, Acio ER, Narula N, et al. Annexin-V imaging for noninvasive detection of cardiac allograft rejection. *Nat Med*. 2001;7:1347–52.

60. Eisen HJ, Eisenberg SB, Saffitz JE, Bolman RM 3rd, Sobel BE, Bergmann SR. Noninvasive detection of rejection of transplanted hearts with indium-111-labeled lymphocytes. *Circulation*. 1987;75:868–76.

61. Hesse B, Mortensen SA, Folke M, Brodersen AK, Aldershvile J, Pettersson G. Ability of antimyosin scintigraphy monitoring to exclude acute rejection during the first year after heart transplantation. *J Heart Lung Transplant*. 1995;14:23–31.

62. Windsor NT, Lloyd KS, Young JB, et al. Dynamics of soluble interleukin-2 receptor levels immediately after heart transplantation. Attenuation of increase by OKT3 therapy. *Transplantation*. 1991;52:78–82.

63. Deng MC, Eisen HJ, Mehra MR, et al. Noninvasive discrimination of rejection in cardiac allograft recipients using gene expression profiling. *Am J Transplant*. 2006;6:150–60.

64. Starling RC, Pham M, Valantine H, et al. Molecular testing in the management of cardiac transplant recipients: initial clinical experience. *J Heart Lung Transplant*. 2006;25:1389–95.

65. Mehra MR. The emergence of genomic and proteomic biomarkers in heart transplantation. *J Heart Lung Transplant*. 2005;24:S213–18.

66. Halloran PF, Reeve J, Kaplan B. Lies, damn lies, and statistics: the perils of the P value. *Am J Transplant*. 2006;6:10–11.

67. Oyer PE, Stinson EB, Jamieson SW, et al. Cyclosporin-A in cardiac allografting: a preliminary experience. *Transpl Proc*. 1983;15:1247–52.

68. Grattan MT, Moreno-Cabral CE, Starnes VA, Oyer PE, Stinson EB, Shumway NE. Eight-year results of cyclosporine-treated patients with cardiac transplants. *J Thorac Cardiovasc Surg*. 1990;99:500–9.

69. Kobashigawa JA, Patel JK. Immunosuppression for heart transplantation: where are we now? *Nat Clin Pract Cardiovasc Med*. 2006;3:203–12.

70. Taylor DO, Barr ML, Radovancevic B, et al. A randomized, multicenter comparison of tacrolimus and cyclosporine immunosuppressive regimens in cardiac transplantation: decreased hyperlipidemia and hypertension with tacrolimus. *J Heart Lung Transplant*. 1999;18:336–45.

71. Radovancevic B, Vrtovec B. Sirolimus therapy in cardiac transplantation. *Transplant Proc*. 2003;35:171S–6S.

72. Dean PG, Lund WJ, Larson TS, et al. Wound-healing complications after kidney transplantation: a prospective, randomized comparison of sirolimus and tacrolimus. *Transplantation*. 2004;77:1555–61.

73. Eisen HJ, Tuzcu EM, Dorent R, et al. Everolimus for the prevention of allograft rejection and vasculopathy in cardiac-transplant recipients. *N Engl J Med*. 2003;349:847–58.

74. Kobashigawa J, Miller L, Renlund D, et al. A randomized active-controlled trial of mycophenolate mofetil in heart transplant recipients. Mycophenolate Mofetil Investigators. *Transplantation*. 1998;66:507–15.

75. Baran DA, Galin ID, Gass AL. Current practices: immunosuppression induction, maintenance, and rejection regimens in contemporary post-heart transplant patient treatment. *Curr Opin Cardiol*. 2002;17:165–70.

76. Lloveras JJ, Escourrou G, Delisle MB, et al. Evolution of untreated mild rejection in heart transplant recipients. *J Heart Lung Transplant*. 1992;11:751–6.

77. Winters GL, Loh E, Schoen FJ. Natural history of focal moderate cardiac allograft rejection. Is treatment warranted? *Circulation*. 1995;91:1975–80.

78. Hosenpud JD, Norman DJ, Pantely GA. Low-dose oral prednisone in the treatment of acute cardiac allograft rejection not associated with hemodynamic compromise. *J Heart Transplant*. 1990;9:292–6.

79. Park MH, Starling RC, Ratliff NB, et al. Oral steroid pulse without taper for the treatment of asymptomatic moderate cardiac allograft rejection. *J Heart Lung Transplant*. 1999;18:1224–7.

80. Costanzo-Nordin MR, McManus BM, Wilson JE, O'Sullivan EJ, Hubbell EA, Robinson JA. Efficacy of photopheresis in the rescue therapy of acute cellular rejection in human heart allografts: a preliminary clinical and immunopathologic report. *Transplant Proc*. 1993;25:881–3.

81. Dall'Amico R, Livi U, Milano A, et al. Extracorporeal photochemotherapy as adjuvant treatment of heart transplant recipients with recurrent rejection. *Transplantation*. 1995;60:45–9.

82. Lehrer MS, Rook AH, Tomaszewski JE, DeNofrio D. Successful reversal of severe refractory cardiac allograft rejection by photopheresis. *J Heart Lung Transplant*. 2001;20:1233–6.

83. Hammond EH, Yowell RL, Nunoda S, et al. Vascular (humoral) rejection in heart transplantation: pathologic observations and clinical implications. *J Heart Transplant*. 1989;8:430–43.

84. Reed EF, Demetris AJ, Hammond E, et al. Acute antibody-mediated rejection of cardiac transplants. *J Heart Lung Transplant*. 2006;25:153–9.

85. Bonnaud EN, Lewis NP, Masek MA, Billingham ME. Reliability and usefulness of immunofluorescence in heart transplantation. *J Heart Lung Transplant*. 1995;14:163–71.

86. Crespo-Leiro MG, Veiga-Barreiro A, Domenech N, et al. Humoral heart rejection (severe allograft dysfunction with no signs of cellular rejection or ischemia): incidence, management, and the value of C4d for diagnosis. *Am J Transplant*. 2005;5:2560–4.

87. Hammond EH, Ensley RD, Yowell RL, et al. Vascular rejection of human cardiac allografts and the role of humoral immunity in chronic allograft rejection. *Transplant Proc*. 1991;23:26–30.

88. Kemnitz J, Restrepo-Specht I, Haverich A, Cremer J. Acute humoral rejection: a new entity in the histopathology of heart transplantation. *J Heart Transplant*. 1990;9:447–9.

89. Lones MA, Czer LS, Trento A, Harasty D, Miller JM, Fishbein MC. Clinical-pathologic features of humoral rejection in cardiac allografts: a study in 81 consecutive patients. *J Heart Lung Transplant*. 1995;14:151–62.

90. Rodriguez ER, Skojec DV, Tan CD, et al. Antibody-mediated rejection in human cardiac allografts: evaluation of immunoglobulins and complement activation products C4d and C3d as markers. *Am J Transplant*. 2005;5:2778–85.

91. Hammond EH, Wittwer CT, Greenwood J, et al. Relationship of OKT3 sensitization and vascular rejection in cardiac transplant patients receiving OKT3 rejection prophylaxis. *Transplantation*. 1990;50:776–82.

92. Ma H, Hammond EH, Taylor DO, et al. The repetitive histologic pattern of vascular cardiac allograft rejection. Increased incidence associated with longer exposure to prophylactic murine monoclonal anti-CD3 antibody (OKT3). *Transplantation*. 1996;62:205–10.

93. Costanzo-Nordin MR, Heroux AL, Radvany R, Koch D, Robinson JA. Role of humoral immunity in acute cardiac allograft dysfunction. *J Heart Lung Transplant*. 1993;12: S143–6.

94. Michaels PJ, Espejo ML, Kobashigawa J, et al. Humoral rejection in cardiac transplantation: risk factors, hemodynamic consequences and relationship to transplant coronary artery disease. *J Heart Lung Transplant*. 2003;22:58–69.

95. Miller LW, Wesp A, Jennison SH, et al. Vascular rejection in heart transplant recipients. *J Heart Lung Transplant*. 1993;12:S147–52.

96. Grattan MT, Moreno-Cabral CE, Starnes VA, Oyer PE, Stinson EB, Shumway NE. Cytomegalovirus infection is associated with cardiac allograft rejection and atherosclerosis. *Jama*. 1989;261:3561–6.

97. Hosenpud JD. Coronary artery disease after heart transplantation and its relation to cytomegalovirus. *Am Heart J*. 1999;138:S469–72.

98. Toyoda M, Petrosian A, Jordan SC. Immunological characterization of anti-endothelial cell antibodies induced by cytomegalovirus infection. *Transplantation*. 1999;68:1311–18.

99. Loy TS, Bulatao IS, Darkow GV, et al. Immunostaining of cardiac biopsy specimens in the diagnosis of acute vascular (humoral) rejection: a control study. *J Heart Lung Transplant*. 1993;12:736–40.

100. McCarthy JF, Cook DJ, Smedira NG, et al. Vascular rejection in cardiac transplantation. *Transplant Proc*. 1999;31:160.

101. Ratkovec RM, Hammond EH, O'Connell JB, et al. Outcome of cardiac transplant recipients with a positive donor-specific crossmatch—preliminary results with plasmapheresis. *Transplantation*. 1992;54:651–5.

102. Cherry R, Nielsen H, Reed E, Reemtsma K, Suciu-Foca N, Marboe CC. Vascular (humoral) rejection in human cardiac allograft biopsies: relation to circulating anti-HLA antibodies. *J Heart Lung Transplant*. 1992;11:24–9.

103. Qian Z, Liu J, Fox-Talbot K, Wasowska BA, Baldwin WM 3rd. A rat model of pregnancy-induced sensitization to transplants. *Transplant Proc*. 2005;37:96–7.

104. Rebibou JM, Chabod J, Alcalay D, et al. Flow cytometric evaluation of pregnancy-induced anti-HLA immunization and blood transfusion-induced reactivation. *Transplantation*. 2002;74:537–40.

105. Petranyi GG, Reti M, Harsanyi V, Szabo J. Immunologic consequences of blood transfusion and their clinical manifestations. *Int Arch Allergy Immunol*. 1997;114:303–15.

106. Karwande SV, Ensley RD, Renlund DG, et al. Cardiac retransplantation: a viable option? The Registry of the International Society for Heart and Lung Transplantation. *Ann Thorac Surg*. 1992;54:840–4.

107. Itescu S, Ankersmit JH, Kocher AA, Schuster MD. Immunobiology of left ventricular assist devices. *Prog Cardiovasc Dis*. 2000;43:67–80.

108. Joyce DL, Southard RE, Torre-Amione G, Noon GP, Land GA, Loebe M. Impact of left ventricular assist device (LVAD)-mediated humoral sensitization on post-transplant outcomes. *J Heart Lung Transplant*. 2005;24:2054–9.

109. Massad MG, Cook DJ, Schmitt SK, et al. Factors influencing HLA sensitization in implantable LVAD recipients. *Ann Thorac Surg*. 1997;64:1120–5.

110. Moazami N, Itescu S, Williams MR, Argenziano M, Weinberg A, Oz MC. Platelet transfusions are associated with the development of anti-major histocompatibility complex class I antibodies in patients with left ventricular assist support. *J Heart Lung Transplant*. 1998;17:876–80.

111. Stringham JC, Bull DA, Fuller TC, et al. Avoidance of cellular blood product transfusions in LVAD recipients does not prevent HLA allosensitization. *J Heart Lung Transplant*. 1999;18:160–5.

112. Taylor DO, Yowell RL, Kfoury AG, Hammond EH, Renlund DG. Allograft coronary artery disease: clinical correlations with circulating anti-HLA antibodies and the immunohistopathologic pattern of vascular rejection. *J Heart Lung Transplant*. 2000;19:518–21.

113. Michaels PJ, Fishbein MC, Colvin RB. Humoral rejection of human organ transplants. *Springer Semin Immunopathol*. 2003;25:119–40.

114. McKenna RM, Takemoto SK, Terasaki PI. Anti-HLA antibodies after solid organ transplantation. *Transplantation*. 2000;69:319–26.

115. Reed EF, Hong B, Ho E, Harris PE, Weinberger J, Suciu-Foca N. Monitoring of soluble HLA alloantigens and anti-HLA antibodies identifies heart allograft recipients at risk of transplant-associated coronary artery disease. *Transplantation*. 1996;61:566–72.

116. Suciu-Foca N, Reed E, Marboe C, et al. The role of anti-HLA antibodies in heart transplantation. *Transplantation*. 1991;51:716–24.

117. Fredrich R, Toyoda M, Czer LS, et al. The clinical significance of antibodies to human vascular endothelial cells after cardiac transplantation. *Transplantation*. 1999;67:385–91.

118. Rose ML. Role of antibodies in rejection. *Current Opinion in Organ Transplantation*. 1999;4:227–233.

119. Sumitran-Holgersson S, Wilczek HE, Holgersson J, Soderstrom K. Identification of the nonclassical HLA molecules, MICA, as targets for humoral immunity associated with irreversible rejection of kidney allografts. *Transplantation*. 2002;74:268–77.

120. Jurcevic S, Ainsworth ME, Pomerance A, et al. Antivimentin antibodies are an independent predictor of transplant-associated coronary artery disease after cardiac transplantation. *Transplantation*. 2001;71:886–92.

121. Laguens RP, Argel MI, Chambo JG, et al. Anti-skeletal muscle glycolipid antibodies in human heart transplantation as markers of acute rejection. Correlation with endomyocardial biopsy. *Transplantation*. 1996;62:211–16.

122. Petrossian GA, Nichols AB, Marboe CC, et al. Relation between survival and development of coronary artery disease and anti-HLA antibodies after cardiac transplantation. *Circulation*. 1989;80:III122–5.

123. Rose EA, Pepino P, Barr ML, et al. Relation of HLA antibodies and graft atherosclerosis in human cardiac allograft recipients. *J Heart Lung Transplant*. 1992;11:S120–3.

124. Shimizu A, Colvin RB. Pathological features of antibody-mediated rejection. *Curr Drug Targets Cardiovasc Haematol Disord*. 2005;5:199–214.

125. Benzaquen LR, Nicholson-Weller A, Halperin JA. Terminal complement proteins C5b-9 release basic fibroblast growth factor and platelet-derived growth factor from endothelial cells. *J Exp Med*. 1994;179:985–92.

126. Baldwin WM 3rd, Kasper EK, Zachary AA, Wasowska BA, Rodriguez ER. Beyond C4d: other complement-related diagnostic approaches to antibody-mediated rejection. *Am J Transplant*. 2004;4:311–18.

127. Hammond ME, Stehlik J, Snow G, et al. Utility of histologic parameters in screening for antibody-mediated rejection of the cardiac allograft: a study of 3,170 biopsies. *J Heart Lung Transplant*. 2005;24:2015–21.

128. Behr TM, Feucht HE, Richter K, et al. Detection of humoral rejection in human cardiac allografts by assessing the capillary deposition of complement fragment C4d in endomyocardial biopsies. *J Heart Lung Transplant*. 1999; 18:904–12.

129. Chantranuwat C, Qiao JH, Kobashigawa J, Hong L, Shintaku P, Fishbein MC. Immunoperoxidase staining for C4d on paraffin-embedded tissue in cardiac allograft endomyocardial biopsies: comparison to frozen tissue immunofluorescence. *Appl Immunohistochem Mol Morphol*. 2004;12:166–71.

130. Vongwiwatana A, Tasanarong A, Hidalgo LG, Halloran PF. The role of B cells and alloantibody in the host response to human organ allografts. *Immunol Rev*. 2003; 196:197–218.

131. Poelzl G, Ullrich R, Huber A, et al. Capillary deposition of the complement fragment C4d in cardiac allograft biopsies is associated with allograft vasculopathy. *Transpl Int*. 2005;18:313–17.

132. Smith RN, Brousaides N, Grazette L, et al. C4d deposition in cardiac allografts correlates with alloantibody. *J Heart Lung Transplant*. 2005;24:1202–10.

133. Baldwin WM 3rd, Samaniego-Picota M, Kasper EK, et al. Complement deposition in early cardiac transplant biopsies is associated with ischemic injury and subsequent rejection episodes. *Transplantation*. 1999;68:894–900.

134. Haas M, Ratner LE, Montgomery RA. C4d staining of perioperative renal transplant biopsies. *Transplantation*. 2002;74:711–17.

135. Williams JM, Holzknecht ZE, Plummer TB, Lin SS, Brunn GJ, Platt JL. Acute vascular rejection and accommodation: divergent outcomes of the humoral response to organ transplantation. *Transplantation*. 2004;78:1471–18.

136. Bach FH, Ferran C, Hechenleitner P, et al. Accommodation of vascularized xenografts: expression of "protective genes" by donor endothelial cells in a host Th2 cytokine environment. *Nat Med*. 1997;3:196–204.

137. Dalmasso AP, Benson BA, Johnson JS, Lancto C, Abrahamsen MS. Resistance against the membrane attack complex of complement induced in porcine endothelial cells with a Gal alpha(1-3)Gal binding lectin: up-regulation of CD59 expression. *J Immunol*. 2000;164:3764–73.

138. Salama AD, Delikouras A, Pusey CD, et al. Transplant accommodation in highly sensitized patients: a potential role for Bcl-xL and alloantibody. *Am J Transplant*. 2001; 1:260–9.

139. Koller H, Steurer W, Mark W, et al. Clearance of C4d deposition after successful treatment of acute humoral rejection in follow-up biopsies: a report of three cases. *Transpl Int*. 2004;17:177–81.

140. Minami K, Murata K, Lee CY, et al. C4d deposition and clearance in cardiac transplants correlates with alloantibody levels and rejection in rats. *Am J Transplant*. 2006;6:923–32.

141. Lepin EJ, Zhang Q, Zhang X, et al. Phosphorylated S6 ribosomal protein: a novel biomarker of antibody-mediated rejection in heart allografts. *Am J Transplant*. 2006;6:1560–71.

142. Behr TM, Richter K, Fischer P, et al. Incidence of humoral rejection in heart transplant recipients treated with tacrolimus or cyclosporine A. *Transplant Proc*. 1998;30:1920–1.

143. Baumann G. Molecular mechanism of immunosuppressive agents. *Transplant Proc*. 1992;24:4–7.

144. Baumann G, Andersen E, Quesniaux V, Eberle MK. Cyclosporine and its analogue SDZ IMM 125 mediate very similar effects on T-cell activation—a comparative analysis in vitro. *Transplant Proc*. 1992;24:43–8.

145. Aranda JM Jr, Scornik JC, Normann SJ, et al. Anti-CD20 monoclonal antibody (rituximab) therapy for acute cardiac humoral rejection: a case report. *Transplantation*. 2002;73: 907–10.

146. Becker YT, Samaniego-Picota M, Sollinger HW. The emerging role of rituximab in organ transplantation. *Transplant Int*. 2006;19:621–8.

147. Jordan SC, Quartel AW, Czer LS, et al. Posttransplant therapy using high-dose human immunoglobulin (intravenous gammaglobulin) to control acute humoral rejection in renal and cardiac allograft recipients and potential mechanism of action. *Transplantation*. 1998;66:800–5.

148. Kaczmarek I, Deutsch MA, Sadoni S, et al. Successful management of antibody-mediated cardiac allograft rejection with combined immunoadsorption and anti-CD20 monoclonal antibody treatment: case report and literature review. *J Heart Lung Transplant*. 2007;26:511–15.

149. Keren A, Hayes HM, O'Driscoll G. Late humoral rejection in a cardiac transplant recipient treated with the anti-CD20 monoclonal antibody rituximab. *Transplant Proc*. 2006;38:1520–2.

150. Kobashigawa JA. Contemporary concepts in noncellular rejection. *Heart Fail Clin*. 2007;3:11–15.

151. Olivari MT, May CB, Johnson NA, Ring WS, Stephens MK. Treatment of acute vascular rejection with immunoadsorption. *Circulation*. 1994;90:II70–3.

152. Wang SS, Chou NK, Ko WJ, et al. Effect of plasmapheresis for acute humoral rejection after heart transplantation. *Transplant Proc*. 2006;38:3692–4.

153. Aziz S, Suzuki K, Thorning D. Mechanism of discordant cardiac xenograft rejection—an alternative view based on ultrastructural observations. Cooper DKC, Kemp E, Reemtsma K, White DJG, editors. *Xenotransplantation. The Transplantation of Organs and Tissues Between Species*. New York: Springer; 1997. pp. 273–86.

154. Cattell V, Jamieson SW. Hyperacute rejection of guinea-pig to rat cardiac xenografts. I. Morphology. *J Pathol*. 1975;115:183–9.

155. Rose AG. Understanding the pathogenesis and the pathology of hyperacute cardiac rejection. *Cardiovasc Pathol*. 2002;11:171–6.

156. Rose AG, Cooper DK. Venular thrombosis is the key event in the pathogenesis of antibody-mediated cardiac rejection. *Xenotransplantation*. 2000;7:31–41.

157. Kemnitz J, Cremer J, Restrepo-Specht I, et al. Hyperacute rejection in heart allografts. Case studies. *Pathol Res Pract*. 1991;187:23–9.

158. Rose AG, Cooper DK, Human PA, Reichenspurner H, Reichart B. Histopathology of hyperacute rejection of the heart: experimental and clinical observations in allografts and xenografts. *J Heart Lung Transplant*. 1991;10:223–34.

159. Forbes RD, Rowan RA, Billingham ME. Endocardial infiltrates in human heart transplants: a serial biopsy analysis comparing four immunosuppression protocols. *Hum Pathol*. 1990;21:850–5.

160. Kottke-Marchant K, Ratliff NB. Endomyocardial lymphocytic infiltrates in cardiac transplant recipients. Incidence and characterization. *Arch Pathol Lab Med*. 1989;113:690–8.

161. Chu KE, Ho EK, de la Torre L, Vasilescu ER, Marboe CC. The relationship of nodular endocardial infiltrates (Quilty lesions) to survival, patient age, anti-HLA antibodies, and coronary artery disease following heart transplantation. *Cardiovasc Pathol*. 2005;14:219–24.

162. Costanzo-Nordin MR, Winters GL, Fisher SG, et al. Endocardial infiltrates in the transplanted heart: clinical significance emerging from the analysis of 5026 endomyocardial biopsy specimens. *J Heart Lung Transplant*. 1993; 12:741–7.

163. Joshi A, Masek MA, Brown BW Jr, Weiss LM, Billingham ME. "Quilty" revisited: a 10-year perspective. *Hum Pathol*. 1995;26:547–57.

164. Stovin PG, al-Tikriti SA. The correlation of various features of rejection in myocardial biopsies after human heart transplantation. *Pathol Res Pract*. 1989;185:836–42.

165. Freimark D, Czer LS, Aleksic I, et al. Pathogenesis of Quilty lesion in cardiac allografts: relationship to reduced endocardial cyclosporine A. *J Heart Lung Transplant*. 1995;14:1197–203.

166. Gajjar NA, Kobashigawa JA, Laks H, Espejo-Vassilakis M, Fishbein MC. FK506 vs. cyclosporin. Pathologic findings in 1067 endomyocardial biopsies. *Cardiovasc Pathol*. 2003;12:73–6.

167. Nakhleh RE, Copenhaver CM, Werdin K, McDonald K, Kubo SH, Strickler JG. Lack of evidence for involvement of Epstein-Barr virus in the development of the "Quilty" lesion of transplanted hearts: an in situ hybridization study. *J Heart Lung Transplant*. 1991;10:504–7.

168. Kemnitz J, Cohnert TR. Lymphoma-like lesion in human orthotopic cardiac allografts. *Am J Clin Pathol*. 1988;89:430.

169. Pardo-Mindan FJ, Lozano MD. "Quilty effect" in heart transplantation: is it related to acute rejection? *J Heart Lung Transplant*. 1991;10:937–41.

170. Smith RN, Chang Y, Houser S, Dec GW, Grazette L. Higher frequency of high-grade rejections in cardiac allograft patients after Quilty B lesions or grade 2/4 rejections. *Transplantation*. 2002;73:1928–32.

171. Yamani MH, Ratliff NB, Starling RC, et al. Quilty lesions are associated with increased expression of vitronectin receptor (alphavbeta3) and subsequent development of coronary vasculopathy. *J Heart Lung Transplant*. 2003;22:687–90.

172. Di Carlo E, D'Antuono T, Contento S, Di Nicola M, Ballone E, Sorrentino C. Quilty effect has the features of lymphoid neogenesis and shares CXCL13-CXCR5 pathway with recurrent acute cardiac rejections. *Am J Transplant*. 2007;7:201–10.

173. Yamani MH, Yang J, Masri CS, et al. Acute cellular rejection following human heart transplantation is associated with increased expression of vitronectin receptor (integrin alphavbeta3). *Am J Transplant*. 2002;2:129–33.

174. Plaza DM, Fernandez D, Builes M, Villegas A, Garcia LF. Cytokine gene polymorphisms in heart transplantation: association of low IL-10 production genotype with Quilty effect. *J Heart Lung Transplant*. 2003;22:851–6.

175. Luthringer DJ, Yamashita JT, Czer LS, Trento A, Fishbein MC. Nature and significance of epicardial lymphoid infiltrates in cardiac allografts. *J Heart Lung Transplant*. 1995;14:537–43.

176. Truell JS, Fishbein MC. Case report of a Quilty lesion within a coronary artery. *Cardiovasc Pathol*. 2006;15:161–4.

177. Winters GL, McManus BM. Consistencies and controversies in the application of the International Society for Heart and Lung Transplantation working formulation for heart transplant biopsy specimens. Rapamycin Cardiac Rejection Treatment Trial Pathologists. *J Heart Lung Transplant*. 1996;15:728–35.

178. Sattar HA, Husain AN, Kim AY, Krausz T. The presence of a CD21+ follicular dendritic cell network distinguishes invasive Quilty lesions from cardiac acute cellular rejection. *Am J Surg Pathol*. 2006;30:1008–13.

179. Grossi P, De Maria R, Caroli A, Zaina MS, Minoli L. Infections in heart transplant recipients: the experience of the Italian heart transplantation program. Italian Study Group on Infections in Heart Transplantation. *J Heart Lung Transplant*. 1992;11:847–66.

180. Hsu RB, Fang CT, Chang SC, et al. Infectious complications after heart transplantation in Chinese recipients. *Am J Transplant*. 2005;5:2011–16.

181. Montoya JG, Giraldo LF, Efron B, et al. Infectious complications among 620 consecutive heart transplant patients at Stanford University Medical Center. *Clin Infect Dis*. 2001;33:629–40.

182. Remington JS, Gaines JD, Griepp RB, Shumway NE. Further experience with infection after cardiac transplantation. *Transplant Proc.* 1972;4:699–705.

183. Hofflin JM, Potasman I, Baldwin JC, Oyer PE, Stinson EB, Remington JS. Infectious complications in heart transplant recipients receiving cyclosporine and corticosteroids. *Ann Intern Med.* 1987;106:209–16.

184. Wagner JA, Ross H, Hunt S, et al. Prophylactic ganciclovir treatment reduces fungal as well as cytomegalovirus infections after heart transplantation. *Transplantation.* 1995;60:1473–7.

185. Miller LW, Naftel DC, Bourge RC, et al. Infection after heart transplantation: a multiinstitutional study. Cardiac Transplant Research Database Group. *J Heart Lung Transplant.* 1994;13:381–92.

186. Smart FW, Naftel DC, Costanzo MR, et al. Risk factors for early, cumulative, and fatal infections after heart transplantation: a multiinstitutional study. *J Heart Lung Transplant.* 1996;15:329–41.

187. Arbustini E, Grasso M, Diegoli M, et al. Histopathologic and molecular profile of human cytomegalovirus infections in patients with heart transplants. *Am J Clin Pathol.* 1992;98:205–13.

188. Chagas disease after organ transplantation – Los Angeles, California, 2006. *MMWR Morb Mortal Wkly Rep.* 2006;55:798–800.

189. Penn I. Occurrence of cancers in immunosuppressed organ transplant recipients. *Clin Transpl.* 1994:99–109.

190. Hunt SA. Malignancy in organ transplantation: heart. *Transplant Proc.* 2002;34:1874–6.

191. Caforio AL, Fortina AB, Piaserico S, et al. Skin cancer in heart transplant recipients: risk factor analysis and relevance of immunosuppressive therapy. *Circulation.* 2000;102:III222–7.

192. Euvrard S, Kanitakis J, Pouteil-Noble C, et al. Comparative epidemiologic study of premalignant and malignant epithelial cutaneous lesions developing after kidney and heart transplantation. *J Am Acad Dermatol.* 1995;33:222–9.

193. Gjersvik P, Hansen S, Moller B, et al. Are heart transplant recipients more likely to develop skin cancer than kidney transplant recipients? *Transplant Int.* 2000;13:S380–1.

194. Jensen P, Moller B, Hansen S. Skin cancer in kidney and heart transplant recipients and different long-term immunosuppressive therapy regimens. *J Am Acad Dermatol.* 2000;42:307.

195. Tan CD, Baldwin WM 3rd, Rodriguez ER. Update on cardiac transplantation pathology. *Arch Pathol Lab Med.* 2007;131:1169–91.

196. Opelz G, Dohler B. Lymphomas after solid organ transplantation: a collaborative transplant study report. *Am J Transplant.* 2004;4:222–30.

197. Opelz G, Henderson R. Incidence of non-Hodgkin lymphoma in kidney and heart transplant recipients. *Lancet.* 1993;342:1514–6.

198. Aull MJ, Buell JF, Trofe J, et al. Experience with 274 cardiac transplant recipients with posttransplant lymphoproliferative disorder: a report from the Israel Penn International Transplant Tumor Registry. *Transplantation.* 2004;78:1676–82.

199. Ho M, Miller G, Atchison RW, et al. Epstein-Barr virus infections and DNA hybridization studies in posttransplantation lymphoma and lymphoproliferative lesions: the role of primary infection. *J Infect Dis.* 1985;152:876–86.

200. Swerdlow AJ, Higgins CD, Hunt BJ, et al. Risk of lymphoid neoplasia after cardiothoracic transplantation. A cohort study of the relation to Epstein-Barr virus. *Transplantation.* 2000;69:897–904.

201. Harris NL, Swerdlow SH, Frizzera G, Knowles DM. Posttransplant lymphoproliferative disorders. In: Jaffe ES, Harris NL, Stein H, Vardiman JW, editors. *World Health Organization Classification of Tumours. Pathology and Genetics of Tumours of Haematopoietic and Lymphoid Tissues.* Lyon France: IARC Press; 2001. pp. 264–269.

202. Eisen HJ, Hicks D, Kant JA, et al. Diagnosis of posttransplantation lymphoproliferative disorder by endomyocardial biopsy in a cardiac allograft recipient. *J Heart Lung Transplant.* 1994;13:241–5.

203. Armitage JM, Kormos RL, Stuart RS, et al. Posttransplant lymphoproliferative disease in thoracic organ transplant patients: ten years of cyclosporine-based immunosuppression. *J Heart Lung Transplant.* 1991;10:877–86.

204. Hanasono MM, Kamel OW, Chang PP, Rizeq MN, Billingham ME, van de Rijn M. Detection of Epstein-Barr virus in cardiac biopsies of heart transplant patients with lymphoproliferative disorders. *Transplantation.* 1995;60:471–3.

205. Hanto DW, Birkenbach M, Frizzera G, Gajl-Peczalska KJ, Simmons RL, Schubach WH. Confirmation of the heterogeneity of posttransplant Epstein-Barr virus-associated B cell proliferations by immunoglobulin gene rearrangement analyses. *Transplantation.* 1989;47:458–64.

206. Kowal-Vern A, Swinnen L, Pyle J, et al. Characterization of postcardiac transplant lymphomas. Histology, immunophenotyping, immunohistochemistry, and gene rearrangement. *Arch Pathol Lab Med.* 1996;120:41–8.

207. Lager DJ, Burgart LJ, Slagel DD. Epstein-Barr virus detection in sequential biopsies from patients with a posttransplant lymphoproliferative disorder. *Mod Pathol.* 1993;6:42–7.

208. Montone KT, Friedman H, Hodinka RL, Hicks DG, Kant JA, Tomaszewski JE. In situ hybridization for Epstein-Barr virus NotI repeats in posttransplant lymphoproliferative disorder. *Mod Pathol.* 1992;5:292–302.

209. Costanzo MR, Naftel DC, Pritzker MR, et al. Heart transplant coronary artery disease detected by coronary angiography: a multiinstitutional study of preoperative donor and recipient risk factors. Cardiac Transplant Research Database. *J Heart Lung Transplant.* 1998;17:744–53.

210. Yeung AC, Davis SF, Hauptman PJ, et al. Incidence and progression of transplant coronary artery disease over 1 year: results of a multicenter trial with use of intravascular ultrasound. Multicenter Intravascular Ultrasound Transplant Study Group. *J Heart Lung Transplant.* 1995;14:S215–20.

211. Billingham ME. Histopathology of graft coronary disease. *J Heart Lung Transplant.* 1992;11:S38–44.

212. Johnson DE, Alderman EL, Schroeder JS, et al. Transplant coronary artery disease: histopathologic correlations with angiographic morphology. *J Am Coll Cardiol.* 1991;17:449–57.

213. Liu G, Butany J. Morphology of graft arteriosclerosis in cardiac transplant recipients. *Hum Pathol.* 1992;23:768–73.

214. Rose AG, Viviers L, Odell JA. Pathology of chronic cardiac rejection: An analysis of the epicardial and intra-myocardial coronary arteries and myocardial alterations in 43 human allografts. *Cardiovasc Pathol.* 1993;2:7–19.

215. Lin H, Wilson JE, Kendall TJ, et al. Comparable proximal and distal severity of intimal thickening and size of epicardial coronary arteries in transplant arteriopathy of human cardiac allografts. *J Heart Lung Transplant.* 1994;13:824–33.

216. Arbustini E, Roberts WC. Morphological observations in the epicardial coronary arteries and their surroundings late after cardiac transplantation (allograft vascular disease). *Am J Cardiol.* 1996;78:814–20.

217. Hruban RH, Beschorner WE, Baumgartner WA, et al. Accelerated arteriosclerosis in heart transplant recipients is associated with a T-lymphocyte-mediated endothelialitis. *Am J Pathol.* 1990;137:871–82.

218. Lin H, Ignatescu M, Wilson JE, et al. Prominence of apolipoproteins B, (a), and E in the intimae of coronary arteries in transplanted human hearts: geographic relationship to vessel wall proteoglycans. *J Heart Lung Transplant.* 1996;15:1223–32.

219. Lin H, Wilson JE, Roberts CR, et al. Biglycan, decorin, and versican protein expression patterns in coronary arteriopathy of human cardiac allograft: distinctness as compared to native atherosclerosis. *J Heart Lung Transplant.* 1996;15:1233–47.

220. McManus BM, Horley KJ, Wilson JE, et al. Prominence of coronary arterial wall lipids in human heart allografts. Implications for pathogenesis of allograft arteriopathy. *Am J Pathol.* 1995;147:293–308.

221. McManus BM, Malcom G, Kendall TJ, et al. Lipid overload and proteoglycan expression in chronic rejection of the human transplanted heart. *Clin Transplant.* 1994;8:336–40.

222. Radio S, Wood S, Wilson J, Lin H, Winters G, McManus B. Allograft vascular disease: comparison of heart and other grafted organs. *Transplant Proc.* 1996;28:496–9.

223. Salomon RN, Hughes CC, Schoen FJ, Payne DD, Pober JS, Libby P. Human coronary transplantation-associated arteriosclerosis. Evidence for a chronic immune reaction to activated graft endothelial cells. *Am J Pathol.* 1991;138:791–8.

224. Neish AS, Loh E, Schoen FJ. Myocardial changes in cardiac transplant-associated coronary arteriosclerosis: potential for timely diagnosis. *J Am Coll Cardiol.* 1992;19:586–92.

225. Winters GL, Schoen FJ. Graft arteriosclerosis-induced myocardial pathology in heart transplant recipients: predictive value of endomyocardial biopsy. *J Heart Lung Transplant.* 1997;16:985–93.

226. Aranda JM Jr, Hill J. Cardiac transplant vasculopathy. *Chest.* 2000;118:1792–800.

227. Ramzy D, Rao V, Brahm J, Miriuka S, Delgado D, Ross HJ. Cardiac allograft vasculopathy: a review. *Can J Surg.* 2005;48:319–27.

228. Sharples LD, Jackson CH, Parameshwar J, Wallwork J, Large SR. Diagnostic accuracy of coronary angiography and risk factors for post-heart-transplant cardiac allograft vasculopathy. *Transplantation.* 2003;76:679–82.

229. Mehra MR, Ventura HO, Chambers R, et al. Predictive model to assess risk for cardiac allograft vasculopathy: an intravascular ultrasound study. *J Am Coll Cardiol.* 1995;26:1537–44.

230. Spes CH, Klauss V, Rieber J, et al. Functional and morphological findings in heart transplant recipients with a normal coronary angiogram: an analysis by dobutamine stress echocardiography, intracoronary Doppler and intravascular ultrasound. *J Heart Lung Transplant.* 1999;18:391–8.

231. Spes CH, Mudra H, Schnaack SD, et al. Dobutamine stress echocardiography for noninvasive diagnosis of cardiac allograft vasculopathy: a comparison with angiography and intravascular ultrasound. *Am J Cardiol.* 1996;78:168–74.

232. Knollmann FD, Bocksch W, Spiegelsberger S, Hetzer R, Felix R, Hummel M. Electron-beam computed tomography in the assessment of coronary artery disease after heart transplantation. *Circulation.* 2000;101:2078–82.

233. Muehling OM, Wilke NM, Panse P, et al. Reduced myocardial perfusion reserve and transmural perfusion gradient in heart transplant arteriopathy assessed by magnetic resonance imaging. *J Am Coll Cardiol.* 2003;42:1054–60.

234. Mehra MR. Contemporary concepts in prevention and treatment of cardiac allograft vasculopathy. *Am J Transplant.* 2006;6:1248–56.

235. Pinney SP, Mancini D. Cardiac allograft vasculopathy: advances in understanding its pathophysiology, prevention, and treatment. *Curr Opin Cardiol.* 2004;19:170–6.

236. Valantine H. Cardiac allograft vasculopathy after heart transplantation: risk factors and management. *J Heart Lung Transplant.* 2004;23:S187–93.

237. Vassalli G, Gallino A, Weis M, et al. Alloimmunity and nonimmunologic risk factors in cardiac allograft vasculopathy. *Eur Heart J.* 2003;24:1180–8.

238. Costanzo-Nordin MR. Cardiac allograft vasculopathy: relationship with acute cellular rejection and histocompatibility. *J Heart Lung Transplant.* 1992;11:S90–103.

239. Hauptman PJ, Nakagawa T, Tanaka H, Libby P. Acute rejection: culprit or coincidence in the pathogenesis of cardiac graft vascular disease? *J Heart Lung Transplant.* 1995;14:S173–80.

240. Hornick P, Smith J, Pomerance A, et al. Influence of acute rejection episodes, HLA matching, and donor/recipient phenotype on the development of 'early' transplant-associated coronary artery disease. *Circulation.* 1997;96:II148–53.

241. Hosenpud JD, Edwards EB, Lin HM, Daily OP. Influence of HLA matching on thoracic transplant outcomes. An analysis from the UNOS/ISHLT Thoracic Registry. *Circulation.* 1996;94:170–4.

242. Jimenez J, Kapadia SR, Yamani MH, et al. Cellular rejection and rate of progression of transplant vasculopathy: a 3-year serial intravascular ultrasound study. *J Heart Lung Transplant.* 2001;20:393–8.

243. Radovancevic B, Poindexter S, Birovljev S, et al. Risk factors for development of accelerated coronary artery disease in cardiac transplant recipients. *Eur J Cardiothorac Surg.* 1990;4:309–12.

244. Vasilescu ER, Ho EK, de la Torre L, et al. Anti-HLA antibodies in heart transplantation. *Transpl Immunol.* 2004;12:177–83.

245. Crisp SJ, Dunn MJ, Rose ML, Barbir M, Yacoub MH. Antiendothelial antibodies after heart transplantation: the

accelerating factor in transplant-associated coronary artery disease? *J Heart Lung Transplant*. 1994;13:81–91.

246. Dunn MJ, Crisp SJ, Rose ML, Taylor PM, Yacoub MH. Anti-endothelial antibodies and coronary artery disease after cardiac transplantation. *Lancet*. 1992;339:1566–70.

247. Hammond EH, Yowell RL, Price GD, et al. Vascular rejection and its relationship to allograft coronary artery disease. *J Heart Lung Transplant*. 1992;11:S111–19.

248. Grauhan O, Patzurek J, Hummel M, et al. Donor-transmitted coronary atherosclerosis. *J Heart Lung Transplant*. 2003;22:568–73.

249. Tuzcu EM, Hobbs RE, Rincon G, et al. Occult and frequent transmission of atherosclerotic coronary disease with cardiac transplantation. Insights from intravascular ultrasound. *Circulation*. 1995;91:1706–13.

250. Gaudin PB, Rayburn BK, Hutchins GM, et al. Peritransplant injury to the myocardium associated with the development of accelerated arteriosclerosis in heart transplant recipients. *Am J Surg Pathol*. 1994;18:338–46.

251. Yamani MH, Tuzcu EM, Starling RC, et al. Myocardial ischemic injury after heart transplantation is associated with upregulation of vitronectin receptor (alpha(v)beta3), activation of the matrix metalloproteinase induction system, and subsequent development of coronary vasculopathy. *Circulation*. 2002;105:1955–61.

252. Everett JP, Hershberger RE, Norman DJ, et al. Prolonged cytomegalovirus infection with viremia is associated with development of cardiac allograft vasculopathy. *J Heart Lung Transplant*. 1992;11:S133–7.

253. Koskinen P, Lemstrom K, Bruggeman C, Lautenschlager I, Hayry P. Acute cytomegalovirus infection induces a subendothelial inflammation (endothelialitis) in the allograft vascular wall. A possible linkage with enhanced allograft arteriosclerosis. *Am J Pathol*. 1994;144:41–50.

254. Koskinen P, Lemstrom K, Bruning H, Daemen M, Bruggeman C, Hayry P. Cytomegalovirus infection induces vascular wall inflammation and doubles arteriosclerotic changes in rat cardiac allografts. *Transplant Proc*. 1995;27:574–5.

255. Koskinen PK, Nieminen MS, Krogerus LA, et al. Cytomegalovirus infection accelerates cardiac allograft vasculopathy: correlation between angiographic and endomyocardial biopsy findings in heart transplant patients. *Transpl Int*. 1993;6:341–7.

256. Valantine HA, Gao SZ, Menon SG, et al. Impact of prophylactic immediate posttransplant ganciclovir on development of transplant atherosclerosis: a post hoc analysis of a randomized, placebo-controlled study. *Circulation*. 1999;100:61–6.

257. Becker DM, Chamberlain B, Swank R, et al. Relationship between corticosteroid exposure and plasma lipid levels in heart transplant recipients. *Am J Med*. 1988;85:632–8.

258. Chamorro CI, Almenar L, Martinez-Dolz L, et al. Do cardiovascular risk factors influence cardiac allograft vasculopathy? *Transplant Proc*. 2006;38:2572–4.

259. Kemna MS, Valantine HA, Hunt SA, Schroeder JS, Chen YD, Reaven GM. Metabolic risk factors for atherosclerosis in heart transplant recipients. *Am Heart J*. 1994;128:68–72.

260. Perrault LP, Mahlberg F, Breugnot C, et al. Hypercholesterolemia increases coronary endothelial dysfunction, lipid content, and accelerated atherosclerosis after heart transplantation. *Arterioscler Thromb Vasc Biol*. 2000;20:728–36.

261. Valantine HA. Role of lipids in allograft vascular disease: a multicenter study of intimal thickening detected by intravascular ultrasound. *J Heart Lung Transplant*. 1995;14:S234–7.

262. Faulk WP, Labarrere CA, Nelson DR, Pitts D. Coronary artery disease in cardiac allografts: association with arterial antithrombin. *Transplant Proc*. 1995;27:1944–6.

263. Labarrere CA, Pitts D, Nelson DR, Faulk WP. Vascular tissue plasminogen activator and the development of coronary artery disease in heart-transplant recipients. *N Engl J Med*. 1995;333:1111–16.

264. Valantine H, Rickenbacker P, Kemna M, et al. Metabolic abnormalities characteristic of dysmetabolic syndrome predict the development of transplant coronary artery disease: a prospective study. *Circulation*. 2001;103:2144–52.

265. Kobashigawa J, Wener L, Johnson J, et al. Longitudinal study of vascular remodeling in coronary arteries after heart transplantation. *J Heart Lung Transplant*. 2000;19:546–50.

266. Tsutsui H, Schoenhagen P, Ziada KM, et al. Early constriction or expansion of the external elastic membrane area determines the late remodeling response and cumulative lumen loss in transplant vasculopathy: an intravascular ultrasound study with 4-year follow-up. *J Heart Lung Transplant*. 2003;22:519–25.

267. Wong C, Ganz P, Miller L, et al. Role of vascular remodeling in the pathogenesis of early transplant coronary artery disease: a multicenter prospective intravascular ultrasound study. *J Heart Lung Transplant*. 2001;20:385–92.

268. Cantor WJ, Daly P, Iwanochko M, Clarke JT, Cusimano RJ, Butany J. Cardiac transplantation for Fabry's disease. *Can J Cardiol*. 1998;14:81–4.

269. Dubrey SW, Burke MM, Hawkins PN, Banner NR. Cardiac transplantation for amyloid heart disease: the United Kingdom experience. *J Heart Lung Transplant*. 2004;23:1142–53.

270. Gries W, Farkas D, Winters GL, Costanzo-Nordin MR. Giant cell myocarditis: first report of disease recurrence in the transplanted heart. *J Heart Lung Transplant*. 1992;11:370–4.

271. Oni AA, Hershberger RE, Norman DJ, et al. Recurrence of sarcoidosis in a cardiac allograft: control with augmented corticosteroids. *J Heart Lung Transplant*. 1992;11:367–9.

272. Scott RL, Ratliff NB, Starling RC, Young JB. Recurrence of giant cell myocarditis in cardiac allograft. *J Heart Lung Transplant*. 2001;20:375–80.

273. Hosenpud JD, DeMarco T, Frazier OH, et al. Progression of systemic disease and reduced long-term survival in patients with cardiac amyloidosis undergoing heart transplantation. Follow-up results of a multicenter survey. *Circulation*. 1991;84:III338–43.

274. Yager JE, Hernandez AF, Steenbergen C, et al. Recurrence of cardiac sarcoidosis in a heart transplant recipient. *J Heart Lung Transplant*. 2005;24:1988–90.

275. Schijman AG, Vigliano C, Burgos J, et al. Early diagnosis of recurrence of Trypanosoma cruzi infection by polymerase chain reaction after heart transplantation of a chronic Chagas' heart disease patient. *J Heart Lung Transplant*. 2000;19:1114–17.

CHAPTER 6

Lung Transplantation Pathology

Dani S. Zander, M.D.

I. INTRODUCTION

For many patients with advanced lung diseases, lung transplantation represents an opportunity to improve daily life and extend lifespan. Since 1963 (1), when the first successful lung transplant procedure was performed, the number of patients choosing this procedure has grown significantly. Current procedural options include four major surgical approaches to lung transplantation: single lung transplantation, bilateral lung transplantation, heart-lung transplantation, and transplantation of lobes of lungs from living donors. The 2007 report of the Registry of the International Society for Heart and Lung Transplantation (ISHLT) indicates that 146 centers performed a total of 2,169 lung transplant procedures on adults in 2005, and these numbers are likely to represent underestimates of the real volumes throughout the world (2). About eighty heart-lung transplantation procedures are performed in adults each year by about forty centers (2). The 2006 Registry report for children indicates that twenty-seven centers performed sixty-seven pediatric lung transplant procedures in 2004, while only four centers reported performing fewer than ten heart-lung transplants in children, with a sharp decline in the number done for cystic fibrosis (CF) as compared to previous years (3).

Among adults, from 1995 to 2006, the major indications for lung transplantation included chronic obstructive pulmonary disease (COPD, 37 percent), idiopathic pulmonary fibrosis (IPF, 19 percent), CF (16 percent), and α_1-anti-trypsin deficiency emphysema (8 percent), while for heart-lung transplantation in adults, the main indication is pulmonary hypertension associated with congenital heart disease (2). Within the last six years, the percentage of lung transplants done for IPF has risen significantly, while those done for COPD have substantially declined. For pediatric recipients, the indications for lung transplantation vary by age. CF is the indication in over half of all pediatric lung transplant recipients, with other diagnoses as follows: 1) for infants, congenital heart disease is the most frequent diagnosis, followed by primary pulmonary hypertension, pulmonary vascular disease, surfactant protein B deficiency, and interstitial pneumonitis; 2) in early childhood (one to five years of age) primary pulmonary hypertension is most frequent, followed by interstitial pneumonitis, congenital heart disease, and IPF; and 3) in late childhood and adolescence, CF is the most common indication, followed by primary pulmonary hypertension (3). Children undergoing heart-lung transplantation are most often between eleven and seventeen years of age, and the primary indications are CF and pulmonary vascular disease (3). Retransplantation for bronchiolitis obliterans syndrome (BOS) and other indications accounted for 7 percent of lung transplantation procedures in children (3). Living donors provide less than 10 percent of all donors for pediatric recipients, a number that has decreased over the past three years (3).

Post-lung transplantation survival rates for adults have shown improvement during the first year after transplantation, but have changed little in successive time periods. Data from the 2007 Registry report indicates 87 percent survival at three months, 78 percent at one year, 62 percent at three years, 50 percent at five years, and 25 percent at ten years (2). Graft failure accounts for 28.3 percent of deaths in the first thirty days after transplantation, followed by infections (20.3 percent), cardiovascular complications (10.8 percent), technical complications (8.2 percent), rejection (5.1 percent), malignancy (0.2 percent), and a variety of causes (27.1 percent) (2). During the period from thirty-one days to one year, infections are the most frequent cause of death (36.4 percent noncytomegalovirus, 3.4 percent cytomegalovirus [CMV]), followed by graft failure (19.2 percent), rejection (6.8 percent), malignancy (5.2 percent), cardiovascular complications (4.2 percent), and technical complications (2.7 percent), and approximately 22.0 percent of deaths classified as other processes (2). After one year, chronic airway rejection (obliterative bronchiolitis [OB]/BOS) remains the most common cause of death, accounting for up to 30 percent of deaths, followed by significant losses due to infections, graft failure, malignancies, and other causes (2). Overall survival in children was similar to that of adults, with substantial improvements noted when the 2000–2004 era was compared to the 1988–1994 period (3). Causes of death were also similar to adults: 1) from one to thirty days after transplantation, graft failure was most frequent, followed by technical issues, cardiovascular issues, and non-CMV infections; 2) from thirty days to one year, infection was the top cause of death, responsible for almost 50 percent of deaths in this period; and 3) after one year, OB/BOS became the most frequent cause of death, responsible for approximately 40 percent of deaths (3).

II. POST-TRANSPLANTATION DIAGNOSTIC EVALUATION

After transplantation, care of the patient includes monitoring of graft functioning and evaluation for complications of transplantation. Assessment of clinical signs and symptoms, pulmonary function testing, radiological evaluation, clinical laboratory and microbiological testing, and monitoring of drug levels are important components of this process. A new assay for immunologic monitoring, the CylexTM ImmuKnow assay, is becoming more widely available and appears quite promising. This test has shown utility for evaluating the effectiveness of therapeutic immunosuppression and the probability of rejection in patients with other types of solid organ transplants, and may have a role in titrating immunosuppressive therapy in lung transplant patients as well (4,5). Testing for anti-HLA antibodies and gastroesophageal reflux also has a place in post-transplant monitoring, since both entities have been associated with poor outcomes (5). Finally, bronchoscopy with collection of biopsy and cytology specimens remains central to follow-up strategies.

Although clinical signs and symptoms are helpful for alerting one to the possibility of a complication, they are not always present. Infections and rejection can trigger symptoms of cough and fever, and shortness of breath may indicate chronic airway rejection, acute rejection (AR) (usually higher grade), or infection. Declines in spirometry, hypoxemia, and infiltrates on chest radiograph, particularly if new or changing, should raise questions about rejection and infection. When suspicions about rejection, infection, or another complication occur, *bronchoscopy* is usually performed and samples are collected for histological and cytological analysis and microbiological testing. Should bronchoscopy be unsuccessful in revealing the cause of the patient's problem, other procedures such as core or fine needle aspiration biopsy, or videoscopic or open lung biopsy can be performed. Many centers also choose to perform surveillance bronchoscopy with biopsy at specified time intervals after transplantation, regardless of whether any indications of graft dysfunction exist. This practice is based upon the theoretical advantage of detecting and treating AR or evolving OB earlier in its course, to potentially reduce the incidence of refractory OB. The utility of this practice has been evaluated in multiple studies looking at rates of development of OB and patient survival, and the results have varied (as have the treatment and biopsy regimens and other variables), so the topic continues to be debated (6–13).

Histological processing of bronchoscopic biopsies should be done using standard formalin fixation and paraffin embedding. Three to five hematoxylin-eosin–stained sections are routinely prepared, and many centers also routinely perform silver staining to evaluate for fungi including *Pneumocystis jiroveci*, although other microbiological, serological, and molecular techniques are also available to detect many of these organisms. A connective tissue stain is also important for facilitating the observation of submucosal fibrosis in small airways, needed for diagnosis of OB. Immunohistochemical staining for CMV can be helpful for interpreting histologically equivocal cases, sometimes occurring after treatment of CMV, and can detect occasional histologically occult cases (14).

Other immunohistochemical, histochemical, and in situ hybridization studies can also be performed, depending upon the differential diagnostic considerations.

Interpretation of biopsies from lung transplant patients should take into account the patient's clinical situation and the results of other pertinent tests and examinations. Clinical and radiographic contextual information can often help one construct a more specific diagnosis or refine interpretations in situations in which the biopsy manifests more than one process. Review of earlier biopsies can also offer insights into the effectiveness of antirejection and other therapies.

Pathological evaluation of transbronchial biopsies should include an assessment of sample adequacy. Since rejection is usually a patchy process, diagnostic sensitivity is influenced by the quantity of alveolar tissue in the biopsy. A minimum of five fragments of well expanded alveolated tissue is recommended for evaluation for AR (15) and lesser volumes should be recognized with a statement to this effect in the pathology report. If features of rejection are not appreciated in the biopsy, this does not preclude the possibility of rejection, since sampling error can occur. Again, correlation with other clinical information is necessary to put the biopsy findings into the proper perspective.

III. EARLY COMPLICATIONS

Complications developing in the first month after transplantation include primary graft dysfunction (PGD), donor-transmitted and other primary infectious pneumonias, and rare cases of hyperacute rejection and symptomatic smoking-related injury in the allograft lung (Table 6.1). Most airway and vascular anastomotic complications also declare themselves during this period, and patients can

TABLE 6.1 Problems of the Early Post-Transplant Period

PGD
Infectious pneumonias, donor transmitted and primary
    Bacterial
    Viral
Rejection
    Antibody mediated (hyperacute or accelerated)
    Acute
Airway anastomotic complications
    Obstructive granulation tissue and stricture
    Anastomotic infections, especially bacterial and fungal
    Bronchomalacia
    Dehiscence
Vascular anastomotic complications
    Pulmonary venous thrombosis
    Pulmonary arterial thrombosis
    Dual pulmonary arterial and venous thrombosis
    Pulmonary artery dissection
Smoking-related respiratory compromise

also experience the onset of AR in these early days after transplantation. Hyperacute rejection and AR will be discussed later in this chapter.

PGD, which refers to the development of a severe acute lung injury syndrome soon after transplantation, is the most common cause of death during the first thirty days after transplantation (2,3,16). Other names used for this process include "primary graft failure," "early graft dysfunction," "severe ischemia reperfusion injury," and "reimplantation response." The hallmark of this condition is poor oxygenation. Physiological changes include worsening gas exchange, decreased pulmonary compliance, and increased pulmonary vascular resistance (17). Grading of PGD is based upon P_aO_2:F_iO_2 and the presence or absence of radiographic infiltrates consistent with pulmonary edema during the first seventy-two hours after final lung reperfusion (16). The incidence of severe PGD appears to lie between 10 and 15 percent, depending upon the criteria for diagnosis, and there is a high associated mortality rate and a long recovery period for survivors (18–20).

In most cases of PGD, the acute injury is believed to stem from *ischemia-reperfusion injury* of the donor lung (17,18,21), but occult infections and rejection may underlie smaller numbers of cases. The pathogenesis of ischemia-reperfusion injury appears to involve ischemia-associated increases in oxidative stress, sodium pump inactivation, intracellular calcium overload, iron release, and induction of cell death (22,23). Upregulation of endothelial cell adhesion molecules during ischemia promotes leukocyte adherence, activation, and extravasation, and a variety of pro- and anti-inflammatory cytokines are released from macrophages, lymphocytes, and other cells (22,24,25) (see Chapter 1). Data also suggest that there is an increased expression of ELR+ CXC chemokines in the lung with ischemia-reperfusion injury and that their interaction with CXCR2 plays a role in the pathogenesis of this complication (26). Increased vascular permeability, complement activation, and accumulation of the vasoconstrictor endothelin-1 occur, leading to increased pulmonary vascular resistance (27,28). These effects may be compounded by other biochemical changes associated with mechanical ventilation, infection, aspiration, brain death, trauma, or hypotension. Histological features are those of diffuse alveolar damage/acute lung injury (Figure 6.1). However, since many infectious pneumonias and rejection can *also* cause diffuse alveolar damage/acute lung injury, careful scrutiny for findings suggesting infection and rejection must be performed before the diffuse alveolar damage/acute lung injury can be attributed to ischemia-reperfusion injury.

Primary and donor-transmitted infections can present in the early post-transplant period, and rapid diagnosis and treatment is crucial. Other cases can present later after transplantation. A recent study found donor-to-host transmission of bacterial or fungal infection in 7.6 percent of lung transplants performed, either due to donor bacteremia or colonization of the graft; 25 percent of donors with bacteremia and 14 percent of colonized grafts were responsible for transmitting infection (29). A discussion and set of recommendations for utilization of donor lungs with infections has recently been published (30). The spectrum of donor-transmitted infectious agents includes bacteria (31,32), CMV (33), adenovirus (34,35), influenza A (36), Epstein-Barr virus (37), fungi (38–41) and toxoplasmosis (in heart-lung transplant recipients, transmitted in the transplanted heart) (42,43). Some cases of tuberculosis in the transplanted lung, probably representing graft-transmitted infections, have also been described (44–47).

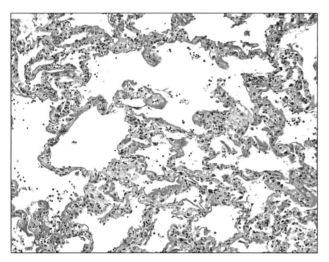

FIGURE 6.1: *Primary graft failure due to ischemia-reperfusion injury: hyaline membranes line alveolar septa and scant inflammatory infiltrate is noted.*

Airway and vascular anastomotic problems usually occur soon after transplantation and occasionally at later points in time. Loss of the bronchial artery blood supply to the donor airways can lead to ischemic airway necrosis if the collateral circulation cannot supply tissue needs. Overall, significant airway anastomotic complications affect 6.8–25.0 percent of lung transplant recipients and include development of obstructive granulation tissue, strictures, infections, bronchomalacia, and dehiscence (48–54). Tall recipients and those receiving lungs from donors with prolonged ventilation are reportedly associated with an increased risk to develop bronchial anastomotic problems (55). In children, preoperative infection with *Pseudomonas cepacia*, postoperative fungal lung infection, and days on mechanical ventilator were found to be significant risk factors (53). Treatment options can include stenting, bronchodilation, laser ablation, bronchoscopic debridement, and/or operative revision (48,49,51,52). Histological changes are influenced by the age of the process and the presence or absence of concurrent infection. Coagulative necrosis of airway mucosa, submucosa, and sometimes cartilage, with ulceration, fibrinous exudates, granulation tissue, fibrosis, and calcification can be seen, depending upon the longevity of the process (Figure 6.2A). With superimposed bacterial or fungal infections (the latter are usually caused by *Candida* or *Aspergillus*), organisms and inflammation can be visible either on the surface of the airway or invading deeper tissues (Figures 6.2B and 6.3).

Significant vascular anastomotic complications occur less often than airway anastomotic complications. Pulmonary venous thrombosis usually presents in the early postoperative period and causes hemorrhagic infarction of the affected lobes. Pulmonary venous thrombosis or stenosis appearing years after lung transplantation, with

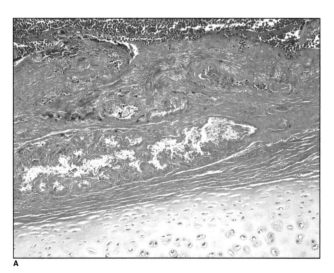

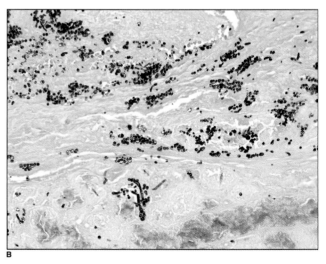

FIGURE 6.2: *Airway anastomotic ischemia with invasive Candida. (A) The mucosa, submucosa, and cartilage demonstrate coagulative necrosis. Aggregates of yeasts infiltrate the necrotic tissues. (B) This Grocott methenamine silver stain highlights the infiltrating yeasts and hyphae at the bronchial anastomosis.*

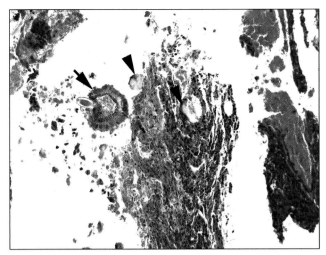

FIGURE 6.3: *Airway anastomotic ischemia with Aspergillus niger colonization: a fruiting head of A. niger (arrow) lies next to fragments of necrotic material and exudate. Oxalate crystals are indicated by arrowheads.*

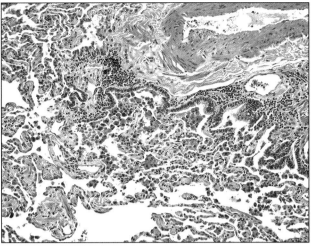

FIGURE 6.4: *Respiratory bronchiolitis: pigmented macrophages fill the lumen of this respiratory bronchiole, and there is associated chronic inflammation. This patient had a slower improvement in respiratory function after transplantation, than was expected.*

development of unilateral pulmonary edema and pleural effusion on the affected side, has also been described (56). Pulmonary arterial and dual arterial and venous obstruction are very rare (57,58). A case of pulmonary artery dissection in a patient transplanted for primary pulmonary hypertension has also been reported (59).

Complications related to the donor's smoking habit are also uncommon. Although screening prevents transplantation of most lungs with significant smoking-related lung disease, in rare cases the degree of COPD can be underestimated and the lungs transplanted. In this setting, postoperative recovery of respiratory function may be slower or less than expected. Respiratory bronchiolitis may be seen on lung biopsy (Figure 6.4).

IV. LUNG ALLOGRAFT REJECTION

Diagnosis and grading of *lung allograft rejection* is essential for patient and graft survival. Bronchoscopy with transbronchial biopsy is generally viewed as having a high sensitivity and specificity for diagnosis of rejection and has therefore become the primary procedure performed to accomplish this important task. The classification and grading of rejection has evolved since the creation of the original *Working Formulation* published in 1990 (60), then revised in 1995 (61), and recently updated again (15). Overall, the scheme has proven itself to be clinically and therapeutically relevant and generally straightforward to apply. Recent studies of interobserver agreement are limited but suggest better agreement on the grading of AR lesions than airway lesions (62–64).

The most recent review of the grading system was undertaken in 2006 under the direction of the ISHLT

and approved by the ISHLT Board of Directors in April, 2007. This multidisciplinary review took into account research done in the decade since the prior revision, as well as comments solicited from the ISHLT membership and from the transplant pathology community. The resulting grading scheme is outlined in Tables 6.2 and 6.3 (15). As previously, alloreactive injury to the donor lung is recognized for its effects on both the vasculature and the airways. As was also true of earlier versions of the Working Formulation, morphological diagnosis of AR is based on perivascular and interstitial mononuclear inflammatory cell infiltrates, which may be accompanied by airway inflammation. Fibrous scarring in bronchioles characterizes the lesion of OB, which is the histological marker of chronic airway rejection, and is sometimes accompanied by accelerated fibrointimal changes in pulmonary arteries and veins (chronic vascular rejection). Grading of airway inflammation has changed in the current version of the *Working Formulation*, however, in two ways: 1) it is now limited to small airways (*lymphocytic bronchiolitis* [LB]), as opposed to the 1996 version which included assessment of bronchial inflammation; and 2) the former airway inflammation grades B1 and B2 have been collapsed into one grade, B1R (low grade), and grade B2R (high grade) includes the former grades B3 and B4. Chronic rejection continues to be histologically defined as OB (grade C), and is categorized as present (C1) or absent (C0), without reference to the presence or absence of inflammatory activity or the degree of airway obstruction observed. Chronic vascular rejection continues to be classified as grade D.

Chronic airway rejection is also diagnosed based upon pulmonary function changes, and in this setting is referred

TABLE 6.2 Grading of Acute Lung Allograft Rejection (15)

Grade (A)	Histological Characteristics
A0 (No AR)	• No mononuclear cell infiltrates, hemorrhage, necrosis
A1 (minimal AR)	• Scattered, infrequent perivascular mononuclear inflammatory cell infiltrates in alveolated lung parenchyma, forming two- to three-cell-thick loose or compact cuffs in the perivascular adventitia, particularly around venules • Inflammatory cell infiltrates include small round, plasmacytoid, and transformed lymphocytes • Eosinophils and endothelialitis are absent • Accompanying LB is less common than in grade A2 and higher grades
A2 (Mild AR)	• More frequent perivascular mononuclear inflammatory cell infiltrates forming loose or compact cuffs around blood vessels, particularly venules, which are readily visible at low magnification • Inflammatory cell infiltrates usually consist of a mixture of small round lymphocytes, activated lymphocytes, and plasmacytoid lymphocytes, often with macrophages and eosinophils • Endothelialitis, that is, subendothelial infiltration by mononuclear cells which may be associated with hyperplastic or regenerative changes in the endothelium, is common • No mononuclear cell infiltration into adjacent alveolar septa or air spaces
A3 (moderate AR)	• Easily recognizable cuffing of venules and arterioles by dense perivascular mononuclear cell infiltrates which extend into perivascular and peribronchiolar alveolar septa and airspaces, either as cells infiltrating singly into alveolar walls or in a more sheet-like pattern with corresponding expansion of the septa; endothelialitis is common • Inflammatory cell infiltrates usually consist of a mixture of small round lymphocytes, activated lymphocytes, and plasmacytoid lymphocytes, and macrophages, eosinophils, and occasional neutrophils are common • Aggregates of macrophages may collect in alveoli adjacent to the zones of alveolar septal infiltration, and type 2 alveolar cell hyperplasia may be seen
A4 (severe AR)	• Diffuse perivascular, interstitial and air space infiltrates of mononuclear cells (similar to spectrum seen in A3); endothelialitis is common • Intra-alveolar necrotic epithelial cells, macrophages, hyaline membranes, hemorrhage, neutrophils, parenchymal necrosis, infarction, or necrotizing vasculitis may be present • There may be a reduction in perivascular infiltrates concomitant with the extension of the inflammatory process into alveolar septa and spaces, with admixture of the lymphoid infiltrates with macrophages

TABLE 6.3 Grading of Small Airway Inflammation in Lung Allografts (15)

Grade	Histological Characteristics
B0, no airway inflammation	• No bronchiolar inflammation
B1R, low-grade small airway inflammation	• Mononuclear cells in the bronchiolar submucosa, which can be infrequent and scattered or form a circumferential band • Occasional eosinophils in the submucosa • No epithelial damage or intraepithelial lymphocytic infiltration
B2R, high-grade small airway inflammation	• Mononuclear cells in the bronchiolar submucosa include large, activated lymphocytes with greater numbers of eosinophils and plasmacytoid cells • Epithelial damage in the form of necrosis, metaplasia, and marked intraepithelial lymphocytic infiltration • May show epithelial ulceration, fibrinopurulent exudate, cellular debris and neutrophils
BX, ungradeable	• Ungradeable due to sampling problems, infection, tangential cutting, artifact, etc.

to as BOS (Table 6.4) (65,66). Diagnosis of chronic airway rejection by physiological means may be more sensitive than histology since physiological measurements may offer a more global analysis of pulmonary function versus the more limited analysis possible from examination of small biopsies. Biopsies may yield tissue that is not necessarily reflective of the majority of the graft condition, or may lack bronchioles to examine for OB, leading to under-diagnosis. As always, the biopsy offers one form of input that must be considered in the context of the whole clinical picture.

i. Clinical and Radiographic Features

Up to 85 percent of lung allograft recipients develop *AR* during the first year after transplantation and all patients remain vulnerable to this complication indefinitely (67–71). AR is usually diagnosed during the first three

TABLE 6.4 Bronchiolitis Obliterans Syndrome (66)

BOS 0: FEV_1 >90% of baseline and FEF_{25-75} >75% of baseline
BOS 0-p: FEV_1 81–90% of baseline and/or
FEF_{25-75} ≤75% of baseline
BOS 1: FEV_1 66–80% of baseline
BOS 2: FEV_1 51–65% of baseline
BOS 3: FEV_1 ≤50% of baseline

months after transplantation and can be as early as three days after transplantation (72). Low-grade fever and cough are common symptoms, and higher grade rejection episodes can be associated with shortness of breath as well. Decline in forced expiratory volume in one second (FEV_1) is typical, and hypoxemia may be evident particularly with higher grade episodes. Chest imaging shows variable changes; it may be normal or show perihilar or lower zone alveolar and interstitial infiltrates, pleural effusions, subpleural edema, and/or peribronchial cuffing (72). Although most episodes of AR will respond to augmented immunosuppressive therapy and the risk of death is low, the greater concern lies in the linkage between AR and chronic airway rejection. AR, particularly when it is high grade and/or persistent or recurrent, is the most important risk factor for development of OB/BOS; other probable risk factors include LB, development of anti-HLA class I or class II antibodies, and medication noncompliance; and other possible risk factors include CMV disease, increased degree of HLA mismatching between donors and recipients, older donor age, longer graft ischemic time, underlying disease, and gastroesophageal reflux with aspiration (9,66,73–86). Other agents that may play a role in development of chronic airway rejection include the respiratory viruses (adenovirus, respiratory syncytial virus, parainfluenza, influenza) (87,88), *Chlamydia pneumoniae* (89), and human herpes virus 6 (90).

Chronic airway rejection can develop as early as sixty days after transplantation but is usually diagnosed between nine and fifteen months after transplantation (91). Transplant patients remain at risk for this complication indefinitely. Among more than 10,000 adult lung transplant patients who survived at least fourteen days, 25 percent had developed BOS by 2.5 years after transplantation, and 50 percent by 5.6 years (2). Among pediatric patients, 32 percent have been diagnosed with BOS by seven years after transplantation (3). Chronic airway rejection remains the most frequent cause of death in adults and children surviving more than one year after transplantation (2,3).

Chronic airway rejection can present following what appears to be a respiratory tract infection or can have a more insidious onset with a nonproductive or minimally productive cough (72). Dyspnea is often progressive and recurrent lower respiratory tract infections can cause exacerbations of symptoms. Many treatment approaches have been tested for their efficacy against established OB/BOS

but have been ineffective in most patients (86). Reports of stabilization or improvement have been published but are difficult to assess due to variations in study design and other factors (9,66,86,92–104). Recent studies looking at statins (105), azithromycin (106–109), and total lymphoid irradiation (110) are promising, but additional work is needed to validate their utility.

ii. Pathological Features of AR

AR is diagnosed and graded based upon the density and distribution of the mononuclear inflammatory cell infiltrates and any associated parenchymal damage (Table 6.2, Figures 6.5–6.10) (15). Although multiple vessels are usually affected, occasionally only a single

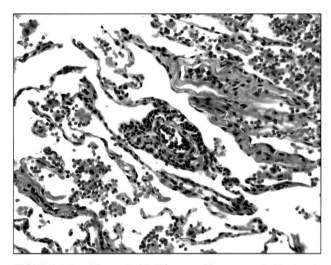

FIGURE 6.5: AR, grade A1: this vessel is surrounded by two to three cell layers of small lymphocytes.

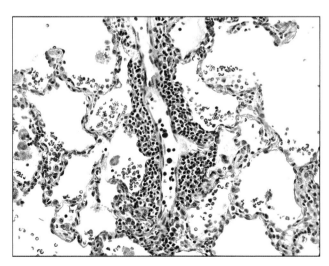

FIGURE 6.6: AR, grade A2: this venule has a cuff of lymphocytes with fewer macrophages and plasma cells. There is no interstitial extension of the inflammatory infiltrate.

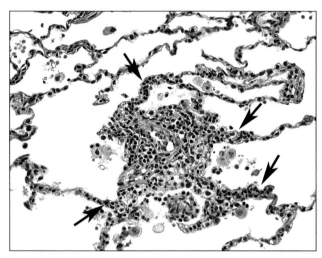

FIGURE 6.7: AR, grade A3: there is dense perivascular cuffing by lymphocytes, which also extend into the alveolar septa (arrows).

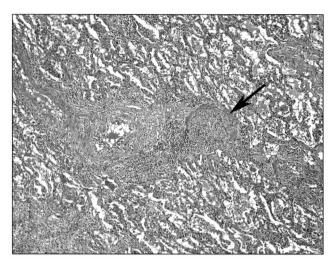

FIGURE 6.9: AR, grade A4, with OB, grade C1: the lung is diffusely infiltrated by mononuclear inflammatory cells with associated early diffuse alveolar damage. A focus of OB (arrow) is also present, made easy to recognize by its position adjacent to an artery.

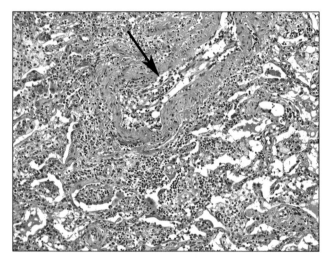

FIGURE 6.8: AR, grade A4: mononuclear inflammatory cells diffusely infiltrate the alveolar septa and airspaces, with associated edema, fibrin deposition, and foamy macrophages. A focus of endothelialitis (arrow) shows marked endothelial vacuolization and hyperplasia.

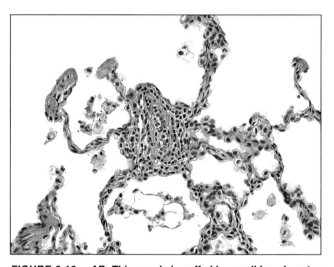

FIGURE 6.10: AR: This venule is cuffed by small lymphocytes that show prominent subendothelial infiltration. Although the thickness of the lymphocyte cuff and the nonactivated state of the lymphocytes fall into the spectrum of grade A1, the intimitis is more characteristic of grade A2. Such lesions can be difficult to classify histologically. Four experienced lung pathologists classified this lesion as borderline A1/A2 (3 people) or A1 (1 person).

vessel is involved; the number of vessels involved, however, does not influence the grading (15). When rejection lesions of multiple grades are observed, the overall grade is determined by the highest grade pattern, not the predominant pattern (15). Mononuclear cell infiltrates around small vessels in the submucosal regions of airways are considered to fall within the spectrum of airway inflammation, and do not by themselves justify a diagnosis of AR (grade A) (15).

AR typically affects *venules*, but other vessels can be involved as well, particularly in high-grade AR. It was the view of the histopathology task force that perivascular infiltrates related to AR should be *circumferential*, and that incomplete vascular cuffing is unlikely to represent AR,

although deeper levels may be helpful to look further for circumferentiality (15). Lymphocytes are the primary inflammatory cell constituents of these infiltrates. They can appear small, activated, or plasmacytoid. Most are T lymphocytes, and are a mixture of CD4+ and CD8+ cells. They can infiltrate the subendothelial region, causing endothelial vacuolization (endothelialitis) (Figure 6.8). Other inflammatory cells participating in AR include plasma cells, macrophages, eosinophils, and neutrophils, particularly in higher rejection grades. High-grade AR demonstrates *extension* of the mononuclear inflammatory cells from the perivascular zones into the alveolar septa and airspaces, with various manifestations of parenchymal injury as outlined in Table 6.2. In many centers, augmentation of immunosuppression is done for AR with a grade of A2 or higher. Grade A1 rejection may prompt similar therapy in some centers and in some clinical settings, but there is less agreement about the handling of this grade of AR. Recent studies supporting a link between grade A1 AR and chronic airway rejection suggest that the treatment threshold should be low (111–113).

LB often accompanies AR lesions, but in some cases may occur without visible AR foci. In this situation, it is partic-

ularly important to exclude infection before ascribing an airway lesion to rejection. Histologically, LB lesions demonstrate submucosal infiltrates of mononuclear inflammatory cells in bronchioles, which may be accompanied by manifestations of epithelial damage (Table 6.3, Figures 6.11 and 6.12) (15). Eosinophils and neutrophils tend to become more conspicuous with high-grade lesions, but a predominance of neutrophils should raise the question of infection.

For reporting, the consensus group recommended continuing the same format that was recommended in the 1996 version of the Working Formulation, that is, stating the AR grade with airway inflammation grade (15). For example, mild AR with low-grade small airway inflammation would be reported as mild AR, grade A2, with airway inflammation, grade B1R. LB without AR would be graded as A0, B1R or A0, B2R depending upon the grade of the airway inflammation.

iii. Differential Diagnosis

The histological findings that define rejection are not specific for rejection and can also occur in other clinicopathological settings. Therefore, correlation of the histological findings with the rest of the patient's clinical picture and radiological and laboratory data is essential. Also complicating matters, in some patients, is the coexistence of multiple pathologies, that is, rejection and infection in the same biopsy, although it is generally not recommended to diagnose rejection in a setting of infection.

Perivascular mononuclear cell infiltrates can be seen with CMV and *P. jiroveci* pneumonia, mycobacterial infection, and post-transplant lymphoproliferative disorders (PTLDs) (114,115). Differentiation between

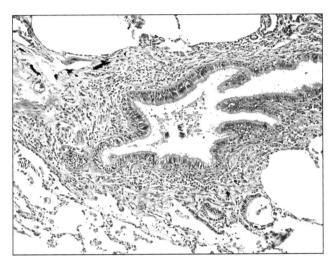

FIGURE 6.11: *LB, grade B1R: there is an infiltrate consisting of lymphocytes and plasma cells in the submucosa of this bronchiole, without infiltration into the overlying epithelium.*

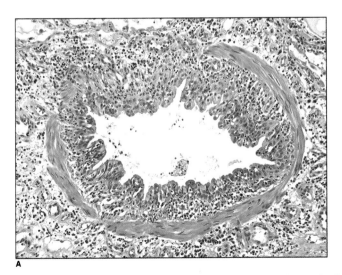

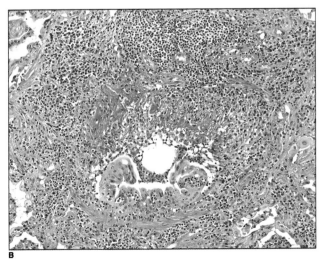

FIGURE 6.12: *LB, grade B2R. (A) The inflammatory infiltrate is circumferential and extends from the submucosa into the epithelium, with epithelial cell dropout, and smaller numbers of neutrophils are also present; (B) this markedly inflamed bronchiole demonstrates necrosis and ulceration with inflammation and reactive changes in the residual epithelium, as well as prominent peribronchiolar lymphoplasmacytic infiltrates.*

these entities is necessary, however, because of the different treatments required for each. Careful morphological examination with performance of appropriate organism and immunohistochemical stains is helpful, as is utilization of microbiological, serological, and molecular testing geared to evaluate for the processes being considered.

Occasionally, it may be necessary to determine whether a case of *diffuse alveolar damage* is caused by AR, infection, or ischemia-reperfusion injury. In this situation, observation of diffuse perivascular, interstitial, and airway-centered lymphocytic infiltrates favors AR, while a hypoinflammatory picture (Figure 6.1) favors one of the other etiologies. Also, diffuse alveolar damage caused by ischemia-reperfusion injury has an onset within hours to three days after transplantation. Many infections are capable of triggering diffuse alveolar damage, so examination for other histological features suggestive of infection, with performance of appropriate organism and immunohistochemical stains, as well as other microbiological, serological, and molecular testing is helpful in order to improve the chances of identifying a causative organism. Observation of acute pneumonia, microabscesses, granulomatous inflammation, prominent eosinophil infiltrates, honeycomb alveolar exudates, viral cytopathic changes, or multinucleated giant cells should raise the question of infection.

LB, particularly when it occurs without accompanying changes of AR, can be problematic. Although some examples are attributable to rejection, the list of potential etiologies for this lesion includes infections with a variety of bacteria, viruses, fungi, *Mycoplasma*, and *Chlamydia*, healing anastomosis or biopsy site, aspiration, asthma, smoking-related injury, and other processes. When bronchiolar neutrophil infiltrates predominate over lymphoid infiltrates, infections with bacteria, *Candida*, or occasionally respiratory viruses should be considered and investigated. It must be kept in mind, however, that neutrophils become more conspicuous with high-grade LB, although the dominant cell type is still the neutrophil. A healing anastomotic or previous biopsy site can display lymphocytic or neutrophilic infiltrates, but hemosiderin-laden macrophages and granulation tissue should raise this consideration, and the bronchoscopist can also supply valuable information about the location of the biopsy site to assist in the resolution of this question. Aspiration should be considered when LB is accompanied by food particles (sometimes with foreign body giant cells) or vacuolated macrophages with open round spaces representing lipid droplets. Lung transplantation predisposes to gastroesophageal reflux and aspiration, and reflux may be important in the genesis of some cases of OB/BOS (5,84,116). In asthma, mononuclear infiltrates are often accompanied by eosinophils, goblet cell hyperplasia, and thickening of the airway basement membrane, findings that should suggest consideration of asthma. The differential diagno-

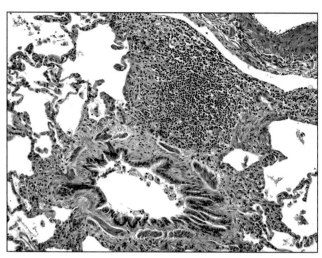

FIGURE 6.13: *Bronchial-associated lymphoid tissue: a lymphoid aggregate lies adjacent to a bronchiole that shows changes of OB (submucosal fibrosis).*

sis of LB also includes bronchial-associated lymphoid tissue (BALT, Figure 6.13), which usually shows better circumscription than LB and is not associated with epithelial injury.

Finally, rare examples of AR demonstrate larger numbers of eosinophils, usually in association with other histological features of high-grade rejection (117). In Yousem's series, this occurred early after transplantation, with leukocytosis and occasional peripheral blood and bronchoalveolar lavage eosinophilia. Distinction of this variant AR presentation from allograft infection is important since four allografts infected with *Aspergillus*, coxsackie A2 virus, and *Pseudomonas maltophilia* also showed prominent graft eosinophilia.

iv. Pathological Features of Chronic Airway Rejection

Although chronic rejection affects all components of the lung, its *small airway* manifestations have the greatest significance to the patient in terms of survival and quality of life. Chronic rejection is histologically defined by the lesion of *obliterative bronchiolitis* (OB, also known as bronchiolitis obliterans). OB is in turn defined by the presence of dense eosinophilic hyaline *fibrosis* in the submucosa of membranous and respiratory bronchioles, which produces partial or complete luminal occlusion (15). The bronchiolar lumen is narrowed by concentric or eccentric areas of subepithelial fibrosis (constrictive bronchiolitis) or can be completely filled by fibrous tissue with loss of epithelium (Figure 6.14). With total fibrous occlusion, the bronchiole may appear inconspicuous, but noticing its location adjacent to a similar sized pulmonary artery can be helpful for recognizing it (Figure 6.9). The fibrosing process may cause fragmentation or replacement of bronchiolar smooth muscle, and the fibrous tissue may extend into

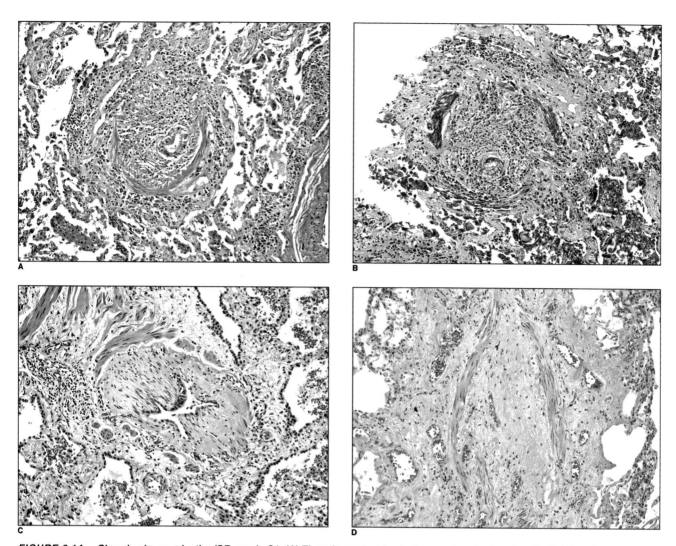

FIGURE 6.14: *Chronic airway rejection/OB, grade C1. (A) There is marked luminal narrowing due to subepithelial fibrosis and inflammation in this terminal bronchiole, and a portion of the smooth muscle has also been replaced by fibrous tissue; (B) this Masson trichrome stain highlights the collagen deposition underlying the inflammation; (C) this bronchiole shows dense fibrosis of the submucosa with minimal inflammation, and a cuboidal epithelial lining; (D) the lumen of this bronchiole is completely filled by dense fibrous tissue.*

peribronchiolar tissues. Variably intense mononuclear inflammatory cell infiltrates, often with some neutrophils, can accompany the fibrous tissue in the airway wall and lumen and cause continuing epithelial damage. Dense neutrophilic infiltrates, however, should raise a question of infection. Mucostasis and foamy macrophages in the small airways and adjacent alveoli are frequently associated with the OB. In the 2006 revision of the Working Formulation, OB is classified as either absent (grade C0) or present (grade C1), with no comment made about inflammatory activity (15).

Bronchiectasis can also be a consequence of rejection usually combined with infection by bacteria or fungi. It is not graded in the current version of the Working Formulation due its lack of specificity for rejection. Histologically, the airway wall demonstrates dense fibrosis with loss of cartilage, smooth muscle, and submucosal glands, and ongoing

inflammation (Figure 6.15). The epithelium can be metaplastic squamous or respiratory, often with reactive changes.

1. Differential Diagnosis

The pathogenesis of OB in lung transplant recipients is not completely understood. In most cases, it is believed to represent the culmination of immunologic injury, but in other cases there is evidence favoring effects of infection and aspiration. In patients who have had both rejection and airway infection, the effects of each are usually not separable. Nonetheless, if a specific, treatable agent or cause can be identified in a biopsy, the pathologist should provide this information so that therapy can be directed appropriately. In cases caused by infections such as adenovirus, however, it is likely that viral cytopathic changes will have disappeared by the time that the OB is detected. Identification of food

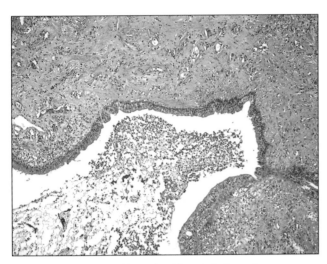

FIGURE 6.15: *Bronchiectasis: this ectatic bronchus demonstrates dense hyaline fibrosis and inflammation with loss of smooth muscle and submucosal glands.*

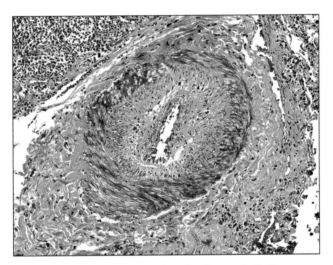

FIGURE 6.16: *Chronic vascular rejection, grade D: the fibrointimal thickening in this vessel is highlighted with a Masson trichrome stain.*

particles and foreign body giant cells is helpful for alerting the clinicians to the occurrence of aspiration.

v. Pathological Features of Chronic Vascular Rejection

Chronic vascular rejection/accelerated graft vascular sclerosis (grade D) refers to fibrointimal thickening of arteries and veins (Figure 6.16). Subendothelial, intimal, and/or medial mononuclear cell infiltrates may also be seen. Similar phlebosclerosis can be found in the lungs of older individuals, so lungs from older donors may have a higher frequency of this change.

vi. Antibody-Mediated Rejection

Although antibody-mediated rejection of lung allografts has been the focus of recent investigation, our understanding

of its incidence, predisposing factors, significance, and therapy needs further growth. Antibody targets include HLA and non-HLA antigens (118–121), and the roles of these antibodies in both AR and OB/BOS need to be more fully elucidated. Evidence is accumulating, however, supporting a role for antibody-mediated rejection in both processes, including associations between these antibodies and high-grade AR, multiple episodes of persistent-recurrent AR, and OB/BOS (81–83,119,122–124).

Histopathological criteria have not yet been established for diagnosis of antibody-mediated rejection in the lung. Pulmonary capillaritis and the spectrum of findings representing "capillary injury" have been suggested by some as potential markers for antibody-mediated rejection (125,126), but it is also recognized that these changes can be seen in infections, diffuse alveolar damage, and severe cellular rejection (15). The ISHLT consensus group did, however, recommend that should there be clinical, immunopathological, or histological suspicion of antibody-mediated rejection, then immunohistochemistry could be performed for C3d, C4d, CD31, and CD68, to provide further information (15). C4d staining is not, unfortunately, a panacea; recent studies have shown conflicting results. Ionescu et al. observed that subendothelial C4d deposition was a marker for the existence of anti-HLA antibodies but was typically patchy and demonstrated low sensitivity and specificity (80), while other investigators found no correlation with diagnosis (127). Bronchoalveolar lavage fluid from lung allograft recipients was analyzed and showed that C4d concentrations higher than 100 ng/ml were correlated with anti-HLA antibodies, but were also found with infection and in asymptomatic patients (128).

In the rare cases of *hyperacute rejection* that occur in lung transplant recipients with preformed antibodies to donor HLA antigens (129–134), these antibodies appear to be central to the catastrophic progression of histological and pathophysiological changes that follow transplantation. Although most patients who have preformed antibodies to donor antigens do not develop the full clinicopathological picture of hyperacute rejection, these antibodies appear to be associated with an increased risk of severe early post-transplant lung dysfunction (131). Clinically, patients with hyperacute rejection develop diffuse pulmonary infiltrates and severe hypoxemia within minutes-days of transplantation, resembling the picture of primary graft failure. The transplanted lung may produce frothy blood-tinged fluid, and hemodynamic instability, thrombocytopenia, and coagulopathy can occur. Although this complication is usually fatal, one patient was successfully treated with plasmapheresis, antithymocyte globulin, and cyclophosphamide, leading to recovery five days postoperatively (132). Intragraft binding of the preformed antibodies to the target donor HLA antigens, which are expressed on alveolar macrophages, endothelial cells, pneumocytes, and respiratory epithelial cells (135–137), is thought to lead to activation of

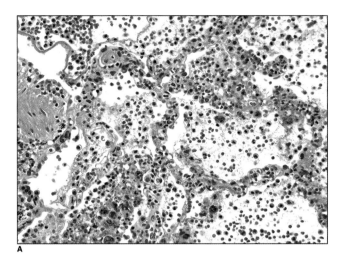
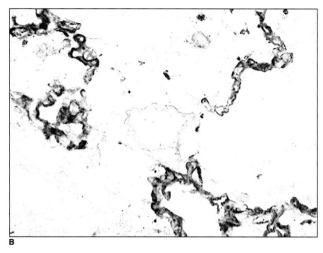

FIGURE 6.17: Hyperacute rejection: (A) early diffuse alveolar damage and hemorrhage are conspicuous, and are accompanied by interstitial neutrophilia and apoptotic cells in the alveolar spaces; (B) capillary walls are outlined by this immunohistochemical stain for C4d, supporting the presence of antibody-mediated (humoral) rejection.

complement, resulting in endothelial and epithelial cell injury, cytokine release, increased vascular permeability, and edema (131,133). Histological features of hyperacute rejection include diffuse alveolar damage, diffuse alveolar hemorrhage, interstitial neutrophilia, small vessel vasculitis, microthrombi, and neutrophil infiltration of airway epithelium (Figure 6.17A) (129–131). Alveolar deposition of IgG can be demonstrated by immunofluorescence and C4d staining of alveolar capillaries may be present (Figure 6.17B).

vii. Pathogenesis of Lung Allograft Rejection

Since the pathogenesis of rejection is discussed more extensively in another chapter (see Chapter 1), only a relatively brief overview is provided here. Immunologic factors are believed to contribute to the development of most cases of OB/BOS, and contributions from nonimmunologic factors may be important in some patients as well. After transplantation, the recipient's CD8+ and CD4+ T cells recognize donor HLA class I and class II antigens, respectively (138–140). Airway epithelial cells and endothelial cells express class I and class II molecules, and there is increased bronchial and bronchiolar class II molecule expression in OB (135–137,141–143), on endothelial cells in a setting of OB (136,141), and on epithelial and endothelial cells in AR (144). Increased CD4+ T-cell alloreactivity toward cells expressing donor HLA molecules appears to be involved in the pathogenesis of OB/BOS (145,146), but the role of CD8+ T cells is less clear. Airway epithelial cells are a primary target of T-lymphocyte–mediated injury during development of OB/BOS (147). Rejection is considered to be primarily a Th1 response, while Th2 responses may also have a role in OB/BOS. AR is associated with local production of proinflammatory

cytokines including tumor necrosis factor-α, interleukin (IL)-1α, IL-1β, IL-1 receptor antagonist (IL-1Ra), IL-2, IL-6, and interferon-γ production (148–151). In OB, higher levels of IL-8 are present (152), and the type 2 cytokine, IL-13, also appears to be important for progression to OB/BOS (153). A recent study also showed an early post-transplant elevation in basal serum levels of proinflammatory chemokines IP-10 and MCP-1 and Th1-cytokines IL-1beta, IL-2, IL-12, and IL-15 in patients with BOS as compared to patients free of BOS and normal subjects, as well as increased development of HLA class II alloantibodies and Th1-predominant donor-specific cellular immunity in patients with BOS (154).

Information about studies linking anti-donor antibodies to AR and OB/BOS is discussed above, in the section devoted to antibody-mediated rejection. In addition, cell culture studies show that anti-HLA antibody binding to HLA molecules on airway epithelial cells induces alterations that are pathogenetically related to the genesis of OB/BOS, including airway epithelial cell proliferation; production of fibrogenic growth factors including heparin-binding epidermal growth factor, platelet-derived growth factor, insulin-like growth factor, and basic fibroblast growth factor; and later airway epithelial cell apoptosis (83,155). An increase in airway epithelial cell apoptosis in a setting of active OB has also been noted by some investigators (156).

In rejection, macrophages expressing adhesion molecules including CD11c, CD31, and CD54 are elevated (151). AR and OB were found to be associated with increased expression of endothelial E-selectin but not intercellular adhesion molecule-1 (ICAM-1/CD54), in one study (157), while the opposite pattern was noted in another study (158). The latter group also reported induction of endothelial cell ICAM-2, lymphocyte function antigen-3, very late antigen-2, and very late antigen-6 molecules in lung transplant rejection (158). Infiltrating inflammatory cells in AR and fibroblasts in active OB demonstrate increased CD44 expression, which may facilitate inflammatory cell migration and fibroblast invasion of extracellular matrix materials (159). Local production of several fibrogenic growth factors has also been demonstrated in the evolution of chronic airway rejection, including platelet-derived growth factor (160,161), transforming growth factor-β (149,161,162), and insulin-like growth factor-1 (163).

Neutrophils are also increased in the airways of patients with chronic airway rejection, exposing the lung to injurious reactive oxygen species and proteases (152,164–167). Bronchoalveolar lavage fluid and tissue ferritin are significantly elevated in transplanted lungs (167,168), and bronchoalveolar lavage fluid NO_2^- levels are elevated with BOS and are strongly linked to the percentage of neutrophils (168), suggesting the potential for significant oxidative stress that is both iron-generated and due to nitric oxide and neutrophil-derived reactive oxygen species, particularly in OB/BOS. Increased expression of the anti-oxidant enzyme heme oxygenase-1 occurs in human lung allografts with AR and OB, and correlates with increased inflammatory/oxidant load as measured by myeloperoxidase expression and ferritin load (167). Significant depletion of total glutathione was noted in alveolar epithelial lining fluid from transplanted lungs, which may predispose to extracellular hydrogen peroxide-mediated toxicity (169).

Finally, recent years have seen numerous publications focused upon chimerism in transplanted organs. In transplanted lungs, there is evidence for at least transient chimerism among lymphocytes and macrophages (170–173), but only recently has evidence emerged supporting the existence of lung parenchymal cell chimerism (i.e., epithelial, endothelial, and mesenchymal cells of recipient karyotype in donor lungs). Most, but not all, studies in humans and animals have shown a low frequency of these cells, usually less than 5 percent of total, which are presumably derived from bone marrow-derived stem cells (174). The significance of these results for patients is not clear, and additional research is needed to determine the potential utility of stem cell–based approaches to treatment of many lung diseases, including those related to lung transplantation.

V. DISEASE RECURRENCE

Although disease recurrence after lung transplantation is unusual, multiple well documented reports exist (Table 6.5). *Sarcoidosis* is the most common disease to recur, and the granulomas appear to consist of cells derived from the recipient (175,176). Likewise, in two cases of recurrent *lymphangioleiomyomatosis*, lesional cells were found to originate from the recipient (177,178). In contrast, *bronchio-*

Table 6.5 Recurrent Diseases in Lung Allografts

Sarcoidosis (175,176,279–288)
Lymphangioleiomyomatosis (178,286,289–295)
Langerhans cell histiocytosis (296–298)
Desquamative interstitial pneumonia (299,300)
Alveolar proteinosis (one case associated with lysinuric protein intolerance) (301,302)
Giant cell interstitial pneumonia (303)
Diffuse panbronchiolitis (304)
Allergic bronchopulmonary aspergillosis (305)
Emphysema in an alpha-1 proteinase inhibitor–deficient cigarette smoking lung transplant recipient (306)
Idiopathic pulmonary hemosiderosis (307)
Intravenous talc granulomatosis [308]
Bilateral diffuse bronchiectasis (309)
Pulmonary veno-occlusive disease (310)
Bronchioloalveolar carcinoma (179,181)

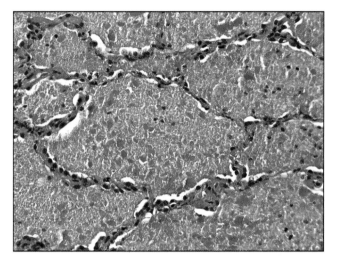

FIGURE 6.18: *Alveolar proteinosis: granular eosinophilic material fills the alveolar spaces.*

loalveolar carcinoma treated by lung transplantation demonstrates a high rate of tumor recurrence within the donor lungs (179–181).

VI. OTHER PULMONARY COMPLICATIONS

Pulmonary alveolar proteinosis is another uncommon complication of lung transplantation, occurring in patients whose histories often include ischemia-reperfusion injury and multiple episodes of rejection and infection (182,183). The histology is identical to alveolar proteinosis arising in other types of patients, and is characterized by accumulation of intra-alveolar eosinophilic granular material in alveoli (Figure 6.18), which is periodic acid-Schiff positive. As with other types of patients, evidence of an infectious process should be sought. *Pulmonary emboli* appear to be more frequent in lung and heart-lung transplant recipients than in the general population, with reported rates of 36.4

percent in patients who died in the first 30 days after transplantation, 20.0 percent for patients who died between 31and 365 days, and 23.8 percent for those patients who died later (184). One report describes a case of graft failure due to embolization of cerebral tissue to the lungs as a consequence of massive cerebral trauma suffered by the donor (185). *Graft transmission of donor malignancies* has been reported for renal cell carcinoma, choriocarcinoma, and glioblastoma multiforme (186,187).

VII. ADDITIONAL FINDINGS IN LUNG ALLOGRAFT SAMPLES

Lung allograft biopsies can demonstrate a variety of other histological changes including intra-alveolar deposition of fibrinous material, *organizing pneumonia* (Figure 6.19), and

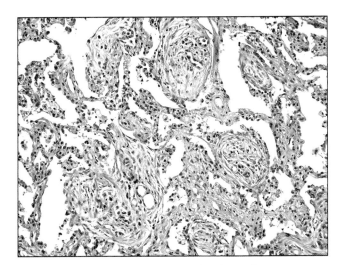

FIGURE 6.19: *Organizing pneumonia: plugs of young connective tissue occupy some of the alveolar spaces.*

accumulation of *hemosiderin-laden macrophages*. These changes are commonly seen with rejection and infection (188–190), and organizing pneumonia can follow ischemia-reperfusion injury (188). Hemosiderin-laden macrophages can also be encountered after a previous infection with a hemorrhagic component, in a biopsy from a previously biopsied area, or in the setting of a bleeding abnormality.

Bronchial-associated lymphoid tissue (BALT, Figure 6.13) is another common finding in lung allograft biopsies that must be histologically differentiated from LB. This can usually be accomplished based on the circumscription of the BALT focus and the lack of associated epithelial injury, versus the less well-bounded inflammatory cell infiltrates in LB, which are in some cases associated with epithelial injury.

Aspiration is common in lung transplant patients due to loss of the cough reflex. Food particles can be seen and are often accompanied by a foreign body giant cell reaction (Figure 6.20A). Aspiration of lipid material can be reflected by the presence of vacuolated macrophages and open round spaces in the tissue, representing the spaces occupied by lipid droplets (Figure 6.20B).

VIII. INFECTIONS IN LUNG TRANSPLANT PATIENTS

Lung transplant recipients are predisposed to infections by multiple factors including immunosuppressive therapies, underlying diseases, and injuries acquired as a consequence of transplantation. The latter may include rejection-associated airway damage and consequences of surgery such as loss or impairment of the cough reflex, which may in turn lead to aspiration and aspiration-related pneumonias, and airway anastomotic ischemia related to the interruption of the bronchial artery blood flow.

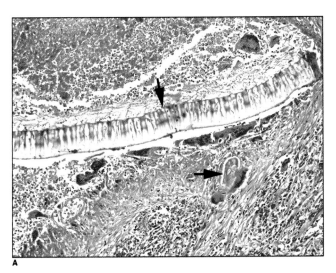

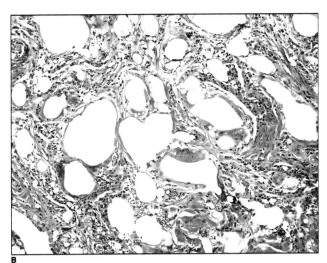

FIGURE 6.20: *Aspiration pneumonia. (A) Aspirated plant material (arrows) with a foreign body giant cell reaction is noted, with a coexisting granulomatous and acute inflammatory response; (B) spaces representing aspirated lipid material (not visible after histological processing) are associated with fibrosis and a foreign body giant cell reaction.*

Hypogammaglobulinemia also appears to be common in lung transplant recipients (191,192). An IgG level of less than 400 mg/dl (normal 717–1410 mg/dl) has been linked to an extremely high risk of bacterial and fungal infections, tissue-invasive CMV, and poorer survival (193). Additionally, development of fungal infections may be fostered by concurrent infections with immunomodulating viruses such as CMV, and bacteria that cause mucociliary injury and ulceration (194).

Distinguishing between infection and rejection remains one of the most important challenges for physicians caring for lung transplant patients. The pathologist plays a key part in this process through interpretation of samples and often through provision of advice about other microbiological, serological, and molecular testing that may be helpful for defining the cause of the patient's decline. The differential diagnosis between infection and rejection is discussed in the section of this chapter focused on rejection, as is the potential role of some infectious agents in the development of OB/BOS. This section is intended to provide general information about the frequencies and pathologies of the more common infectious agents affecting this patient group. A broad overview of the types of injury associated with these agents is provided in Table 6.6, and more detailed information can be obtained from a number of pulmonary pathology texts.

In lung transplant patients, infections can involve the allograft or a remaining native lung, and transmission from the donor via the graft or blood can occur (see Early Complications). For lung transplant patients overall, bacterial infections are most common and peak during the first month after transplantation (195–201). *Pseudomonas aeruginosa, Klebsiella pneumoniae, Escherichia coli, Staphylococcus aureus, Streptococcus* sp., and *Enterobacter cloacae* are the most common bacterial pathogens (202). Observation of prominent neutrophilic infiltrates in airways and alveoli (acute bronchopneumonia, Figure 6.21) should prompt consideration of a bacterial infection. *Nocardia* infection was reported in 2.1 percent of lung transplant recipients, often involves the native lung, and typically occurs more than one year after transplantation (196,203,204). *Chlamydia pneumoniae* was recently found in the lavage fluid

TABLE 6.6 Patterns of Injury Associated with Infections

Category	Patterns of Injury
Bacteria	Airway anastomotic infection Acute bronchitis and bronchopneumonia, abscesses Diffuse alveolar damage
Viruses	Diffuse alveolar damage Interstitial pneumonia Interstitial microabscesses (CMV) Granulomatous reaction (CMV) Acute and/or necrotizing airway infection (bronchitis, bronchiolitis, and/or bronchopneumonia) (respiratory viruses, HSV) Necrotizing hemorrhagic nodules (HSV, VZV) Giant cell pneumonia (RSV, parainfluenza, measles) OB (adenovirus, other respiratory viruses)
Candida	Airway anastomotic infection Acute bronchitis and bronchopneumonia, microabscesses Diffuse alveolar damage
Aspergillus	Airway anastomotic infection Airway colonization and invasive airway infection Colonization of a parenchymal cavity Chronic necrotizing aspergillosis Invasive fungal pneumonia Diffuse alveolar damage Bronchocentric granulomatous infection Eosinophilic pneumonia
Pneumocystis jiroveci	Interstitial pneumonia, occasionally with granuloma formation Diffuse alveolar damage
Other fungal species	Airway anastomotic infection Abscess Granulomatous infection Invasive fungal pneumonia
Mycobacteria	Granulomatous infection, variable neutrophils
Toxoplasma gondii	Necrotizing pneumonia

HSV, herpes simplex virus; VZV, varicella zoster virus; RSV, respiratory syncytial virus.

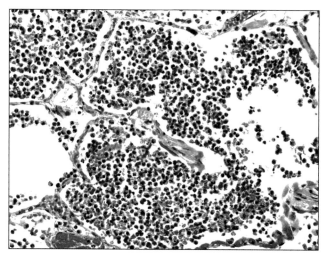

FIGURE 6.21: *Acute bronchopneumonia: neutrophils fill the alveolar spaces in this case of bacterial pneumonia.*

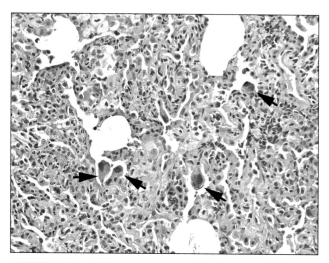

FIGURE 6.22: *CMV pneumonia: infected cells (arrows) demonstrate cytomegaly, nucleomegaly, and intranuclear and intracytoplasmic inclusions.*

of 25 percent of the lung transplant recipients studied more than thirty days after lung transplantation, five of whom had pneumonia and eight of whom had BOS (205). Diffuse alveolar damage caused by *Mycoplasma hominis* was encountered in one lung transplant recipient (206).

Among the viruses, CMV is the most frequent infecting agent, with other viruses accounting for smaller numbers of infections (33,196,198,207–210). The incidence of CMV pneumonia after transplantation is reported between 15 and 55 percent, and as many as 15 percent of cases of CMV pneumonia in lung transplant patients are asymptomatic (33). CMV disease can occur due to reactivation of latent virus or due to primary infection, including some cases of transmission in the allograft. Seronegative recipients receiving lungs from seropositive donors are at greatest risk for acquiring CMV pneumonia after transplantation (72), and treatment of rejection with augmented immunosuppression also predisposes to infection and pneumonia (211). Most cases of CMV infection are recognized between 14 and 100 days after transplantation (72), and the diagnosis is usually easily made on biopsy material showing the appropriate viral cytopathic changes (cytomegaly, nucleomegaly, nuclear and cytoplasmic inclusions, Figure 6.22) and an appropriate host response (Table 6.6). In questionable cases, particularly those from patients who have been treated for CMV, immunohistochemistry is of value. Microbiological and molecular methods are also readily available for diagnosis of this infection. Fortunately, the prevalence and mortality due to CMV infection have declined recently due to use of ganciclovir (198), and the incidence of *herpes simplex virus* pneumonia (Figure 6.23) has also been markedly reduced with routine acyclovir or ganciclovir prophylaxis (72).

In contrast, *community respiratory viral infections* (adenovirus, influenza, parainfluenza, respiratory syncytial virus,

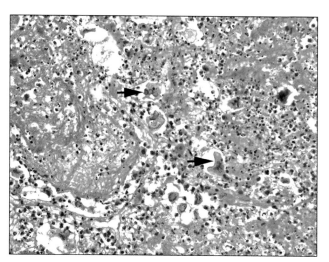

FIGURE 6.23: *Herpes simplex virus pneumonia: multinucleated giant cells (arrows) with ground glass chromatin are visible in a background of necrotizing pneumonia.*

rhinovirus, coronavirus, human metapneumovirus) are increasingly recognized as causes of significant pneumonias in lung transplant patients, but still appear to be less frequent than CMV (212–216). Adenovirus affects more children than adults and is associated with a particularly high risk of death, graft loss, and eventual development of OB (35,217,218). Adenovirus causes a severe necrotizing pneumonia and diffuse alveolar damage, and can be recognized by its characteristic smudge cells and other inclusions (Figure 6.24) (35,217). Influenza, parainfluenza (Figure 6.25), and respiratory syncytial virus (Figure 6.26) are also capable of causing a severe pneumonia but are less likely to take a fatal course than adenovirus. Influenza infections have been associated with features of AR (215) and with subsequent development of OB (219).

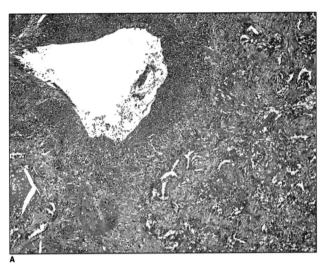

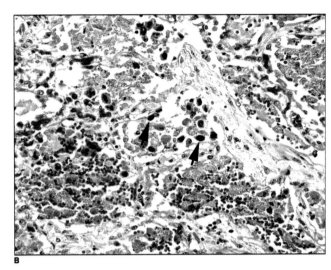

A

B

FIGURE 6.24: Adenovirus pneumonia. (A) Necrotizing bronchiolitis and diffuse alveolar damage are shown; (B) smudge cells (arrows) are characteristic of this virus.

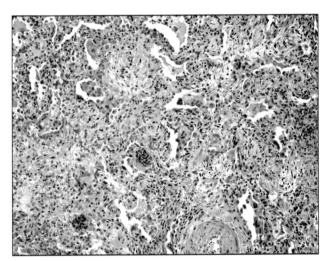

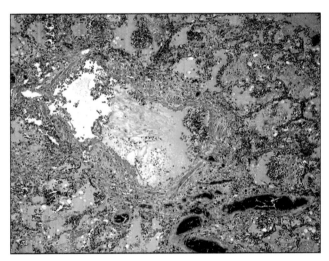

FIGURE 6.25: Parainfluenza pneumonia: there is a background of organizing diffuse alveolar damage with scattered multinucleated giant cells characteristic of parainfluenza. The differential diagnosis for these histological findings also includes respiratory syncytial virus and measles pneumonia.

FIGURE 6.26: Respiratory syncytial virus pneumonia: this bronchiole demonstrates a hypoinflammatory necrotizing bronchiolitis, with loss of epithelium and replacement by fibrinous exudate. In contrast, bronchiolitis due to rejection will have many more lymphocytes. Pulmonary edema is also noted.

Respiratory tract infections with respiratory syncytial virus and parainfluenza usually resolve but can take a more aggressive course in some patients (212,220). Rhinovirus (221,222), coronavirus (221,222), and human metapneumovirus (222–225) have also been identified in lung transplant recipients with symptomatic respiratory tract illnesses, and more information is needed to determine their importance in this patient group.

Fungal infections range from colonizations to localized and more extensive pulmonary invasive forms and examples of disseminated invasive disease. Overall, *Candida* and *Aspergillus* account for most fungal colonizations and infections, but other species have also been reported

(196,226–229). *Candida* and *Aspergillus* are the most frequent fungal causes of airway anastomotic infections arising early after transplantation (54,196,210,230–233). Between one and six months after transplantation, infections occur with opportunistic fungi (*Aspergillus, Pneumocystis,* zygomycetes, *Cryptococcus*) and occasional examples of geographically restricted endemic fungi, usually in patients living in endemic areas (194). After six months, fungal infections are usually associated with chronic airway rejection or mechanical abnormalities of airways.

Aspergillus represents a particular problem for lung transplant patients. An aggregated analysis of published information determined rates of 26, 4, and 5 percent for

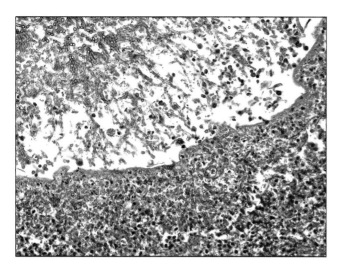

FIGURE 6.27: *Aspergillus infections: airway invasion by the fungus is noted in this bronchus from a patient who had chronic rejection and bronchiectasis. The hyphae are thin, septate, branching, and have parallel walls.*

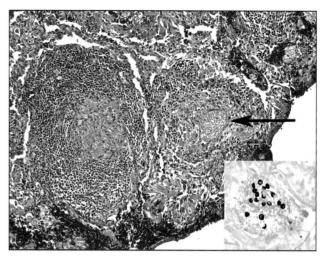

FIGURE 6.28: *Pneumocystis jiroveci pneumonia: This case shows the typical eosinophilic honeycomb exudate (arrow) with an associated granulomatous reaction. In the inset, the characteristic cysts are shown, highlighted by a Grocott methenamine silver stain. Several contain a dot or have a cup-shaped appearance.*

airway colonization, isolated tracheobronchitis, and invasive pneumonia, respectively, in lung transplant patients (234). Over half of the infections were discovered in the first six months after transplantation, but the incidence of progression from airway colonization to invasive disease was low (approximately 3 percent). In the pooled published data, 82 percent of patients with isolated tracheobronchitis responded to antifungal therapy and/or surgical debridement, and 41 percent with invasive pneumonia or disseminated disease survived. *Aspergillus* infection can manifest a variety of clinical and histological presentations (Table 6.6, Figure 6.27) including unusual presentations such as bronchocentric mycosis (235) and acute eosinophilic pneumonia (117). *Scedosporium apiospermum* can be a persistent colonizer or an occasional cause of an invasive airway anastomotic infection or pneumonia (236). Zygomycetes rarely cause invasive pneumonias (228,237–239) or airway anastomotic infection (54) in lung transplant recipients. *Pneumocystis jiroveci* (Figure 6.28) prophylaxis has substantially reduced the development of significant infections with this organism (240), but occasional examples of this infection continue to be seen (241).

Pulmonary and pleural mycobacterial infections appear to be uncommon in the lung transplant patient population, with an estimated frequency of 2.6–9.1 percent (242–245). In this patient group, non-tuberculous mycobacteria are more common than *M. tuberculosis*, and *M. avium* complex is most frequent among the non-tuberculous mycobacteria (33). Other agents isolated have included *M. abscessus, M. asiaticum, M. kansasii, M. chelonae,* and *M. fortuitum* (246–252).

Pulmonary toxoplasmosis is a rare complication occurring in heart-lung transplant recipients who presumably acquired their infections from their cardiac allografts. It

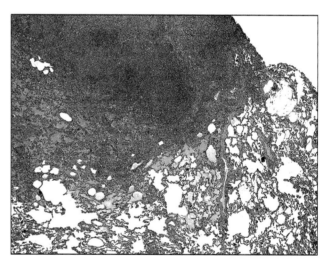

FIGURE 6.29. *PTLD: the nodular appearance of this lesion is obvious at low power.*

has been largely eliminated due to antimicrobial prophylaxis in *T. gondii*–mismatched patients (253).

IX. POST-TRANSPLANT LYMPHOPROLIFERATIVE DISORDERS

PTLDs occur in 2.5–6.1 percent of lung transplant patients (254–256). Pulmonary presentation with nodular disease (Figure 6.29), often in the allograft, is typical and may be accompanied by an ulcerative bronchitis, but extrapulmonary origin also occurs (255,257,258). Although cases arise most often in the first year after transplantation, patients remain at risk for this complication indefinitely. In solid organ transplant recipients, the majority of PTLDs are

B-cell lymphomas that are derived from host cells and contain Epstein-Barr virus (259–267). Therapeutic strategies have included reduction of immunosuppression and more recently, the anti-CD20 antibody rituximab has shown efficacy against many of these tumors (256,268,269).

PTLDs manifest a spectrum of morphologies and have evolved through multiple histological classification systems (270–274). The 2001 World Health Organization classification system is shown in Table 6.7 (274) (see Chapter 10). Early lesions are usually polyclonal, and the other lesions are usually monoclonal B-cell proliferations. Early lesions usually affect lymph nodes, while pulmonary lesions more commonly fall into the polymorphic or monomorphic PTLD categories. Polymorphic PTLD lesions typically consist of nodules that replace the normal lung architecture and consist of a mixture of small

TABLE 6.7 Classification of PTLDs (274)

Early lesions
  Reactive plasmacytic hyperplasia
  Infectious mononucleosis-like

Polymorphic PTLD

Monomorphic PTLD
  B-cell neoplasms
  Diffuse large B-cell lymphoma (immunoblastic, centroblastic, anaplastic)
  Burkitt/Burkitt-like lymphoma
  Plasma cell myeloma
  Plasmacytoma-like lesion
  T-cell neoplasms
  Peripheral T-cell lymphoma, not otherwise specified
  Other types

Hodgkin's lymphoma and Hodgkin's lymphoma–like PTLD

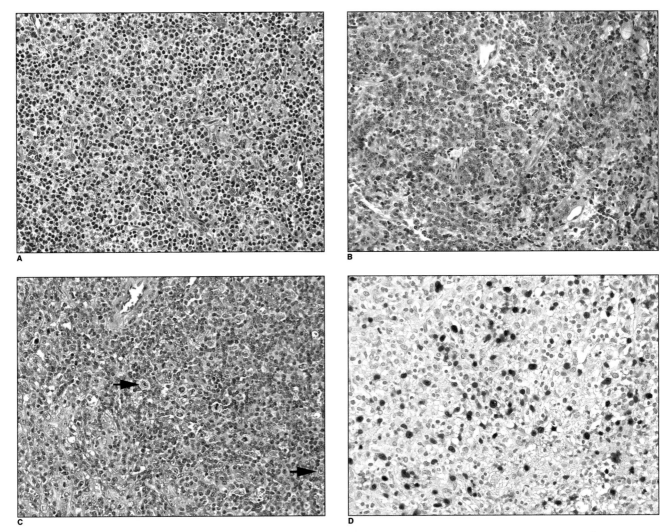

FIGURE 6.30: PTLDs: (A) polymorphic case includes atypical large lymphoid cells admixed with smaller and other activated lymphocytes, plasma cells, and histiocytes; (B) monomorphic example has the histology of a diffuse large cell lymphoma; (C) Hodgkin's-like case shows occasional mononuclear Reed-Sternberg variant cells (arrows) in a background of lymphocytes; (D) Epstein-Barr virus RNA is present in the blue-stained nuclei in this tumor (EBER1 in situ hybridization).

lymphocytes, large lymphocytes, immunoblasts, plasma-cytoid lymphocytes, and plasma cells (Figure 6.30A). Monomorphic PTLD lesions are comprised of sheets of large transformed atypical lymphocytes often resembling diffuse large B-cell lymphomas (Figure 6.30B). Necrosis associated with angiocentric infiltration can be seen in some cases. Fewer cases have also been classified as Burkitt/Burkitt-like lymphoma, plasma cell myeloma, plasma-cytoma-like lesions, peripheral T-cell lymphoma, NK-cell type lymphoma, Hodgkin's lymphoma, and Hodgkin's lymphoma–like PTLD (Figure 6.30C).

Immunohistochemical staining, flow cytometry, and molecular testing can be used to evaluate the phenotype and clonality of the lymphoid cells and search for the presence of Epstein-Barr virus. In polymorphic PTLDs, the lymphocytes include a mixture of CD20+ B and CD3+ T lymphocytes. Immunoglobulin light chain expression by B lymphocytes and plasma cells can show a polyclonal or monoclonal pattern. In most monomorphic PTLDs, the large atypical lymphocytes are B cells that express CD19, CD20, and CD79a. CD43 and CD45RO expression may also be seen and occasional cases may express CD30. A monoclonal pattern of kappa and lambda light chain expression is usually observed. In both polymorphous and monomorphous PTLDs, polymerase chain reaction analysis of the immunoglobulin heavy chain gene will usually reveal a clonal gene rearrangement. Epstein-Barr virus can also be identified in atypical lymphocytes in most polymorphic and monomorphic PTLD cases. EBER1 in situ hybridization (Figure 6.30D) is more sensitive than immunohistochemical staining for EBV-LMP1, but a positive result with either of these methodologies provides strong support for a diagnosis of PTLD. If Epstein-Barr virus is present and the histology is not conclusive, another biopsy may be diagnostic. In the occasional sample taken from the periphery of a lesion, where one may see perivascular mononuclear cell infiltrates similar to AR, detection of Epstein-Barr virus can favor a diagnosis of PTLD (115). Given the availability of adequate tissue, however, most cases will be relatively straightforward to diagnose.

X. OTHER POST-TRANSPLANT MALIGNANCIES

In adult lung transplant patients, the percentage of individuals diagnosed with a malignancy increases with longer survival. The 2007 ISHLT Registry data indicate that 3.7 percent of one-year survivors, 12.4 percent of five-year survivors, and 25.0 percent of ten-year survivors have at least one malignancy (2). Lymphoid neoplasms are the most common malignancy during the first two years after transplantation, followed by skin and other cancers (2). In five- and ten-year survivors, skin neoplasms are most common, followed by lymphoid neoplasms and other types of cancers (2). In the first year after transplantation, lymphoma and other cancers each caused 1.6 percent of

deaths, while in later years 9.3 percent of all deaths were due to malignancies (2). Cutaneous malignancies are primarily squamous cell carcinomas, some of which may take a more aggressive course with local invasion or regional metastasis (275). Individuals with significant smoking histories who receive a single lung transplant may be at increased risk of developing lung cancer in the native lung as compared to recipients of bilateral lung transplants; 6.9 percent of single lung transplant recipients developed a non–small-cell lung cancer in one series (276), while the incidence was 2.4 percent either at the time of transplantation or following transplantation in another series (277). Kaposi's sarcoma and transitional cell carcinoma of the urinary tract were increased in lung transplant recipients in another series (278). In children, lymphoma is responsible for less than 4 percent of deaths during the first five years after transplantation and 10 percent of deaths in subsequent years, while other malignancies are rare (3).

REFERENCES

1. Hardy, J.D., Webb, W.R., Dalton, M.L., Jr., Walker, G.R., Jr. 1963. Lung homotransplantation in man. *JAMA*, 186: 1065–74.
2. Trulock, E.P., Christie, J.D., Edwards, L.B., Boucek, M.M., Aurora, P., Taylor, D.O., Dobbels, F., Rahmel, A.O., Keck, B.M., Hertz, M.I. 2007. Registry of the International Society for Heart and Lung Transplantation: twenty-fourth official adult lung and heart-lung transplantation report-2007. *J Heart Lung Transplant*, 26: 782–95.
3. Waltz, D.A., Boucek, M.M., Edwards, L.B., Keck, B.M., Trulock, E.P., Taylor, D.O., Hertz, M.I. 2006. Registry of the International Society for Heart and Lung Transplantation: ninth official pediatric lung and heart-lung transplantation report – 2006. *J Heart Lung Transplant*, 25: 904–11.
4. Kowalski, R., Post, D., Schneider, M.C., Britz, J., Thomas, J., Deierhoi, M., Lobashevsky, A., Redfield, R., Schweitzer, E., Heredia, A. et al. 2003. Immune cell function testing: an adjunct to therapeutic drug monitoring in transplant patient management. *Clin Transplant*, 17: 77–88.
5. Visner, G.A., Goldfarb, S.B. 2007. Posttransplant monitoring of pediatric lung transplant recipients. *Curr Opin Pediatr*, 19: 321–6.
6. Kukafka, D.S., O'Brien, G.M., Furukawa, S., Criner, G.J. 1997. Surveillance bronchoscopy in lung transplant recipients. *Chest*, 111: 377–381.
7. Chakinala, M.M., Trulock, E.P. 2003. Acute allograft rejection after lung transplantation: diagnosis and therapy. *Chest Surg Clin N Am*, 13: 525–42.
8. Dransfield, M.T., Garver, R.I., Weill, D. 2004. Standardized guidelines for surveillance bronchoscopy reduce complications in lung transplant recipients. *J Heart Lung Transplant*, 23: 110–14.
9. Bando, K., Paradis, I.L., Similo, S., Konishi, H., Komatsu, K., Zullo, T.G., Yousem, S.A., Close, J.M., Zeevi, A., Duquesnoy, R.J. 1995. Obliterative bronchiolitis after lung and heart-lung transplantation. An analysis of risk factors and management. *J Thorac Cardiovasc Surg*, 110: 4–13.

10. Swanson, S.J., Mentzer, S.J., Reilly, J.J., Bueno, R., Lukanich, J.M., Jaklitsch, M.T., Kobzik, L., Ingenito, E.P., Fuhlbrigge, A., Donovan, C. et al. 2000. Surveillance transbronchial lung biopsies: implication for survival after lung transplantation. *J Thorac Cardiovasc Surg*, 119: 27–37.

11. Valentine, V.G., Taylor, D.E., Dhillon, G.S., Knower, M.T., McFadden, P.M., Fuchs, D.M., Kantrow, S.P. 2002. Success of lung transplantation without surveillance bronchoscopy. *J Heart Lung Transplant*, 21: 319–26.

12. Glanville, A.R. 2006. The role of bronchoscopic surveillance monitoring in the care of lung transplant recipients. *Semin Respir Crit Care Med*, 27: 480–91.

13. Benden, C., Harpur-Sinclair, O., Ranasinghe, A.S., Hartley, J.C., Elliott, M.J., Aurora, P. 2007. Surveillance bronchoscopy in children during the first year after lung transplantation: is it worth it? *Thorax*, 62: 57–61.

14. Arbustini, E., Morbini, P., Grasso, M., Diegoli, M., Fasani, R., Porcu, E., Banchieri, N., Perfetti, V., Pederzolli, C., Grossi, P. et al. 1996. Human cytomegalovirus early infection, acute rejection, and major histocompatibility class II expression in transplanted lung. Molecular, immunocytochemical, and histopathologic investigations. *Transplantation*, 61: 418–427.

15. Stewart, S., Fishbein, M.C., Snell, G.I., Berry, G.J., Boehler, A., Burke, M.M., Glanville, A., Gould, F.K., Magro, C.M., Marboe, C.C., McNeil, K.D., Reed E.F., Reinsmoen, N.L., Scott, JP., Studer, S.M., Tazelaar H.D., Wallwork J.L., Westall G., Zamora M.R., Zeevi, A. Yousem, S.A. 2007. Revision of the 1996 Working Formulation for the standardization of nomenclature in the diagnosis of lung rejection. *J Heart Lung Transplant*, 26(12):1229–42.

16. Christie, J.D., Carby, M., Bag, R., Corris, P., Hertz, M., Weill, D. 2005. Report of the ISHLT Working Group on Primary Lung Graft Dysfunction part II: definition. A consensus statement of the International Society for Heart and Lung Transplantation. *J Heart Lung Transplant*, 24: 1454–9.

17. Carter, Y.M., Davis, R.D. 2006. Primary graft dysfunction in lung transplantation. *Semin Respir Crit Care Med*, 27: 501–7.

18. Christie, J.D., Bavaria, J.E., Palevsky, H.I., Litzky, L., Blumenthal, N.P., Kaiser, L.R., Kotloff, R.M. 1998. Primary graft failure following lung transplantation. *Chest*, 114: 51–60.

19. Thabut, G., Vinatier, I., Stern, J.B., Leseche, G., Loirat, P., Fournier, M., Mal, H. 2002. Primary graft failure following lung transplantation: predictive factors of mortality. *Chest*, 121: 1876–82.

20. Christie, J.D., Kotloff, R.M., Pochettino, A., Arcasoy, S.M., Rosengard, B.R., Landis, J.R., Kimmel, S.E. 2003. Clinical risk factors for primary graft failure following lung transplantation. *Chest*, 124: 1232–41.

21. Sleiman, C., Mal, H., Fournier, M., Duchatelle, J.P., Icard, P., Groussard, O., Jebrak, G., Mollo, J.L., Raffy, O., Roue, C. 1995. Pulmonary reimplantation response in single-lung transplantation. *Eur Respir J*, 8: 5–9.

22. de Perrot, M., Liu, M., Waddell, T.K., Keshavjee, S. 2003. Ischemia-reperfusion-induced lung injury. *Am J Respir Crit Care Med*, 167: 490–511.

23. Unruh, H.W. 1995. Lung preservation and lung injury. *Chest Surg Clin N Am*, 5: 91–106.

24. Serrick, C., Adoumie, R., Giaid, A., Shennib, H. 1994. The early release of interleukin-2, tumor necrosis factor-alpha and interferon-gamma after ischemia reperfusion injury in the lung allograft. *Transplantation*, 58: 1158–62.

25. De Perrot, M., Sekine, Y., Fischer, S., Waddell, T.K., McRae, K., Liu, M., Wigle, D.A., Keshavjee, S. 2002. Interleukin-8 release during early reperfusion predicts graft function in human lung transplantation. *Am J Respir Crit Care Med*, 165: 211–5.

26. Belperio, J.A., Keane, M.P., Burdick, M.D., Gomperts, B.N., Xue, Y.Y., Hong, K., Mestas, J., Zisman, D., Ardehali, A., Saggar, R. et al. 2005. CXCR2/CXCR2 ligand biology during lung transplant ischemia-reperfusion injury. *J Immunol*, 175: 6931–9.

27. Shennib, H., Serrick, C., Saleh, D., Adoumie, R., Stewart, D.J., Giaid, A. 1995. Alterations in bronchoalveolar lavage and plasma endothelin-1 levels early after lung transplantation. *Transplantation*, 59: 994–8.

28. Abraham, D., Taghavi, S., Riml, P., Paulus, P., Hofmann, M., Baumann, C., Kocher, A., Klepetko, W., Aharinejad, S. 2002. VEGF-A and -C but not -B mediate increased vascular permeability in preserved lung grafts. *Transplantation*, 73: 1703–6.

29. Ruiz, I., Gavalda, J., Monforte, V., Len, O., Roman, A., Bravo, C., Ferrer, A., Tenorio, L., Roman, F., Maestre, J. et al. 2006. Donor-to-host transmission of bacterial and fungal infections in lung transplantation. *Am J Transplant*, 6: 178–82.

30. Garrity, E.R., Jr., Boettcher, H., Gabbay, E. 2005. Donor infection: an opinion on lung donor utilization. *J Heart Lung Transplant*, 24: 791–7.

31. Ciulli, F., Tamm, M., Dennis, C., Biocina, B., Mullins, P., Wells, F.C., Large, S.R., Wallwork, J. 1993. Donor-transmitted bacterial infection in heart-lung transplantation. *Transplant Proc*, 25: 1155–6.

32. Jones, S.D., Fullerton, D.A., Zamora, M.R., Badesch, D.B., Campbell, D.N., Grover, F.L. 1994. Transmission of Lactobacillus pneumonia by a transplanted lung. *Ann Thorac Surg*, 58: 887–9.

33. Stewart, S. 2007. Pulmonary infections in transplantation pathology. *Arch Pathol Lab Med*, 131: 1219–31.

34. Koutlas, T.C., Bridges, N.D., Gaynor, J.W., Nicolson, S.C., Steven, J.M., Spray, T.L. 1997. Pediatric lung transplantation—are there surgical contraindications? *Transplantation*, 63: 269–74.

35. Bridges, N.D., Spray, T.L., Collins, M.H., Bowles, N.E., Towbin, J.A. 1998. Adenovirus infection in the lung results in graft failure after lung transplantation. *J Thorac Cardiovasc Surg*, 116: 617–23.

36. Meylan, P.R., Aubert, J.D., Kaiser, L. 2007. Influenza transmission to recipient through lung transplantation. *Transpl Infect Dis*, 9: 55–7.

37. Haque, T., Thomas, J.A., Falk, K.I., Parratt, R., Hunt, B.J., Yacoub, M., Crawford, D.H. 1996. Transmission of donor Epstein-Barr virus (EBV) in transplanted organs causes lymphoproliferative disease in EBV-seronegative recipients. *J Gen Virol*, 77: 1169–72.

38. Kanj, S.S., Welty-Wolf, K., Madden, J., Tapson, V., Baz, M.A., Davis, R.D., Perfect, J.R. 1996. Fungal infections in lung and heart-lung transplant recipients. Report of 9 cases and review of the literature. *Medicine (Baltimore)*, *75*: 142–56.

39. Tripathy, U., Yung, G.L., Kriett, J.M., Thistlethwaite, P.A., Kapelanski, D.P., Jamieson, S.W. 2002. Donor transfer of pulmonary coccidioidomycosis in lung transplantation. *Ann Thorac Surg*, *73*: 306–8.

40. Miller, M.B., Hendren, R., Gilligan, P.H. 2004. Posttransplantation disseminated coccidioidomycosis acquired from donor lungs. *J Clin Microbiol*, *42*: 2347–9.

41. Shah, S.S., Karnak, D., Shah, S.N., Budev, M., Machuzak, M., Gildea, T.R., Mehta, A.C. 2007. Broncholith caused by donor-acquired histoplasmosis in a lung transplant recipient. *J Heart Lung Transplant*, *26*: 407–10.

42. Wreghitt, T.G., Hakim, M., Gray, J.J., Balfour, A.H., Stovin, P.G., Stewart, S., Scott, J., English, T.A., Wallwork, J. 1989. Toxoplasmosis in heart and heart and lung transplant recipients. *J Clin Pathol*, *42*: 194–199.

43. Couvreur, J., Tournier, G., Sardet-Frismand, A., Fauroux, B. 1992. Heart or heart-lung transplantation and toxoplasmosis. *Presse Med.*, *21*: 1569–74.

44. Ridgeway, A.L., Warner, G.S., Phillips, P., Forshag, M.S., McGiffin, D.C., Harden, J.W., Harris, R.H., Benjamin, W.H., Jr, Zorn, G.L., Jr, Dunlap, N.E. 1996. Transmission of Mycobacterium tuberculosis to recipients of single lung transplants from the same donor. *Am J Respir Crit Care Med*, *153*: 1166–8.

45. Schulman, L.L., Scully, B., McGregor, C.C., Austin, J.H. 1997. Pulmonary tuberculosis after lung transplantation. *Chest*, *111*: 1459–62.

46. Lee, J., Yew, W.W., Wong, C.F., Wong, P.C., Chiu, C.S. 2003. Multidrug-resistant tuberculosis in a lung transplant recipient. *J Heart Lung Transplant*, *22*: 1168–73.

47. Shitrit, D., Bendayan, D., Saute, M., Kramer, M.R. 2004. Multidrug resistant tuberculosis following lung transplantation: treatment with pulmonary resection. *Thorax*, *59*: 79–80.

48. Date, H., Trulock, E.P., Arcidi, J.M., Sundaresan, S., Cooper, J.D., Patterson, G.A. 1995. Improved airway healing after lung transplantation. An analysis of 348 bronchial anastomoses. *J Thorac Cardiovasc Surg*, *110*: 1424–32.

49. Kshettry, V.R., Kroshus, T.J., Hertz, M.I., Hunter, D.W., Shumway, S.J., Bolman, R.M. 1997. Early and late airway complications after lung transplantation: incidence and management. *Ann Thorac Surg*, *63*: 1576–83.

50. Kaditis, A.G., Gondor, M., Nixon, P.A., Webber, S., Keenan, R.J., Kaye, R., Kurland, G. 2000. Airway complications following pediatric lung and heart-lung transplantation. *Am J Respir Crit Care Med*, *162*: 301–9.

51. Alvarez, A., Algar, J., Santos, F., Lama, R., Aranda, J.L., Baamonde, C., Lopez-Pujol, J., Salvatierra, A. 2001. Airway complications after lung transplantation: a review of 151 anastomoses. *Eur J Cardiothorac Surg*, *19*: 381–7.

52. Mulligan, M.S. 2001. Endoscopic management of airway complications after lung transplantation. *Chest Surg Clin N Am*, *11*: 907–15.

53. Choong, C.K., Sweet, S.C., Zoole, J.B., Guthrie, T.J., Mendeloff, E.N., Haddad, F.J., Schuler, P., De la Morena, M.,

Huddleston, C.B. 2006. Bronchial airway anastomotic complications after pediatric lung transplantation: incidence, cause, management, and outcome. *J Thorac Cardiovasc Surg*, *131*: 198–203.

54. McGuire, F.R., Grinnan, D.C., Robbins, M. 2007. Mucormycosis of the bronchial anastomosis: a case of successful medical treatment and historic review. *J Heart Lung Transplant*, *26*: 857–61.

55. Van De Wauwer, C., Van Raemdonck, D., Verleden, G.M., Dupont, L., De Leyn, P., Coosemans, W., Nafteux, P., Lerut, T. 2007. Risk factors for airway complications within the first year after lung transplantation. *Eur J Cardiothorac Surg*, *31*: 703–10.

56. Liguori, C., Schulman, L.L., Weslow, R.G., DiTullio, M.R., McGregor, C.C., Smith, C.R., Homma, S. 1997. Late pulmonary venous complications after lung transplantation. *J Am Soc Echocardiogr*, *10*: 763–67.

57. Clark, S.C., Levine, A.J., Hasan, A., Hilton, C.J., Forty, J., Dark, J.H. 1996. Vascular complications of lung transplantation. *Ann Thorac Surg*, *61*: 1079–82.

58. Fadel, B.M., Abdulbaki, K., Nambiar, V., Al Amri, M., Shahid, M., Khouqeer, F., Canver, C. 2007. Dual thrombosis of the pulmonary arterial and venous anastomotic sites after single lung transplantation: role of transesophageal echocardiography in diagnosis and management. *J Am Soc Echocardiogr*, *20*: 438 e9–12.

59. Sakamaki, Y., Minami, M., Ohta, M., Takahashi, T., Matsumiya, G., Miyoshi, S., Matsuda, H. 2006. Pulmonary artery dissection complicating lung transplantation for primary pulmonary hypertension. *Ann Thorac Surg*, *81*: 360–2.

60. Berry, G.J., Brunt, E.M., Chamberlain, D., Hruban, R.H., Sibley, R.K., Stewart, S., Tazelaar, H.D. 1990. A working formulation for the standardization of nomenclature in the diagnosis of heart and lung rejection: Lung Rejection Study Group. The International Society for Heart Transplantation. *J Heart Transplant*, *9*: 593–601.

61. Yousem, S.A., Berry, G.J., Cagle, P.T., Chamberlain, D., Husain, A.N., Hruban, R.H., Marchevsky, A., Ohori, N.P., Ritter, J., Stewart, S. et al. 1996. Revision of the 1990 working formulation for the classification of pulmonary allograft rejection: Lung Rejection Study Group. *J Heart Lung Transplant*, *15*: 1–15.

62. Chakinala, M.M., Ritter, J., Gage, B.F., Aloush, A.A., Hachem, R.H., Lynch, J.P., Patterson, G.A., Trulock, E.P. 2005. Reliability for grading acute rejection and airway inflammation after lung transplantation. *J Heart Lung Transplant*, *24*: 652–7.

63. Colombat, M., Groussard, O., Lautrette, A., Thabut, G., Marrash-Chahla, R., Brugiere, O., Mal, H., Leseche, G., Fournier, M., Degott, C. 2005. Analysis of the different histologic lesions observed in transbronchial biopsy for the diagnosis of acute rejection. Clinicopathologic correlations during the first 6 months after lung transplantation. *Hum Pathol*, *36*: 387–94.

64. Stephenson, A., Flint, J., English, J., Vedal, S., Fradet, G., Chittock, D., Levy, R.D. 2005. Interpretation of transbronchial lung biopsies from lung transplant recipients: inter- and intraobserver agreement. *Can Respir J*, *12*: 75–7.

65. Cooper, J.D., Billingham, M., Egan, T., Hertz, M.I., Higenbottam, T., Lynch, J., Mauer, J., Paradis, I., Patterson, G.A., Smith, C. 1993. A working formulation for the standardization of nomenclature and for clinical staging of chronic dysfunction in lung allografts. International Society for Heart and Lung Transplantation. *J Heart Lung Transplant*, 12: 713–16.

66. Estenne, M., Maurer, J.R., Boehler, A., Egan, J.J., Frost, A., Hertz, M., Mallory, G.B., Snell, G.I., Yousem, S. 2002. Bronchiolitis obliterans syndrome 2001: an update of the diagnostic criteria. *J Heart Lung Transplant*, 21: 297–310.

67. Baz, M.A., Layish, D.T., Govert, J.A., Howell, D.N., Lawrence, C.M., Davis, R.D., Tapson, V.F. 1996. Diagnostic yield of bronchoscopies after isolated lung transplantation. *Chest*, 110: 84–8.

68. DeVito Dabbs, A., Hoffman, L.A., Iacono, A.T., Wells, C.L., Grgurich, W., Zullo, T.G., McCurry, K.R., Dauber, J.H. 2003. Pattern and predictors of early rejection after lung transplantation. *Am J Crit Care*, 12: 497–507.

69. Palmer, S.M., Baz, M.A., Sanders, L., Miralles, A.P., Lawrence, C.M., Rea, J.B., Zander, D.S., Edwards, L.J., Staples, E.D., Tapson, V.F. et al. 2001. Results of a randomized, prospective, multicenter trial of mycophenolate mofetil versus azathioprine in the prevention of acute lung allograft rejection. *Transplantation*, 71: 1772–6.

70. McNeil, K., Glanville, A.R., Wahlers, T., Knoop, C., Speich, R., Mamelok, R.D., Maurer, J., Ives, J., Corris, P.A. 2006. Comparison of mycophenolate mofetil and azathioprine for prevention of bronchiolitis obliterans syndrome in de novo lung transplant recipients. *Transplantation*, 81: 998–1003.

71. Trulock, E.P., Edwards, L.B., Taylor, D.O., Boucek, M.M., Keck, B.M., Hertz, M.I. 2005. Registry of the International Society for Heart and Lung Transplantation: twenty-second official adult lung and heart-lung transplant report – 2005. *J Heart Lung Transplant*, 24: 956–67.

72. Nizami, I., Frost, A.E. 2000. Clinical diagnosis of transplant-related problems. In *Diagnostic Pulmonary Pathology*. Cagle, P.T., ed. Marcel Dekker, Inc., New York, pp. 485–99.

73. Reichenspurner, H., Girgis, R.E., Robbins, R.C., Yun, K.L., Nitschke, M., Berry, G.J., Morris, R.E., Theodore, J., Reitz, B.A. 1996. Stanford experience with obliterative bronchiolitis after lung and heart-lung transplantation. *Ann Thorac Surg*, 62: 1467–72.

74. Girgis, R.E., Tu, I., Berry, G.J., Reichenspurner, H., Valentine, V.G., Conte, J.V., Ting, A., Johnstone, I., Miller, J., Robbins, R.C. et al. 1996. Risk factors for the development of obliterative bronchiolitis after lung transplantation. *J Heart Lung Transplant*, 15: 1200–8.

75. Kroshus, T.J., Kshettry, V.R., Savik, K., John, R., Hertz, M.I., Bolman, R.M. 1997. Risk factors for the development of bronchiolitis obliterans syndrome after lung transplantation. *J Thorac Cardiovasc Surg*, 114: 195–202.

76. Heng, D., Sharples, L.D., McNeil, K., Stewart, S., Wreghitt, T., Wallwork, J. 1998. Bronchiolitis obliterans syndrome: incidence, natural history, prognosis, and risk factors. *J Heart Lung Transplant*, 17: 1255–63.

77. Husain, A.N., Siddiqui, M.T., Holmes, E.W., Chandrasekhar, A.J., McCabe, M., Radvany, R., Garrity, E.R. 1999. Analysis of risk factors for the development of bronchiolitis obliterans syndrome. *Am J Respir Crit Care Med*, 159: 829–33.

78. Schulman, L.L., Weinberg, A.D., McGregor, C.C., Suciu-Foca, N.M., Itescu, S. 2001. Influence of donor and recipient HLA locus mismatching on development of obliterative bronchiolitis after lung transplantation. *Am J Respir Crit Care Med*, 163: 437–42.

79. Chalermskulrat, W., Neuringer, I.P., Schmitz, J.L., Catellier, D.J., Gurka, M.J., Randell, S.H., Aris, R.M. 2003. Human leukocyte antigen mismatches predispose to the severity of bronchiolitis obliterans syndrome after lung transplantation. *Chest*, 123: 1825–31.

80. Ionescu, D.N., Girnita, A.L., Zeevi, A., Duquesnoy, R., Pilewski, J., Johnson, B., Studer, S., McCurry, K.R., Yousem, S.A. 2005. C4d deposition in lung allografts is associated with circulating anti-HLA alloantibody. *Transpl Immunol*, 15: 63–8.

81. Jaramillo, A., Smith, M.A., Phelan, D., Sundaresan, S., Trulock, E.P., Lynch, J.P., Cooper, J.D., Patterson, G.A., Mohanakumar, T. 1999. Development of ELISA-detected anti-HLA antibodies precedes the development of bronchiolitis obliterans syndrome and correlates with progressive decline in pulmonary function after lung transplantation. *Transplantation*, 67: 1155–61.

82. Palmer, S.M., Davis, R.D., Hadjiliadis, D., Hertz, M.I., Howell, D.N., Ward, F.E., Savik, K., Reinsmoen, N.L. 2002. Development of an antibody specific to major histocompatibility antigens detectable by flow cytometry after lung transplant is associated with bronchiolitis obliterans syndrome. *Transplantation*, 74: 799–804.

83. Reznik, S.I., Jaramillo, A., Zhang, L., Patterson, G.A., Cooper, J.D., Mohanakumar, T. 2000. Anti-HLA antibody binding to HLA class I molecules induces proliferation of airway epithelial cells: a potential mechanism for bronchiolitis obliterans syndrome. *J Thorac Cardiovasc Surg*, 119: 39–45.

84. Verleden, G.M., Dupont, L.J., Van Raemdonck, D.E. 2005. Is it bronchiolitis obliterans syndrome or is it chronic rejection: a reappraisal? *Eur Respir J*, 25: 221–4.

85. D'Ovidio, F., Mura, M., Tsang, M., Waddell, T.K., Hutcheon, M.A., Singer, L.G., Hadjiliadis, D., Chaparro, C., Gutierrez, C., Pierre, A. et al. 2005. Bile acid aspiration and the development of bronchiolitis obliterans after lung transplantation. *J Thorac Cardiovasc Surg*, 129: 1144–52.

86. Knoop, C., Estenne, M. 2006. Acute and chronic rejection after lung transplantation. *Semin Respir Crit Care Med*, 27: 521–33.

87. Billings, J.L., Hertz, M.I., Savik, K., Wendt, C.H. 2002. Respiratory viruses and chronic rejection in lung transplant recipients. *J Heart Lung Transplant*, 21: 559–66.

88. Vilchez, R.A., Dauber, J., Kusne, S. 2003. Infectious etiology of bronchiolitis obliterans: the respiratory viruses connection – myth or reality? *Am J Transplant*, 3: 245–9.

89. Kotsimbos, T.C., Snell, G.I., Levvey, B., Spelman, D.W., Fuller, A.J., Wesselingh, S.L., Williams, T.J., Ostergaard, L. 2005. Chlamydia pneumoniae serology in donors and

recipients and the risk of bronchiolitis obliterans syndrome after lung transplantation. *Transplantation, 79*: 269–75.

90. Neurohr, C., Huppmann, P., Leuchte, H., Schwaiblmair, M., Bittmann, I., Jaeger, G., Hatz, R., Frey, L., Uberfuhr, P., Reichart, B. et al. 2005. Human herpesvirus 6 in bronchalveolar lavage fluid after lung transplantation: a risk factor for bronchiolitis obliterans syndrome? *Am J Transplant, 5*: 2982–91.

91. Paradis, I., Yousem, S., Griffith, B. 1993. Airway obstruction and bronchiolitis obliterans after lung transplantation. *Clin Chest Med, 14*: 751–63.

92. Iacono, A.T., Keenan, R.J., Duncan, S.R., Smaldone, G.C., Dauber, J.H., Paradis, I.L., Ohori, N.P., Grgurich, W.F., Burckart, G.J., Zeevi, A. et al. 1996. Aerosolized cyclosporine in lung recipients with refractory chronic rejection. *Am J Respir Crit Care Med, 153*: 1451–5.

93. Snell, G.I., Esmore, D.S., Williams, T.J. 1996. Cytolytic therapy for the bronchiolitis obliterans syndrome complicating lung transplantation. *Chest, 109*: 874–8.

94. Dusmet, M., Maurer, J., Winton, T., Kesten, S. 1996. Methotrexate can halt the progression of bronchiolitis obliterans syndrome in lung transplant recipients. *J Heart Lung Transplant, 15*: 948–54.

95. Ross, D.J., Lewis, M.I., Kramer, M., Vo, A., Kass, R.M. 1997. FK 506 'rescue' immunosuppression for obliterative bronchiolitis after lung transplantation. *Chest, 112*: 1175–9.

96. Kesten, S., Chaparro, C., Scavuzzo, M., Gutierrez, C. 1997. Tacrolimus as rescue therapy for bronchiolitis obliterans syndrome. *J Heart Lung Transplant, 16*: 905–912.

97. Date, H., Lynch, J.P., Sundaresan, S., Patterson, G.A., Trulock, E.P. 1998. The impact of cytolytic therapy on bronchiolitis obliterans syndrome. *J Heart Lung Transplant, 17*: 869–75.

98. Diamond, D.A., Michalski, J.M., Lynch, J.P., Trulock, E.P. 1998. Efficacy of total lymphoid irradiation for chronic allograft rejection following bilateral lung transplantation. *Int J Radiat Oncol Biol Phys, 41*: 795–800.

99. Paradis, I. 1998. Bronchiolitis obliterans: pathogenesis, prevention, and management. *Am J Med Sci, 315*: 161–78.

100. O'Hagan, A.R., Stillwell, P.C., Arroliga, A., Koo, A. 1999. Photopheresis in the treatment of refractory bronchiolitis obliterans complicating lung transplantation. *Chest, 115*: 1459–62.

101. Salerno, C.T., Park, S.J., Kreykes, N.S., Kulick, D.M., Savik, K., Hertz, M.I., Bolman, R.M., 3rd. 1999. Adjuvant treatment of refractory lung transplant rejection with extracorporeal photopheresis. *J Thorac Cardiovasc Surg, 117*: 1063–9.

102. Verleden, G.M., Buyse, B., Delcroix, M., Fabri, R., Vanhaecke, J., Van Raemdonck, D., Lerut, T., Demedts, M. 1999. Cyclophosphamide rescue therapy for chronic rejection after lung transplantation. *J Heart Lung Transplant, 18*: 1139–42.

103. Boehler, A., Estenne, M. 2000. Obliterative bronchiolitis after lung transplantation. *Curr Opin Pulm Med, 6*: 133–9.

104. Cairn, J., Yek, T., Banner, N.R., Khaghani, A., Hodson, M.E., Yacoub, M. 2003. Time-related changes in pulmonary function after conversion to tacrolimus in bronchiolitis obliterans syndrome. *J Heart Lung Transplant, 22*: 50–7.

105. Johnson, B.A., Iacono, A.T., Zeevi, A., McCurry, K.R., Duncan, S.R. 2003. Statin use is associated with improved function and survival of lung allografts. *Am J Respir Crit Care Med, 167*: 1271–8.

106. Gerhardt, S.G., McDyer, J.F., Girgis, R.E., Conte, J.V., Yang, S.C., Orens, J.B. 2003. Maintenance azithromycin therapy for bronchiolitis obliterans syndrome: results of a pilot study. *Am J Respir Crit Care Med, 168*: 121–5.

107. Verleden, G.M., Dupont, L.J. 2004. Azithromycin therapy for patients with bronchiolitis obliterans syndrome after lung transplantation. *Transplantation, 77*: 1465–7.

108. Shitrit, D., Bendayan, D., Gidon, S., Saute, M., Bakal, I., Kramer, M.R. 2005. Long-term azithromycin use for treatment of bronchiolitis obliterans syndrome in lung transplant recipients. *J Heart Lung Transplant, 24*: 1440–3.

109. Yates, B., Murphy, D.M., Forrest, I.A., Ward, C., Rutherford, R.M., Fisher, A.J., Lordan, J.L., Dark, J.H., Corris, P.A. 2005. Azithromycin reverses airflow obstruction in established bronchiolitis obliterans syndrome. *Am J Respir Crit Care Med, 172*: 772–5.

110. Fisher, A.J., Rutherford, R.M., Bozzino, J., Parry, G., Dark, J.H., Corris, P.A. 2005. The safety and efficacy of total lymphoid irradiation in progressive bronchiolitis obliterans syndrome after lung transplantation. *Am J Transplant, 5*: 537–43.

111. Hachem, R.R., Khalifah, A.P., Chakinala, M.M., Yusen, R.D., Aloush, A.A., Mohanakumar, T., Patterson, G.A., Trulock, E.P., Walter, M.J. 2005. The significance of a single episode of minimal acute rejection after lung transplantation. *Transplantation, 80*: 1406–13.

112. Khalifah, A.P., Hachem, R.R., Chakinala, M.M., Yusen, R.D., Aloush, A., Patterson, G.A., Mohanakumar, T., Trulock, E.P., Walter, M.J. 2005. Minimal acute rejection after lung transplantation: a risk for bronchiolitis obliterans syndrome. *Am J Transplant, 5*: 2022–30.

113. Malouf, M.A., Hopkins, P.M., Singleton, L., Chhajed, P.N., Plit, M.L., Glanville, A.R. 2004. Sexual health issues after lung transplantation: importance of cervical screening. *J Heart Lung Transplant, 23*: 894–7.

114. Tazelaar, H.D. 1991. Perivascular inflammation in pulmonary infections: implications for the diagnosis of lung rejection. *J Heart Lung Transplant, 10*: 437–41.

115. Rosendale, B., Yousem, S.A. 1995. Discrimination of Epstein-Barr virus-related posttransplant lymphoproliferations from acute rejection in lung allograft recipients. *Arch Pathol Lab Med, 119*: 418–23.

116. Davis, R.D., Jr., Lau, C.L., Eubanks, S., Messier, R.H., Hadjiliadis, D., Steele, M.P., Palmer, S.M. 2003. Improved lung allograft function after fundoplication in patients with gastroesophageal reflux disease undergoing lung transplantation. *J Thorac Cardiovasc Surg, 125*: 533–42.

117. Yousem, S.A. 1992. Graft eosinophilia in lung transplantation. *Hum Pathol, 23*: 1172–7.

118. Otten, H.G., van den Bosch, J.M., van Ginkel, W.G., van Loon, M., van de Graaf, E.A. 2006. Identification of non-HLA target antigens recognized after lung transplantation. *J Heart Lung Transplant, 25*: 1425–30.

119. Reinsmoen, N.L., Nelson, K., Zeevi, A. 2004. Anti-HLA antibody analysis and crossmatching in heart and lung transplantation. *Transpl Immunol, 13*: 63–71.

120. Appel, J.Z., 3rd, Hartwig, M.G., Cantu, E., 3rd, Palmer, S.M., Reinsmoen, N.L., Davis, R.D. 2006. Role of flow cytometry to define unacceptable HLA antigens in lung transplant recipients with HLA-specific antibodies. *Transplantation*, *81*: 1049–57.

121. Jaramillo, A., Naziruddin, B., Zhang, L., Reznik, S.I., Smith, M.A., Aloush, A.A., Trulock, E.P., Patterson, G.A., Mohanakumar, T. 2001. Activation of human airway epithelial cells by non-HLA antibodies developed after lung transplantation: a potential etiological factor for bronchiolitis obliterans syndrome. *Transplantation*, *71*: 966–76.

122. Sundaresan, S., Mohanakumar, T., Smith, M.A., Trulock, E.P., Lynch, J., Phelan, D., Cooper, J.D., Patterson, G.A. 1998. HLA-A locus mismatches and development of antibodies to HLA after lung transplantation correlate with the development of bronchiolitis obliterans syndrome. *Transplantation*, *65*: 648–53.

123. Girnita, A.L., McCurry, K.R., Iacono, A.T., Duquesnoy, R., Corcoran, T.E., Awad, M., Spichty, K.J., Yousem, S.A., Burckart, G., Dauber, J.H. et al. 2004. HLA-Specific antibodies are associated with high-grade and persistent-recurrent lung allograft acute rejection. *J Heart Lung Transplant*, *23*: 1135–41.

124. Girnita, A.L., Duquesnoy, R., Yousem, S.A., Iacono, A.T., Corcoran, T.E., Buzoianu, M., Johnson, B., Spichty, K.J., Dauber, J.H., Burckart, G. et al. 2005. HLA-specific antibodies are risk factors for lymphocytic bronchiolitis and chronic lung allograft dysfunction. *Am J Transplant*, *5*: 131–8.

125. Badesch, D.B., Zamora, M., Fullerton, D., Weill, D., Tuder, R., Grover, F., Schwarz, M.I. 1998. Pulmonary capillaritis: a possible histologic form of acute pulmonary allograft rejection. *J Heart Lung Transplant*, *17*: 415–22.

126. Magro, C.M., Deng, A., Pope-Harman, A., Waldman, W.J., Bernard Collins, A., Adams, P.W., Kelsey, M., Ross, P. 2002. Humorally mediated posttransplantation septal capillary injury syndrome as a common form of pulmonary allograft rejection: a hypothesis. *Transplantation*, *74*: 1273–80.

127. Wallace, W.D., Reed, E.F., Ross, D., Lassman, C.R., Fishbein, M.C. 2005. C4d staining of pulmonary allograft biopsies: an immunoperoxidase study. *J Heart Lung Transplant*, *24*: 1565–70.

128. Miller, G.G., Destarac, L., Zeevi, A., Girnita, A., McCurry, K., Iacono, A., Murray, J.J., Crowe, D., Johnson, J.E., Ninan, M. et al. 2004. Acute humoral rejection of human lung allografts and elevation of C4d in bronchoalveolar lavage fluid. *Am J Transplant*, *4*: 1323–30.

129. Frost, A.E., Jammal, C.T., Cagle, P.T. 1996. Hyperacute rejection following lung transplantation. *Chest*, *110*: 559–62.

130. Choi, J.K., Kearns, J., Palevsky, H.I., Montone, K.T., Kaiser, L.R., Zmijewski, C.M., Tomaszewski, J.E. 1999. Hyperacute rejection of a pulmonary allograft. Immediate clinical and pathologic findings. *Am J Respir Crit Care Med*, *160*: 1015–8.

131. Scornik, J.C., Zander, D.S., Baz, M.A., Donnelly, W.H., Staples, E.D. 1999. Susceptibility of lung transplants to preformed donor-specific HLA antibodies as detected by flow cytometry. *Transplantation*, *68*: 1542–6.

132. Bittner, H.B., Dunitz, J., Hertz, M., Bolman, M.R., 3rd, Park, S.J. 2001. Hyperacute rejection in single lung transplantation–case report of successful management by means of plasmapheresis and antithymocyte globulin treatment. *Transplantation*, *71*: 649–51.

133. Takemoto, S.K., Zeevi, A., Feng, S., Colvin, R.B., Jordan, S., Kobashigawa, J., Kupiec-Weglinski, J., Matas, A., Montgomery, R.A., Nickerson, P. et al. 2004. National conference to assess antibody-mediated rejection in solid organ transplantation. *Am J Transplant*, *4*: 1033–41.

134. Masson, E., Stern, M., Chabod, J., Thevenin, C., Gonin, F., Rebibou, J.M., Tiberghien, P. 2007. Hyperacute rejection after lung transplantation caused by undetected low-titer anti-HLA antibodies. *J Heart Lung Transplant*, *26*: 642–5.

135. Yousem, S.A., Curley, J.M., Dauber, J., Paradis, I., Rabinowich, H., Zeevi, A., Duquesnoy, R., Dowling, R., Zenati, M., Hardesty, R. et al. 1990. HLA-class II antigen expression in human heart-lung allografts. *Transplantation*, *49*: 991–5.

136. Milne, D.S., Gascoigne, A.D., Wilkes, J., Sviland, L., Ashcroft, T., Malcolm, A.J., Corris, P.A. 1994. MHC class II and ICAM-1 expression and lymphocyte subsets in transbronchial biopsies from lung transplant recipients. *Transplantation*, *57*: 1762–6.

137. Devouassoux, G., Pison, C., Drouet, C., Pin, I., Brambilla, C., Brambilla, E. 2001. Early lung leukocyte infiltration, HLA and adhesion molecule expression predict chronic rejection. *Transpl Immunol*, *8*: 229–36.

138. Reinsmoen, N.L., Bolman, R.M., Savik, K., Butters, K., Hertz, M. 1992. Differentiation of class I- and class II-directed donor-specific alloreactivity in bronchoalveolar lavage lymphocytes from lung transplant recipients. *Transplantation*, *53*: 181–9.

139. Rogers, N.J., Leckler, R.I. 2001. Allorecognition. *Am J Transplant*, *1*: 97–102.

140. Heeger, P.S. 2003. T cell allorecognition and transplant rejection: a summary and update. *Am J Transplant*, *3*: 525–33.

141. Taylor, P.M., Rose, M.L., Yacoub, M.H. 1989. Expression of MHC antigens in normal human lungs and transplanted lungs with obliterative bronchiolitis. *Transplantation*, *48*: 506–10.

142. Mauck, K.A., Hosenpud, J.D. 1996. The bronchial epithelium: a potential allogeneic target for chronic rejection after lung transplantation. *J Heart Lung Transplant*, *15*: 709–14.

143. Smith, C.R., Jaramillo, A., Duffy, B.F., Mohanakumar, T. 2000. Airway epithelial cell damage mediated by antigen-specific T cells: implications in lung allograft rejection. *Hum Immunol*, *61*: 985–92.

144. Hasegawa, S., Ockner, D.M., Ritter, J.H., Patterson, G.A., Trulock, E.P., Cooper, J.D., Wick, M.R. 1995. Expression of class II major histocompatibility complex antigens (HLA-DR) and lymphocyte subset immunotyping in chronic pulmonary transplant rejection. *Arch Pathol Lab Med*, *119*: 432–9.

145. Duncan, S.R., Leonard, C., Theodore, J., Lega, M., Girgis, R.E., Rosen, G.D., Theofilopoulos, A.N. 2002. Oligoclonal CD4(+) T cell expansions in lung transplant recipients with obliterative bronchiolitis. *Am J Respir Crit Care Med*, *165*: 1439–44.

146. Lu, K.C., Jaramillo, A., Mendeloff, E.N., Huddleston, C.B., Sweet, S.C., Patterson, G.A., Mohanakumar, T. 2003. Concomitant allorecognition of mismatched donor HLA class I- and class II-derived peptides in pediatric lung transplant recipients with bronchiolitis obliterans syndrome. *J Heart Lung Transplant, 22*: 35–43.

147. Jaramillo, A., Fernandez, F.G., Kuo, E.Y., Trulock, E.P., Patterson, G.A., Mohanakumar, T. 2005. Immune mechanisms in the pathogenesis of bronchiolitis obliterans syndrome after lung transplantation. *Pediatr Transplant, 9*: 84–93.

148. Sundaresan, S., Alevy, Y.G., Steward, N., Tucker, J., Trulock, E.P., Cooper, J.D., Patterson, G.A., Mohanakumar, T. 1995. Cytokine gene transcripts for tumor necrosis factor-alpha, interleukin-2, and interferon-gamma in human pulmonary allografts. *J Heart Lung Transplant, 14*: 512–18.

149. Magnan, A., Mege, J.L., Escallier, J.C., Brisse, J., Capo, C., Reynaud, M., Thomas, P., Meric, B., Garbe, L., Badier, M. et al. 1996. Balance between alveolar macrophage IL-6 and TGF-beta in lung-transplant recipients. Marseille and Montreal Lung Transplantation Group. *Am J Respir Crit Care Med, 153*: 1431–6.

150. Iacono, A., Dauber, J., Keenan, R., Spichty, K., Cai, J., Grgurich, W., Burckart, G., Smaldone, G., Pham, S., Ohori, N.P. et al. 1997. Interleukin 6 and interferon-gamma gene expression in lung transplant recipients with refractory acute cellular rejection: implications for monitoring and inhibition by treatment with aerosolized cyclosporine. *Transplantation, 64*: 263–9.

151. Rizzo, M., SivaSai, K.S., Smith, M.A., Trulock, E.P., Lynch, J.P., Patterson, G.A., Mohanakumar, T. 2000. Increased expression of inflammatory cytokines and adhesion molecules by alveolar macrophages of human lung allograft recipients with acute rejection: decline with resolution of rejection. *J Heart Lung Transplant, 19*: 858–65.

152. Slebos, D.J., Postma, D.S., Koeter, G.H., Van Der Bij, W., Boezen, M., Kauffman, H.F. 2004. Bronchoalveolar lavage fluid characteristics in acute and chronic lung transplant rejection. *J Heart Lung Transplant, 23*: 532–40.

153. Keane, M.P., Gomperts, B.N., Weigt, S., Xue, Y.Y., Burdick, M.D., Nakamura, H., Zisman, D.A., Ardehali, A., Saggar, R., Lynch, J.P., 3rd, et al. 2007. IL-13 is pivotal in the fibro-obliterative process of bronchiolitis obliterans syndrome. *J Immunol, 178*: 511–9.

154. Bharat, A., Narayanan, K., Street, T., Fields, R.C., Steward, N., Aloush, A., Meyers, B., Schuessler, R., Trulock, E.P., Patterson, G.A. et al. 2007. Early posttransplant inflammation promotes the development of alloimmunity and chronic human lung allograft rejection. *Transplantation, 83*: 150–8.

155. Jaramillo, A., Smith, C.R., Zhang, L., Patterson, G.A., Mohanakumar, T. 2003. Anti-HLA antibody binding to HLA class I molecules induces production of fibrogenic growth factors and apoptotic cell death: a possible mechanism for bronchiolitis obliterans syndrome. *Hum Immunol, 64*: 521–9.

156. Hansen, P.R., Holm, A.M., Svendsen, U.G., Olsen, P.S., Andersen, C.B. 2000. Apoptosis and formation of peroxynitrite in the lungs of patients with obliterative bronchiolitis. *J Heart Lung Transplant, 19*: 160–6.

157. Shreeniwas, R., Schulman, L.L., Narasimhan, M., McGregor, C.C., Marboe, C.C. 1996. Adhesion molecules (E-selectin and ICAM-1) in pulmonary allograft rejection. *Chest, 110*: 1143–9.

158. Steinhoff, G., Behrend, M., Richter, N., Schlitt, H.J., Cremer, J., Haverich, A. 1995. Distinct expression of cell-cell and cell-matrix adhesion molecules on endothelial cells in human heart and lung transplants. *J Heart Lung Transplant, 14*: 1145–55.

159. Zander, D.S., Baz, M.A., Massey, J.K. 1999. Patterns and significance of CD44 expression in lung allografts. *J Heart Lung Transplant, 18*: 646–53.

160. Hertz, M.I., Henke, C.A., Nakhleh, R.E., Harmon, K.R., Marinelli, W.A., Fox, J.M., Kubo, S.H., Shumway, S.J., Bolman, R.M., Bitterman, P.B. 1992. Obliterative bronchiolitis after lung transplantation: a fibroproliferative disorder associated with platelet-derived growth factor. *Proc Natl Acad Sci, 89*: 10385–9.

161. Bergmann, M., Tiroke, A., Schafer, H., Barth, J., Haverich, A. 1998. Gene expression of profibrotic mediators in bronchiolitis obliterans syndrome after lung transplantation. *Scand Cardiovasc J, 32*: 97–103.

162. El-Gamel, A., Sim, E., Hasleton, P., Hutchinson, J., Yonan, N., Egan, J., Campbell, C., Rahman, A., Sheldon, S., Deiraniya, A. et al. 1999. Transforming growth factor beta (TGF-beta) and obliterative bronchiolitis following pulmonary transplantation. *J Heart Lung Transplant, 18*: 828–37.

163. Charpin, J.M., Stern, M., Grenet, D., Israel-Biet, D. 2000. Insulinlike growth factor-1 in lung transplants with obliterative bronchiolitis. *Am J Respir Crit Care Med, 161*: 1991–8.

164. Riise, G.C., Andersson, B.A., Kjellstrom, C., Martensson, G., Nilsson, F.N., Ryd, W., Schersten, H. 1999. Persistent high BAL fluid granulocyte activation marker levels as early indicators of bronchiolitis obliterans after lung transplant. *Eur Respir J, 14*: 1123–30.

165. Riise, G.C. 2000. On interleukin-8, neutrophil activation, and bronchiolitis obliterans syndrome in lung transplantation. *Transplantation, 70*: 265–6.

166. Elssner, A., Vogelmeier, C. 2001. The role of neutrophils in the pathogenesis of obliterative bronchiolitis after lung transplantation. *Transpl Infect Dis, 3*: 168–76.

167. Lu, F., Zander, D.S., Visner, G.A. 2002. Increased expression of heme oxygenase-1 in human lung transplantation. *J Heart Lung Transplant, 21*: 1120–6.

168. Reid, D., Snell, G., Ward, C., Krishnaswamy, R., Ward, R., Zheng, L., Williams, T., Walters, H. 2001. Iron overload and nitric oxide-derived oxidative stress following lung transplantation. *J Heart Lung Transplant, 20*: 840–9.

169. Baz, M.A., Tapson, V.F., Roggli, V.L., Van Trigt, P., Piantadosi, C.A. 1996. Glutathione depletion in epithelial lining fluid of lung allograft patients. *Am J Respir Crit Care Med, 153*: 742–6.

170. Yousem, S.A., Sonmez-Alpan, E. 1991. Use of a biotinylated DNA probe specific for the human Y chromosome in the evaluation of the allograft lung. *Chest, 99*: 275–9.

171. Bittmann, I., Dose, T., Baretton, G.B., Muller, C., Schwaiblmair, M., Kur, F., Lohrs, U. 2001. Cellular chimerism of the lung after transplantation. An interphase cytogenetic study. *Am J Clin Pathol, 115*: 525–33.

172. Wiebe, B.M., Mortensen, S.A., Petterson, G., Svendsen, U.G., Andersen, C.B. 2001. Macrophage and lymphocyte chimerism in bronchoalveolar lavage cells from human lung allograft recipients. *Apmis*, 109: 435–40.

173. Rothmeier, C., Roux, E., Spiliopoulos, A., Gerbase, M., Nicod, L.P. 2001. Early chimerism of macrophages and lymphocytes in lung transplant recipients is predictive of graft tolerance. *Transplantation*, 71: 1329–33.

174. Zander, D.S. in press. Stem cells in non-neoplastic lung disorders. In *Molecular Pathology of Lung Diseases*. Zander, D.S., Popper, H., Jagidar, J., Haque, A., Cagle, P.T., Barrios, R., eds. Springer.

175. Milman, N., Andersen, C.B., Burton, C.M., Iversen, M. 2005. Recurrent sarcoid granulomas in a transplanted lung derive from recipient immune cells. *Eur Respir J*, 26: 549–52.

176. Ionescu, D.N., Hunt, J.L., Lomago, D., Yousem, S.A. 2005. Recurrent sarcoidosis in lung transplant allografts: granulomas are of recipient origin. *Diagn Mol Pathol*, 14: 140–5.

177. Bittmann, I., Rolf, B., Amann, G., Lohrs, U. 2003. Recurrence of lymphangioleiomyomatosis after single lung transplantation: new insights into pathogenesis. *Hum Pathol*, 34: 95–8.

178. Karbowniczek, M., Astrinidis, A., Balsara, B.R., Testa, J.R., Lium, J.H., Colby, T.V., McCormack, F.X., Henske, E.P. 2003. Recurrent lymphangiomyomatosis after transplantation: genetic analyses reveal a metastatic mechanism. *Am J Respir Crit Care Med*, 167: 976–82.

179. Garver, R.I., Jr., Zorn, G.L., Wu, X., McGiffin, D.C., Young, K.R., Jr., Pinkard, N.B. 1999. Recurrence of bronchioloalveolar carcinoma in transplanted lungs. *N Engl J Med*, 340: 1071–4.

180. Paloyan, E.B., Swinnen, L.J., Montoya, A., Lonchyna, V., Sullivan, H.J., Garrity, E. 2000. Lung transplantation for advanced bronchioloalveolar carcinoma confined to the lungs. *Transplantation*, 69: 2446–8.

181. Zorn, G.L., Jr., McGiffin, D.C., Young, K.R., Jr., Alexander, C.B., Weill, D., Kirklin, J.K. 2003. Pulmonary transplantation for advanced bronchioloalveolar carcinoma. *J Thorac Cardiovasc Surg*, 125: 45–8.

182. Yousem, S.A. 1997. Alveolar lipoproteinosis in lung allograft recipients. *Hum Pathol*, 28: 1383–6.

183. Gal, A.A., Bryan, J.A., Kanter, K.R., Lawrence, E.C. 2004. Cytopathology of pulmonary alveolar proteinosis complicating lung transplantation. *J Heart Lung Transplant*, 23: 135–8.

184. Burns, K.E., Iacono, A.T. 2004. Pulmonary embolism on postmortem examination: an under-recognized complication in lung-transplant recipients? *Transplantation*, 77: 692–8.

185. Rosendale, B.E., Keenan, R.J., Duncan, S.R., Hardesty, R.L., Armitage, J.A., Griffith, B.P., Yousem, S.A. 1992. Donor cerebral emboli as a cause of acute graft dysfunction in lung transplantation. *J Heart Lung Transplant*, 11: 72–6.

186. Buell, J.F., Trofe, J., Hanaway, M.J., Lo, A., Rosengard, B., Rilo, H., Alloway, R., Beebe, T., First, M.R., Woodle, E.S. 2001. Transmission of donor cancer into cardiothoracic transplant recipients. *Surgery*, 130: 660–6.

187. Armanios, M.Y., Grossman, S.A., Yang, S.C., White, B., Perry, A., Burger, P.C., Orens, J.B. 2004. Transmission of glioblastoma multiforme following bilateral lung transplantation from an affected donor: case study and review of the literature. *Neuro-oncol*, 6: 259–63.

188. Yousem, S.A., Duncan, S.R., Griffith, B.P. 1992. Interstitial and airspace granulation tissue reactions in lung transplant recipients. *Am J Surg Pathol*, 16: 877–84.

189. Chaparro, C., Chamberlain, D., Maurer, J., Winton, T., Dehoyos, A., Kesten, S. 1996. Bronchiolitis obliterans organizing pneumonia (BOOP) in lung transplant recipients. *Chest*, 110: 1150–4.

190. Siddiqui, M.T., Garrity, E.R., Husain, A.N. 1996. Bronchiolitis obliterans organizing pneumonia-like reactions: a nonspecific response or an atypical form of rejection or infection in lung allograft recipients? *Hum Pathol*, 27: 714–19.

191. Kawut, S.M., Shah, L., Wilt, J.S., Dwyer, E., Maani, P.A., Daly, T.M., O'Shea, M.K., Sonett, J.R., Arcasoy, S.M. 2005. Risk factors and outcomes of hypogammaglobulinemia after lung transplantation. *Transplantation*, 79: 1723–6.

192. Yip, N.H., Lederer, D.J., Kawut, S.M., Wilt, J.S., D'Ovidio, F., Wang, Y., Dwyer, E., Sonett, J.R., Arcasoy, S.M. 2006. Immunoglobulin G levels before and after lung transplantation. *Am J Respir Crit Care Med*, 173: 917–21.

193. Goldfarb, N.S., Avery, R.K., Goormastic, M., Mehta, A.C., Schilz, R., Smedira, N., Pien, L., Haug, M.T., Gordon, S.M., Hague, L.K. et al. 2001. Hypogammaglobulinemia in lung transplant recipients. *Transplantation*, 71: 242–6.

194. Kubak, B.M. 2002. Fungal infection in lung transplantation. *Transpl Infect Dis*, 4 Suppl 3: 24–31.

195. Maurer, J.R., Tullis, D.E., Grossman, R.F., Vellend, H., Winton, T.L., Patterson, G.A. 1992. Infectious complications following isolated lung transplantation. *Chest*, 101: 1056–9.

196. Kramer, M.R., Marshall, S.E., Starnes, V.A., Gamberg, P., Amitai, Z., Theodore, J. 1993. Infectious complications in heart-lung transplantation. Analysis of 200 episodes. *Arch Intern Med*, 153: 2010–16.

197. Horvath, J., Dummer, S., Loyd, J., Walker, B., Merrill, W.H., Frist, W.H. 1993. Infection in the transplanted and native lung after single lung transplantation. *Chest*, 104: 681–5.

198. Paradis, I.L., Williams, P. 1993. Infection after lung transplantation. *Semin Respir Infect*, 8: 207–15.

199. Chan, C.C., Abi-Saleh, W.J., Arroliga, A.C., Stillwell, P.C., Kirby, T.J., Gordon, S.M., Petras, R.E., Mehta, A.C. 1996. Diagnostic yield and therapeutic impact of flexible bronchoscopy in lung transplant recipients. *J Heart Lung Transplant*, 15: 196–205.

200. Husain, A.N., Siddiqui, M.T., Reddy, V.B., Yeldandi, V., Montoya, A., Garrity, E.R. 1996. Postmortem findings in lung transplant recipients. *Mod Pathol*, 9: 752–61.

201. Zander, D.S., Baz, M.A., Visner, G.A., Staples, E.D., Donnelly, W.H., Faro, A., Scornik, J.C. 2001. Analysis of early deaths after isolated lung transplantation. *Chest*, 120: 225–32.

202. Deusch, E., End, A., Grimm, M., Graninger, W., Klepetko, W., Wolner, E. 1993. Early bacterial infections in lung transplant recipients. *Chest*, 104: 1412–16.

203. Roberts, S.A., Franklin, J.C., Mijch, A., Spelman, D. 2000. Nocardia infection in heart-lung transplant recipients at Alfred Hospital, Melbourne, Australia, 1989-1998. *Clin Infect Dis, 31*: 968–72.

204. Husain, S., McCurry, K., Dauber, J., Singh, N., Kusne, S. 2002. Nocardia infection in lung transplant recipients. *J Heart Lung Transplant, 21*: 354–9.

205. Glanville, A.R., Gencay, M., Tamm, M., Chhajed, P., Plit, M., Hopkins, P., Aboyoun, C., Roth, M., Malouf, M. 2005. Chlamydia pneumoniae infection after lung transplantation. *J Heart Lung Transplant, 24*: 131–6.

206. Lyon, G.M., Alspaugh, J.A., Meredith, F.T., Harrell, L.J., Tapson, V., Davis, R.D., Kanj, S.S. 1997. Mycoplasma hominis pneumonia complicating bilateral lung transplantation: case report and review of the literature. *Chest, 112*: 1428–32.

207. Douglas, R.G., Jr, Anderson, S., Weg, J.G., Williams, T., Jenkins, D.E., Knight, V., Beall, A.C., Jr. 1969. Herpes simplex virus pneumonia. Occurrence in an allotransplanted lung. *JAMA, 210*: 902–4.

208. Fend, F., Prior, C., Margreiter, R., Mikuz, G. 1990. Cytomegalovirus pneumonitis in heart-lung transplant recipients: histopathology and clinicopathologic considerations. *Hum Pathol, 21*: 918–26.

209. Smyth, R.L., Higenbottam, T.W., Scott, J.P., Wreghitt, T.G., Stewart, S., Clelland, C.A., McGoldrick, J.P., Wallwork, J. 1990. Herpes simplex virus infection in heart-lung transplant recipients. *Transplantation, 49*: 735–9.

210. Husain, A.N., Siddiqui, M.T., Montoya, A., Chandrasekhar, A.J., Garrity, E.R. 1996. Post-lung transplant biopsies: an 8-year Loyola experience. *Mod Pathol, 9*: 126–32.

211. Smyth, R.L., Scott, J.P., Borysiewicz, L.K., Sharples, L.D., Stewart, S., Wreghitt, T.G., Gray, J.J., Higenbottam, T.W., Wallwork, J. 1991. Cytomegalovirus infection in heart-lung transplant recipients: risk factors, clinical associations, and response to treatment. *J Infect Dis, 164*: 1045–50.

212. Wendt, C.H., Fox, J.M., Hertz, M.I. 1995. Paramyxovirus infection in lung transplant recipients. *J Heart Lung Transplant, 14*: 479–85.

213. Palmer, S.M., Jr, Henshaw, N.G., Howell, D.N., Miller, S.E., Davis, R.D., Tapson, V.F. 1998. Community respiratory viral infection in adult lung transplant recipients. *Chest, 113*: 944–50.

214. Billings, J.L., Hertz, M.I., Wendt, C.H. 2001. Community respiratory virus infections following lung transplantation. *Transpl Infect Dis, 3*: 138–48.

215. Vilchez, R., McCurry, K., Dauber, J., Iacono, A., Keenan, R., Griffith, B., Kusne, S. 2002. Influenza and parainfluenza respiratory viral infection requiring admission in adult lung transplant recipients. *Transplantation, 73*: 1075–8.

216. Vilchez, R.A., Dauber, J., McCurry, K., Iacono, A., Kusne, S. 2003. Parainfluenza virus infection in adult lung transplant recipients: an emergent clinical syndrome with implications on allograft function. *Am J Transplant, 3*: 116–20.

217. Ohori, N.P., Michaels, M.G., Jaffe, R., Williams, P., Yousem, S.A. 1995. Adenovirus pneumonia in lung transplant recipients. *Hum Pathol, 26*: 1073–9.

218. Simsir, A., Greenebaum, E., Nuovo, G., Schulman, L.L. 1998. Late fatal adenovirus pneumonitis in a lung transplant recipient. *Transplantation, 65*: 592–4.

219. Garantziotis, S., Howell, D.N., McAdams, H.P., Davis, R.D., Henshaw, N.G., Palmer, S.M. 2001. Influenza pneumonia in lung transplant recipients: clinical features and association with bronchiolitis obliterans syndrome. *Chest, 119*: 1277–80.

220. Vilchez, R.A., McCurry, K., Dauber, J., Iacono, A., Keenan, R., Zeevi, A., Griffith, B., Kusne, S. 2001. The epidemiology of parainfluenza virus infection in lung transplant recipients. *Clin Infect Dis, 33*: 2004–8.

221. Kumar, D., Erdman, D., Keshavjee, S., Peret, T., Tellier, R., Hadjiliadis, D., Johnson, G., Ayers, M., Siegal, D., Humar, A. 2005. Clinical impact of community-acquired respiratory viruses on bronchiolitis obliterans after lung transplant. *Am J Transplant, 5*: 2031–6.

222. Gerna, G., Vitulo, P., Rovida, F., Lilleri, D., Pellegrini, C., Oggionni, T., Campanini, G., Baldanti, F., Revello, M.G. 2006. Impact of human metapneumovirus and human cytomegalovirus versus other respiratory viruses on the lower respiratory tract infections of lung transplant recipients. *J Med Virol, 78*: 408–16.

223. Raza, K., Ismailjee, S.B., Crespo, M., Studer, S.M., Sanghavi, S., Paterson, D.L., Kwak, E.J., Rinaldo, C.R., Jr., Pilewski, J.M., McCurry, K.R. et al. 2007. Successful outcome of human metapneumovirus (hMPV) pneumonia in a lung transplant recipient treated with intravenous ribavirin. *J Heart Lung Transplant, 26*: 862–4.

224. Dare, R., Sanghavi, S., Bullotta, A., Keightley, M.C., George, K.S., Wadowsky, R.M., Paterson, D.L., McCurry, K.R., Reinhart, T.A., Husain, S. et al. 2007. Diagnosis of human metapneumovirus infection in immunosuppressed lung transplant recipients and children evaluated for pertussis. *J Clin Microbiol, 45*: 548–52.

225. Larcher, C., Geltner, C., Fischer, H., Nachbaur, D., Muller, L.C., Huemer, H.P. 2005. Human metapneumovirus infection in lung transplant recipients: clinical presentation and epidemiology. *J Heart Lung Transplant, 24*: 1891–901.

226. Judson, M.A. 1993. Clinical aspects of lung transplantation. *Clin Chest Med, 14*: 335–57.

227. Davis, R.D., Jr, Pasque, M.K. 1995. Pulmonary transplantation. *Ann Surg, 221*: 14–28.

228. Grossi, P., Farina, C., Fiocchi, R., Dalla Gasperina, D. 2000. Prevalence and outcome of invasive fungal infections in 1,963 thoracic organ transplant recipients: a multicenter retrospective study. Italian Study Group of Fungal Infections in Thoracic Organ Transplant Recipients. *Transplantation, 70*: 112–6.

229. Tamm, M., Malouf, M., Glanville, A. 2001. Pulmonary scedosporium infection following lung transplantation. *Transpl Infect Dis, 3*: 189–94.

230. Marchevsky, A., Hartman, G., Walts, A., Ross, D., Koerner, S., Waters, P. 1991. Lung transplantation: the pathologic diagnosis of pulmonary complications. *Mod Pathol, 4*: 133–8.

231. Patel, S.R., Kirby, T.J., McCarthy, P.M., Meeker, D.P., Stillwell, P., Rice, T.W., Kavuru, M.S., Mehta, A.C.

1993. Lung transplantation: the Cleveland Clinic experience. *Cleve Clin J Med*, 60: 303–19.

232. Nunley, D.R., Gal, A.A., Vega, J.D., Perlino, C., Smith, P., Lawrence, E.C. 2002. Saprophytic fungal infections and complications involving the bronchial anastomosis following human lung transplantation. *Chest*, 122: 1185–91.

233. Helmi, M., Love, R.B., Welter, D., Cornwell, R.D., Meyer, K.C. 2003. Aspergillus infection in lung transplant recipients with cystic fibrosis: risk factors and outcomes comparison to other types of transplant recipients. *Chest*, 123: 800–8.

234. Mehrad, B., Paciocco, G., Martinez, F.J., Ojo, T.C., Iannettoni, M.D., Lynch, J.P., 3rd. 2001. Spectrum of Aspergillus infection in lung transplant recipients: case series and review of the literature. *Chest*, 119: 169–75.

235. Tazelaar, H.D., Baird, A.M., Mill, M., Grimes, M.M., Schulman, L.L., Smith, C.R. 1989. Bronchocentric mycosis occurring in transplant recipients. *Chest*, 96: 92–5.

236. Castiglioni, B., Sutton, D.A., Rinaldi, M.G., Fung, J., Kusne, S. 2002. Pseudallescheria boydii (Anamorph Scedosporium apiospermum). Infection in solid organ transplant recipients in a tertiary medical center and review of the literature. *Medicine (Baltimore)*, 81: 333–48.

237. Hunstad, D.A., Cohen, A.H., St Geme, J.W., 3rd. 1999. Successful eradication of mucormycosis occurring in a pulmonary allograft. *J Heart Lung Transplant*, 18: 801–4.

238. Zander, D.S., Cicale, M.J., Mergo, P. 2000. Durable cure of mucormycosis involving allograft and native lungs. *J Heart Lung Transplant*, 19: 615–8.

239. Mattner, F., Weissbrodt, H., Strueber, M. 2004. Two case reports: fatal Absidia corymbifera pulmonary tract infection in the first postoperative phase of a lung transplant patient receiving voriconazole prophylaxis, and transient bronchial Absidia corymbifera colonization in a lung transplant patient. *Scand J Infect Dis*, 36: 312–4.

240. Chaparro, C., Kesten, S. 1997. Infections in lung transplant recipients. *Clin Chest Med*, 18: 339–51.

241. Fishman, J.A. 2001. Prevention of infection caused by Pneumocystis carinii in transplant recipients. *Clin Infect Dis*, 33: 1397–405.

242. Kesten, S., Chaparro, C. 1999. Mycobacterial infections in lung transplant recipients. *Chest*, 115: 741–5.

243. Morales, P., Briones, A., Torres, J.J., Sole, A., Perez, D., Pastor, A. 2005. Pulmonary tuberculosis in lung and heart-lung transplantation: fifteen years of experience in a single center in Spain. *Transplant Proc*, 37: 4050–5.

244. Bravo, C., Roldan, J., Roman, A., Degracia, J., Majo, J., Guerra, J., Monforte, V., Vidal, R., Morell, F. 2005. Tuberculosis in lung transplant recipients. *Transplantation*, 79: 59–64.

245. Bonvillain, R.W., Valentine, V.G., Lombard, G., LaPlace, S., Dhillon, G., Wang, G. 2007. Post-operative infections in cystic fibrosis and non-cystic fibrosis patients after lung transplantation. *J Heart Lung Transplant*, 26: 890–7.

246. Malouf, M.A., Glanville, A.R. 1999. The spectrum of mycobacterial infection after lung transplantation. *Am J Respir Crit Care Med*, 160: 1611–6.

247. Trulock, E.P., Bolman, R.M., Genton, R. 1989. Pulmonary disease caused by Mycobacterium chelonae in a heart-lung transplant recipient with obliterative bronchiolitis. *Am Rev Respir Dis*, 140: 802–5.

248. Paciocco, G., Martinez, F.J., Kazerooni, E.A., Bossone, E., Lynch, J.P., 3rd. 2000. Tuberculous pneumonia complicating lung transplantation: case report and review of the literature. *Monaldi Arch Chest Dis*, 55: 117–21.

249. Schulman, L.L., Htun, T., Staniloae, C., McGregor, C.C., Austin, J.H. 2000. Pulmonary nodules and masses after lung and heart-lung transplantation. *J Thorac Imaging*, 15: 173–9.

250. Sanguinetti, M., Ardito, F., Fiscarelli, E., La Sorda, M., D'Argenio, P., Ricciotti, G., Fadda, G. 2001. Fatal pulmonary infection due to multidrug-resistant Mycobacterium abscessus in a patient with cystic fibrosis. *J Clin Microbiol*, 39: 816–9.

251. Baldi, S., Rapellino, M., Ruffini, E., Cavallo, A., Mancuso, M. 1997. Atypical mycobacteriosis in a lung transplant recipient. *Eur Respir J*, 10: 952–4.

252. Fairhurst, R.M., Kubak, B.M., Shpiner, R.B., Levine, M.S., Pegues, D.A., Ardehali, A. 2002. Mycobacterium abscessus empyema in a lung transplant recipient. *J Heart Lung Transplant*, 21: 391–4.

253. Wreghitt, T.G., Gray, J.J., Pavel, P., Balfour, A., Fabbri, A., Sharples, L.D., Wallwork, J. 1992. Efficacy of pyrimethamine for the prevention of donor-acquired Toxoplasma gondii infection in heart and heart-lung transplant patients. *Transpl Int*, 5: 197–200.

254. Paranjothi, S., Yusen, R.D., Kraus, M.D., Lynch, J.P., Patterson, G.A., Trulock, E.P. 2001. Lymphoproliferative disease after lung transplantation: comparison of presentation and outcome of early and late cases. *J Heart Lung Transplant*, 20: 1054–63.

255. Ramalingam, P., Rybicki, L., Smith, M.D., Abrahams, N.A., Tubbs, R.R., Pettay, J., Farver, C.F., Hsi, E.D. 2002. Posttransplant lymphoproliferative disorders in lung transplant patients: the Cleveland Clinic experience. *Mod Pathol*, 15: 647–56.

256. Reams, B.D., McAdams, H.P., Howell, D.N., Steele, M.P., Davis, R.D., Palmer, S.M. 2003. Posttransplant lymphoproliferative disorder: incidence, presentation, and response to treatment in lung transplant recipients. *Chest*, 124: 1242–9.

257. Yousem, S.A., Randhawa, P., Locker, J., Paradis, I.L., Dauber, J.A., Griffith, B.P., Nalesnik, M.A. 1989. Posttransplant lymphoproliferative disorders in heart-lung transplant recipients: primary presentation in the allograft. *Hum Pathol*, 20: 361–9.

258. Egan, J.J., Hasleton, P.S., Yonan, N., Rahman, A.N., Deiraniya, A.K., Carroll, K.B., Woodcock, A.A. 1995. Necrotic, ulcerative bronchitis, the presenting feature of lymphoproliferative disease following heart-lung transplantation. *Thorax*, 50: 205–7.

259. Ho, M., Jaffe, R., Miller, G., Breinig, M.K., Dummer, J.S., Makowka, L., Atchison, R.W., Karrer, F., Nalesnik, M.A., Starzl, T.E. 1988. The frequency of Epstein-Barr virus infection and associated lymphoproliferative syndrome after transplantation and its manifestations in children. *Transplantation*, 45: 719–27.

260. Randhawa, P.S., Jaffe, R., Demetris, A.J., Nalesnik, M., Starzl, T.E., Chen, Y.Y., Weiss, L.M. 1992. Expression of Epstein-Barr virus-encoded small RNA (by the EBER-1

gene) in liver specimens from transplant recipients with post-transplantation lymphoproliferative disease. *N Engl J Med*, 327: 1710–4.

261. Chadburn, A., Suciu-Foca, N., Cesarman, E., Reed, E., Michler, R.E., Knowles, D.M. 1995. Post-transplantation lymphoproliferative disorders arising in solid organ transplant recipients are usually of recipient origin. *Am J Pathol*, 147: 1862–70.

262. Larson, R.S., Scott, M.A., McCurley, T.L., Vnencak-Jones, C.L. 1996. Microsatellite analysis of posttransplant lymphoproliferative disorders: determination of donor/recipient origin and identification of putative lymphomagenic mechanism. *Cancer Res*, 56: 4378–81.

263. Le Frere-Belda, M.A., Martin, N., Gaulard, P., Zafrani, E.S. 1997. Donor or recipient origin of post-transplantation lymphoproliferative disorders: evaluation by in situ hybridization. *Mod Pathol*, 10: 701–7.

264. Ng, I.O., Shek, T.W., Thung, S.N., Ye, M.M., Lo, C.M., Fan, S.T., Lee, J.M., Chan, K.W., Cheung, A.N. 2000. Microsatellite analysis in post-transplantation lymphoproliferative disorder to determine donor/recipient origin. *Mod Pathol*, 13: 1180–5.

265. Petit, B., Le Meur, Y., Jaccard, A., Paraf, F., Robert, C.L., Bordessoule, D., Labrousse, F., Drouet, M. 2002. Influence of host-recipient origin on clinical aspects of posttransplantation lymphoproliferative disorders in kidney transplantation. *Transplantation*, 73: 265–71.

266. Gulley, M.L., Swinnen, L.J., Plaisance, K.T., Jr., Schnell, C., Grogan, T.M., Schneider, B.G. 2003. Tumor origin and CD20 expression in posttransplant lymphoproliferative disorder occurring in solid organ transplant recipients: implications for immune-based therapy. *Transplantation*, 76: 959–64.

267. Peterson, M.R., Emery, S.C., Yung, G.L., Masliah, E., Yi, E.S. 2006. Epstein-Barr virus-associated posttransplantation lymphoproliferative disorder following lung transplantation is more commonly of host origin. *Arch Pathol Lab Med*, 130: 176–80.

268. Oertel, S.H., Verschuuren, E., Reinke, P., Zeidler, K., Papp-Vary, M., Babel, N., Trappe, R.U., Jonas, S., Hummel, M., Anagnostopoulos, I. et al. 2005. Effect of anti-CD 20 antibody rituximab in patients with post-transplant lymphoproliferative disorder (PTLD). *Am J Transplant*, 5: 2901–6.

269. Knoop, C., Kentos, A., Remmelink, M., Garbar, C., Goldman, S., Feremans, W., Estenne, M. 2006. Post-transplant lymphoproliferative disorders after lung transplantation: first-line treatment with rituximab may induce complete remission. *Clin Transplant*, 20: 179–87.

270. Frizzera, G., Hanto, D.W., Gajl-Peczalska, K.J., Rosai, J., McKenna, R.W., Sibley, R.K., Holahan, K.P., Lindquist, L.L. 1981. Polymorphic diffuse B-cell hyperplasias and lymphomas in renal transplant recipients. *Cancer Res*, 41: 4262–79.

271. Nalesnik, M.A., Jaffe, R., Starzl, T.E., Demetris, A.J., Porter, K., Burnham, J.A., Makowka, L., Ho, M., Locker, J. 1988. The pathology of posttransplant lymphoproliferative disorders occurring in the setting of cyclosporine A-prednisone immunosuppression. *Am J Pathol*, 133: 173–92.

272. Knowles, D.M., Cesarman, E., Chadburn, A., Frizzera, G., Chen, J., Rose, E.A., Michler, R.E. 1995. Correlative morphologic and molecular genetic analysis demonstrates three distinct categories of posttransplantation lymphoproliferative disorders. *Blood*, 85: 552–65.

273. Harris, N.L., Ferry, J.A., Swerdlow, S.H. 1997. Posttransplant lymphoproliferative disorders: Summary of Society for Hematopathology Workshop. *Semin Diagn Pathol*, 14: 8–14.

274. Harris, N.L., Swerdlow, S.H., Frizzera, G., al., e.2001. Post-transplant lymphoproliferative disorders. In *Pathology and Genetics of Tumours of Haematopoietic and Lymphoid Tissue*. Jaffe, E.S., Harris, N.L., Stein, H., Vardiman, J.W., eds. IARC Press, Lyon France, pp. 264–9.

275. Veness, M.J., Quinn, D.I., Ong, C.S., Keogh, A.M., Macdonald, P.S., Cooper, S.G., Morgan, G.W. 1999. Aggressive cutaneous malignancies following cardiothoracic transplantation: the Australian experience. *Cancer*, 85: 1758–64.

276. Dickson, R.P., Davis, R.D., Rea, J.B., Palmer, S.M. 2006. High frequency of bronchogenic carcinoma after single-lung transplantation. *J Heart Lung Transplant*, 25: 1297–301.

277. Arcasoy, S.M., Hersh, C., Christie, J.D., Zisman, D., Pochettino, A., Rosengard, B.R., Blumenthal, N.P., Palevsky, H.I., Bavaria, J.E., Kotloff, R.M. 2001. Bronchogenic carcinoma complicating lung transplantation. *J Heart Lung Transplant*, 20: 1044–53.

278. Amital, A., Shitrit, D., Raviv, Y., Bendayan, D., Sahar, G., Bakal, I., Kramer, M.R. 2006. Development of malignancy following lung transplantation. *Transplantation*, 81: 547–51.

279. Johnson, B.A., Duncan, S.R., Ohori, N.P., Paradis, I.L., Yousem, S.A., Grgurich, W.F., Dauber, J.H., Griffith, B.P. 1993. Recurrence of sarcoidosis in pulmonary allograft recipients. *Am Rev Respir Dis*, 148: 1373–7.

280. Bjortuft, O., Foerster, A., Boe, J., Geiran, O. 1994. Single lung transplantation as treatment for end-stage pulmonary sarcoidosis: recurrence of sarcoidosis in two different lung allografts in one patient. *J Heart Lung Transplant*, 13: 24–29.

281. Kazerooni, E.A., Jackson, C., Cascade, P.N. 1994. Sarcoidosis: recurrence of primary disease in transplanted lungs. *Radiology*, 192: 461–4.

282. Martinez, F.J., Orens, J.B., Deeb, M., Brunsting, L.A., Flint, A., Lynch, J.P. 1994. Recurrence of sarcoidosis following bilateral allogeneic lung transplantation. *Chest*, 106: 1597–9.

283. Carre, P., Rouquette, I., Durand, D., Didier, A., Dahan, M., Fournial, G., Leophonte, P. 1995. Recurrence of sarcoidosis in a human lung allograft. *Transplant Proc*, 27: 1686.

284. Martel, S., Carre, P.C., Carrera, G., Pipy, B., Leophonte, P.J. 1996. Tumour necrosis factor-alpha gene expression by alveolar macrophages in human lung allograft recipient with recurrence of sarcoidosis. Toulouse Lung Transplantation Group. *Eur Respir J*, 9: 1087–9.

285. Yeatman, M., McNeil, K., Smith, J.A., Stewart, S., Sharples, L.D., Higenbottam, T., Wells, F.C., Wallwork, J. 1996. Lung transplantation in patients with systemic diseases: an

eleven-year experience at Papworth Hospital. *J Heart Lung Transplant*, *15*: 144–9.

286. Pigula, F.A., Griffith, B.P., Zenati, M.A., Dauber, J.H., Yousem, S.A., Keenan, R.J. 1997. Lung transplantation for respiratory failure resulting from systemic disease. *Ann Thorac Surg*, *64*: 1630–4.

287. Klemen, H., Husain, A.N., Cagle, P.T., Garrity, E.R., Popper, H.H. 2000. Mycobacterial DNA in recurrent sarcoidosis in the transplanted lung–a PCR-based study on four cases. *Virchows Arch*, *436*: 365–9.

288. Collins, J., Hartman, M.J., Warner, T.F., Muller, N.L., Kazerooni, E.A., McAdams, H.P., Slone, R.M., Parker, L.A. 2001. Frequency and CT findings of recurrent disease after lung transplantation. *Radiology*, *219*: 503–9.

289. Nine, J.S., Yousem, S.A., Paradis, I.L., Keenan, R., Griffith, B.P. 1994. Lymphangioleiomyomatosis: recurrence after lung transplantation. *J Heart Lung Transplant*, *13*: 714–9.

290. O'Brien, J.D., Lium, J.H., Parosa, J.F., Deyoung, B.R., Wick, M.R., Trulock, E.P. 1995. Lymphangiomyomatosis recurrence in the allograft after single-lung transplantation. *Am J Respir Crit Care Med*, *151*: 2033–6.

291. Boehler, A., Speich, R., Russi, E.W., Weder, W. 1996. Lung transplantation for lymphangioleiomyomatosis. *N Engl J Med*, *335*: 1275–80.

292. Bittmann, I., Dose, T.B., Muller, C., Dienemann, H., Vogelmeier, C., Lohrs, U. 1997. Lymphangioleiomyomatosis: recurrence after single lung transplantation. *Hum Pathol*, *28*: 1420–3.

293. Collins, J., Muller, N.L., Kazerooni, E.A., McAdams, H.P., Leung, A.N., Love, R.B. 1999. Lung transplantation for lymphangioleiomyomatosis: role of imaging in the assessment of complications related to the underlying disease. *Radiology*, *210*: 325–32.

294. Pechet, T.T., Meyers, B.F., Guthrie, T.J., Battafarano, R.J., Trulock, E.P., Cooper, J.D., Patterson, G.A. 2004. Lung transplantation for lymphangioleiomyomatosis. *J Heart Lung Transplant*, *23*: 301–8.

295. Chen, F., Bando, T., Fukuse, T., Omasa, M., Aoyama, A., Hamakawa, H., Fujinaga, T., Shoji, T., Sakai, H., Hanaoka, N. et al. 2006. Recurrent lymphangioleiomyomatosis after living-donor lobar lung transplantation. *Transplant Proc*, *38*: 3151–3.

296. Habib, S.B., Congleton, J., Carr, D., Partridge, J., Corrin, B., Geddes, D.M., Banner, N., Yacoub, M., Burke, M. 1998. Recurrence of recipient Langerhans' cell histiocytosis following bilateral lung transplantation. *Thorax*, *53*: 323–5.

297. Gabbay, E., Dark, J.H., Ashcroft, T., Milne, D., Gibson, G.J., Healy, M., Corris, P.A. 1998. Recurrence of Langerhans' cell granulomatosis following lung transplantation. *Thorax*, *53*: 326–7.

298. Dauriat, G., Mal, H., Thabut, G., Mornex, J.F., Bertocchi, M., Tronc, F., Leroy-Ladurie, F., Dartevelle, P., Reynaud-Gaubert, M., Thomas, P. et al. 2006. Lung transplantation for pulmonary langerhans' cell histiocytosis: a multicenter analysis. *Transplantation*, *81*: 746–50.

299. King, M.B., Jessurun, J., Hertz, M.I. 1997. Recurrence of desquamative interstitial pneumonia after lung transplantation. *Am J Respir Crit Care Med*, *156*: 2003–5.

300. Verleden, G.M., Sels, F., Van Raemdonck, D., Verbeken, E.K., Lerut, T., Demedts, M. 1998. Possible recurrence of desquamative interstitial pneumonitis in a single lung transplant recipient. *Eur Respir J*, *11*: 971–4.

301. Parker, L.A., Novotny, D.B. 1997. Recurrent alveolar proteinosis following double lung transplantation. *Chest*, *111*: 1457–8.

302. Santamaria, F., Brancaccio, G., Parenti, G., Francalanci, P., Squitieri, C., Sebastio, G., Dionisi-Vici, C., D'Argenio, P., Andria, G., Parisi, F. 2004. Recurrent fatal pulmonary alveolar proteinosis after heart-lung transplantation in a child with lysinuric protein intolerance. *J Pediatr*, *145*: 268–72.

303. Frost, A.E., Keller, C.A., Brown, R.W., Noon, G.P., Short, H.D., Abraham, J.L., Pacinda, S., Cagle, P.T. 1993. Giant cell interstitial pneumonitis. Disease recurrence in the transplanted lung. *Am Rev Respir Dis*, *148*: 1401–4.

304. Baz, M.A., Kussin, P.S., Van Trigt, P., Davis, R.D., Roggli, V.L., Tapson, V.F. 1995. Recurrence of diffuse panbronchiolitis after lung transplantation. *Am J Respir Crit Care Med*, *151*: 895–8.

305. Fitzsimons, E.J., Aris, R., Patterson, R. 1997. Recurrence of allergic bronchopulmonary aspergillosis in the posttransplant lungs of a cystic fibrosis patient. *Chest*, *112*: 281–2.

306. Mal, H., Guignabert, C., Thabut, G., d'Ortho, M.P., Brugiere, O., Dauriat, G., Marrash-Chahla, R., Rangheard, A.S., Leseche, G., Fournier, M. 2004. Recurrence of pulmonary emphysema in an alpha-1 proteinase inhibitor-deficient lung transplant recipient. *Am J Respir Crit Care Med*, *170*: 811–4.

307. Calabrese, F., Giacometti, C., Rea, F., Loy, M., Sartori, F., Di Vittorio, G., Abudureheman, A., Thiene, G., Valente, M. 2002. Recurrence of idiopathic pulmonary hemosiderosis in a young adult patient after bilateral single-lung transplantation. *Transplantation*, *74*: 1643–5.

308. Cook, R.C., Fradet, G., English, J.C., Soos, J., Muller, N.L., Connolly, T.P., Levy, R.D. 1998. Recurrence of intravenous talc granulomatosis following single lung transplantation. *Can Respir J*, *5*: 511–4.

309. Chen, F., Hasegawa, S., Bando, T., Kitaichi, M., Hiratsuka, T., Kawashima, M., Hanaoka, N., Yoshimura, T., Tanaka, F., Trulock, E.P. et al. 2006. Recurrence of bilateral diffuse bronchiectasis after bilateral lung transplantation. *Respirology*, *11*: 666–8.

310. Izbicki, G., Shitrit, D., Schechtman, I., Bendayan, D., Fink, G., Sahar, G., Saute, M., Ben-Gal, T., Kramer, M.R. 2005. Recurrence of pulmonary veno-occlusive disease after heart-lung transplantation. *J Heart Lung Transplant*, *24*: 635–7.

CHAPTER 7

Pancreas Transplantation Pathology

Cinthia B. Drachenberg, M.D.
John C. Papadimitriou, M.D., Ph.D.

I. INTRODUCTION

Diabetes mellitus (DM), characterized by hyperglycemia, is the result of insufficient or defective insulin secretion and/ or insulin activity. Although DM can result from multiple causes, the vast majority of patients can be classified as two types: DM type 1, typically resulting from immune-mediated destruction of the insulin producing β cells, and DM type 2, which is much more common, and results from resistance to insulin action compounded with an inadequate compensatory insulin secretory response (1). Over time, patients with DM develop extensive microvascular pathology that can lead to complications such as renal failure, retinopathy, and systemic neuropathy. These chronic complications are associated with a marked increase in morbidity and mortality and have a significant impact on patient overall quality of life. In addition, patients with DM, particularly type 1, may have life-threatening acute complications such as diabetic ketoacidosis and severe hypoglycemia (1).

Treatment for DM type 1 consists of frequent, self-adjusted insulin administration (intensive insulin therapy). This type of treatment is costly and requires rigorous monitoring of blood glucose and interval testing of HbA1c. Despite significant improvement in glucose control, exogenous insulin therapy does not achieve complete normalization of HbA1c in most cases, and although the risk of secondary complications is decreased, it is not eliminated. In addition, insulin therapy carries a significant risk for hypoglycemia (2).

Given the limitations of intensive insulin therapy, there is a need for the development of other therapeutic options for DM, such as pancreas or islet transplantation. Although the slow advancement in the optimization of these treatments has precluded their widespread use, it is clear that successful pancreas and islet transplantation are the only options that can provide complete normalization of the glucose metabolism with prevention of the development of secondary complications (3–6). As of 2004, more than 23,000 pancreas transplants were reported to the International Pancreas Transplant Registry, approximately 17,000 in the United States and 6,000 in other countries, predominantly in Europe (7).

i. Indications for Pancreas Transplantation

The surgical and immunosuppression-dependent risks of pancreas transplantation are considered justified in insulin-dependent diabetic patients with episodic hypoglycemic unawareness, or if there is rapid progression of the secondary diabetic complications. Marked improvement in the quality of life is reported by most patients with a functioning pancreas transplant (8).

The vast majority of pancreas transplants are done in patients with DM type 1, in whom a successful procedure results in normalization of the glucose metabolism and disappearance of the acute complications of the disease.

Pancreas transplantation also results in prevention, stabilization, and, in some cases, reversal of some of the long-term renal and neural complications of diabetes (3–6). Pancreas transplantation is also indicated in a minority of patients with insulin-dependent DM type 2, this category representing only 4–6 percent of patients undergoing pancreas transplantation (7).

There are three pancreas transplant types, depending on the patient's kidney function. In patients with uremia/ end stage renal disease, a simultaneous pancreas-kidney (SPK) transplant is the treatment of choice, or alternatively the pancreas can be transplanted after a successful (previous) kidney transplant (pancreas after kidney, PAK). In contrast, a pancreas transplant alone (PTA) is used in nonuremic diabetic patients (9).

In addition, pancreas transplantation is very rarely indicated in patients that have undergone surgical resection of the native pancreas (e.g., for a benign tumor) or if there is advanced chronic pancreatitis leading to exocrine as well as endocrine pancreas deficiency. In patients with pancreatectomy for benign disease, pancreas or islet autotransplantation should be considered before allotransplantation in order to avoid the need for immunosuppression (10).

Results of pancreas transplantation have continuously improved since the late 1980s, with reported one-year graft survival rates of 85 percent for SPK, 78 percent for PAK, and 77 percent for PTA. Patient survival is excellent, in the order of 95–96 percent at one year in all pancreas transplant types (11). The improved graft outcomes are attributed to decreases in the technical and immunological failure rates, newer and more specific immunosuppression, better diagnosis of rejection, and improved treatment of infections. In recent years the risk of graft loss to acute rejection in technically successful transplants has decreased to 2, 8, and 10 percent at one year for SPK, PAK, and PTA cases, respectively. It is in the category of PTA that most dramatic improvements has been achieved, resulting in a progressive proportional increase in the number of PTA that now represent 35 percent of all pancreas transplants. Pancreas biopsies play their most decisive role with PTA, since there is a higher risk of rejection (7,11,12).

The slower progress made with pancreas transplantation in comparison to other organ transplants is to a large extent related to the more challenging technical problems inherent to the organ itself. Specifically, over time there has been increasing evidence for the need to improve management of pancreatic exocrine secretions. Secondarily, the manner of venous drainage has also attracted careful consideration (13).

ii. Brief History of Pancreas Transplantation/Surgical Techniques

The first pancreas transplant was done in 1966 at the University of Minnesota, simultaneously with a kidney transplant (SPK) (14). The pancreas exocrine secretions were managed by duct ligation, based on animal studies indicating that this would result in diffuse atrophy of the exocrine parenchyma allowing for the preservation of a vascularized endocrine component. The postoperative course, however, was complicated by a pancreatic fistula formation and pancreatitis. The patient was insulin free for six days but died a week later due to a pulmonary embolism (14). After this initial experience, a dozen pancreas transplantations were done in the following years at the University of Minnesota with the exocrine secretions managed by cutaneous graft duodenostomy (n = 4) and enteric drainage (n = 8) (15). Venous drainage was most commonly directed through the iliac veins (systemic drainage). In the 1970s and 1980s, a variety of surgical techniques were tried by different centers, including enteric drainage, ureteral drainage, open duct drainage, and duct injection with synthetic polymers, but results were in general poor resulting from both acute rejection and technical complications. Initially, segmental pancreas transplantation was preferred over whole organ transplantation (16).

By the early 1980s, only 105 pancreas transplants had been performed worldwide with equivalent proportions done in the United States and Europe. In 1983, a new technique was developed at the University of Wisconsin, based on the use of whole pancreas transplants and drainage of the exocrine secretions to the urinary bladder (Figure 7.1) (17). Bladder drained pancreas transplants attained general acceptance in the 1990s and this technique was used in more than 80–90 percent of cases. Unfortunately, significant complications such as hematuria, urine leaks, recurrent urinary tract infections, urethritis, and reflux pancreatitis were present in up to 25 percent of patients, eventually requiring conversion to enteric drainage. A major advantage of bladder drainage (pancreaticoduodenocystostomy technique) was the diagnostic use of the decrease in urinary amylase for the detection of acute rejection (see clinical diagnosis of rejection). In the 1990s, a marked decrease in the immunological rates of graft losses were reported, related to the availability of more potent immunosuppressive drugs leading to further improvement in graft outcomes. Also, further refinements of the surgical techniques allowed for a return to preferred enteric drainage in order to avoid the common complications seen with bladder drainage (Figure 7.2). Currently, enteric drainage is the most commonly used method to treat the exocrine secretions in SPK patients in whom elevations in creatinine are proposed as surrogate markers of pancreas rejection. Bladder drainage is still preferred by some for patients with solitary pancreas transplants, in order to take advantage of the diagnostic use of urinary amylase. In enteric drained transplants, venous drainage is preferably done into the portal vein (rather than in the iliac veins) to more closely resemble the physiological status (Figure 7.2) (13).

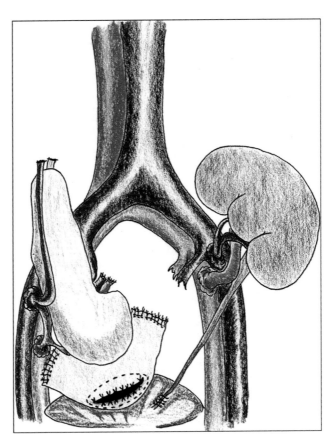

FIGURE 7.1: *Schematic representation of pancreas and kidney transplants. The pancreatic exocrine secretions are drained in the urinary bladder and its venous drainage is systemic (iliac veins).*

II. DIAGNOSIS OF ACUTE ALLOGRAFT REJECTION

i. Clinical Diagnosis of Acute Allograft Rejection

Clinical symptoms are unusual in acute pancreas rejection so that the diagnosis relies heavily on laboratory methods indicating abnormalities in the exocrine secretions (i.e., amylase, lipase) and/or the endocrine function (e.g., blood glucose). Abnormalities in the exocrine secretions indicate acute acinar cell injury that is common in cell-mediated rejection (18–25). In pancreas, transplants with exocrine drainage into the urinary bladder, serial measurements of amylasuria are useful for monitoring of acute rejection, if there is a decrease of more than 25 percent or more than 50 percent from baseline levels (17,22,24,25). However, decreased urine amylase is not specific and can also be seen in several situations including acute pancreatitis, graft thrombosis, and duct obstruction. When correlated with biopsy findings, decrease in urinary amylase had a specificity of 30 percent and a positive predictive value of 53 percent (20,21).

Increase in serum amylase and lipase are general markers of acinar cell injury and while useful for monitoring pancreas patients (increase in acute rejection), also do so in acute pancreatitis and other inflammatory processes

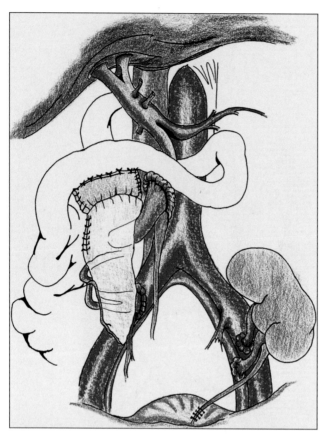

FIGURE 7.2: Schematic representation of pancreas and kidney transplants. The pancreatic exocrine secretions are drained into a loop of small intestine (enteric drainage) and the venous drainage is to the portal system (portal venous drainage).

diagnostic value is questionable since isolated rejection of one of these organs is not uncommon and may occur in up to 30 percent of cases (31).

Acute rejection occurs earlier and is more common in PTA recipients (31). Similarly, graft loss from irreversible rejection occurs more frequently with PTA than with the other transplant types (9,15, and 30 percent versus 2,3, and 7 percent at one, two, and five years, respectively, in SPK) (7). The availability of the percutaneous pancreas biopsy technique in these recipients, in whom the renal function is not available as a "sentinel," has significantly improved the outcomes in PTA (12,31,32). It is important to emphasize that timely and accurate diagnosis of acute pancreatic rejection is of paramount importance to prevent graft sclerosis. Episodes of acute rejection, and particularly late acute rejection, significantly increase the risk for graft loss due to chronic rejection (30,33–39).

ii. Histological Diagnosis of Acute Rejection

Overall, the clinical markers of acute pancreas rejection have been shown to correlate with biopsy proven acute allograft rejection in approximately 80 percent of instances (32).

Due to the nonspecific nature of the laboratory tests, needle core biopsies have become the gold standard for diagnosis of rejection (18,19,23,31,40–54).

III. PANCREAS ALLOGRAFT BIOPSIES

The percutaneous needle biopsy technique was described by Allen et al. in the early 1990s (18). Needle core biopsies are usually done under ultrasound or computer tomographic guidance, with eighteen- or twenty-gauge needles (50–53). Adequate tissue can be obtained in 88–90 percent of instances (32,44,47,49,51–54). Significant complications have been reported in 2–3 percent of cases (i.e., bleeding), none leading to graft loss (49,51).

In patients with intestinal drainage, bowel loops are often interposed between the abdominal wall and the graft, interfering in the performance of percutaneous needle biopsies. This problem is circumvented with the use of the laparoscopic biopsy technique as an alternative to the percutaneous biopsy (55,56). Open (surgical) biopsies are only done in selected cases when all the other methods fail to provide tissue adequate for diagnosis (45,46).

In patients with bladder drainage, cystoscopic transduodenal pancreas biopsies can provide clinically useful information in the same manner as percutaneous core biopsies, but adequate pancreatic tissue is only obtained in 57–80 percent of cases (57–63). Features of acute rejection can be recognized sometimes in samples containing only duodenal tissue, but a negative duodenal biopsy does not rule out pancreas rejection (see duodenal graft pathology) (60,61,64). Since the development of the percutaneous biopsy technique,

of the pancreas. In acute rejection, a rapid increase in serum amylase and lipase is more characteristically associated with severe rejection; however, there is significant variability from patient to patient and the overall level of the pancreatic enzymes does not show good correlation with the lower rejection grades (23).

In contrast to abnormalities of the exocrine parameters (amylase and lipase) that are usually present in most forms of acute rejection, endocrine abnormalities such as hyperglycemia are relatively rare and occur only in severe, often irreversible acute rejection typically associated with extensive parenchymal necrosis (23,26). In addition to severe rejection, hyperglycemia can be caused by other processes (i.e., recurrence of autoimmune disease, islet cell drug toxicity, chronic rejection) (27,28).

The development of chronic rejection/graft sclerosis leads to progressive impairment of glucose homeostasis that is usually accompanied by a gradual decrease in the levels of amylase and lipase in urine and/or serum (29,30).

In patients with SPK transplants, monitoring of renal function by serial serum creatinine levels is often used as a surrogate for rejection in both organs. Although this method is widely used in clinical practice, its absolute

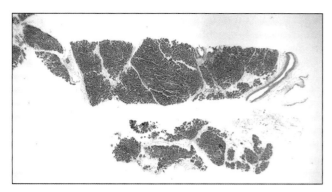

FIGURE 7.3: *Low-power view of a needle core biopsy of the pancreas. The lobular tissue is separated by fibrous septa containing vessels and ducts but no inflammation. The acinar lobules are compact without evidence of acinar loss. The periphery of the lobules is more or less regular (i.e., there is no significant fragmentation of the lobules in the interface with the connective tissue).*

cystoscopic biopsies are rarely used due to their more invasive nature. This procedure is also more costly (46).

i. Needle Core Biopsy Adequacy

Although the adequacy of any particular biopsy sample is ultimately determined by the examining pathologist, it is recommended that pancreas graft biopsies contain at least three lobular areas and their associated interlobular septa (Figure 7.3). The latter typically contain veins and branches of the pancreatic duct. Arterial branches that follow separate courses, more or less embedded within the acinar components, are sampled with more difficulty. In contrast, due to the diagnostic importance ascribed to the arterial lesions, it is recommended that absence of arterial branches be specifically stated in the pathology report.

ii. Guidelines for Processing Pancreas Allograft Biopsies

For best diagnostic yield, it is recommended that at least two hematoxylin and eosin (H&E)–stained sections are examined from two different levels of the core. Five to ten adjacent/intervening unstained sections should be available in order to perform additional stains as needed (i.e., cytomegalovirus (CMV) stain).

Masson's trichrome stain can aid in the identification of specific structures or pathological changes (i.e., arterial walls, fibrinoid necrosis) and is also indicated in biopsies with suspected chronic rejection to demonstrate incipient interacinar fibrosis (65).

In patients biopsied due to hyperglycemia, it is essential to perform stains for insulin and glucagon to identify selective loss of beta cells indicating recurrence of autoimmune disease (66).

It is recommended that C4d immunostain is performed in all biopsies. This stain is particularly indicated in the absence of other findings if the biopsy is performed for

hyperglycemia, in patients with increased risk of humoral rejection (i.e., retransplantation) and if there is margination of neutrophils or other inflammatory cells in the interacinar capillaries (67,68).

iii. Correlation between Pancreas and Kidney Rejection in SPK

Animal studies have shown that acute rejection in kidney and pancreas grafts often occur together (synchronously) (69–72). Interestingly, even in synchronous rejection, the histological grade or severity of rejection may be discordant between the two organs (69,73).

In clinical practice, it is often assumed that SPK transplants are usually rejected synchronously, of at least in "tandem" with the kidney rejection preceding the pancreas rejection (71,72,74,75). Despite the general acceptance of this generalization, the occurrence of asynchronous rejection has been amply documented (31,77) in SPK recipients. In a large study, based on concurrent biopsies of both organs, the pancreas and kidney showed synchronous rejection in 65 percent of episodes, with the pancreas and kidney being selectively involved in 22 and 13 percent of instances, respectively. The possibility of isolated rejection in one of the organs in more than a third of cases, underscores the need for selective renal or pancreatic biopsy evaluation even in patients with SPK (31,32).

iv. Protocol Biopsies

There are very few studies describing the histological findings in protocol biopsies. These are defined as biopsies performed at specified time points, regardless of graft function. In the prospective study of Stratta et al. (76) done in the cyclosporine era, mild rejection was identified in more than half of the patients (54 percent) in the first months posttransplantation. Despite treatment with steroids, 60 percent of these patients went on to develop recurrent biopsy-proven rejection within two months. The authors concluded that patients with rejection should have undergone standard treatment with antilymphocytic antibodies to prevent subsequent episodes of rejection and that protocol biopsies identified patients at risk of acute rejection (76).

In contrast, a retrospective study evaluating protocol biopsies with Maryland grade II (minimal) rejection concluded that these rarely progress to more severe degrees of inflammation (43).

In a recent study, Rogers et al. found acute rejection in 50 percent of protocol PTA biopsies done in the first and second months after transplantation. Aggressive treatment of rejection in their cohort of PTA recipients significantly improved outcomes, comparable to results in the SPK transplants done at the same period (78). This specific study group consisted of twenty solitary pancreas transplants recipients that underwent biopsy the first month after transplantation with repeat biopsy at two months if the first biopsy was negative. The patients had been induced with depleting antibody, and maintenance immunosuppression consistent of tacrolimus and Mycophendate Mofetil (MMF) (77).

The conclusions of Stratta et al. and Rogers et al. are supported by a study of thirty patients with normal graft function biopsied at a mean of 15.4 months (two days to seven years), at the time of laparotomy for reasons unrelated to the pancreas graft function. Most of these biopsies (83 percent) showed no evidence of rejection. Of the five patients with histological, albeit subclinical, evidence of mild rejection, four went on to develop accelerated chronic rejection and lost their grafts between fourteen and twenty months after transplantation. (78).

V. ACUTE ALLOGRAFT REJECTION

i. Immunological Aspects

The mechanisms of acute allograft rejection in the pancreas are not different from those in other solid transplants (see chapter 1), although, the dual nature of the pancreas (i.e., exocrine and endocrine) justifies some special considerations. In the early post-transplantation period, most histopathological manifestations are related to the surgical trauma that invariably leads to some degree of pancreatitis (infiltration by neutrophils and macrophages with variable degrees of cell necrosis) (80–83). Soon after implantation, the events related to antigen presentation are started, followed by T-cell activation, generation of a large array of cytokines and the capability for cell-mediated or humoral rejection.

Graft rejection depends highly on the degree of incompatibility between recipient and donor major histocompatibility complex (MHC) antigens (80). The MHC class I and II molecules are differentially expressed in exocrine and endocrine pancreatic tissues. Variations are also noted between a normal pancreas and a pancreas that is being rejected. In the normal pancreas, class I antigens are expressed weakly on islet cells and strongly on ductal epithelium. By contrast, the acinar cells are negative for class I molecules (84). Under normal circumstances, expression of class II antigens has not been demonstrated in any cell compartment (84). but experimental studies have shown that in acute rejection, acinar cells overexpress class I and class II antigens. The latter are also expressed in ductal epithelium and endothelial cells, whereas class I antigens are expressed on the β cells (85). Class II alloantibodies have also been associated with an increased risk of humoral rejection and graft loss (86).

Although overlaps in the mechanisms of acute rejection do exist, the morphological findings are generally classified as "cell mediated" or "antibody mediated" (80,87). Morphologically, these categories are characterized by tissue infiltration by the effector inflammatory cells and by antibody/complement deposition in the vascular walls,

respectively. In each of these pathways, the graft injury results from both antigen-specific immune damage and other nonspecific factors (80,87).

As with other types of solid organ transplants, the principal effectors in pancreas allograft cell-mediated rejection are T lymphocytes, monocytes, and eosinophils. Cytotoxic T lymphocytes (CTLs) lyse target cells through specific antigen recognition pathways. As described in Chapter 1, CTLs release lytic molecules that cause among other effects, complement-like osmotic cell injury of the target cell (i.e., perforins, granzyme A and B, granulysin). Also, induction of apoptosis occurs through the former mechanism or when the CTL's Fas transmembrane glycoprotein binds to the Fas-ligand on the target cell. Well-developed, uncontrolled acute cell-mediated rejection is characterized by extensive inflammatory cell graft infiltration that invariably results in rapid or occasionally more protracted graft destruction (80,88).

In antibody-mediated rejection, deposition of antibodies in the vascular walls cause direct injury by activation of the complement cascade and also through antibody-dependent, cell-mediated toxicity (ADCC) (86,89). Therefore, vascular injury and necrosis, development of thrombosis, and secondary ischemic parenchymal necrosis are characteristic of the more severe forms of antibody-mediated rejection (i.e., hyperacute rejection) (80,87,89). Although initially thought to be only associated with immediate effects, more protracted forms of antibody-mediated rejection (acute versus hyperacute, and active chronic) are now being recognized. Neutrophils are recruited in abundance in antibody-mediated rejection through the release of complement chemokines. Neutrophils can be present also in the more severe forms of cell-mediated rejection as well as in any form of severe parenchymal injury (80,87).

Different rejection patterns for the exocrine and endocrine components of the pancreas likely reflect variations of MHC expression, as well as other factors such as type and quality of the microvasculature and differential sensitivity to ischemia. Experience with animal and clinical studies have shown that the acinar lobules are the primary target of cell-mediated rejection, with less common involvement of the arterial walls. Acinar damage/dropout and chronic vascular injury both lead to a fibrogenic reaction that represents the main feature of chronic rejection (90). The islets are not directly affected in cell-mediated acute rejection (19,40,69,72,91–93). On the contrary, documented cases of humoral rejection have presented with hyperglycemia, suggesting that the islets may be more susceptible to microvascular injury associated to antibody deposition in this form of rejection (67,68,94).

ii. Morphological Features of Acute Allograft Rejection

Both in small and larger animal models, acute rejection of pancreas is manifested by inflammatory infiltrates in the interstitium, consistent involvement of small veins and variable more heterogeneous involvement of ducts (40,90, 91,95). Acinar inflammation and cell damage including apoptosis are also characteristic of acute rejection (40,71, 90,96,97). The severe, more advanced forms of acute rejection manifest with intimal arteritis, necrotizing vasculitis, thrombosis, and eventually parenchymal necrosis (90,91). Although islets appear not to be the primary target in cell-mediated rejection, extensive parenchymal necrosis can be associated with secondary islet involvement and hyperglycemia (40,70,90,91,98).

An examination of the first series of explanted pancreas allografts provided a glimpse of the spectrum of pathological changes that can be seen in these organs. Two weeks after implantation the first pancreas allograft showed significant architectural disarray and fibrosis, likely secondary

to the ligation of the pancreatic duct. In addition, there was a moderate amount of mononuclear cells in the interlobular septa and focally in the acini, consistent with acute cell-mediated rejection. The islets were normal (14). The dozen cases done subsequently demonstrated that in contrast to cases with duct ligation, unrestricted drainage of the exocrine secretions allowed for maintenance of the exocrine pancreatic structure. From the experience with cases drained externally (cutaneous graft duodenostomy), it was concluded that inflammation of the exposed segment of the graft duodenum correlated with pancreas rejection (15).

In the following decades, seminal studies involving sequential and random samples consistently demonstrated similar histological findings as those seen in animal models (Figures 7.4–7.10) (42,99). The negative impact of intimal and transmural arteritis for the outcome of the graft was

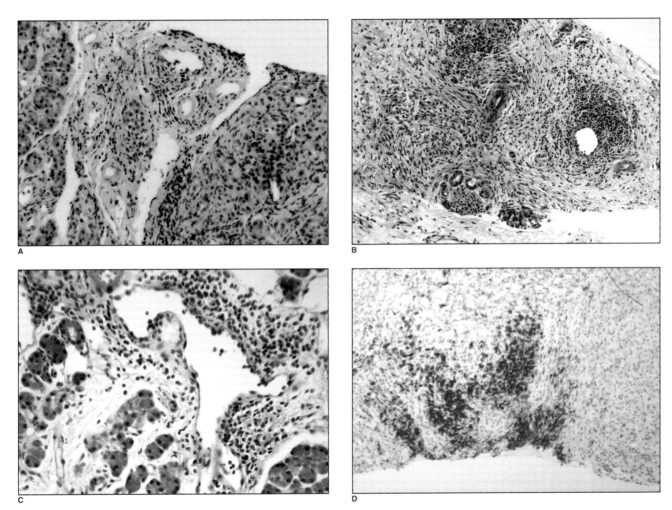

FIGURE 7.4: *(A) Acute cell-mediated allograft rejection. This connective tissue septa contains active inflammation with involvement of a vein (venulitis) and a small duct. The inflammation extends to the adjacent lobule to the right. (B) Marked fibrous expansion of a septal area in a patient with three previous episodes of biopsy proven and treated acute cell-mediated rejection . There is marked mononuclear inflammation cuffing a vein but with out definite venulitis (right). On the top left, residual atrophic acinar tissue shows persistent lymphocytic inflammation suggesting ongoing cell-mediated rejection. An islet in the bottom center is normal. (C) Mononuclear cuffing of a vein with questionable subendothelial lifting and endothelial cell damage. In the complete absence of any other finding this biopsy could be classified as indeterminate for acute rejection. (D) CD3 stain in a patient with acute cell-mediated allograft rejection demonstrates that the vast majority of the septal infiltrates consist of T lymphocytes. This is in contrast with cases of EBV-related PTLD.*

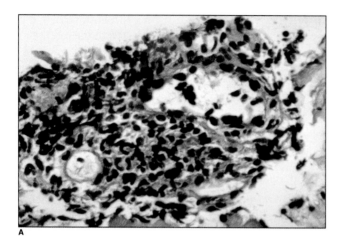

A

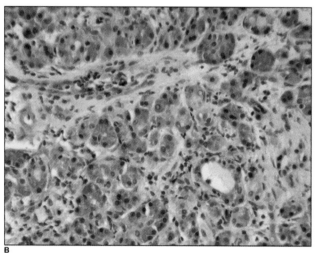

B

FIGURE 7.5: (A) Venulitis. High-power view of vein cuffed by activated (blastic) lymphocytes. Note endothelial cell damage: lifting of the endothelial lining and sloughing. Nuclear enlargement indicates endothelial cell activation. (B) Subtle venulitis in a thin connective tissue septa (upper left) and incipient inflammation of a small duct (lower right). Note relatively sparse acinar inflammation in the slightly edematous connective tissue (left corner) and in the acini located above the small duct (right center).

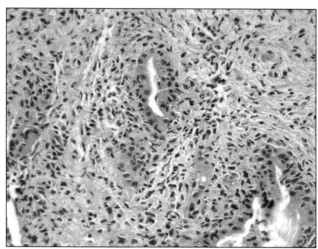

FIGURE 7.6: Inflamed septal area with pronounced ductitis, defined as permeation of the ductal epithelium by the inflammatory cells. There is also evidence of epithelial damage (loss of polarity, eosinophilic change in the cytoplasm, anisonucleosis).

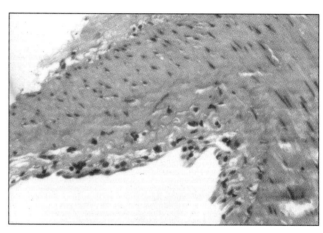

FIGURE 7.7: High-power view of arterial segment with intimal arteritis defined as subendothelial accumulation of inflammatory cells with lifting and partial sloughing of the endothelial lining.

widely recognized, and accordingly, arterial involvement was used as a marker of severe rejection in the grading schema proposed by Nakhleh and Sutherland, based on a comparison of histological material from failed and functioning allografts (100). In subsequent years, routine availability of needle core biopsies allowed for the recognition of the full spectrum of pathological changes in biopsies from well-functioning and rejecting allografts (18,31,36, 53,54,60,63,64,76,100). Based on the previous available studies and a systematic comparison of the histological changes in protocol and indication biopsies, a schema for grading acute rejection was developed at the University of Maryland which comprised six grades (0–V) (26). The latter schema emphasized progressive changes ranging from lack of inflammation (grade 0), to isolated involvement of

fibrous septa (grade I) and septal structures (grade II), to acinar (grade III) and arterial involvement (grade IV). Parenchymal necrosis defined the most severe form of rejection (grade V). The Maryland grading schema had overall good correlation with ultimate graft outcomes and response to treatment (103). It is notable, however, that long-term outcomes and response to antirejection treatment between grades II and III were remarkably similar, both likely reflecting grafts with milder forms of acute rejection in contrasts to the higher grades (IV and V) (23).

In 2003, a plan was made at the Banff conference on allograft pathology to reevaluate and update the currently available grading schema. A multidisciplinary group of physicians with particular expertise in the field was first convened for this purpose for the 2005 Banff

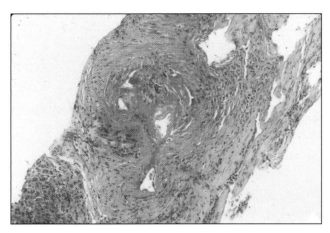

FIGURE 7.8: *Necrotizing arteritis (in a patient whose rejection was refractory to antirejection treatment). The wall of a distorted artery is completely replaced by bright red amorphous material indicating fibrinoid necrosis. Note the presence of inflammation in the fibrotic connective tissue around the artery and in the adjacent acinar tissue (lower left), consistent with the history of ongoing rejection.*

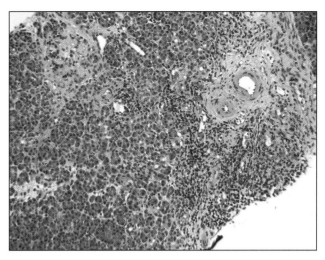

FIGURE 7.10: *Acute cell-mediated allograft rejection manifesting as septal inflammation with early acinar involvement (right low center).*

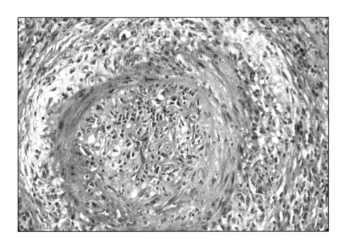

FIGURE 7.9: *Arterial cross-section with transmural inflammation and necrosis (arteritis) in the lower half of its circumference. Note slit-like lumen and neo-intima formation (left of center) resulting from severe expansion of the subendothelial areas due to accumulation of inflammatory cells and loose fibroblastic-myofibroblastic proliferation. The latter features indicate that in addition to the acute injury (arteritis) there is a subacute to chronic component.*

conference, following the successful model used for the development of the Banff schemas for grading rejection in the kidney and liver (104,105). This concerted effort was aimed to synthesize the previously published data, and the collective experience accumulated by pathologists, nephrologists, and surgeons since pathological evaluation of pancreas samples became standard for pancreas transplantation. The resulting working proposal (Table 7.1) is the result of extensive consensus discussions that culminated at the 2007 Banff conference on allograft pathology (La Coruña Spain).

VI. CHRONIC ALLOGRAFT REJECTION/GRAFT SCLEROSIS

i. Pathogenetic Aspects

In the first months after transplantation, graft losses are more often related to surgical complications, idiopathic thrombosis, acute rejection, and peripancreatic infections, (7,29,30,106) but after the first year, chronic rejection—with or without superimposed acute rejection—accounts for the majority of graft losses (30). In contrast to acute rejection that presents with sudden graft dysfunction and can be prevented or successfully treated in the majority of cases, chronic rejection is characterized by a slowly, progressive decline in graft function and does not respond well to treatment (106).

Clear association has been found between acute rejection and chronic rejection in pancreas allograft recipients. Repeated, higher grade, and late (more than one year) episodes of acute rejection are all associated with an increased risk of chronic rejection and graft loss. In many cases, progressive fibrosis and acinar loss are observed over a prolonged period of time in serial biopsies (36,165).

It is unclear if in the pancreas similar mechanisms operate for the propagation of tissue damage once a critical amount of parenchymal mass is lost, as is the case in the kidney. It is conceivable that in addition to immune-mediated acinar cell and vascular injury, other factors play a role in the pathogenesis of graft sclerosis. The main histological findings in chronic rejection (septal fibrosis, acinar loss) are very similar to those of chronic pancreatitis in native organs. In native pancreas fibrosis, microcirculatory disturbances have been heavily implicated (83,108). These appear to play a very important role also in chronic allograft rejection/sclerosis (109).

TABLE 7.1 Banff Pancreas Acute Allograft Rejection Working Grading Schema[#*]

1. Normal: Absent inflammation or inactive septal, mononuclear inflammation not involving ducts, veins, arteries, or acini. There is no graft sclerosis. The fibrous component is limited to normal septa and its amount is proportional to the size of the enclosed structures (ducts and vessels). The acinar parenchyma shows no signs of atrophy or injury.

2. Indeterminate: Septal inflammation that appears active but the overall features do not fulfill the criteria for mild cell-mediated acute rejection.

3. Cell-mediated rejection
   Type (grade)
   Acute cell-mediated rejection
   Grade I/Mild acute cell-mediated rejection
   Active septal inflammation (activated, blastic lymphocytes, ± eosinophils) involving septal structures: venulitis (subendothelial accumulation of inflammatory cells and endothelial damage in septal veins, ductitis (epithelial inflammation and damage of ducts). Neural/perineural inflammation.
   and/or
   Focal acinar inflammation. No more than 2 inflammatory foci per lobule with absent or minimal acinar cell injury.

   Grade II/moderate acute cell-mediated rejection
   Multifocal (but not confluent or diffuse) acinar inflammation (≥ 3 foci per lobule) with spotty (individual) acinar cell injury and dropout.
   and/or
   Minimal intimal arteritis.

   Grade III/severe acute cell-mediated rejection
   Diffuse (widespread, extensive) acinar inflammation with focal or diffuse multicellular /confluent acinar cell necrosis.
   and/or
   Moderate or severe intimal arteritis.
   and/or
   Transmural inflammation—necrotizing arteritis.
   Chronic active cell-mediated rejection: Chronic allograft arteriopathy (arterial intimal fibrosis with mononuclear cell infiltration in fibrosis, formation of neo-intima).

4. Antibody-mediated rejection = C4d positivity[**] + confirmed donor-specific antibodies + graft dysfunction.
   Type
   Hyperacute rejection: Immediate graft necrosis (≤1 hour) due to preformed antibodies in recipient's blood.
   Accelerated antibody-mediated rejection: Severe, fulminant form of antibody-mediated rejection with morphological similarities to hyperacute rejection but occurring later (within hours or days of transplantation).
   Acute antibody-mediated rejection: Specify percentage of biopsy surface (focal or diffuse). Associated histological findings: ranging from none to neutrophilic or mononuclear cell margination (capillaritis), thrombosis, vasculitis, parenchymal necrosis.
   Chronic active antibody-mediated rejection: Features of categories 4 and 5.

5. Chronic allograft rejection/graft sclerosis
   Stage I (mild graft sclerosis)
   Expansion of fibrous septa; the fibrosis occupies less than 30 percent of the core surface but the acinar lobules have eroded, irregular contours. The central lobular areas are normal.
   Stage II (moderate graft sclerosis)
   The fibrosis occupies 30–60 percent of the core surface. The exocrine atrophy affects the majority of the lobules in their periphery (irregular contours) and in their central areas (thin fibrous strands criss-cross between individual acin).
   Stage III (severe graft sclerosis)
   The fibrotic areas predominate and occupy more than 60 percent of the core surface with only isolated areas of residual acinar tissue and/or islets present.

6. Other histological diagnosis: Pathological changes not considered to be due to acute and/or chronic rejection, e.g., CMV pancreatitis, PTLD.

\# Categories 2–6 may be diagnosed concurrently and should be listed in the diagnosis in the order of their clinicopathological significance.

* See text for morphological definition of lesions.

** If there are no donor-specific antibodies or these data are unknown, identification of histological features of antibody-mediated rejection may be diagnosed as "suspicious for acute antibody-mediated rejection," particularly if there is graft dysfunction.

As is the case with other organ transplants, pancreas allograft fibrosis most likely represents the end effect of cumulative injury (or injuries) of diverse origins, immunological and nonimmunological. Accordingly, the presence of graft sclerosis is not synonymous with chronic rejection, particularly in patients in whom a clear history of preceding episodes of acute rejection cannot be elicited. The use of the more encompassing term chronic pancreas allograft rejection/graft sclerosis is therefore recommended (30).

ii. Clinical Diagnosis of Chronic Rejection/Graft Sclerosis

The clinical presentation of chronic rejection/graft sclerosis is nonspecific, with loss of glycemic control being the main feature. Hyperglycemia may develop progressively or may be unmasked by infection or other physiologic stresses (106). In addition, the exocrine tissue markers (e.g., blood or urinary amylase) progressively decrease and eventually disappear when extensive fibrosis develops in the graft (30).

Development of hyperglycemia due to chronic rejection indicates that the mass of functioning beta cells is significantly decreased and it heralds a short graft life (65,106).

Pancreas graft sclerosis can be demonstrated by imaging studies, indicating progressive decrease in graft size on ultrasound and magnetic resonance imaging studies, or there may be evidence of decreased parenchymal perfusion. In general, there is no clinical marker for the monitoring of progressive loss of pancreas functional reserve, comparable to the serial measurements of serum creatinine or glomerular filtration rate in kidney transplantation, but progressive decline in C-peptide levels correlates roughly with loss of functional beta cell mass (106).

In the early post-transplantation period, severe peripancreatic infections with abscess formation may lead to the observation of septal fibrosis resembling chronic rejection/graft sclerosis in biopsies obtained from the periphery of the graft. In those cases, the deeper parenchymal areas are not affected and resolution of the infection may allow for a normal graft life span.

iii. Morphological Features of Chronic Rejection/Graft Sclerosis

Similar to animal models and to the clinical experience with other organs, pancreas chronic rejection is manifested histologically with progressive fibrosis arising from expansion of the fibrous septa leading to large areas of fibrosis intervening between atrophic acinar lobules (Figure 7.11). With progression of graft sclerosis, the exocrine lobules appear fragmented by proliferating fibroblastic bundles randomly interspersed between the acini. All exocrine tissue is eventually lost, with some areas becoming unrecognizable except for occasional residual islets embedded in the dense scar tissue. Although in most patients disappear-

ance of the acinar component forecasts progressive disappearance of islets as well, in a minority of patients, glycemic control has been maintained for some time even after extensive fibrosis had replaced the exocrine tissue (30).

Narrowing of the arterial branches due to proliferative intimal endarteritis/transplant arteriopathy is also characteristic of the process (Figure 7.12) (30,65,90,95). The role of chronic vascular injury in pancreas chronic rejection/graft sclerosis is unequivocal. Recent or organized thrombi are routinely seen in pancreatectomies for chronic rejection. Late thrombosis leading to graft failure is typically superimposed on intimal arteritis or transplant arteriopathy (30). In patients with long-term grafts, immunosuppression with calcineurin inhibitors may be associated with widespread arteriolar hyalinosis, but it is not clearly established if this contributes to the process of graft sclerosis (Figure 7.13) (111). Furthermore, in patients with generalized atherosclerotic disease, atheroemboli have been demonstrated to lodge in the pancreas allograft causing late pancreatitis and further ischemic compromise (Figure 7.14) (112).

VII. PANCREAS ALLOGRAFT REJECTION BANFF 2007 WORKING GRADING SCHEMA

This schema includes six diagnostic categories that cover the range of histopathological changes that can occur in pancreas allografts. Similar to other transplanted organs, two main forms of allograft rejection are recognized: cell mediated and antibody mediated (87). For each of these rejection types, acute and chronic histological manifestations are identified. For cell-mediated acute rejection and chronic allograft rejection/graft sclerosis, which are by far the most common diagnostic findings seen in pancreas allograft biopsies, the schema specifically defines severity grades (mild—grade I, moderate—grade II, and severe—grade III). These two parallel nomenclatures (i.e., mild/grade I) have the same clinical connotation, being therefore amenable to be used according to the preference of the pathologist rendering the biopsy diagnosis (i.e., mild cell-mediated acute rejection versus cell-mediated acute rejection grade I).

The diagnosis and grading of rejection are based on the global assessment of the biopsy. As this is a working grading schema, it is possible that in the future, numerical scores will be added to further describe the histological lesions as in the kidney Banff grading schema or similar to the liver histology activity index (105).

Specific histological features utilized in the 2007 Banff grading schema (Table 7.1): 1) Septal inflammatory infiltrates, predominantly mononuclear, including "blastic" (activated) lymphocytes and variable numbers of eosinophils. Eosinophils may be the predominant cell type in occasional cases (Figure 7.15); 2) venulitis, defined as subendothelial accumulation of inflammatory cells and endothelial damage observed in septal veins (Figure 7.16); 3) ductitis, defined as epithelial infiltration of branches of

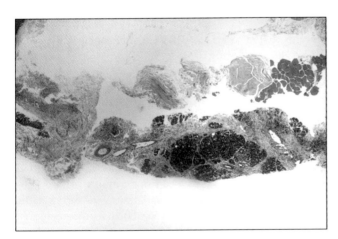

FIGURE 7.11: Low power view of needle core biopsy with marked lymphoid infiltrates in expanded septal areas. Severe episodes of acute rejection or undertreated cell-mediated rejection results in progressive fibrosis. Note the fragmentation of the acinar contours that typically occurs in association with progression of the septal fibrosis.

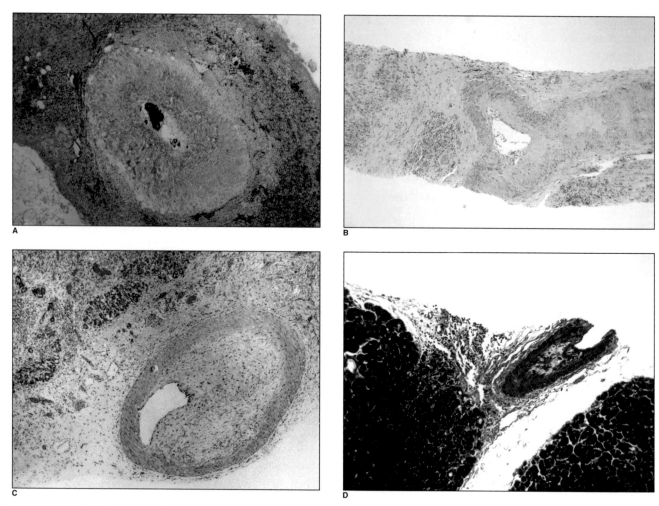

FIGURE 7.12: *(A) Cross section of thickened artery with features of chronic active T-cell–mediated rejection characterized by intimal fibrosis with infiltrating mononuclear cells in the fibrotic area. Note formation of neo-intima. (B) Focus of intimal arteritis and focal, sparse inflammation of subendothelial areas of fibrosis in an artery with significant fibrous narrowing. The septal areas are markedly expanded due to fibrosis with only rare remaining acini present (left of center). (C) Asymmetric narrowing of artery with marked luminal narrowing and features of chronic active T-cell–mediated rejection infiltrating mononuclear cells in the fibrotic areas. (D) Variant of chronic active cell-mediated rejection with accumulation of subendothelial foam cells with formation of neo-intima.*

the pancreatic ducts by mononuclear or eosinophilic inflammation and evidence of ductal epithelial cell damage (Figure 7.17); 4) neural and perineural inflammation of intrinsic parenchymal nerve branches; 5) acinar inflammation, defined by the presence of inflammatory infiltrates with similar characteristics as the septal infiltrates amidst the exocrine acini (Figure 7.18–7.22); 6) single cell and confluent acinar cell necrosis/apoptosis in association with the acinar inflammation; 7) intimal arteritis defined as infiltration by mononuclear cells under the arterial endothelium (Figure 7.7); 8) necrotizing arteritis defined as transmural inflammation with focal or circumferential fibrinoid necrosis (Figure 7.8); and 9) C4d-positive staining in interacinar and islet capillaries and small vessels as a feature of antibody-mediated rejection, if in association with donor-specific antibodies in serum. Neutrophil and macrophage margination in interacinar capillaries is considered a feature likely to be associated with acute anti-

body-mediated rejection, if occurring concurrently with C4d positivity (Figure 7.23–7.25).

i. Histological Features Defining the Severity of Acute Rejection

Intimal arteritis and necrotizing arteritis define the more severe forms of acute pancreas rejection because these arterial lesions are more refractory to antirejection treatment and are known to carry an increased risk for immediate and subsequent graft thrombosis/loss and transplant arteriopathy (30). In contrast, inflammation confined to the septa and septal structures (veins, ducts) is considered a milder form of rejection that is usually responsive to antirejection treatment and less likely to result in irreversible sequelae (33).

The new Banff pancreas grading schema characterizes moderate and severe rejection forms by arterial involvement, as well as by the extent of acinar inflammation (focal

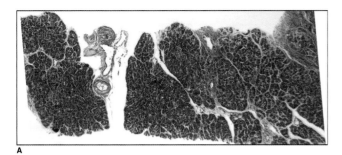

A

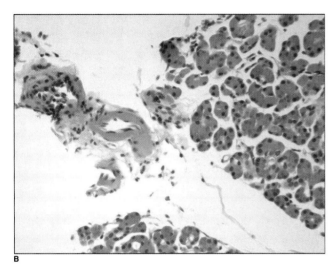

B

FIGURE 7.13: *(A) Medium power view of a needle core biopsy from a patient with a well-functioning graft fifty-two months after transplantation. Note absence of inflammation or significant fibrosis, although two arterioles show circumferential hyalinosis likely related to calcineurin inhibitor toxicity. (B) Well-functioning graft with arteriolar hyalinosis. There is no significant inflammation. Based on findings in adjacent sections, the structure to the left is a tangentially cut vessel without inflammation.*

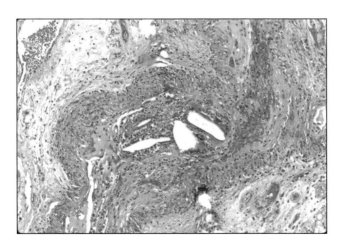

FIGURE 7.14: *Artery occluded by atheroembolus found in pancreas biopsy from a patient with acute increase in serum amylase and lipase. There was no evidence of acute rejection.*

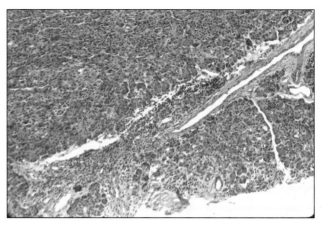

FIGURE 7.15: *Early cell-mediated acute allograft rejection with inflammation mostly confined to the connective tissue septa.*

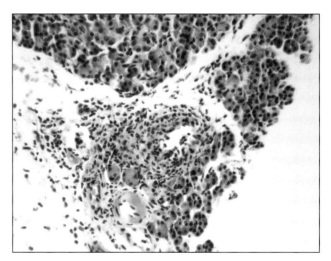

FIGURE 7.16: *Typical example of venulitis, characterizing early cell-mediated acute allograft rejection.*

versus multifocal diffuse) and the presence and extent of acinar cell injury. This is based on evidence that extensive acinar injury and damage can lead to fibrosis and accelerated graft loss if untreated or undertreated (113).

1. Diagnostic Categories: Specific Considerations

1. Normal: Inflammatory infiltrates are absent, or very sparse, inactive, mononuclear cells (i.e., small lymphocytes, rare plasma cells). If there is slight inflammation, it is focal and confined to the septa with lack of involvement of any of the septal structures (vessels, ducts, nerves) (Figures 7.26–7.28).

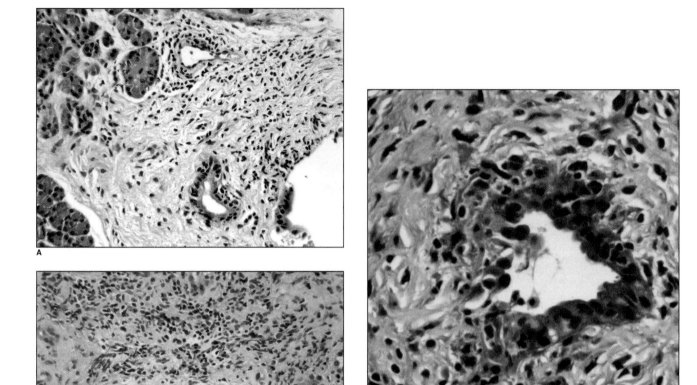

FIGURE 7.17: *(A) Mild cell-mediated acute allograft rejection. There is mild cuffing of the vein but the predominant lesion is ductitis with prominent cell damage including apoptosis (lower right of center) and epithelial sloughing in the larger duct. (B) Ductitis in acute cell-mediated rejection. Epithelial cell degeneration and reactive/regenerative atypia is noted in association with the intraepithelial inflammation. (C) Marked epithelial damage secondary to acute cell-mediated allograft rejection resulted in sloughing of the ductal epithelium. Only few epithelial cells with reactive changes are noted in the lower segment of the ductal circumference.*

An adequate biopsy with these histological characteristics essentially rules out a diagnosis of cell-mediated acute rejection. Accordingly, these type of findings are often encountered in protocol biopsies of well-functioning grafts (26,78).

It should be emphasized, however, that "normal" appearing biopsies may be also encountered under other clinical circumstances. Specifically, in patients biopsied for hyperglycemia, the differential diagnosis includes three main processes: 1) late phase of recurrent autoimmune disease, that is, after resolution of isletitis (27,114). This process can only be recognized by the evaluation of immunohistochemical stains for insulin and glucagon demonstrating selective loss of beta cells. 2) Drug toxicity that is primarily characterized by vacuolization and damage of

islet cells (28). C) Acute antibody-mediated rejection. It is noteworthy that an essentially normal biopsy was found in the first well-documented case of acute antibody-mediated rejection (Figure 7.29) (68). It is then advisable that negative biopsies in patients with graft dysfunction should be stained for C4d to rule out antibody-mediated rejection.

2. Indeterminate for rejection: This category is defined by the presence of focal septal inflammation that displays features of activation (blastic changes, some eosinophils), but the overall features do not fulfill the criteria for mild rejection (i.e., partial cuffing of a septal vein or duct but lacking any evidence of endothelial or epithelial involvement) (Figure 7.31–7.33). These histological features can be seen in protocol biopsies of well-functioning grafts as well as in

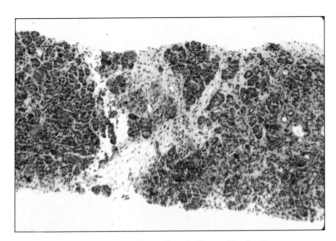

FIGURE 7.18: *Acute cell-mediated allograft rejection manifesting predominantly as acinar inflammation. The latter is patchy, involving clusters of acini (lower center and left).*

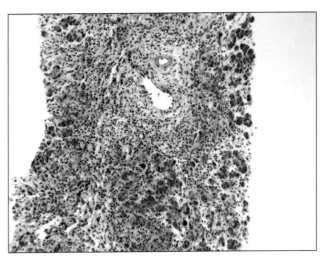

FIGURE 7.19: *Representative field of a biopsy showing moderate acute cell-mediated rejection. The inflammation involves the septal areas as well as the acinar areas in a diffuse manner. Only few areas in the biopsy were free of inflammation.*

patients biopsied for graft dysfunction. Similar to the "borderline" category in the kidney, these changes may represent early as well as treated acute rejection, or alternatively may be entirely nonspecific (23,26,78).

The treatment of patients with biopsies showing "indeterminate" features may vary depending on the indication for biopsy, and ultimately depends on clinical judgment. In accordance with the heterogeneous nature of the indeterminate histological changes, response to treatment varies significantly in comparison to biopsies with definite acute cell-mediated rejection that are usually responsive to treatment (23).

3. Cell-mediated acute rejection is graded as mild, moderate, or severe (grades I, II, and III, respectively), based on the identification of lesions that have been shown to prognosticate progressively worse outcomes (23,26,33,42,100).

a) Mild cell-mediated acute rejection (grade I): This grade is defined by the presence of septal inflammatory infiltrates that have features of activation ("blastic" lymphocytes, variable numbers of eosinophils) but also involve septal structures (veins, ducts) and with varying degrees of focal acinar inflammation. These findings may vary between septal areas, however, *any* degree of venulitis (subendothelial accumulation of inflammatory cells and endothelial damage in septal veins) or ductitis (epithelial inflammation and damage of pancreatic ducts) is sufficient for the diagnosis of mild, grade I, cell-mediated rejection. Inflammation of peripheral nerve branches coursing through the parenchyma is also a feature of rejection, although this is a rare finding due to the scarcity of these structures in biopsy material.

Focal acinar inflammation in biopsies with the features described above (mild, grade I) is not uncommon and is typically seen in the interface between the septal connective tissue and the acinar lobules (e.g., periphery of the exocrine

areas). In some cases (due to sampling), the foci of acinar inflammation appear to be completely separate of the septal inflammation within "deeper" areas of the lobules.

Mild cell-mediated rejection grade I also includes cases in which due to sampling, septal involvement is not present and only focal acinar inflammation is evident. In any case, the acinar inflammation should be clearly focal (i.e., no more than two inflammatory foci per lobule as defined below) in mild grade I rejection, and should be lacking evidence of acinar cell injury (apoptosis, necrosis).

Recognition of an acinar inflammatory lesion/focus is not difficult at medium to high power; however, in order to avoid ambiguity, the grading schema provides a specific definition (collection of at least ten lymphocytes/eosinophils within an acinar area), particularly for cases in which the septal inflammation is mild or absent and the diagnosis of mild (grade I) cell-mediated rejection will hinge on the acinar lesions only. The composition of the acinar inflammation is typically similar to that of the septal infiltrates (mixture of activated and small lymphocytes with variable numbers of eosinophils).

Biopsies with the features defining this rejection grade are occasionally found in patients with well-functioning grafts (23,77,78). but are more commonly seen in biopsies performed for graft dysfunction (typically increase in amylase/lipase in serum, or decrease in urinary amylase in bladder drained grafts). The main histological differential diagnosis in this category is CMV pancreatitis, which is often patchy in nature (Figures 7.34–7.38) (115).

b) Moderate cell-mediated acute rejection (grade II): This grade can be defined by two histological features that may be identified either in isolation or concurrently.

Multifocal acinar inflammation. The most common presentation of this grade consists of multiple foci (three

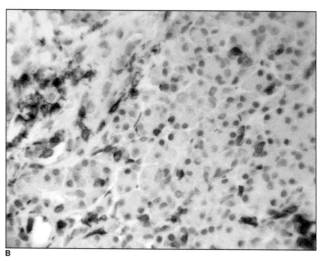

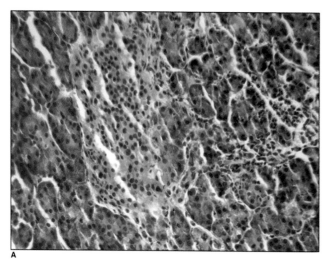

FIGURE 7.20: (A) High-power view of a focus of acinar inflammation, (right) composed of lymphocytes and eosinophils. Islets are not targeted in cell-mediated rejection, although there are few eosinophils in the right upper part of the islet in continuity with the acinar inflammation. (B) CD3 stain highlighting demonstrates tight association between T-lymphocytes—main effectors in cell-mediated rejection—and the acinar cells. The latter, together with ductal epithelium and endothelium of arteries and veins are the main targets in acute cell-mediated rejection.

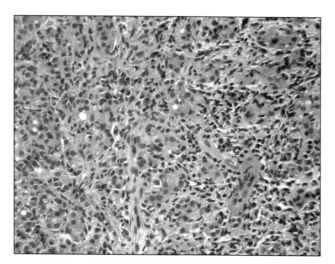

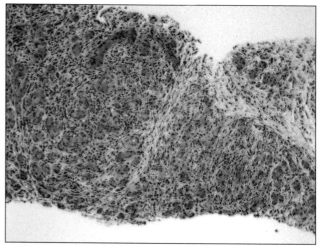

FIGURE 7.21: Marked inflammation in cell-mediated allograft rejection. Numerous acinar cells show cytoplasmic vacuolization.

FIGURE 7.22: Masson's trichrome stain of biopsy represented in Figure 7.21 shows incipient interacinar fibrosis.

of more foci per lobule) of acinar inflammation and associated spotty (individual) acinar cell injury and dropout. The acinar inflammatory involvement in this grade should be identified with ease at medium power; however, the involvement should *not* be confluent or diffuse. From a practical point of view, completely un-inflamed acinar/exocrine areas should be easily identified between the inflamed foci. Absence of confluent inflammation will differentiate this grade from the next higher category. Significant acinar inflammation is always associated with evidence of acinar cell injury, (116,117) but in this grade the latter should be spotty (isolated). Specifically, acinar

cell injury may appear as any of the following: cellular dropout (empty spaces equaling the size of individual cells), cytoplasmic swelling and vacuolization, nuclear pyknosis, apoptotic bodies, or single cell lytic necrosis (Figure 7.39).

Minimal intimal arteritis. Alternatively, depending on sampling variations, the category of moderate cell-mediated rejection grade II can be defined by the sole presence of mild, focal intimal arteritis defined by the presence of rare, occasional but clearly defined subendothelial (intimal) mononuclear cells. The latter changes may or may not be accompanied by the complete constellation of inflammatory changes described earlier in the septa and lobules (Figure 7.40).

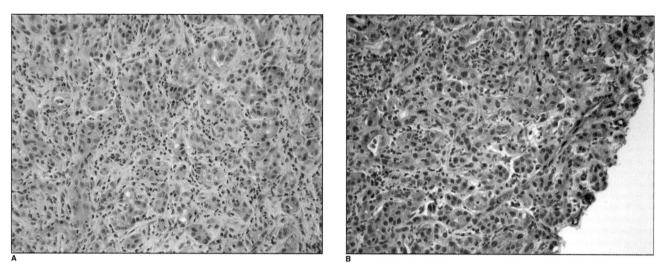

FIGURE 7.23:   (A) Acinar inflammation in acute antibody-mediated allograft rejection, predominantly consisting of neutrophils accumulating in capillaries and interstitium. (B) Acute antibody-mediated rejection (see Figure 7.23A). C4d stain demonstrates complement deposition in microvasculature.

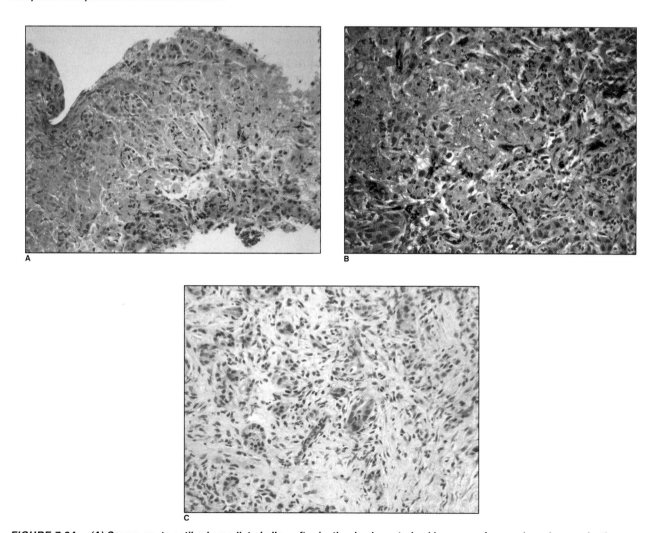

FIGURE 7.24:   (A) Severe acute antibody-mediated allograft rejection is characterized by areas of parenchymal necrosis, the extent of which is variable, mostly depending on the size and number of vessels affected by necrosis and thrombosis. (B) C4d stain is strongly positive in a case of acute antibody-mediated rejection. Note infiltrating neutrophils and area of necrosis (upper left). (C) Follow-up biopsy three weeks after biopsy represented in Figure 7.23A shows progression of fibrosis with more pronounced loss of the acinar component. The pancreatectomy specimen is represented in Figure 7.47.

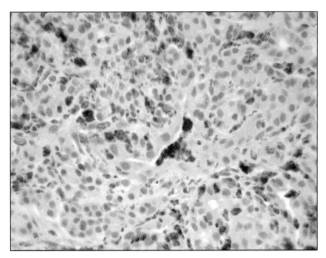

FIGURE 7.25: *In addition to neutrophils, acute antibody-mediated allograft rejection may be characterized by accumulation of interstitial and intracapillary macrophages, highlighted here with CD68 stain.*

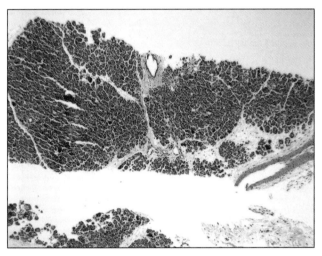

FIGURE 7.26: *Protocol biopsy at three months after transplantation in a well-functioning pancreas allograft. No inflammation is present.*

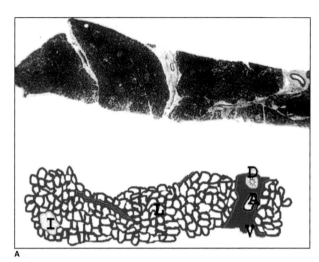

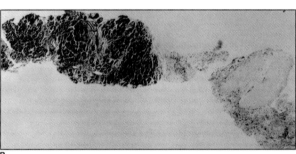

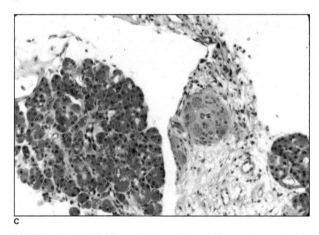

FIGURE 7.27: *(A) Microphotograph and diagram representing a normal proportion of connective tissue in a protocol biopsy of a well-functioning graft twelve months after transplantation. The periphery of the lobules is smooth and the acinar component is compact with total absence of interacinar connective tissue. A minimum of three lobular areas and associated septa are necessary to consider a biopsy negative for acute rejection. (B) The normal pancreas is not encapsulated, but rather surrounded by poorly defined connective tissue that may become prominent after transplantation due to reactive and reparative mechanisms. Needle biopsies may demonstrate a variety of changes in the peripancreatic connective tissue, including fat necrosis (extreme right). The latter is more commonly seen early after transplantation. (C) Ganglion cell clusters may be identified rarely in pancreas allograft biopsies. These should not be confused with cytomegalovirus cytopathic changes.*

From a clinical point of view, biopsies with features of moderate cell-mediated rejection grade II are typically found in patients with graft dysfunction (e.g., increase in amylase/lipase in serum or decrease in urinary amylase in bladder drained grafts).

c) Severe cell-mediated acute rejection (grade III): This grade can be defined by three histological features that may be identified ether in isolation or concurrently.

Severe acinar inflammation and acinar cell damage. This entity is characterized by confluent/diffuse (widespread, extensive) acinar inflammation with associated focal or diffuse multicellular/confluent acinar cell necrosis. The inflammation may be predominantly lymphoid or may contain abundant eosinophils or variable amounts of neutrophils. By definition, there should be none or only rare,

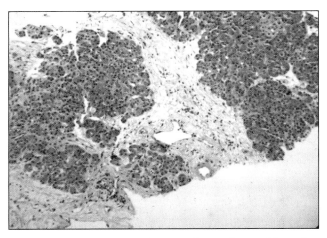

FIGURE 7.28: *Representative area of a needle core biopsy in a patient with a well-functioning graft. There are very sparse inflammatory cells in the septa and mild interstitial edema. These findings are nonspecific; there is no evidence of acute cell-mediated rejection.*

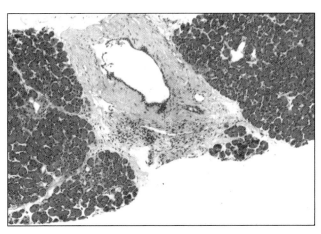

FIGURE 7.30: *Single focus of septal inflammation sparing vein and duct found in a biopsy of a patient with fluctuating serum amylase and lipase. The inflammation appears inactive and is likely nonspecific. The patient was treated with bolus steroids with no clear response.*

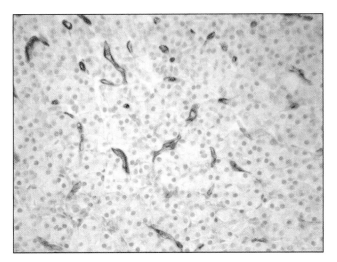

FIGURE 7.29: *C4d stain in biopsy performed for increased serum amylase. A diagnosis of mild cell-mediated rejection was made based on septal changes not depicted here; the exocrine component was histologically normal on routine stains. Amylase and lipase normalized after treatment with bolus steroids. Despite C4d positivity and proven HLA type II donor-specific antibodies the graft continues to function well sixty-six months after transplantation.*

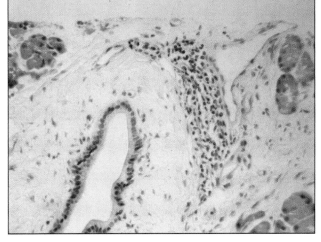

FIGURE 7.31: *One of several foci of septal inflammation sparing veins and ducts in a biopsy performed for increase in amylase and lipase. This histological picture is compatible with a diagnosis of "indeterminate" for acute rejection.*

focal areas of completely un-inflamed acinar/exocrine parenchyma (Figure 7.39).

Moderate or severe intimal arteritis, defined as easily identifiable (i.e., more than six to eight) lymphocytes within the intima of an involved muscular artery, is by itself sufficient to justify a diagnosis of severe cell-mediated rejection grade III (Figure 7.41). Moderate or severe intimal arteritis is usually associated with some evidence of intimal injury (i.e., endothelial cell hypertrophy, fibrin leakage, coating neutrophils, and/or macrophages and activation of intimal myofibroblasts).

Necrotizing arteritis. Transmural arterial inflammation leading to complete or partial circumferential necrosis also defines severe cell-mediated rejection. Transmural fibrinoid arterial necrosis is, however, more often associated with antibody-mediated rejection. C4d staining and search for donor-specific antibodies is therefore necessary to rule out humoral rejection if necrotizing arteritis is identified (Figure 7.42).

Each of the three lesions used to define severe cell-mediated rejection portend poor outcome to the graft because they are associated with or lead to irreversible parenchymal damage. The short- and long-term impact to the organ will depend on the extent of acinar damage

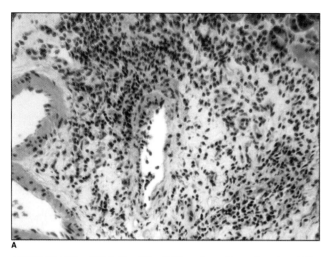

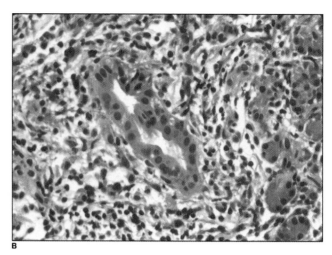

FIGURE 7.32: *(A) Active (blastic) lymphocytic and eosinophilic septal inflammation with early venulitis in acute cell-mediated allograft rejection. (B) Pancreatic duct surrounded and focally permeated by prominent septal inflammation with features of activation (blastic transformation), including occasional markedly atypical nuclei (top left).*

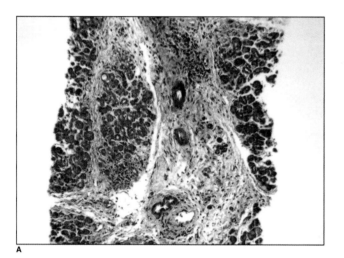

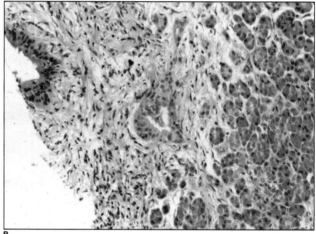

FIGURE 7.33: *(A and B) Biopsies performed two and three weeks after the biopsies represented in Figure 7. 32A, B, respectively, shows features found in "treated" acute rejection. The histological findings are more difficult to be classified and may fall in the categories of "indeterminate" for rejection or mild rejection. Note incipient septal fibrosis with early fragmentation of the periphery of the exocrine lobules.*

and the size and the number of the arteries affected by intimal arteritis or necrosis.

Confluent acinar inflammation and necrosis is invariably followed by some degree of secondary collagenization of the interacinar areas and eventual loss or disappearance of the exocrine component in the affected area. Changes of this nature markedly alter the microvascular environment of the graft on which the islets depend to maintain an adequate function (83,108,118,119).

Similar to other solid organ transplants, intimal arteritis is associated with an increased risk of immediate or delayed thrombosis (Figure 7.43). This lesion is also a precursor of transplant arteriopathy (30). Transmural arteritis/vasculitis is associated with an immediate likelihood of thrombosis and secondary parenchymal infarction.

Biopsies with histological findings corresponding to this category are characteristically associated with graft dysfunction/failure, often including hyperglycemia (23,26).

d) Chronic active cell-mediated rejection: This diagnosis is characterized by the presence of "active" transplant arteriopathy. The lesion consists of narrowing of the arterial lumen by a subendothelial proliferation of fibroblasts, myofibroblasts, and smooth muscle cells with superimposed evidence of ongoing inflammatory activity. The latter consists of infiltration of the subintimal fibrous proliferation by mononuclear cells, typically T cells and macrophages (Figure 7.12). Although rarely seen in needle biopsies due to sampling issues, this lesion is consistently present in pancreatectomies from failed grafts due to chronic rejection (30,120).

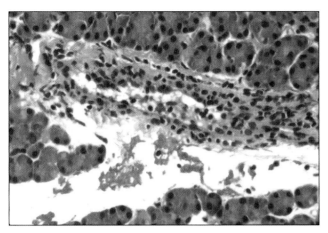

FIGURE 7.34: *Septal inflammation confined to septal/ perivenular area, however, diagnostic of acute rejection due to the presence of marked endothelial damage (lifting, vacuolization and focal sloughing). The inflammation has features of activation (blastic changes), and there are eosinophils.*

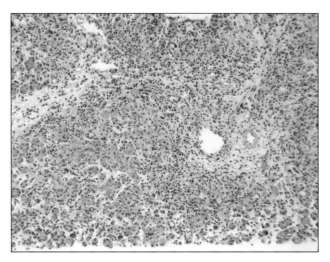

FIGURE 7.36: *Moderate acute cell-mediated allograft rejection. In contrast to the biopsy in Figure 7.35, the inflammation involves extensively the periphery of the acinar lobules, as well as areas more distant from the septa.*

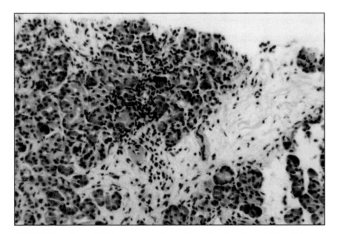

FIGURE 7.35: *Mild acute cell-mediated rejection defined by focal but active acinar inflammation in the interface with the septal connective tissue. The biopsy was from a patient with a bladder-drained pancreas allograft who presented with decrease in urine amylase. Amylase levels normalized after antirejection treatment.*

The entity of "active transplant arteriopathy" is included in the grading schema because according to clinical and experimental studies, this lesion represents an intermediate stage between intimal arteritis and chronic transplant arteriopathy. The extent of the histological changes and the amount of inflammatory infiltrates correlates with suboptimal immunosuppression (120). The identification of this lesion has clinical impact potentially, as the process of ongoing cell-mediated vascular injury leading to further arterial narrowing may be halted with optimization of the immunosuppression treatment (120).

4. Antibody-mediated acute rejection

Acute antibody-mediated rejection: The category of antibody-mediated rejection in the pancreas is poorly characterized because only few bona fide cases have been reported to date (78,94). The process has three specific defining features, namely the presence of C4d positivity in interacinar capillaries and islet capillaries and small veins; the identification of donor specific antibodies in serum; and graft dysfunction (68). In the absence of graft dysfunction or if donor-specific antibodies are not found, a diagnosis of "suspicious for acute antibody-mediated rejection" may be considered; however, the significance of C4d positivity in that setting is currently unknown.

Antibody-mediated rejection is acute, when graft dysfunction is sudden, and there is no histological evidence of underlying chronic injury (i.e., fibrosis). This scenario typically occurs in the early post-transplantation period. The spectrum of histopathological changes varies significantly, from completely normal H&E histology (68) to interacinar neutrophilic and/or macrophagic inflammation (much like capillaritis in the kidney), to vascular fibrinoid necrosis and associated parenchymal necrosis (94).

The threshold of positivity for the C4d stain (i.e., percentage of positive interacinar capillaries) is not determined to this point. The current recommendation is to report the positive C4d staining, specifying the percentage of biopsy surface marked by the staining. The need for correlation with serological studies (donor specific antibodies) should be also stated in the pathology report.

Similarly, there is no general agreement with respect to the best technique for C4d staining (122). Most likely, similarly to the kidney, the immunofluorescence technique will prove to be more sensitive, although C4d staining of formalin-fixed, paraffin-embedded sections is widely used with acceptable results (Figures 7.23 and 7.24) (121,122).

All cases reported cases of antibody-mediated rejection have presented clinically with hyperglycemia, suggesting

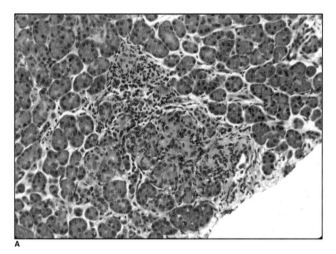 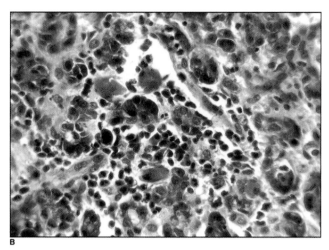

A   **B**

FIGURE 7.37: (A) Medium power view of a focus of acinar inflammation in mild acute cell-mediated rejection. Note that the inflammation is confined and the surrounding areas show normal acini. (B) High-power view of an inflammatory focus demonstrating the intimate association between the activated appearing inflammatory infiltrates and the acinar cells. The inflammation is mixed composed of lymphocytes, eosinophils and some plasma cells.

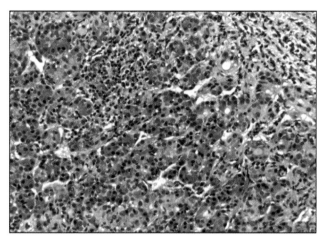

FIGURE 7.38: Septal and acinar inflammation in acute cell-mediated allograft rejection with a predominance of eosinophils.

that compromise of the islet microvasculature plays an important pathogenic role, (78,94) differentiating it from the cell-mediated injury where the islets remain largely spared of direct immune damage.

Hyperacute/accelerated allograft rejection: As it is the case in other organs, routine pretransplant cross-matching has virtually eliminated this entity. Early experience with transplantation and experimental studies have shown that this catastrophic form of humoral rejection is character-ized by extensive immunoglobulin vascular deposition (typically IgG), leading to necrosis of arteries and veins with secondary massive and immediate thrombosis. Graft necrosis/failure is immediate in hyperacute rejection (74). In addition to hyperacute rejection, this diagnostic cate-gory contemplates the possibility of severe humoral rejec-tion presenting with clinically attenuated features. Several

cases of so-called accelerated rejection, delayed hyperacute rejection and so forth have occurred despite negative pretransplant cross-matching but with post-transplant documentation of existing donor-specific antibodies (30). Morphologically, the findings in these cases were similar to those of hyperacute rejection (generalized immunoglobulin and complement vascular deposition, thrombosis, and necrosis), but the event occurs within few hours (rather than within minutes) after transplantation (Figure 7.44). This clinical presentation resembles graft thrombosis attributed to technical failure and needs to be differentiated from it. Whereas hyperacute rejection is exceedingly rare (<.01 percent of pancreas transplants), accelerated rejection was found in 2.5 percent of pancreatectomies in a com-bined clinicopathological study (30).

Chronic active antibody-mediated rejection: Humoral mechanisms have been clearly implicated in the develop-ment of chronic rejection (86,87). A diagnosis of chronic active antibody-mediated rejection is applied to biopsies showing features of chronic rejection/graft sclerosis (see category 6), together with C4d-positive staining in the majority of parenchymal capillaries and small vessels (87). This scenario has been well described in the report of Carbajal et al (67). Vascular fibrinoid necrosis, with recent or organized thrombosis, is supportive of ongoing antibody-mediated rejection. As with all situations when humoral rejection is suspected, correlation with the pres-ence of donor specific antibodies is required for diagnosis (67,68,87,94).

5. Grading of chronic allograft rejection/graft sclerosis: Histological grading of chronic rejection/graft sclerosis in the pancreas, has been shown to correlate with graft survival, that is, mild fibrosis is associated with lengthy graft survival, and severe fibrosis heralds a limited time of

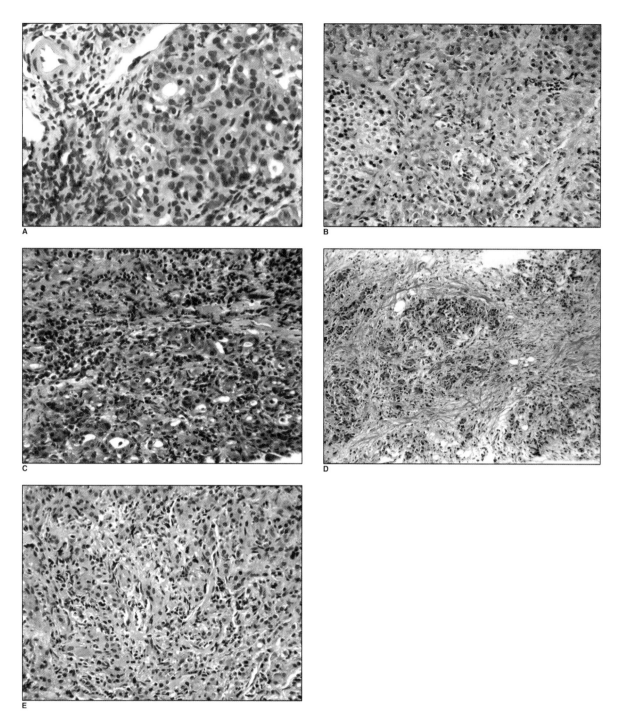

FIGURE 7.39: *(A) Moderate acute cell-mediated allograft rejection defined by multifocal acinar inflammation and single cell (spotty) acinar cell damage. Only a small area of the biopsy is depicted here at high magnification in order to appreciate acinar cell vacuolization and occasional cell undergoing apoptosis (center left). (B) Medium-power view of areas of multicellular acinar cell damage. Note marked acinar cell vacuolization and dissolution of the acinar architecture (lower center). An islet mostly free of inflammation is seen to the left. (C) Representative area of biopsy with severe acute cell-mediated rejection defined by extensive inflammation of septa and acini and evidence of acinar cell damage. Note dissolution of the acinar architecture in the lower right areas and secondary infiltration by neutrophils. C4d stain was negative. (D) Diffuse acinar inflammation and multicellular acinar cell damage are precursors of acinar atrophy/fibrosis as observed in this biopsy obtained six weeks after the biopsy represented in Figure 7.39B. (E) Another example of multicellular acinar cell damage characterized by disappearance of the acinar architecture and accumulation of amorphous eosinophilic material.*

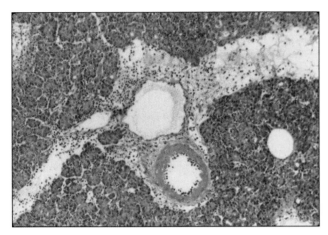

FIGURE 7.40: *Moderate acute cell-mediated allograft rejection defined by the presence of mild intimal arteritis. Marked septal edema and mild septal inflammation are also present.*

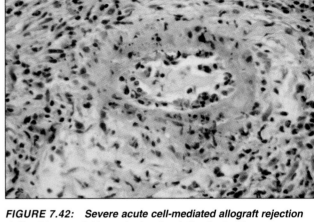

FIGURE 7.42: *Severe acute cell-mediated allograft rejection defined by arterial branch showing intimal arteritis, transmural inflammation, and fibrinoid necrosis. C4d stain was negative.*

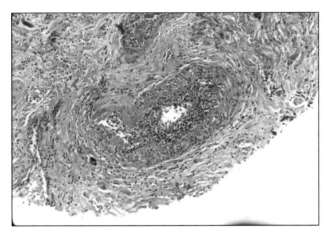

FIGURE 7.41: *Severe intimal arteritis with marked narrowing of the lumen.*

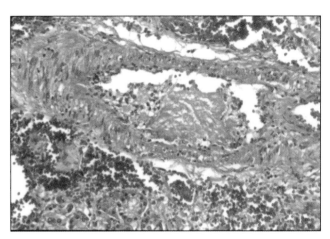

FIGURE 7.43: *Vascular involvement in acute rejection markedly increases the risk of thrombosis as observed in this artery showing intimal arteritis (best appreciated in the extreme left of the vessel) and an associated recent thrombus.*

remaining graft function (65). Furthermore, despite its notoriously patchy nature, the progression of pancreas allograft fibrosis can be reliably assessed in core biopsies through a semiquantitative grading schema that is both simple and reproducible. Grading is based on the semiquantitative determination of the proportion of sclerotic/fibrotic areas versus the remaining acinar/lobular tissue (65).

Three grades are recognized in this diagnostic category: mild graft sclerosis – chronic grade I; moderate graft sclerosis – chronic grade II; and severe graft sclerosis – chronic grade III, based on the identification of less than 30 percent, 30–60 percent, and more than 60 percent of fibrosis in the biopsy core, respectively (Figures 7.45–7.47).

Transplant arteriopathy closely parallels the degree of fibrosis. Despite their major physiopathological importance, the vascular lesions are not used for grading of chronic rejection/graft sclerosis, because vascular disease that is fully appreciated in pancreatectomy specimens appears only sporadically in needle core biopsies (123).

Similarly, evaluation of endocrine islets is not used for grading because their disappearance does not follow a predictable course in relationship to that of graft fibrosis (110).

Inflammatory infiltrates associated with ongoing acinar cell injury, venulitis, and/or intimal arteritis and ductal inflammation indicate active cell-mediated allograft rejection. Acute cell-mediated rejection and chronic rejection/graft sclerosis should be graded independently based on the key histological features respectively specified on each of these categories.

6. Other histological diagnosis: A variety of other pathological processes affecting the pancreas allografts have histopathological manifestations. Identification of any of these processes may be achieved in isolation or concurrently with other diagnostic categories in the schema.

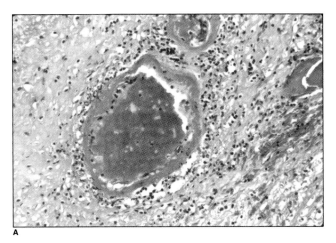
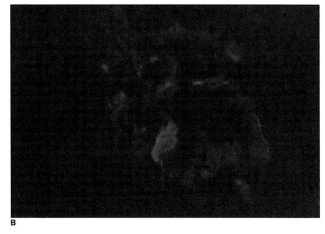

A   B

FIGURE 7.44: *(A) Severe, accelerated acute antibody-mediated allograft rejection is rare and presents with acute graft failure within hours or days of transplantation. Histologically, there is diffuse fibrinoid necrosis of the vasculature and associated thrombosis as represented in the picture. (B) IgG deposition in arteries (same case as Figure 7.44A).*

VIII. OTHER FORMS OF PANCREAS GRAFT PATHOLOGY

i. Surgical Complications

1. Graft Thrombosis

Of the surgical complications that are grouped together under the category of technical failure (leaks, bleeding, thrombosis, infections, and pancreatitis), thrombosis continues to be the leading cause of nonimmunological graft loss with higher rates seen in PAK and PTA cases with enteric drainage (7,124).

Thrombosis in large- and medium-size vessels of the pancreas is routinely found in pancreatectomy specimens performed at any time after transplantation (30). Pancreas graft thrombosis occurs in different settings, including:

• Thrombosis in otherwise normal pancreas: this is the prime example of early graft thrombosis leading to graft loss for "technical Failure." In these grafts, the only pathological changes consist of recent vascular thrombosis and bland ischemic parenchymal necrosis. There is no underlying vascular pathology or any other specific histological change (Figure 7.48) (30). Lack of obvious histological changes does not rule out ultrastructural or subtle functional damage in these organs since older donor age and longer cold ischemia times are associated with increased risk for early thrombosis. The pancreas intrinsically has a low blood flow compared to other solid organs. Perioperative inflammation and edema, as well as microvascular and endothelial damage relating to donor/procurement factors and organ preservation, all contribute to further compromise of the blood flow. Similarly, factors associated with ischemic pancreatitis, such as longer cold ischemia times, have been associated with increased incidence of early graft thrombosis (7,124).

• Thrombosis in association with acute rejection may occur at any time after transplantation and is typically the result of vascular injury due to cell-mediated acute rejection (Figures 7.43 and 7.44). Accordingly, the most common underlying lesion in this form of thrombosis is intimal arteritis. More unusual is the presence of underlying transmural inflammation and/or necrotizing arteritis. Thrombosis is also a characteristic feature of the different variants of humoral rejection including the so-called accelerated rejection described above.

• Late graft thrombosis is a recognized cause of late graft loss. This process is also associated to underlying vascular pathology that may be immune mediated (acute or chronic active cell-mediated vascular rejection) or may be nonimmune related (i.e., atherosclerosis) (30).

2. Post-transplantation (ischemic) Pancreatitis

A significant number of patients with pancreas transplants require early re-laparotomy due to surgical complications. The most common reasons for re-laparotomy are intra-abdominal infections and graft pancreatitis, pancreas graft thrombosis, and anastomotic leak. The need for re-laparotomy is associated with a decrease in patient and graft survival (125).

Graft pancreatitis in the early post-transplantation period is secondary to ischemic injury, which causes dissolution of the cellular structures and spillage of pancreatic cell contents leading to acute inflammation. The incidence and severity of graft pancreatitis correlates with the length of cold ischemia time and is directly related to disturbances of the microcirculation in the reperfusion period (126–130). Grafts from older donors appear to have a higher probability to develop graft pancreatitis presumably due to vascular quality issues (126–128). Less common causes

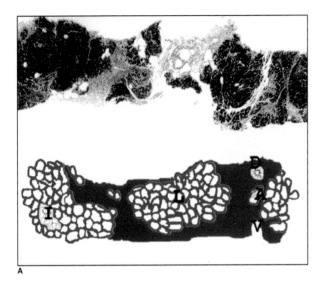

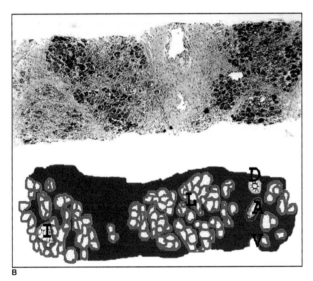

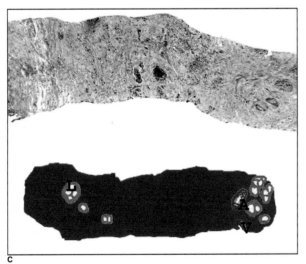

FIGURE 7.45: *(A, B and C) Low-power photomicrographs and corresponding diagrams showing mild, moderate, and severe chronic rejection/graft sclerosis (stages I, II, and III, respectively) characterized by progressive increase in fibrosis and acinar atrophy.*

of graft pancreatitis are impairment of drainage of exocrine secretions (130).

The morphology of post-transplant graft pancreatitis is similar to that of native pancreatitis. The main histological features being infiltration by neutrophils and macrophages, enzymatic necrosis of fat and parenchyma, and edema of the interlobular septa (131). The more severe forms of graft pancreatitis appear with extensive hemorrhagic necrosis (Figure 7.49).

Ischemia-reperfusion injury not only plays an important role in the development of graft pancreatitis but also appears to be causally related to vascular thrombosis after pancreas transplantation. Massive thrombosis of large blood vessels is associated with extensive coagulation necrosis of the graft and rapid loss of graft function. In contrast, thrombosis in small blood vessels is associated with patchy coagulation necrosis of acinar tissue. These findings may be subtle and do overlap with those of acute pancreatitis (30).

Mild ischemia-reperfusion injury can be identified histologically in most samples obtained within the first week post-transplantation. This is characterized by spotty acinar cell dropout, spotty apoptosis, flattening of the acinar cells, and otherwise minimal inflammation (81,130). Another manifestation of ischemia is the presence of marked acinar and islet cell cytoplasmic swelling and vacuolization. In this setting, islet cell ballooning and spotty islet cell dropout may occur that should be distinguished from islet drug toxicity (28).

3. Post-transplant Infectious Pancreatitis/Peripancreatitis/ Fluid Collection/Peripancreatic Abscess

Infectious peripancreatitis is a relatively common early complication of pancreas transplantation often secondary to ischemic graft pancreatitis (Figure 7.50) (132–134).

Infected intra-abdominal fluid collections are treated conservatively with percutaneous drainage and antibiotics; however, abdominal exploration for drainage and debridement is often required (135,137). Needle biopsies obtained from the grafted pancreas during these surgical procedures show characteristic features. The pancreas parenchyma shows variable degrees of mixed inflammation, predominantly septally located. The inflammation is composed of lymphocytes, eosinophils, neutrophils, and less numerous plasma cells. A typical finding in these biopsies is the presence of dissecting bundles of active, tissue culture–like, connective tissue with abundant fibroblasts (Figure 7.51). The fibrous bands run between the exocrine lobules giving the biopsy a "cirrhotic" appearance. The fibrosis becomes more pronounced as time passes if the peripancreatic infected fluid collection persists. The periphery of the acinar lobules usually shows some involvement by the inflammation. Typically, however, the acinar parenchyma shows proportionally little inflammation and acinar damage (65).

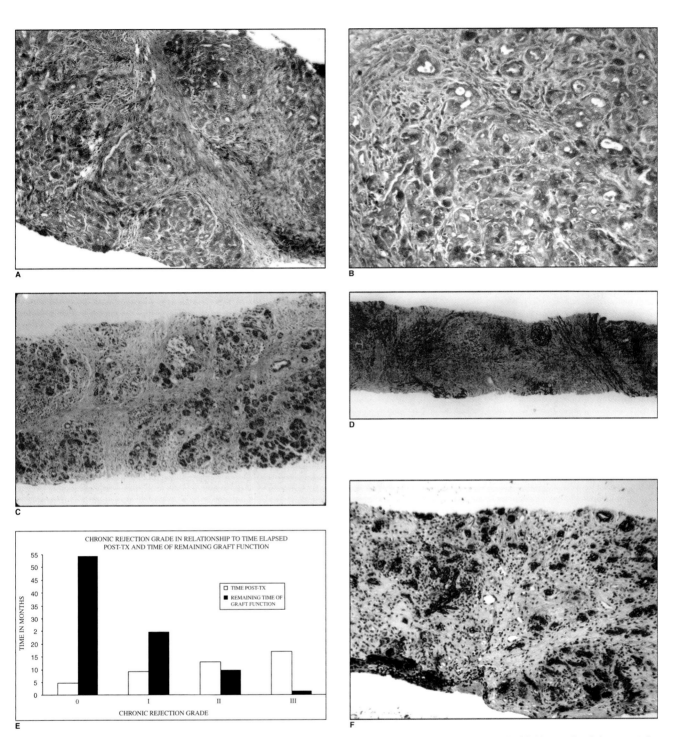

FIGURE 7.46: *(A, B, C, and D) Progressive degrees of fibrosis can be appreciated in biopsies stained with Masson's trichrome stain. A: Incipient septal fibrosis with minimal extension to the acini. B: High-power view of acinar area with incipient periacinar fibrosis. C: Moderate fibrosis with expansion of fibrous septa and "fragmentation" of the lobules due to periacinar and intraacinar fibrosis. D: Diffuse fibrosis with essential disappearance of the exocrine component and replacement by fibrous tissue and inflammatory infiltrates. (E) Graph demonstrating the relationship between the grade of chronic rejection/graft sclerosis and shortened graft survival. (F) Cytokeratin stain highlighting marked architectural distortion of the exocrine parenchyma that mainly consists of residual ductules.*

The main differential diagnosis in biopsies from grafts with intra-abdominal/peripancreatic abscesses is with acute and with chronic rejection. In order to distinguish each of this process, the availability of clinical information is of utmost importance. Thus, typical cases of post transplant peripancreatitis are diagnosed within days or few weeks post-transplantation in patients who had clinical evidence of infection (i.e., fever). Correlation with microbiological

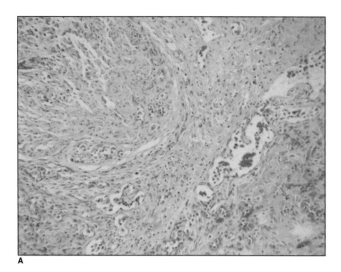

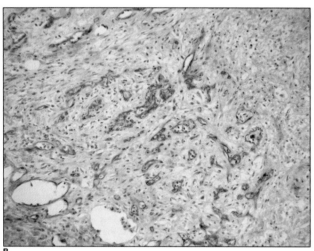

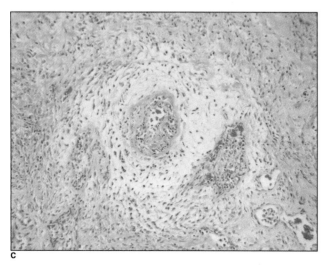

FIGURE 7.47: (A, B, and C) Pancreatectomy for graft failure secondary to acute and chronic antibody-mediated rejection resulting in graft loss two months after transplantation. (A) Complete loss of exocrine and endocrine structures with prominent residual vascular structures. (B) C4d stain stains strongly the capillary size vessels. (C) Larger vessels showed fibrinoid necrosis and thrombosis with recanalization. Previous biopsies on this patient are represented on Figures 7.23 and 7.24.

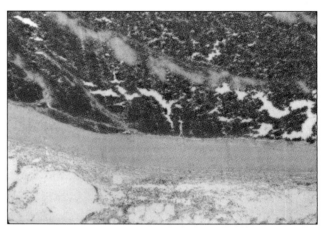

FIGURE 7.48: Thrombosed artery due to "technical failure." The arteries were normal except for the presence of recent thrombi. The patient underwent pancreatectomy twenty-four hours after transplantation.

studies is useful confirming the infectious nature of the inflammation.

From the morphological point of view, the inflammation in acute cell-mediated rejection is not typically associated with active fibrosis (or any active septal fibroblastic proliferation). A feature useful to differentiate fibrosis secondary to peripancreatitis from chronic rejection/graft sclerosis is the evaluation of the acinar lobules. The latter are essentially preserved in peripancreatitis, whereas extensive atrophy of the central parts of the exocrine lobules is found in chronic rejection/graft sclerosis (64).

Although the degree of septal fibrosis seen in biopsies from patients that require one or more re-laparotomies may be very pronounced, these changes are usually confined to the periphery (surface) of the graft and therefore superficial fibrotic biopsies may not represent the status of the whole organ.

Necrotizing infectious duodeno-pancreatitis with abscess formation can present at any time after transplantation but occur more often in the first months after transplantation. A variety of organisms can be cultured from these grafts, most commonly being enterobacteria (Enterobacter cloacae, Proteus mirabilis) and methicillin-resistant Staphylococcus aureus). Fungal infections, more often from Candida species and mixed bacterial/fungal infection, are not uncommon (125,136,137). Necrotizing pancreatitis can be rarely secondary to CMV infection (138).

Anastomotic leak: Infection, ischemia, and poor surgical technique may lead to dehiscence of the anastomosis between the duodenal cuff and the urinary bladder or small intestine (125). Pathological examination of grafts resected for this reason may show specific causes such as CMV-related perforation, or may only show nonspecific changes such as necrosis in the area around the anastomosis and acute inflammation. The adjacent peritoneal surfaces typically show acute fibrinous or purulent serositis.

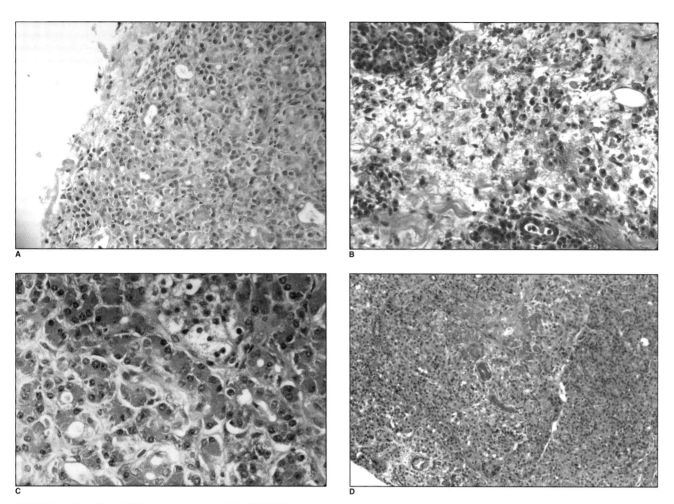

FIGURE 7.49: *(A and B) Ischemic pancreatitis. (A) Mild ischemic pancreatitis characterized by clusters of neutrophils in the connective tissue septa and nearby acini. (B) More pronounced acute pancreatitis shows areas of fat necrosis with scattered lipid laded macrophages, septal (interstitial) edema, and patchy hemorrhages. (C) Ischemic injury is manifested as acinar and islet cell vacuolization with spotty cell dropout. The acinar changes are better appreciated in the bottom half of the image. (D) Ischemic injury and ischemic pancreatitis are associated with an increased risk of thrombosis. Focal acinar necrosis with thrombosis of small associated vessels was found in this needle core biopsy performed forty-eight hours before a pancreatectomy showing diffuse arterial and venous thrombosis but no evidence of cell-mediated or humoral rejection.*

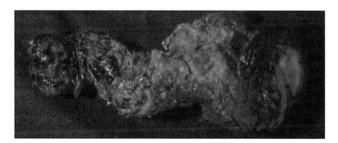

FIGURE 7.50: *Graft pancreatectomy for severe bacterial peripancreatitis and extensive formation of peripancreatic abscesses.*

ii. Viral Infections

1. CMV Infection

The use of newer more potent immunosuppressive drugs such as tacrolimus and mycophenolate mofetil is potentially associated with an increase in all types of infections (bacterial, fungal, and viral). Antiviral drugs are used prophylactically in many transplant centers to prevent CMV infection. There is evidence that prophylaxis for CMV delays the infection and reduces its severity (139–142).

Although the incidence of CMV disease in kidney-pancreas transplants may be up to 22 percent in donor-positive, recipient-negative cases, the actual diagnosis of CMV graft pancreatitis is rare. Klassen et al. reported biopsy-proven CMV pancreatitis in four patients with the diagnosis made eighteen weeks to forty-four months after transplantation. With prolonged ganciclovir treatment, clinical and histological resolution of the infection was achieved in all patients (115).

The clinical presentation of CMV graft pancreatitis is indistinguishable from acute rejection, for example, increase in serum amylase and lipase. Similarly, on percutaneous needle biopsies, both acute allograft rejection

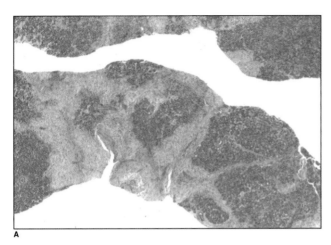
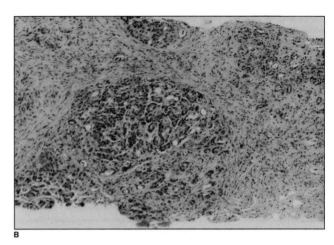

FIGURE 7.51: *Biopsies obtained at the time of laparotomy for exploration and "washout" in patients with peripancreatic infections or fluid collections often show reactive changes in the pancreatic parenchyma. These consist of active fibroblastic proliferation of fibrous septa that may appear markedly expanded separating adjacent exocrine lobules. The connective tissue bands typically have mixed inflammation that may resemble acute rejection. Venulitis, ductal inflammation, and acinar inflammation in areas away from the septa are usually absent. (B) The areas of pancreas in the periphery of the graft and in direct continuity with the infection may become atrophic in a manner that may resemble chronic rejection/graft sclerosis. The most important distinguishing factor is the clinical history (i.e., recent transplantation and evidence of peripancreatic infection or fluid collection).*

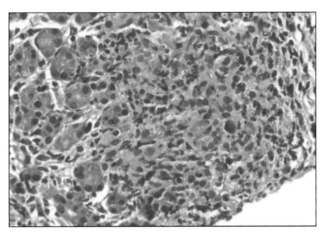

FIGURE 7.52: *CMV infection. Focus of dense acinar inflammation composed predominantly of mononuclear cells (lymphocytes and macrophages). The viral cytopathic changes are subtle (note occasional atypical nuclei center right). Careful search for viral cytopathic changes is necessary in any transplant biopsy before a diagnosis of rejection is rendered.*

and mild CMV pancreatitis may present with modest, predominantly lymphocytic acinar inflammation (115). In addition, venous endothelial inflammation resembling venulitis may also occur in CMV infection. Eosinophils are more common in rejection but may be present in small numbers in CMV infection as well. Neutrophils may be present in association with areas of necrosis or acinar cell damage in both rejection and CMV pancreatitis. Due to the morphological similarities between rejection and CMV infection, evidence of viral cytopathic changes should be sought systematically in all graft biopsies, independent of the clinical setting (Figure 7.52) Multiple tissue

sections and CMV stains should be performed if deemed necessary to ruled out the viral infection (115).

Severe cases of CMV infection may present with intractable gastrointestinal hemorrhage and/or duodenal-cuff perforation (139–142). Necrotizing CMV infection with abscess formation (143). and development of a CMV-related arteriovenous fistula (144). have been reported.

2. EBV-Related Post-Transplant Lymphoproliferative Disorder (PTLD)

PTLD occurs in 1–3 percent of pancreas transplant recipients (145–149). As described in Chapter 10, most PTLD are EBV related, and of B-cell lineage. The time of occurrence after transplantation appears to depend on the intensity of immunosuppression and varies from a few weeks to several years after transplantation. Very rare PTLD are of T-cell lineage and these tend to occur later after transplantation (150).

EBV-related PTLD include a wide range of processes from benign hyperplastic to overtly malignant lymphoid proliferations. On the most benign end of the spectrum (plasmacytic hyperplasia), the patients present with generalized type of symptoms and lymphadenopathy rather than with graft dysfunction and therefore graft biopsies usually play no role in the diagnostic workup. Pancreatic graft involvement is not unusual in the other forms of PTLD (polymorphic B-cell hyperplasia/lymphoma, immunoblastic lymphoma), as previously reported in the kidney. Graft involvement by monomorphic PTLD/lymphoma is recognized by the presence of monomorphic atypical immunoblasts of B-cell immunophenotype. Extensive parenchymal infiltration and geographic areas of necrosis are common in these cases (Figure 7.53) (150).

In contrast, polymorphic PTLD involving the pancreas allograft may be difficult to differentiate from acute cellular rejection. The differentiation between these two processes is very difficult in the earlier stages of polymorphic PTLD, particularly if there is a component of concurrent acute rejection (145). Evaluation of T- and B-cell markers (e.g., CD3, CD20) can aid by the identification of the predominant cellular component in different areas of the biopsy. Acute rejection is characterized by a predominant population of T cells (typically more than 75 percent) and a minor population of B cells that form aggregates no larger than 200–300 μm. In contrast, the identification of large, confluent, nodular B-cell aggregates are consistent with graft involvement by PTLD (145). The presence of marked cytological atypia in infiltrates predominantly composed of immunoblastic and plasmacytoid cells also favors PTLD. Eosinophils are present in variable proportions both in acute rejection and in PTLD. Immunoglobulin light chain restriction can be demonstrated in patients with polymorphic B-cell hyperplasia and is typically found in lymphoma.

EBV-related PTLD is confirmed with in situ hybridization for EBV-encoded RNAs that marks a significant proportion of the atypical cells. Also, stains for LMP-1 (EBV latent membrane protein) are usually positive in a variable proportion of the cells (Figure 7.53).

Other minor features of pancreas allograft involvement by EBV-related PTLD have been described. All sizes of veins are consistently infiltrated by the atypical B cells with associated lifting and damage of the endothelium similar to that seen in acute rejection. Also, nerves and adjacent soft tissues are usually extensively infiltrated by the lymphoproliferative process. With respect to the arteries, if concurrent cell-mediated rejection is present in the form of intimal arteritis, the subendothelial infiltrates are predominantly composed of T cells, in contrast to the predominant population of B cells seen in the areas of PTLD. In the absence of vascular rejection the arterial walls appear to be consistently resistant to permeation by the atypical B-cell infiltrates.

Lastly, the random involvement seen in cases of PTLD with areas of parenchyma that may be completely free of infiltrates contrasts with the more diffuse involvement of the pancreas seen in the severe forms of cell-mediated acute rejection (26,145).

iii. Islet Graft Pathology

1. Nonspecific Islet Pathology

There is no experimental or clinical evidence that endocrine islets are principally targeted in cell-mediated alloimmune reactions. Islet pathology in acute and chronic allograft rejection is in essence nonspecific, secondary to the overall degree of acute parenchymal injury (primarily

directed to exocrine pancreas) and ensuing fibrosis/sclerosis (65). The pathological findings consist of islet inflammation and occasional necrosis, in a degree proportional to the severity of acute rejection. The inflammation is therefore random and the cells infiltrating the islets are similar to the surrounding inflammatory infiltrates, more or less representing a "spillover" phenomenon (64,92).

In long-term pancreas allografts, islet distribution and morphology to a large extent reflects ongoing injury and repair. Extensive collagenization in chronic rejection leads to fragmentation of exocrine lobules as well as of islets that acquire irregular shapes and may consist of only few cell clusters with irregular distribution, nevertheless still containing a mixture of both insulin and glucagon producing cells. Conversely in some grafts, aggregates of large but otherwise normal appearing islets may reflect compensatory hyperplasia (93). Insulinomas or other islet cell tumors have not been described in whole pancreas allografts (151).

Islet cell atypia and hyperchromasia is seen in less than 5 percent of cases independently of the cause of the biopsy and is of unknown etiology or significance (92,93).

2. Recurrence of Type I DM

Type 1 diabetes is an autoimmune disease that can as such recur after pancreas transplantation. Recurrence of autoimmune disease is, however, a rare process that has been well documented in approximately a dozen cases (114,152,153). This process is characterized by selective autoimmune-mediated destruction of beta cells in an analogous manner as occurs in type 1 diabetes in the native pancreas. The diagnosis of recurrent disease is made with the combination of sudden or progressive lack of glycemic control associated with selective loss of the insulin producing beta cells in the graft and persistence of the other types of islet cells, particularly the glucagon producing alpha cells. In some cases, the active phase of beta cell destruction has been demonstrated, consisting of mononuclear cell infiltration (isletitis) (153). Similar to the disease in the native pancreas, the inflammation is centered in islets still containing beta cells and the isletitis resolves when beta cells disappear. An additional similarity between the native and graft disease is the occasional accumulation of amorphous eosinophilic deposits composed of amylin, within the diseased islets (Figure 7.54) (153,154).

The first reported cases of recurrent DM occurred in transplants from identical twins or HLA-identical siblings that were not immunosuppressed or which received minimal immunosuppression. In nonimmunosuppressed patients, disease recurrence occurred within weeks after transplantation. In some cases, isletitis resolved after introduction or increase in immunosuppression (27,114). HLA-mismatched transplants from cadaveric donors are also susceptible to recurrence of the autoimmune diabetes with selective beta cell destruction but this occurs rarely.

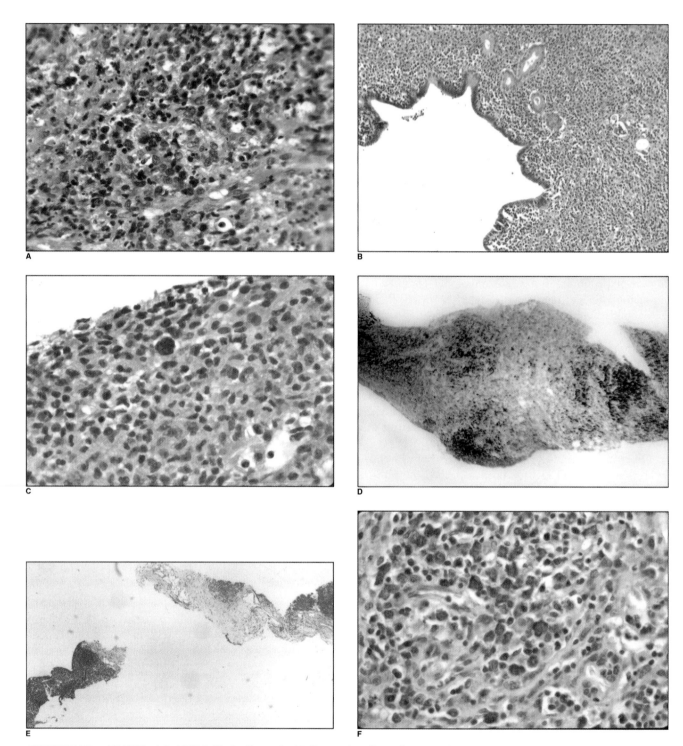

FIGURE 7.53:   (A) EBV-related PTLD. Markedly atypical inflammation distending septal area. The presence of necrosis (abundant nuclear fragments) is helpful for the diagnosis of PTLD. (B) EBV-related PTLD. Pancreatic duct surrounded by dense inflammatory infiltrates. (C) High-magnification view of monomorphic EBV-related PTLD. (D) CD20 stain highlights large, nodular, and expansile B-cell aggregates in a needle core biopsy from a patient with early graft involvement by EBV-related PTLD. (E) In rare occasions, pancreas transplant needle core biopsies may contain benign lymphoid tissue from the peripancreatic tissues (left lower corner) -that should not be confused with a lymphoproliferative disorder. (F) LMP-1 (EBV latent membrane protein-1) highlights numerous positive cells in a case of polymorphous EBV-related PTLD. (G) In situ hybridization for EBER (EBV-encoded RNAs) is confirmatory of a diagnosis of EBV-related PTLD.

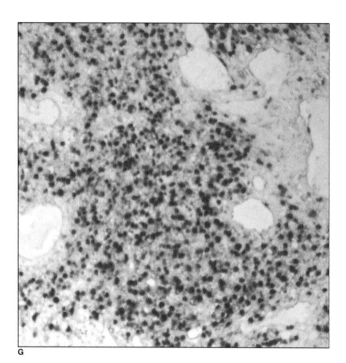

G

FIGURE 7.53: (Continued)

The rarity of recurrent type I DM in whole pancreas transplantation has been attributed to the inclusion of donor lymphoid tissue with the transplanted pancreas. This would lead to modulatory effects from recipient chimerism for a donor T cell subset (RT6.2) (155).

In addition to the clinical and histological findings, the diagnosis of recurrent autoimmune disease is aided by the demonstration of islet cell autoantibodies in serum (GAD 65 and IA-2); however, these may also be found in patients with no clinical evidence of autoimmune disease recurrence. In a study comparing patients with chronic graft failure versus patients with well-functioning grafts, islet cell autoantibodies before transplantation and at the time of graft failure were significantly higher in the former group. Also, patients with failed grafts showed an increase in autoantibodies at the time of loss of graft function (156).

From the pathological point of view, it is important to emphasize that the active destructive phase consisting of isletitis with progressive and selective loss of beta cells is transient. In the inactive phase (after the disappearance of beta cells and associated isletitis), the pancreas may superficially look normal or may show fibrosis. The diagnosis can only be made with the immunohistochemical demonstration of lack of insulin-producing cells in islets. After a prolonged period of time, the islets as a whole can disappear (30,92,157).

3. Islet Cell Drug Toxicity

In the pre-cyclosporine era, post-transplant DM occurred in almost half of renal transplant patients secondary to the use of large doses of corticosteroids. Older age, higher body weight, family history of abnormal glucose metabolism, and

African-American or Hispanic descent are associated with higher incidence of post-transplant DM. The latter is believed to result from a combination of insulin resistance with a relative deficiency of insulin production. Insulin resistance results from decreased insulin receptor number and affinity, impaired glucose uptake, and probable inhibition of insulin secretion by beta cells (1).

The use of cyclosporine and tacrolimus has markedly improved the outcome in pancreas transplantation. In addition to nephrotoxicity, hirsutism/alopecia, neurological, and gastrointestinal side effects, both of these drugs can cause abnormalities in glucose metabolism. Hyperglycemia is more commonly seen in patients receiving tacrolimus. In animal studies, cyclosporine administration has been associated with reduction in insulin secretion, diminished beta cell density, decreased insulin synthesis, and defective insulin secretion. Similar morphological findings have been seen also with tacrolimus (158). The incidence of hyperglycemia in patients receiving cyclosporine and tacrolimus is reported to be 11–19 percent and 15–29 percent, respectively. Most patients had also received steroids, and this represents a confounding factor (159).

The morphological findings in biopsies from patients with clinical evidence of drug toxicity consist of cytoplasmic swelling and vacuolization of islet cells. The islets appear optically clear and stand out from the more eosinophilic acinar parenchyma. In more severe cases, islet cell dropout with formation of empty spaces (lacunae) and can be seen if there is confluent islet cell dropout. Rarely, intra-islet apoptotic cell fragments can be identified (Figure 7.55) (28).

Immunoperoxidase stains for insulin and glucagon show diminished staining for insulin in beta cells in comparison to controls. This is the light microscopic counterpart of the marked loss of insulin dense core granules seen in beta cells by electron microscopy. The latter study shows preservation of the peripheral non-beta cells in the islets has been demonstrated. The histological changes as well as the clinical findings are reversible with reduction or discontinuation of the drug. Hyperglycemia and the histological evidence of drug toxicity are worsened with the concurrent use of pulse steroids to treat acute rejection (28). Islet toxicity should be less common under the current steroid sparing immunosuppression protocols.

4. Nesidioblastosis

In native pancreas this is a regenerative change leading to differentiation of adult pancreatic ductal epithelium into insulin-producing cells (Figure 7.56). Nesidioblastosis was demonstrated in one animal model of pancreas transplantation (160).

In systematic studies of pancreas graft biopsies, nesidioblastosis was found in approximately 4 percent of samples, with or without evidence of graft rejection. In most instances, the change was associated with documented previous

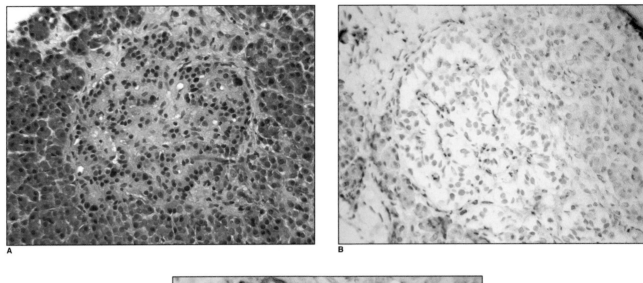

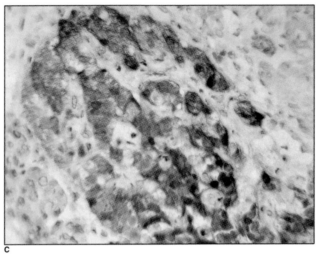

FIGURE 7.54:   (A, B and C): Recurrence of diabetes mellitus in pancreas allograft. (A) On H&E stain, the islet is only remarkable for focal accumulation of amorphous eosinophilic material consistent with amylin as it occurs in diabetes mellitus in the native pancreas. The acinar tissue is normal. (B) Negative insulin stain. The absence of isletitis is consistent with the complete loss of beta cells. (C) Glucagon stain highlights remaining alpha cells that represent the vast majority of the islet cells.

injury (i.e., ischemic pancreatitis) and subsequent regenerative changes. The process had no discernible clinical significance (91,92). Nesidioblastosis has been associated with hypoglycemia in one report (161).

iv. Duodenal Graft Pathology

In whole organ pancreas allografts, the exocrine drainage anastomosis is typically done through a segment of the graft duodenum. In patients with urinary bladder drainage, histological samples of the duodenal graft can be obtained by the cystoscopic biopsy technique. Duodenal tissue can be also obtained fortuitously through the percutaneous route.

Acute rejection in the duodenum most commonly occurs concurrently with pancreas rejection, but rejection can also occur independently in each of these organs (60).

Mild acute duodenal rejection is manifested by an increase in the inflammatory cells in the lamina propria with mild villous blunting and apoptosis of epithelial cells (see Chapter 8). Severe rejection has confluent epithelial necrosis with total loss of the epithelial lining. Necrosis can extend to all layers, including the muscularis propria. Arterial involvement (i.e., intimal arteritis, vasculitis) are diagnostic of rejection and may be seen also in the duodenum (60). A case of perforation due to duodenal rejection has been reported (162).

Other forms of duodenal pathology amenable to being diagnosed with cystoscopic biopsies are ischemic and infectious duodenal ulcers (i.e., CMV, bacterial, fungal), Foley catheter trauma and bladder tumors, and so forth (163). Recurrent urological complications may require

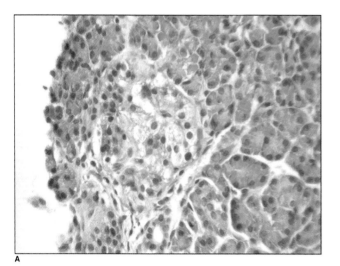

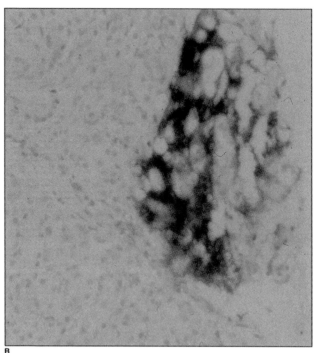

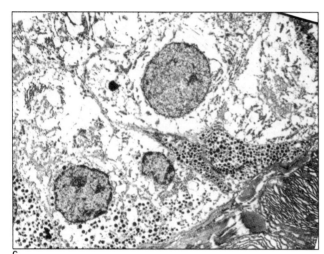

FIGURE 7.55: *(A) Calcineurin inhibitor islet cell toxicity is characterized by marked islet cell vacuolization and occasional islet cell apoptosis or dropout. The biopsy was obtained in a patient presenting with hyperglycemia and high levels of FK506 (tacrolimus). Note the lack of vacuolization of acinar cells and lack of inflammation. (B) Insulin staining of islets with calcineurin inhibitor islet cell toxicity result in a weaker, "washed-out" pattern of staining. (C) On electron microscopic evaluation there is marked vacuolization and loss of neuroendocrine granules in the beta (insulin-producing) cells with preservation of the abundant neuroendocrine granulos in the alpha (glucagon-producing) cells (lower half of image).*

conversion of a bladder-drained pancreas transplant to enteric drainage (7,101).

IX. GROSS AND MICROSCOPIC EVALUATION OF FAILED ALLOGRAFTS

Graft pancreatectomy specimens usually consist of the whole pancreas and attached portion of duodenum. The latter is present in continuity either with a loop of recipient's small intestine or a patch of urinary bladder wall (Figures 7.1 and 7.2) Macroscopic evaluation of an explanted pancreas can be best accomplished if the pathologist understands the complexity of the technical issues in pancreas transplantation (see section on history of surgical techniques).

Systematic histological evaluation of failed grafts is necessary for accurate classification of the cause of graft loss.

Minimum histological sampling should include cross sections of all large vessels and several sections from the parenchyma to include an adequate number of medium sized and small vessels. The number of histological sections depends on each case, usually ranging from four to ten sections to allow for the most important structures to be sampled. Specific guidelines for gross and microscopic evaluation:

• Large arteries and veins: evaluate for thrombosis (recent and organized), intimal arteritis, transplant vasculopathy, donor atherosclerosis, and so forth.
• Random samples from parenchyma (viable and necrotic, usually three to five sections): evaluate for evidence of ischemia/pancreatitis, acute rejection, chronic rejection, presence of infectious organisms, and so forth.
• Area of anastomosis: evaluate for dehiscence (leak) and serositis.

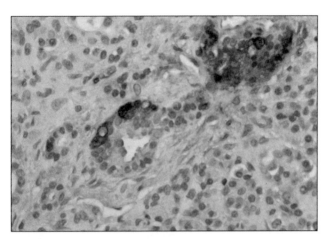

FIGURE 7.56: *Nesidioblastosis. Insulin-producing cells in pancreatic duct, appearing after severe ischemic injury. This likely represents a reactive/regenerative phenomenon.*

- Samples from any other lesions: masses (i.e., PTLD, cysts, abscesses, lymph nodes).

Ancillary studies:

- Immunoperoxidase stains for insulin and glucagon should be performed to evaluate for selective destruction of beta cells due to recurrence of autoimmune disease. These cases may show near normal parenchyma with no significant evidence of fibrosis/acinar loss such as it is seen in chronic rejection.
- C4d stain is necessary to determine if there is a component of humoral rejection present.
- Frozen tissue samples for immunofluorescence stains for immunoglobulins and complement in cases suspected to represent hyperacute/accelerated acute rejection.
- Electron microscopy: may be used to demonstrate selective beta cell loss in recurrence of diabetes type 1 or beta cell degeneration in calcineurin inhibitor toxicity.

X. OTHER COMPLICATIONS OF PANCREAS TRANSPLANTATION WITH HISTOPATHOLOGICAL MANIFESTATIONS

Thrombotic microangiopathy is a well-known complication of transplantation and has been described in SPK patients. Clinicopathological evidence of pancreas involvement is typically lacking, even in patients with systemic manifestations of the process (164).

Graft-versus-host disease secondary to pancreas transplantation has been well documented but is rare with an overall incidence of less than 0.5 percent (165). The diagnosis is based on the characteristic clinical and pathological findings secondary to gastrointestinal, hepatic, and skin involvement (see another chapter). The presence of donor HLA or DNA material in the affected organs or in peripheral blood confirms the diagnosis.

Polyomavirus infection: Polyomavirus nephropathy is considered one of the main causes of renal graft loss in SPK (166). Since the infection is confined to the kidney allograft, the diagnosis relies on the demonstration of viral cytopathic changes in a renal biopsy. Urinary cytology and viral loads in blood are useful additional tools for diagnosis.

Gastrointestinal drug toxicity: Chronic diarrhea is one of the common side effects of mycophenolate mofetil use. The most typical pathological changes in colonic biopsies performed in this context show strong similarities to those changes seen in other immunosuppressive states, namely, increased crypt cell apoptosis. Florid cases resemble intestinal acute graft-versus-host disease. Dose reduction or discontinuation of the drug lead to clinical and histological improvement (167).

i. Adenovirus

Adenovirus has been associated with hemorrhagic cystitis in renal transplant patients and in rare occasions renal parenchyma involvement has been demonstrated (adenovirus pyelonephritis). There has been only one report of adenovirus infection in a combined kidney-pancreas transplant recipient. Adenovirus type 11 was demonstrated in some renal tubules but the pancreas allograft continued to have normal function and apparently was not affected (168).

ii. Neoplasia

A single case of pancreatic adenocarcinoma originating in a pancreas allograft has been reported. (169).

REFERENCES

1. Pirart J: Diabetes mellitus and its degenerative complications: a prospective study of 4,400 patients observered between 1947 and 1973 (Parts 1 & 2). *Diabetes Care* 1978, 1:168–88, 252–63.
2. Hirsch IB, Farkas-Hirsch R, Skyler JS: Intensive insulin therapy for treatment of type I diabetes. *Diabetes Care* 1990, 13:1265–83.
3. Paty BW, Lanz K, Kendall DM, et al.: Restored hypoglycemic counterregulation is stable in successful pancreas transplant recipients for up to 19 years after transplantation. *Transplantation* 2001, 72:1103–7.
4. Secchi A, Di Carlo V, Martinenghi S, et al.: Effect of pancreas transplantation on life expectancy, kidney function and quality of life in uraemic type 1 (insulin-dependent) diabetic patients. *Diabetologia* 1991, 34 Suppl. 1:S141–4.
5. Sudan D, Sudan R, Stratta R: Long-term outcome of simultaneous kidney-pancreas transplantation: analysis of 61 patients with more than 5 years follow-up. *Transplantation* 2000, 69:550–5.
6. Robertson RP, Davis C, Larsen J, et al.: Pancreas and islet transplantation in type 1 diabetes. *Diabetes Care* 2006, 29:935.

7. Gruessner AC, Sutherland DE: Pancreas transplant outcomes for United States (US) and non-US cases as reported to the United Network for Organ Sharing (UNOS) and the International Pancreas Transplant Registry (IPTR) as of June 2004. *Clin Transplant* 2005, 19:433–55.

8. Voruganti L, Sells R: Quality of life of diabetic patients after combined pancreatic-renal transplantation. *Clin Transpl* 1989, 3:78–82.

9. Gruessner RW, Sutherland DE, Gruessner AC: Mortality assessment for pancreas transplants. *Am J Transplant* 2004, 4:2018–26.

10. Gruessner RW, Manivel C, Dunn DL, et al.: Pancreaticoduodenal transplantation with enteric drainage following native total pancreatectomy for chronic pancreatitis: a case report. *Pancreas* 1991, 6:479–88.

11. Andreoni KA, Brayman KL, Guidinger MK, et al.: Kidney and pancreas transplantation in the United States, 1996-2005. *Am J Transplant* 2007, 7:1359–75.

12. Kuo PC, Johnson LB, Schweitzer EJ, et al.: Solitary pancreas allografts. The role of percutaneous biopsy and standardized histologic grading of rejection. *Arch Surg* 1997, 132:52–7.

13. Stratta RJ, Gaber AO, Shokouh-Amiri MH, et al.: A prospective comparison of systemic-bladder versus portal-enteric drainage in vascularized pancreas transplantation. *Surgery* 2000, 127:217–26.

14. Kelly WD, Lillehei RC, Merkel FK, et al.: Allotransplantation of the pancreas and duodenum along with the kidney in diabetic nephropathy. *Surgery* 1967, 61:827–37.

15. Lillehei RC, Simmons RL, Najarian JS, et al.: Pancreaticoduodenal allotransplantation: experimental and clinical experience. *Ann Surg* 1970, 172:405–36.

16. Gruessner R, Sutherland D: *Transplantation of the Pancreas: History of Pancreas Transplantation*. Springer; 1st edition (April 27, 2004) Chapter 11.

17. Sollinger HW, Odorico JS, Knechtle SJ, et al.: Experience with 500 simultaneous pancreas-kidney transplants. *Ann Surg* 1998, 228:284–96.

18. Allen RD, Wilson TG, Grierson JM, et al.: Percutaneous biopsy of bladder-drained pancreas transplants. *Transplantation* 1991, 51:1213–6.

19. Bartlett ST, Kuo PC, Johnson LB, et al.: Pancreas transplantation at the University of Maryland. *Clin Transpl* 1996: 271–80.

20. Benedetti E, Najarian JS, Gruessner AC, et al.: Correlation between cystoscopic biopsy results and hypoamylasuria in bladder-drained pancreas transplants. *Surgery* 1995, 118:864–72.

21. Moukarzel M, Benoit G, Charpentier B, et al.: Is urinary amylase a reliable index for monitoring whole pancreas endocrine graft function? *Transplant Proc* 1992, 24:925–6.

22. Nankivell BJ, Allen RD, Bell B, et al.: Factors affecting urinary amylase excretion after pancreas transplantation. *Transplant Proc* 1990, 22:2156–7.

23. Papadimitriou JC, Drachenberg CB, Wiland A, et al.: Histologic grading of acute allograft rejection in pancreas needle biopsy: correlation to serum enzymes, glycemia, and response to immunosuppressive treatment. *Transplantation* 1998, 66:1741–5.

24. Prieto M, Sutherland DE, Fernandez-Cruz L, et al.: Urinary amylase monitoring for early diagnosis of pancreas allograft rejection in dogs. *J Surg Res* 1986, 40: 597–604.

25. Prieto M, Sutherland DE, Fernandez-Cruz L, et al.: Experimental and clinical experience with urine amylase monitoring for early diagnosis of rejection in pancreas transplantation. *Transplantation* 1987, 43:73–9.

26. Drachenberg CB, Papadimitriou JC, Klassen DK, et al.: Evaluation of pancreas transplant needle biopsy: reproducibility and revision of histologic grading system. *Transplantation* 1997, 63:1579–86.

27. Sutherland DE, Goetz FC, Sibley RK: Recurrence of disease in pancreas transplants. *Diabetes* 1989, 38 Suppl. 1:85–7.

28. Drachenberg CB, Klassen DK, Weir MR, et al.: Islet cell damage associated with tacrolimus and cyclosporine: morphological features in pancreas allograft biopsies and clinical correlation. *Transplantation* 1999, 68:396–402.

29. Humar A, Khwaja K, Ramcharan T, et al.: Chronic rejection: the next major challenge for pancreas transplant recipients. *Transplantation* 2003, 76:918–23.

30. Drachenberg CB, Papadimitriou JC, Farney A, et al.: Pancreas transplantation: the histologic morphology of graft loss and clinical correlations. *Transplantation* 2001, 71: 1784–91.

31. Bartlett ST, Schweitzer EJ, Johnson LB, et al.: Equivalent success of simultaneous pancreas kidney and solitary pancreas transplantation. A prospective trial of tacrolimus immunosuppression with percutaneous biopsy. *Ann Surg* 1996, 224:440–9; discussion 9–52.

32. Klassen DK, Hoen-Saric EW, Weir MR, et al.: Isolated pancreas rejection in combined kidney pancreas tranplantation. *Transplantation* 1996, 61:974–7.

33. Papadimitriou JC: Diffuse acinar inflammation is the most important histological predictor of chronic rejection in pancreas allografts. *Transplantation* 2006, 82:223.

34. Tesi RJ, Henry ML, Elkhammas EA, et al.: The frequency of rejection episodes after combined kidney-pancreas transplant—the impact on graft survival. *Transplantation* 1994, 58:424–30.

35. Stegall MD: Surveillance biopsies in solitary pancreas transplantation. *Acta Chir Austriaca* 2001, 33:6.

36. Stratta RJ: Late acute rejection after pancreas transplantation. *Transplant Proc* 1998, 30:646.

37. Stratta RJ: Graft failure after solitary pancreas transplantation. *Transplant Proc* 1998, 30:289.

38. Stratta RJ: Patterns of graft loss following simultaneous kidney-pancreas transplantation. *Transplant Proc* 1998, 30:288.

39. Basadonna GP, Matas AJ, Gillingham KJ, et al.: Early versus late acute renal allograft rejection: impact on chronic rejection. *Transplantation* 1993, 55:993–5.

40. Allen RD, Grierson JM, Ekberg H, et al.: Longitudinal histopathologic assessment of rejection after bladder-drained canine pancreas allograft transplantation. *Am J Pathol* 1991, 138:303–12.

41. Atwell TD, Gorman B, Larson TS, et al.: Pancreas transplants: experience with 232 percutaneous US-guided biopsy procedures in 88 patients. *Radiology* 2004, 231: 845–9.

42. Boonstra JG, van der Pijl JW, Smets YF, et al.: Interstitial and vascular pancreas rejection in relation to graft survival. *Transpl Int* 1997, 10:451–6.

43. Casey ET, Smyrk TC, Burgart LJ, et al.: Outcome of untreated grade II rejection on solitary pancreas allograft biopsy specimens. *Transplantation* 2005, 79:1717–22.

44. Kuhr CS, Davis CL, Barr D, et al.: Use of ultrasound and cystoscopically guided pancreatic allograft biopsies and transabdominal renal allograft biopsies: safety and efficacy in kidney-pancreas transplant recipients. *J Urol* 1995, 153:316–21.

45. Laftavi MR, Gruessner AC, Bland BJ, et al.: Significance of pancreas graft biopsy in detection of rejection. *Transplant Proc* 1998, 30:642–4.

46. Laftavi MR, Gruessner AC, Bland BJ, et al.: Diagnosis of pancreas rejection: cystoscopic transduodenal versus percutaneous computed tomography scan-guided biopsy. *Transplantation* 1998, 65:528–32.

47. Lee BC, McGahan JP, Perez RV, et al.: The role of percutaneous biopsy in detection of pancreatic transplant rejection. *Clin Transplant* 2000, 14:493–8.

48. Papadimitriou JC: Role of histopathology evaluation in pancreas transplantation. *Current Opinion in Organ Transplantation* 2002, 7:185–90.

49. Klassen DK, Weir MR, Cangro CB, et al.: Pancreas allograft biopsy: safety of percutaneous biopsy-results of a large experience. *Transplantation* 2002, 73:553–5.

50. Klassen DK, Weir MR, Schweitzer EJ, et al.: Isolated pancreas rejection in combined kidney-pancreas transplantation: results of percutaneous pancreas biopsy. *Transplant Proc* 1995, 27:1333–4.

51. Aideyan OA, Schmidt AJ, Trenkner SW, et al.: CT-guided percutaneous biopsy of pancreas transplants. *Radiology* 1996, 201:825–8.

52. Bernardino M, Fernandez M, Neylan J, et al.: Pancreatic transplants: CT-guided biopsy. *Radiology* 1990, 177:709–11.

53. Gaber AO, Gaber LW, Shokouh-Amiri MH, et al.: Percutaneous biopsy of pancreas transplants. *Transplantation* 1992, 54:548–50.

54. Gaber LW, Stratta RJ, Lo A, et al.: Role of surveillance biopsies in monitoring recipients of pancreas alone transplants. *Transplant Proc* 2001, 33:1673–4.

55. Silver JM, Vitello JM, Benedetti E: Laparoscopic-guided biopsy of pancreatic transplant allograft. *J Laparoendosc Adv Surg Tech A* 1997, 7:319–22.

56. Kayler LK, Merion RM, Rudich SM, et al.: Evaluation of pancreatic allograft dysfunction by laparoscopic biopsy. *Transplantation* 2002, 74:1287–9.

57. Perkins JD, Munn SR, Marsh CL, et al.: Safety and efficacy of cystoscopically directed biopsy in pancreas transplantation. *Transplant Proc* 1990, 22:665–6.

58. Jones JW, Nakhleh RE, Casanova D, et al.: Cystoscopic transduodenal pancreas transplant biopsy: a new needle. *Transplant Proc* 1994, 26:527–8.

59. Lowell JA, Bynon JS, Nelson N, et al.: Improved technique for transduodenal pancreas transplant biopsy. *Transplantation* 1994, 57:752–3.

60. Nakhleh RE, Benedetti E, Gruessner A, et al.: Cystoscopic biopsies in pancreaticoduodenal transplantation. Are duodenal biopsies indicative of pancreas dysfunction? *Transplantation* 1995, 60:541–6.

61. Nakhleh RE, Sutherland DE, Benedetti E, et al.: Diagnostic utility and correlation of duodenal and pancreas biopsy tissue in pancreaticoduodenal transplants with emphasis on therapeutic use. *Transplant Proc* 1995, 27:1327–8.

62. Casanova D, Gruessner R, Brayman K, et al.: Retrospective analysis of the role of pancreatic biopsy (open and transcystoscopic technique) in the management of solitary pancreas transplants. *Transplant Proc* 1993, 25:1192–3.

63. Carpenter HA, Engen DE, Munn SR, et al.: Histologic diagnosis of rejection by using cystoscopically directed needle biopsy specimens from dysfunctional pancreatoduodenal allografts with exocrine drainage into the bladder. *Am J Surg Pathol* 1990, 14:837–46.

64. Drachenberg CB, Papadimitriou JC: The inflamed pancreas transplant: histological differential diagnosis. *Semin Diagn Pathol* 2004, 21:255–9.

65. Papadimitriou JC, Drachenberg CB, Klassen DK, et al.: Histological grading of chronic pancreas allograft rejection/graft sclerosis. *Am J Transplant* 2003, 3:599–605.

66. Tyden G, Reinholt FP, Sundkvist G, et al.: Recurrence of autoimmune diabetes mellitus in recipients of cadaveric pancreatic grafts. *N Engl J Med* 1996, 335:860–3.

67. Carbajal R, Karam G, Renaudin K, et al.: Specific humoral rejection of a pancreas allograft in a recipient of pancreas after kidney transplantation. *Nephrol Dial Transplant* 2007, 22:942–4.

68. Melcher ML, Olson JL, Baxter-Lowe LA, et al.: Antibody-mediated rejection of a pancreas allograft. *Am J Transplant* 2006, 6:423–8.

69. Gruessner RW, Nakhleh R, Tzardis P, et al.: Differences in rejection grading after simultaneous pancreas and kidney transplantation in pigs. *Transplantation* 1994, 57:1021–8.

70. Nakhleh RE, Sutherland DE, Tzardis P, et al.: Correlation of rejection of the duodenum with rejection of the pancreas in a pig model of pancreaticoduodenal transplantation. *Transplantation* 1993, 56:1353–6.

71. Severyn W, Olson L, Miller J, et al.: Studies on the survival of simultaneous canine renal and segmental pancreatic allografts. *Transplantation* 1982, 33:606–12.

72. Vogt P, Hiller WF, Steiniger B, et al.: Differential response of kidney and pancreas rejection to cyclosporine immunosuppression. *Transplantation* 1992, 53:1269–72.

73. Gruessner RW, Sutherland DE, Troppmann C, et al.: The surgical risk of pancreas transplantation in the cyclosporine era: an overview. *J Am Coll Surg* 1997, 185:128–44.

74. Hawthorne WJ, Allen RD, Greenberg ML, et al.: Simultaneous pancreas and kidney transplant rejection: separate or synchronous events? *Transplantation* 1997, 63:352–8.

75. Reinholt FP, Tyden G, Bohman SO, et al.: Pancreatic juice cytology in the diagnosis of pancreatic graft rejection. *Clin Transpl* 1988, 2:127–33.

76. Stratta RJ, Taylor RJ, Grune MT, et al.: Experience with protocol biopsies after solitary pancreas transplantation. *Transplantation* 1995, 60:1431–7.

77. Rogers J, Iskandar S, Farney A, et al.: Surveillance pancrease biopsies in solitary pancreas transplantation: A shot in the dark. *Am J Transplant* 2007, 7, Suppl. 2:251.

78. Drachenberg CB, Papadimitriou JC, Schweitzer E, et al.: Histological findings in "incidental" intraoperative pancreas allograft biopsies. *Transplant Proc* 2004, 36:780–1.

79. Benz S, Pfeffer F, Adam U, et al.: Impairment of pancreatic microcirculation in the early reperfusion period during simultaneous pancreas-kidney transplantation. *Transpl Int* 1998, 11 Suppl. 1:S433–5.

80. Dallman M: Immunobiology of graft rejection. In: Ginns LC, Cosimi AB, Morris PJ, eds. *Transplantation* 1988:23–42.

81. Benz S, Schnabel R, Morgenroth K, et al.: Ischemia/reperfusion injury of the pancreas: a new animal model. *J Surg Res* 1998, 75:109–15.

82. Troppmann C, Gruessner AC, Papalois BE, et al.: Delayed endocrine pancreas graft function after simultaneous pancreas-kidney transplantation. Incidence, risk factors, and impact on long-term outcome. *Transplantation* 1996, 61:1323–30.

83. Uhlman D, Ludwig S, Geissler F, et al.: Importance of microcirculatory distrubances in teh pathogenesis of pancreatitis. *Zentralbl Chir* 2001, 126:873–8.

84. Daar AS, Fuggle SV, Fabre JW, et al.: The detailed distribution of HLA-A, B, C antigens in normal human organs. *Transplantation* 1984, 38:287–92.

85. Steiniger B, Klempnauer J, Wonigeit K: Altered distribution of class I and class II MHC antigens during acute pancreas allograft rejection in the rat. *Transplantation* 1985, 40:234–9.

86. Pelletier RP, Hennessy PK, Adams PW, et al.: Clinical significance of MHC-reactive alloantibodies that develop after kidney or kidney-pancreas transplantation. *Am J Transplant* 2002, 2:134–41.

87. Solez K, Colvin RB, Racusen LC, et al.: Banff '05 Meeting Report: differential diagnosis of chronic allograft injury and elimination of chronic allograft nephropathy ('CAN'). *Am J Transplant* 2007, 7:518–26.

88. Le Moine A, Goldman M, Abramowicz D: Multiple pathways to allograft rejection. *Transplantation* 2002, 73:1373–81.

89. Hawthorne WJ, Griffin AD, Lau H, et al.: Experimental hyperacute rejection in pancreas allotransplants. *Transplantation* 1996, 62:324–9.

90. Steiniger B, Klempnauer J: Distinct histologic patterns of acute, prolonged, and chronic rejection in vascularized rat pancreas allografts. *Am J Pathol* 1986, 124:253–62.

91. Dietze O, Konigsrainer A, Habringer C, et al.: Histological features of acute pancreatic allograft rejection after pancreaticoduodenal transplantation in the rat. *Transpl Int* 1991, 4:221–6.

92. Drachenberg CB, Papadimitriou JC, Klassen DK, et al.: Distribution of alpha and beta cells in pancreas allograft biopsies: correlation with rejection and other pathologic processes. *Transplant Proc* 1998, 30:665–6.

93. Drachenberg CB, Papadimitriou JC, Weir MR, et al.: Histologic findings in islets of whole pancreas allografts: lack of evidence for recurrent cell-mediated diabetes mellitus. *Transplantation* 1996, 62:1770–2.

94. Papadimitriou JC: Antibody mediated rejection in pancreas allografts. *Ninth Banff Conference on Allograft Pathology* 2007.

95. Carpenter HA, Engen DE, Munn SR, et al.: Histologic features of rejection in cystoscopically directed needle biopsies of pancreatoduodenal allografts in dogs and humans. *Transplant Proc* 1990, 22:707–8.

96. Knoop M, McMahon RF, Jones CJ, et al.: Apoptosis in pancreatic allograft rejection – ultrastructural observations. *Exp Pathol* 1991, 41:219–24.

97. Dubernard JM, Traeger J, Touraine JL, et al.: Rejection of human pancreatic allografts. *Transplant Proc* 1980, 12:103–6.

98. Oberhuber G, Schmid T, Thaler W, et al.: The pattern of rejection after combined stomach, small bowel, and pancreas transplantation in the rat. *Transpl Int* 1993, 6:296–8.

99. Sibley RK: Pancreas transplantation. In: Sale GEed. *The pathology of organ transplantation.* Boston, MA: Butterworths 1990, 179.

100. Nakhleh RE, Sutherland DE: Pancreas rejection. Significance of histopathologic findings with implications for classification of rejection. *Am J Surg Pathol* 1992, 16:1098–107.

101. Boudreaux JP, Nealon WH, Carson RC, et al.: Pancreatitis necessitating urinary undiversion in a bladder-drained pancreas transplant. *Transplant Proc* 1990, 22:641–2.

102. Sutherland DE, Casanova D, Sibley RK: Role of pancreas graft biopsies in the diagnosis and treatment of rejection after pancreas transplantation. *Transplant Proc* 1987, 19:2329–31.

103. Papadimitriou JC, Wiland A, Drachenberg CB, et al.: Effectiveness of immunosuppressive treatment for recurrent or refractory pancreas allograft rejection: correlation with histologic grade. *Transplant Proc* 1998, 30:3945.

104. Racusen LC, Solez K, Colvin RB, et al.: The Banff 97 working classification of renal allograft pathology. *Kidney Int* 1999, 55:713–23.

105. Banff schema for grading liver allograft rejection: an international consensus document. *Hepatology* 1997, 25:658–63.

106. Klassen D: Chronic rejection in pancreas transplantation. *Graft* 1998, Suppl. II:74–6.

107. Brayman K, Morel P, Chau C, et al.: Influence of rejection episodes on the relationship between exocrine and endocrine function in bladder-drained pancreas transplants. *Transplant Proc* 1992, 24:921–3.

108. Schilling MK, Redaelli C, Reber PU, et al.: Microcirculation in chronic alcoholic pancreatitis: a laser Doppler flow study. *Pancreas* 1999, 19:21–5.

109. Nakhleh RE, Gruessner RW: Ischemia due to vascular rejection causes islet loss after pancreas transplantation. *Transplant Proc* 1998, 30:539–40.

110. Gruessner R: Immunobiology, Diagnosis, and Treatment of Pancreas Allograft Rejection. *Pancreas Transplantation* 2004, Gruessner RWG and and Sutherland DER Ed.:349–80.

111. Burke GW, Ciancio G, Cirocco R, et al.: Microangiopathy in kidney and simultaneous pancreas/kidney recipients treated with tacrolimus: evidence of endothelin and cytokine involvement. *Transplantation* 1999, 68:1336–42.

112. Matsukuma S, Suda K, Abe H: Histopathological study of pancreatic ischemic lesions induced by cholesterol emboli: fresh and subsequent features of pancreatic ischemia. *Hum Pathol* 1998, 29:41–6.

113. Eight Banff Conference on Allograft Pathology, 2005, Edmonton Canada.

114. Sibley RK, Sutherland DE, Goetz F, et al.: Recurrent diabetes mellitus in the pancreas iso- and allograft. A light and

electron microscopic and immunohistochemical analysis of four cases. *Lab Invest* 1985, 53:132–44.

115. Klassen DK, Drachenberg CB, Papadimitriou JC, et al.: CMV allograft pancreatitis: diagnosis, treatment, and histological features. *Transplantation* 2000, 69:1968–71.

116. Noronha IL, Oliveira SG, Tavares TS, et al.: Apoptosis in kidney and pancreas allograft biopsies. *Transplantation* 2005, 79:1231–5.

117. Boonstra JG, Wever PC, Laterveer JC, et al.: Apoptosis of acinar cells in pancreas allograft rejection. *Transplantation* 1997, 64:1211–3.

118. Henderson JR, Moss MC: A morphometric study of the endocrine and exocrine capillaries of the pancreas. *Q J Exp Physiol* 1985, 70:347–56.

119. Olsson R, Carlsson PO: The pancreatic islet endothelial cell: emerging roles in islet function and disease. *Int J Biochem Cell Biol* 2006, 38:492–7.

120. Wieczorek G, Bigaud M, Menninger K, et al.: Acute and chronic vascular rejection in nonhuman primate kidney transplantation. *Am J Transplant* 2006, 6:1285–96.

121. Bohmig GA, Regele H, Exner M, et al.: C4d-positive acute humoral renal allograft rejection: effective treatment by immunoadsorption. *J Am Soc Nephrol* 2001, 12:2482–9.

122. Nadasdy GM, Bott C, Cowden D, et al.: Comparative study for the detection of peritubular capillary C4d deposition in human renal allografts using different methodologies. *Hum Pathol* 2005, 36:1178–85.

123. Sharma S, Green KB: The pancreatic duct and its arterio-venous relationship: an underutilized aid in the diagnosis and distinction of pancreatic adenocarcinoma from pancreatic intraepithelial neoplasia. A study of 126 pancreatectomy specimens. *Am J Surg Pathol* 2004, 28:613–20.

124. Troppmann C, Gruessner AC, Benedetti E, et al.: Vascular graft thrombosis after pancreatic transplantation: univariate and multivariate operative and nonoperative risk factor analysis. *J Am Coll Surg* 1996, 182:285–316.

125. Troppmann C, Gruessner AC, Dunn DL, et al.: Surgical complications requiring early relaparotomy after pancreas transplantation: a multivariate risk factor and economic impact analysis of the cyclosporine era. *Ann Surg* 1998, 227:255–68.

126. Grewal HP, Garland L, Novak K, et al.: Risk factors for post-implantation pancreatitis and pancreatic thrombosis in pancreas transplant recipients. *Transplantation* 1993, 56:609–12.

127. Gruessner RW, Dunn DL, Gruessner AC, et al.: Recipient risk factors have an impact on technical failure and patient and graft survival rates in bladder-drained pancreas transplants. *Transplantation* 1994, 57:1598–606.

128. Gruessner RW, Troppmann C, Barrou B, et al.: Assessment of donor and recipient risk factors on pancreas transplant outcome. *Transplant Proc* 1994, 26:437–8.

129. Obermaier R, Benz S, Kortmann B, et al.: Ischemia/reperfusion-induced pancreatitis in rats: a new model of complete normothermic in situ ischemia of a pancreatic tail-segment. *Clin Exp Med* 2001, 1:51–9.

130. Schulak JA, Franklin WA, Stuart FP, et al.: Effect of warm ischemia on segmental pancreas transplantation in the rat. *Transplantation* 1983, 35:7–11.

131. Busing M, Hopt UT, Quacken M, et al.: Morphological studies of graft pancreatitis following pancreas transplantation. *Br J Surg* 1993, 80:1170–3.

132. Hesse UJ, Sutherland DE, Simmons RL, et al.: Intra-abdominal infections in pancreas transplant recipients. *Ann Surg* 1986, 203:153–62.

133. Patel BK, Garvin PJ, Aridge DL, et al.: Fluid collections developing after pancreatic transplantation: radiologic evaluation and intervention. *Radiology* 1991, 181:215–20.

134. Knight RJ, Bodian C, Rodriguez-Laiz G, et al.: Risk factors for intra-abdominal infection after pancreas transplantation. *Am J Surg* 2000, 179:99–102.

135. Hiatt JR, Fink AS, King W, 3rd, et al.: Percutaneous aspiration of peripancreatic fluid collections: a safe method to detect infection. *Surgery* 1987, 101:523–30.

136. Letourneau JG, Hunter DW, Crass JR, et al.: Percutaneous aspiration and drainage of abdominal fluid collections after pancreatic transplantation. *AJR Am J Roentgenol* 1988, 150:805–9.

137. Nobrega J, Halvorsen RA, Letourneau JG, et al.: Cystic central necrosis of transplanted pancreas. *Gastrointest Radiol* 1990, 15:202–4.

138. Fernandez-Cruz L, Sabater L, Gilabert R, et al.: Native and graft pancreatitis following combined pancreas-renal transplantation. *Br J Surg* 1993, 80:1429–32.

139. Humar A, Uknis M, Carlone-Jambor C, et al.: Cytomegalovirus disease recurrence after ganciclovir treatment in kidney and kidney-pancreas transplant recipients. *Transplantation* 1999, 67:94–7.

140. Ishibashi M, Bosshard S, Fukuuchi F, et al.: Incidence of CMV infection in simultaneous pancreas and kidney transplantation: comparative study of two surgical procedures of segmental pancreas versus whole bladder-drained pancreas. *Transplant Proc* 1996, 28:2859–60.

141. Keay S: CMV infection and disease in kidney and pancreas transplant recipients. *Transpl Infect Dis* 1999, 1 Suppl. 1: 19–24.

142. Lo A, Stratta RJ, Egidi MF, et al.: Patterns of cytomegalovirus infection in simultaneous kidney-pancreas transplant recipients receiving tacrolimus, mycophenolate mofetil, and prednisone with ganciclovir prophylaxis. *Transpl Infect Dis* 2001, 3:8–15.

143. Backman L, Brattstrom C, Reinholt FP, et al.: Development of intrapancreatic abscess – a consequence of CMV pancreatitis? *Transpl Int* 1991, 4:116–21.

144. Fernandez JA, Robles R, Ramirez P, et al.: Arterioenteric fistula due to cytomegalovirus infection after pancreas transplantation. *Transplantation* 2001, 72:966–8.

145. Drachenberg CB, Abruzzo LV, Klassen DK, et al.: Epstein-Barr virus-related posttransplantation lymphoproliferative disorder involving pancreas allografts: histological differential diagnosis from acute allograft rejection. *Hum Pathol* 1998, 29:569–77.

146. Heyny-von Haussen R, Klingel K, Riegel W, et al.: Post-transplant lymphoproliferative disorder in a kidney-pancreas transplanted recipient: simultaneous development of clonal lymphoid B-cell proliferation of host and donor origin. *Am J Surg Pathol* 2006, 30:900–5.

147. Keay S, Oldach D, Wiland A, et al.: Posttransplantation lymphoproliferative disorder associated with OKT3 and decreased antiviral prophylaxis in pancreas transplant recipients. *Clin Infect Dis* 1998, 26:596–600.

148. Rehbinder B, Wullstein C, Bechstein WO, et al.: Epstein-barr virus-associated posttransplant lymphoproliferative disorder of donor origin after simultaneous pancreas-kidney transplantation limited to pancreas allograft: a case report. *Am J Transplant* 2006, 6:2506–11.

149. Kroes AC, van der Pijl JW, van Tol MJ, et al.: Rapid occurrence of lymphoproliferative disease after pancreas-kidney transplantation performed during acute primary Epstein-Barr virus infection. *Clin Infect Dis* 1997, 24:339–43.

150. Paya CV, Fung JJ, Nalesnik MA, et al.: Epstein-Barr virus-induced posttransplant lymphoproliferative disorders. ASTS/ASTP EBV-PTLD Task Force and The Mayo Clinic Organized International Consensus Development Meeting. *Transplantation* 1999, 68:1517–25.

151. Dombrowski F, Klingmuller D, Pfeifer U: Insulinomas derived from hyperplastic intra-hepatic islet transplants. *Am J Pathol* 1998, 152:1025–38.

152. Petruzzo P, Andreelli F, McGregor B, et al.: Evidence of recurrent type I diabetes following HLA-mismatched pancreas transplantation. *Diabetes Metab* 2000, 26:215–8.

153. Ruiz P: Recurrence of Type 1 Diabetes in pancreas transplantation. *Ninth Banff Conference on Allograft Pathology* 2007.

154. Gong W, Liu ZH, Zeng CH, et al.: Amylin deposition in the kidney of patients with diabetic nephropathy. *Kidney Int* 2007, 72:213–8.

155. Bartlett ST, Schweitzer EJ, Kuo PC, et al.: Prevention of autoimmune islet allograft destruction by engraftment of donor T cells. *Transplantation* 1997, 63:299–303.

156. Braghi S, Bonifacio E, Secchi A, et al.: Modulation of humoral islet autoimmunity by pancreas allotransplantation influences allograft outcome in patients with type 1 diabetes. *Diabetes* 2000, 49:218–24.

157. Sibley RK: Morphologic features of chronic rejection in kidney and less commonly transplanted organs. *Clin Transplant* 1994, 8:293–8.

158. Hirano Y, Fujihira S, Ohara K, et al.: Morphological and functional changes of islets of Langerhans in FK506-treated rats. *Transplantation* 1992, 53:889–94.

159. Gruessner RW, Burke GW, Stratta R, et al.: A multicenter analysis of the first experience with FK506 for induction and rescue therapy after pancreas transplantation. *Transplantation* 1996, 61:261–73.

160. Dudek RW, Lawrence IE, Jr., Hill RS, et al.: Induction of islet cytodifferentiation by fetal mesenchyme in adult pancreatic ductal epithelium. *Diabetes* 1991, 40:1041–8.

161. Semakula C, Pambuccian S, Gruessner R, et al.: Clinical case seminar: hypoglycemia after pancreas transplantation: association with allograft nesidiodysplasia and expression of islet neogenesis-associated peptide. *J Clin Endocrinol Metab* 2002, 87:3548–54.

162. Esterl RM, Stratta RJ, Taylor RJ, et al.: Rejection with duodenal rupture after solitary pancreas transplantation: an unusual cause of severe hematuria. *Clin Transplant* 1995, 9:155–9.

163. Hakim NS, Gruessner AC, Papalois BE, et al.: Duodenal complications in bladder-drained pancreas transplantation. *Surgery* 1997, 121:618–24.

164. Rangel EB, Gonzalez AM, Linhares MM, et al.: Thrombotic microangiopathy after simultaneous pancreas-kidney transplantation. *Clin Transplant* 2007, 21:241–5.

165. Weinstein A, Dexter D, KuKuruga DL, et al.: Acute graft-versus-host disease in pancreas transplantation: a comparison of two case presentations and a review of the literature. *Transplantation* 2006, 82:127–31.

166. Gaber LW, Egidi MF, Lo A, et al.: Renal pathology and clinical presentations of polyomavirus nephropathy in simultaneous kidney pancreas transplant recipients compared with kidney transplant recipients. *Transplant Proc* 2004, 36:1095–6.

167. Papadimitriou JC, Cangro CB, Lustberg A, et al.: Histologic features of mycophenolate mofetil-related colitis: a graft-versus-host disease-like pattern. *Int J Surg Pathol* 2003, 11:295–302.

168. Mathur S, Squiers E, Tatum A, et al.: Adenovirus infection of the renal allograft with sparing of pancreas graft function in the recipient of a combined kidney-pancreas transplant. *Transplantation* 2000, 65(1):138–41.

169. Roza AM, Johnson C, Juckett M, et al.: Adenocarcinoma arising in a transplanted pancreas. *Transplantation* 2001, 72:1156–7.

CHAPTER 8

The Pathology of Intestinal and Multivisceral Transplantation

Phillip Ruiz, M.D., Ph.D.

Andreas Tzakis, M.D.

Hidenori Takahashi, M.D.

I. INTRODUCTION AND BACKGROUND

The past 20 years has witnessed an evolution in the area of intestinal and multivisceral transplantation such that these once rare procedures are now routinely employed in the therapy of intestinal failure (1,2). Enteral feeding remains a mainstay in the maintenance of persons with short gut syndrome; however, this therapy is incumbent with numerous and often life-threatening complications, high costs, and altered quality-of-life issues (3). By comparison, the successful implementation of an intestinal (ITx) or multivisceral (MVTx) transplant potentially allows the recipient a reacquisition of a functionary alimentary tract with minimal or no dietary restrictions, improved growth and development, and an opportunity for a more normal lifestyle (4). Of course, the introduction of an intestinal or multivisceral graft into a recipient represents a massive histoincompatible antigenic challenge to the host, with the gut containing a noteworthy lymphoid and nonlymphoid parenchymal cellular mass. As a result, ITx and MVTx, as with most other solid organ allografts, require significant and typically indefinite use of powerful immunosuppressive agents in order to maintain the viability of the grafts in the face of a sustained and vigorous immune-mediated attack from the host. The induction of such an immunosuppressed state places the recipient at high risk for infections and the development of malignancies; moreover, the drugs themselves often leave direct toxicities on several organ systems (e.g., renal, neurological) (5).

Nonetheless, successful implementation of ITX and MVTx has become more frequent with the advent of improved and constantly evolving immunosuppression, better surgical techniques, and enhanced clinical management (6,7). As well, our increased understanding of the mechanisms involved in intestinal graft rejection (see Chapter 1) has allowed the design of interventional protocols that often now protect the recipient and graft from immunologically based injury. There are a variety of underlying conditions with compromised gut function resulting in "short gut syndrome" that has been treated with intestinal or multivisceral transplantation. The main failure in these particular circumstances is a loss of the absorptive function of the intestines, ultimately resulting in malnourishment of the recipient. Some of these conditions are listed in Table 8.1 (8). Pediatric and adult patients are each treated by this procedure, and the disorders compromising gut function are often conspicuously different according to the age group (Table 8.1). A majority of these patients are maintained by enteral feeding prior to transplantation.

A variety of animal models utilizing orthotopic and heterotopic gut transplantation have been studied and have been instrumental in helping to improve the procedures and therapies in a clinical situation (9). The experience gained in these models has helped identify complications that can occur at all levels as well as the effectiveness of immunosuppressive therapies and refinement of surgical techniques. The surgical procedures utilized in intestinal and multivisceral transplantation have evolved and been refined over the past three decades from when these surgeries were first attempted (4,7). Pretransplant donor and recipient screening procedures as well as post-transplant immunosuppression protocols have likewise improved. All of these variables, along with a fundamental increased knowledge base of gut physiology and immunology, have greatly contributed to improved graft and patient survival. However, ITx and MVTx, while significantly improved, remain frequently susceptible to a variety of complications, some that are listed in Table 8.2.

Monitoring of intestinal graft function and patient status has evolved over the past two decades and the pathologist, whether by biopsy evaluation or coordination of laboratory analysis, can play a central role in the clinical team's vigilance of post-transplant complications (10–12). In this regard, the field of transplant pathology as it pertains to gastrointestinal (GI) transplantation has evolved into a discipline that combines traditional histological examination with clinical laboratory support and evolving molecular techniques.

The surgical implementation of an intestinal allograft can be performed as an isolated graft or as part of an abdominal organ bloc that can include stomach, small and large intestine, liver, pancreas and spleen (the latter scenario known as multivisceral transplantation). Providing an isolated intestine (ITx) or multivisceral graft

TABLE 8.1 Primary Diseases of Patients Receiving Intestinal or Multivisceral Transplants*

Disease	%
Pediatric	
Gastroschisis	22
Volvulus	17
Necrotizing enterocolitis	12
Psuedoobstruction	9
Intestinal atresia	8
Aganglionosis/hirschsprung	7
Retransplant	7
Microvillous inclusion	6
Other causes	4
Malabsorption	3
Short gut other	3
Tumor	1
Other	1
Adult	
Ischemia	25
Crohn's disease	13
Trauma	9
Short gut other	9
Volvulus	8
Motility	8
Desmoids	8
Retransplant	6
Miscellaneous	6
Other tumor	5
Gardner's syndrome	3

* Experience described from the Small Bowel Transplant Registry.

TABLE 8.2 List of Potential Complications after Intestinal Transplantation

Complications
    Acute rejection
    Chronic rejection
    Infection
    PTLD
    GVHD
    Renal dysfunction
    Pancreatitis
    Bowel perforation
    Anastomotic leakage
    Others

(MVTx) depends upon the underlying pathological conditions compromising gut function in the recipient. In recent years, the use of MVTx has increased with graft and patient survival being comparable to isolated intestinal transplantation (4,7). From the pathologist's perspective, the use of MVTx requires that there be an expanded knowledge of surgical allografts not typically encountered or discussed (i.e., stomach, colon) and an awareness of likelihood of pathological changes depending upon which area of alimentary tract is sampled (e.g., duodenal versus ileal). These patients have an exteriorized ostomy through which endoscopy is often performed—typically, biopsies obtained from the ostomy site are not as useful in evaluating graft function due to nonspecific inflammatory processes and distorted histological architecture, thus they are discouraged.

II. HISTOPATHOLOGICAL EVALUATIONS

Histopathological evaluation of allografts and medical laboratory support are critical to all stages of clinical intestinal and multivisceral transplantation, including the pretransplant phases and continuously through the evaluation and maintenance of long-term surviving grafts. The great majority of tissue samples taken from selected regions of ITx and MVTx allografts are visualized by endoscopy and sampling of mucosal areas is the norm. Biopsies from intestinal and gastric allografts are technically obtained in a fashion similar to biopsies from the native organ counterparts. It is important that the endoscopist have some experience with GI transplants in order to determine which regions to biopsy and that there be communication with the pathologist regarding the type of changes seen in the mucosa. Submucosal areas of allografts are only evaluated when there is surgical revision of problematic areas or when grafts are explanted to be replaced. As with biopsies obtained from any transplanted organ, it is imperative that the transplant pathologist have a reasonable clinical history of the recipient (e.g., date of transplant, native disease or problem that necessitated the transplantation, current clinical symptoms), what were the previous biopsy results (if any), and as mentioned above, an impression of the endoscopic appearance of the organ. Biopsies should be noted from which area they are taken such as lesional, perilesional, and noninvolved areas since there can be a gamut of different histological changes between adjacent regions. A majority of the problems affecting GI transplants are urgent and could rapidly lead to allograft dysfunction and potential graft loss. Thus, processing and evaluation of allograft biopsies should be as expeditious as possible and available seven days a week.

One or two fragments per area should be placed immediately in an appropriate fixative (typically buffered formalin) and should remain for at least one hour before processing. The paraffin sections are typically cut at 0.5 cm and multiple levels are encouraged since processes such as rejection may be focal and not diffusely distributed. Hematoxylin and eosin (H&E) stains are used for the initial evaluation. The histology laboratory should be capable of performing special stains, immunohistochemical stains (e.g., to infectious agents such as cytomegalovirus [CMV], adenovirus), and in situ hybridization techniques for viruses such as Epstein-Barr virus (EBV); it is useful to have a molecular pathology laboratory that can perform viral load measurements (e.g., to EBV) and that can measure antigen receptor rearrangement studies for T and B cells when evaluating the possibility of post-transplant lymphoproliferative disease (PTLD).

III. DONOR ORGANS AND PRESERVATION INJURY

The field of small bowel and multivisceral transplantation, as with other solid organ allografts, is continuously refining organ procurement methodologies and surgical techniques to help address the continual shortage of suitable donors and to allow for more organs to be used. However, unlike other allografts such as kidney and liver in which pretransplant biopsies are obtained when there is a questionable clinical history or the organ appears grossly suspicious, it is not typical that the pathologist is asked to evaluate a donor bowel or stomach prior to being transplanted. Clinical history of the donor, gross appearance, and size of the recipient abdominal cavity (e.g., pediatric age) usually screen the majority of the donor candidates for any potential problems. The pathologist often does examine residual donor tissue left from the operation and in our experience there have not been any significant pathological changes aside from minimal ischemic injury, as would be expected from graft preservation.

Transplantation of organs necessitates that there be a preservation of organs in cold solutions followed by a warm reperfusion of the grafts upon vascular anastomosis with the recipient blood supply. Following implantation and revascularization of the donor organs, there often is some degree of preservation-associated or ischemia reperfusion (I/R) injury to the allograft. Physiologically, the gut may respond by a reduction in motility and this may be the result of an inflammatory response throughout the bowel instigated by the reduced blood flow to the organ (13). In the large majority of the cases, these I/R changes are mild and have no considerable consequence to the organ's short-term function, although there may be significant effects on the allograft organ's eventual susceptibility to immune-mediated injury and physiological operation (14). Moreover, there is now increasing evidence that cadaveric organs, even obtained under the most optimal conditions and histologically unremarkable, are not transcriptionally silent. For example, cadaveric organs can show a marked increase in several groups of genes associated with inflammation and transport after harvesting (15). The implication of these changes remains unknown and currently bowel allografts have not been extensively studied; however, it remains possible that these changes in the harvested organs likely impact long-term graft function. With the shortage now experienced in the donor pool, there has been an increase in the number of "marginal" donors (e.g., grafts from older donors or donation following cardiac death) used as a source of transplanted organs. These suboptimal sources of organs are more susceptible to I/R injury, and there is an increased incidence of primary nonfunction or delayed graft function and complications such as rejection (15–19).

Morphology: Mucosal biopsies obtained in the early post-transplant period are the ones that characteristically demonstrate preservation injury changes (12,20). In small bowel and colon, these changes in a case of mild preservation injury include diffuse edema and swelling of the villi without a significant increase in the inflammatory cell infiltrate, some vascular congestion, and a separation of the surface epithelial lining from the underlying lamina propria (Figures 8.1 and 8.2). More severe I/R injury shows additional changes such as epithelial cell necrosis that can extend from the surface of the mucosa to the deep submucosa. Experimental models of I/R injury in rats demonstrate transmural necrosis of the small intestine

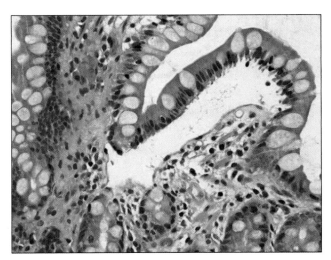

FIGURE 8.1: *Preservation injury (original magnification 200×, H&E): small intestinal biopsy several days after transplant shows swelling of the villi without a significant increase in the inflammatory cell infiltrate, some vascular congestion, and a separation of the surface epithelial lining from the underlying lamina propria.*

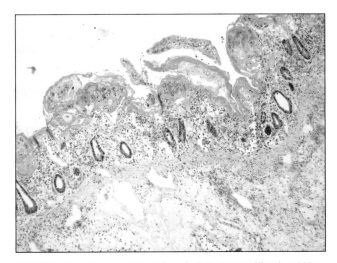

FIGURE 8.2: *Preservation injury (original magnification 100×, H&E): example of more severe I/R injury with epithelial cell necrosis, extending from the surface of the mucosa to the deep submucosa.*

(21); clinical correlates with these latter changes are uncommon but can be evident when there is I/R injury along with prolonged vascular compromise (Figure 8.3). In the latter scenario, the allograft tissues show ischemic changes similar to bowel ischemia in native organs. At this point, we are not aware of the effects of I/R injury to GI transplants to enduring organ function and survival, and no pathognomonic changes are yet known in long-standing allografts that had early I/R injury. To date, there is little experience with morphology of stomach allografts undergoing I/R injury.

IV. ACUTE REJECTION

The detection and effective treatment of acute rejection in recipients of small bowel and multivisceral transplants is a continuous challenge that clinicians face to achieve successful long-term function of the grafted organs. Despite the implementation of potent immunosuppressive drugs that have altered the natural history, severity, and frequency of allograft acute rejection, this immune-based response by the host to the graft remains as the most important complication in GI transplantation (Table 8.2). The mechanisms involved in cell-mediated and humoral-based forms of acute rejection are similar to other organ systems (22,23) and are discussed in a previous chapter (see chapter 1). Essentially, T cells and B cells originating from the host, along with natural killer cells and macrophages, are centrally important in the genesis and culmination of immunological pathways that recognize the allogeneic small bowel (22,24,25). The targets in bowel for immune effector cells are numerous and include enterocytes and their progenitors, vascular endothelial cells, muscle, and neural cells. Injury or death of these various cell populations leads to the consequences clinically manifested in allograft rejection of the bowel such as

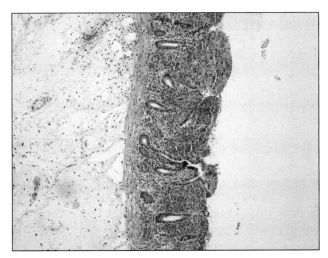

FIGURE 8.3: *Preservation injury (original magnification 40×, H&E): I/R injury along with prolonged vascular compromise.*

malabsorption, dysmotility, and ischemia (4,7). Due to the large antigenic mass present in the GI allograft, acute rejection of the bowel can progress rapidly if untreated, ultimately leading to the dreaded complications of exfoliative severe rejection and translocation of luminal bacteria, the latter scenario evolving to sepsis. It thus becomes imperative that diagnosing acute rejection in small bowel and multivisceral transplantation be done expeditiously and accurately since the clinical consequences are ominous if rejection continues unabated in the host. As with other biopsies of GI allografts, there should be clinical and endoscopic correlation when considering the potential diagnosis of acute rejection. Itx or MVTx patients undergoing acute rejection can display a constellation of symptoms that can include increased fecal output (early on from their stoma), fever, and swelling; these symptoms are not specific and other processes such as infection can also induce similar effects. In this regard, the biopsy can be crucial in distinguishing these processes. The phenomenon of *subclinical rejection* (SCR) has been described in several other transplants including liver (26,27) and kidney (28,29). By definition, SCR is the situation where a biopsy displays the morphological characteristics associated with acute rejection in the absence of clinical symptoms (30). Therefore, this is usually picked up when biopsies are taken as part of protocol surveillance and the patients are clinically stable. Currently, many investigators feel that SCR is potentially an important entity since patients with it can have a higher rate of eventual graft loss (e.g., kidney) (29,31) and some protocols are now addressing whether or not to treat cases of SCR with additional immunosuppression (32). In addition, transcriptional information from these cases shows similar sets of genes as compared to acutely rejecting grafts. We have recently described SCR in small bowel allografts (33) and found it to be at a high frequency when considering the total number of biopsies in our experience. These cases of SCR were discovered in biopsies taken during protocol surveillance when patients were clinically quiescent and displayed most often changes compatible with grade 1 acute rejection. Interestingly, patients experiencing SCR in bowel allografts had a higher rate of eventual graft loss (33). Future studies will address whether to treat these patients and how protocol surveillance biopsies should be performed and at what frequency in the post-transplant period.

Less invasive approaches than biopsy for diagnosing intragraft acute rejection (e.g., immunophenotypical analysis of peripheral T lymphocytes, serum and urine levels of numerous cytokines) (34–37) as of yet have not gained clinical popularity due to a lack of optimal specificity and sensitivity. The amino acid *citrulline* appears to represent a specific marker of intestinal mass (38,39) and serial measurements of peripheral blood levels of this analyte (beginning three months after transplantation) appear to be able to discriminate whether or not there is injury

occurring in the allograft (40–42). However, specificity in detecting acute (or chronic) rejection with citrulline alone does not appear possible; future algorithms with other markers of inflammation may yield more diagnostic specificity to the use of citrulline. Currently, histopathological examination of GI allograft biopsies remains as the most reliable and definitive method to diagnose rejection.

Morphology: The spectrum of histopathological findings associated with acute rejection in post transplant biopsies is wide (10–12) and sometimes related to the time elapsed after the transplant. As with other organ allografts, the classification of acute rejection in small bowel and multivisceral transplantation utilizes terms that originate from basic immunology (hyperacute rejection, accelerated acute rejection, acute vascular rejection [AVR], etc.) but which may not reflect the histopathological findings observed in the tissue specimen.

i. Hyperacute and Accelerated Acute Rejection

Hyperacute and accelerated acute rejection are terms that describe the uncommon clinical setting in which an allograft organ is severely rejected within minutes to hours (*hyperacute rejection*) or a few days (*accelerated acute rejection*) following implantation. It has been demonstrated that this phenomenon occurs in the presensitized patient and is secondary to a severe humoral response (antibody mediated) in which the vasculature is the main target and vascular injury, thrombosis, and ischemic lesions characterize it histologically. Experimental evidence of these forms of rejection in bowel allografts exist (43) but documented clinical cases of hyperacute rejection in small bowel transplants are not commonly encountered. In this regard, a completion of cross-matching of recipient sera with donor cells before GI transplantation has not been the norm but this may be changing since we (manuscript in press) and others (personal communication, University of Pittsburgh) have found hyperacute rejection episodes in bowel associated with the presence of pretransplant donor-specific antibodies. In our case, the donor graft upon anastomosis immediately turned dusky in color and hyperemic, resembling changes seen in other solid organ grafts experiencing hyperacute rejection. Morphologically, there was extensive mucosal congestion and necrosis with neutrophils and margination around vessels. The congestion extended into the submucosa and was not present on the preimplantation biopsy. Native tissue was unremarkable. Remarkably, these patients have the capacity to overcome this severe form of humoral acute rejection if there is appropriate intervention with plasmapheresis, treatment with anti-CD20 antibody (among other immunosuppression) and close monitoring. Our patient with hyperacute rejection displayed a full recovery (normal graft morphology and asymptomatic) that coincided with decreasing titers of anti-donor antibodies and normal endoscopic appearance). However, as mentioned, we are now considering implementation of cross-match information being completed before the GI transplant based on this recent experience.

We have also found rare instances of an accelerated AVR that occurred in the first several days following small bowel transplantation in which there was presensitization with alloantibody and which morphologically demonstrated features of AVR described below, but not to the degree seen for hyperacute rejection.

ii. Acute Vascular (Humoral) Rejection

AVR in human small bowel and multivisceral transplantation is an entity whose frequency and severity have typically not been well understood. It is generally accepted that antibodies directed to alloantigens (i.e., humoral response), initiates the sequelae associated with AVR (44,45), depending upon the type and level of the antibody, as well as the type of transplant scenario. However, the cell-mediated arm of the immune response (T-cell–mediated vasculitis) can also be an underlying cause of vasculitis in bowel allograft vessels (46–49), thus, distinguishing the etiology of this form of rejection cannot be done without adjunct techniques and information. Severe forms of AVR in small bowel transplants have been described (50) and are often associated with alloantibody post transplant sensitization of the recipient to donor antigens and subsequent rises in titers of pretransplant antibodies that were present at very low amounts before the transplant. The graft demonstrates extensive inflammatory changes with the principal lesion being *vasculitis* of large to small arterial branches (Figures 8.4 and 8.5). The morphology of this vasculitis tends to be an infiltration of the intimal layer of the artery by a mixture of acute and chronic inflammatory cells, with

subintimal edema and endothelial injury. C4d may be present in these vessels (Figure 8.6) but there may be cell-mediated immune processes also participating in this lesion. The vasculitis progresses with transmural inflammation and fibrin deposition; left unchecked, this process can evolve into necrosis of the artery with severe ischemic injury to the graft. For unknown reasons, severe vasculitis

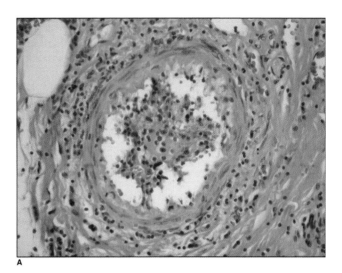

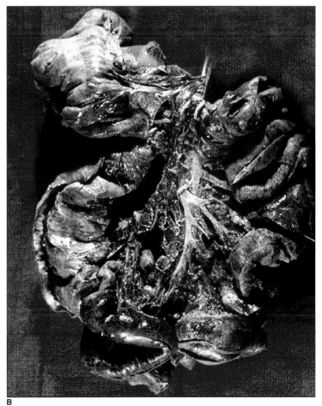

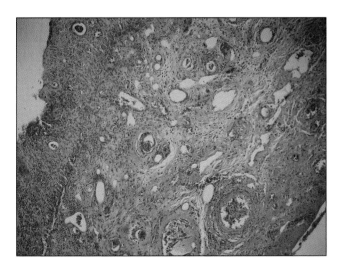

FIGURE 8.4: *AVR (original magnification 100×, H&E): The intestinal allograft showed loss of crypts and diffuse fibrosis in lamina propria and submucosa. Medium- to large-sized vessels showed severe vasculitis. These findings indicated moderate to severe AVR with concurrent chronic rejection.*

FIGURE 8.5: *AVR (A: original magnification 200×, H&E): severe vasculitis in medium- to large-sized vessels. (B) Gross photomicrograph of bowel explant with segmental necrosis secondary to mesenteric artery thrombus, formed as a result of vascular rejection.*

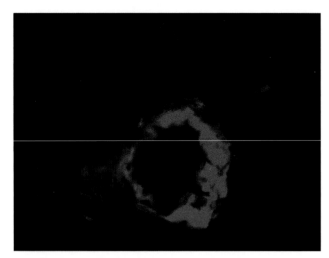

FIGURE 8.6: AVR (original magnification 400×, immunofluorescence staining for C4d): immunofluorescence staining of a small bowel allograft suspected to have AVR shows positive staining of C4d in the microvasculature of the mucosa.

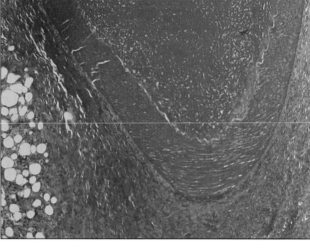

FIGURE 8.7: AVR (original magnification 100×, H&E): example of sclerosing mesenteritis. Medium- to large-sized vessels are effaced from an intense fibrinoid necrosis.

can occasionally involve selective arteries in the graft more severely than others. For example, mesenteric arteries can undergo vascular rejection in some patients and this can lead to *sclerosing mesenteritis* (Figures 8.7 and 8.8) (51). This latter phenomenon is uncommon but when encountered in ITx and MVTx, alloantibody measurements in the recipient should be performed, along with immunohisto-chemical staining for T cells and other inflammatory cell populations. Stomach and colon allografts can demon-strate the severe vasculitis patterns as seen in the small bowel but as implied above; there can be notable differ-ences in the severity and distribution of vascular lesions according to the site of the allografts (52). The differential diagnosis for this form of severe vasculitis only involving the transplant includes infectious agents (such as fungal or viral agents), therefore, special stains and cultures should also be performed. Other causes of vasculitis such as drugs, cancer, autoimmune processes are not typically causative in these allografts and would be distributed in native organs and not limited to the allograft.

For the pathologist, large vessel vasculitis is not encountered in mucosal biopsies but is identified in explants or rejected organs or autopsies. Table 8.3 shows our grading system for vasculitis lesions during AVR in small bowel transplants (comment: a similar grading scheme has not been developed for stomach or colon allografts). As noted above, extensive necrosis of the graft and eventual loss of the transplant can be the result with this form of AVR. However, less severe forms of AVR can also occur in small bowel transplants and at a higher frequency than previously believed. In this regard, we have characterized changes identifying early, mild or evolving AVR that can occur isolated or in con-junction with cell-mediated acute rejection (53). The

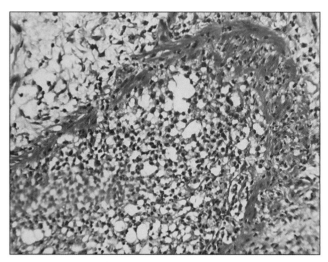

FIGURE 8.8: AVR (original magnification 200×, H&E): section of mesentery showing large artery with transmural vasculitis.

morphological changes can occur in the mucosa and appear associated in many cases with preexisting or de novo alloantibody formation. These changes can occur at any point in the life of the allograft, but most partic-ularly in the early stages. The pathological changes occur in the microvasculature of the bowel mucosa and can range from mild vascular congestion in a small portion of the biopsy to diffuse, significant congestion and eryth-rocyte extravasation (Figures 8.9 and 8.10. see scoring system, Table 8.4). The villous region and lamina pro-pria are the areas principally involved with these changes, and while the smaller vessels are principally affected, there may be no evidence of any significant vasculitis. There may or may not be any significant increase in chronic inflammatory cells and usually there is interstitial

TABLE 8.3 Vasculitis Lesions in AVR

Grade	Histopathological Findings	
0	No inflammatory changes	
1	Mild inflammatory changes	Rare vessels with adherent inflammatory cells and no evidence of necrosis or fibrin deposition
2	Moderate inflammatory changes	>50% of vessels showing inflammatory changes but no evidence of necrosis or transmural inflammation
3	Severe inflammatory changes	Transmural inflammation with necrosis and fibrin deposition

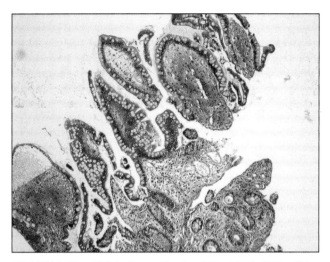

FIGURE 8.10: *(Original magnification 200×, H&E): AVR, mild. Patient with positive cross-match and clinical evidence of rejection. Mild nonspecific inflammatory changes but marked congestion of the microvasculature with erythrocyte extravasation.*

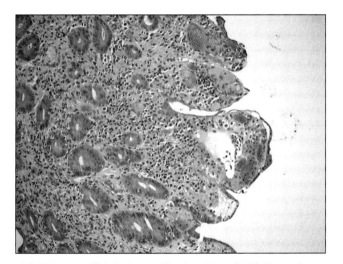

FIGURE 8.9: *(Original magnification 100×, H&E): Example of indeterminate for acute rejection with vascular component. Significant congestion and erythrocyte extravasation in villi are present.*

TABLE 8.4 Scoring System for the Evaluation of Microvascular Changes during AVR in GI Allograft Mucosal Biopsies

Grade	Histopathological Findings*
0	No significant congestion or extravasation
1	10–40% of the tissue shows changes
2	40–70% of the tissue shows changes
3	70% or greater portion of the tissues shows changes

* Capillaries, small venous and arterial branches in the lamina propria and the submucosa are evaluated for the presence of dilatation and erythrocyte congestion. In addition, the surrounding interstitium is assessed for the presence of extravasated erythrocytes and edema. Scoring is calculated and based on the percentage of the overall biopsy.

edema but preservation of epithelial structures. These milder forms of AVR are similar in colon allografts; no literature or published experience for stomach allografts is currently available.

Typically, supplementary tests are not performed for evaluation of humoral based forms of acute rejection. If the humoral rejection is suspected or was previously diagnosed we have solicited additional tissue to be placed in appropriate preservative media such as Michel's or Zeus fixative; this tissue is then evaluated by an immunofluorescence panel for the presence of immunoglobulins (IgG, IgA, IgM) and complement components (C3, C4, C4d, C1q), fibrinogen and other immunoreactants as needed. We have found immunoglobulins to be deposited along vessels and within interstitium along with complement components. As in other transplanted organs undergoing humoral rejection (54) there can be deposition of C4d in vessels; we have found C4d in small arteries and small capillaries in patients with acute humoral rejection (Figure 8.11) (53). At this point, there is no strict correlation with C4d staining since many cases with humoral rejection have not had the immunofluorescence evaluation. Immunoperoxidase staining for C4d using a polyclonal antibody has been tried in our lab and others with the advantage being that formalin-fixed paraffin-embedded biopsy material can be used. Successful staining is possible but in our hands this technique is not yet optimized for bowel so that immunofluorescence still appears more sensitive. These more subtle forms of AVR are not specific histopathological findings and can be found in ischemia, nonspecific enteritis, viral infections and mechanical vascular problems. Therefore, it is necessary to incorporate the clinical history and lab values (e.g., anti-donor antibody titers), lesion distribution (allograft versus native tissue), other morphological

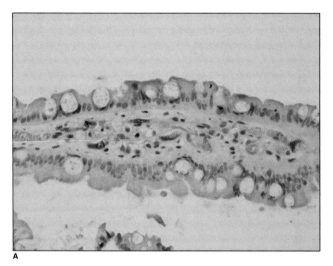
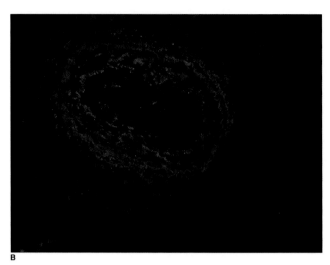

FIGURE 8.11 *AVR (A: original magnification 200×, immunohistochemistry): immunoperoxidase staining for C4d appears positive in capillary in the villi. (B: original magnification 200×) immunofluorescent staining for C3 appears positive in the vessels.*

findings (e.g., the presence of an acute inflammatory cell infiltrate or superficial epithelial changes with enteritis) and culture results. Moreover, there should be correlation of symptom and pathology resolution with increased immunosuppression along with lowering of antibody levels.

iii. Acute Cellular Rejection

Acute cellular rejection (ACR) is the most common form of acute rejection in small bowel, stomach, and colon transplants and may be present simultaneously with AVR, infections, or other complications. This form of rejection is primarily the consequence of the recipient's T-cell–mediated response to donor alloantigens (55,56) and is represented by a predominant lymphocyte-rich chronic inflammatory cell infiltrate that is distributed within the interstitial regions of the organs and that injures specific tissue elements. In the bowel and stomach, these elements are principally cells within crypts, glandular structures and lining the surface epithelium; however, muscle, endothelial and nerve cells may also be affected. These target cells upon being attacked by the host effector immune response can be affected functionally with little morphological change, they can become reactive or undergo metaplastic changes (particularly in stomach) or they may undergo apoptosis. If there is sufficient cell death and there is also vascular compromise from the alloimmune response to the vessels, then there may be extensive necrosis. Detailed molecular mechanisms of ACR remain unclear but it is clearly a multifactorial process in which both CD4+ and CD8+ T cells are involved (57), analogous to other forms of allograft rejection. One of the main features in ACR in intestinal allografts is *crypt epithelial cell apoptosis*. It appears that CD8+ cytotoxic T cells induce target cell apoptosis through two distinct mechanisms, the granzyme B/Perforin-dependent granule-exocytosis path-

way and Fas and Fas ligand–mediated cytotoxicity, and both processes are involved in ACR in the intestinal allograft (57–60). In this regard, upregulation of granzyme B and perforin mRNA expression is a possible marker for ACR and antibody-mediated rejection (59–61). Interestingly, even in the absence of CD8+ T cells, crypt epithelial cell apoptosis and acute allograft rejection can occur in animal experimental models (57,58), implying that there may be additional mechanisms that cause ACR in the intestinal allograft.

As with other solid organ allografts (62,63), it has been recognized that there is a benefit to grading acute rejection in GI transplantation. A majority of the classification systems that have been employed involve small bowel transplants since that is the greatest experience of different centers to date. A classification system for stomach has been developed at the University of Miami (64) but no formal one for colon is as yet utilized. In 2003 at the Eighth International Small Bowel Transplant Symposium, an international group of pathologists and clinicians experienced in small bowel transplant morphology met to derive a unified grading scheme for ACR in small bowel allografts (Table 8.5) (10). This scheme is now widely used and has been employed at our institution for greater than 2,500 biopsies. To date, there appears to be good correlation between the morphological grading system and the clinical symptoms displayed by the recipient. Initial interobserver studies between different institutions (unpublished data) has been very good. However, as mentioned above, cases of clinically silent (subclinical) rejection do occur.

It is critical that the evaluating pathologist be very familiar with the normal histological changes present in different regions of the small intestine since there are often only subtle changes present in the early stages of ACR or when there is ACR in the face of significant immunosuppression such as Campath (alemtuzmab) induction therapy (65–67).

TABLE 8.5 Characteristics of ACR in Small Intestinal Allograft

Grade	Score	Description	Histopathological Findings
0	0	No evidence of acute rejection	Unremarkable histological changes that are essentially similar to normal native intestine.
IND	1	Indeterminate for acute rejection	A minor amount of epithelial cell injury or destruction; increase in crypt epithelial cell apoptosis, but with less than six apoptotic bodies per 10 crypts; increased inflammatory infiltrate in lamina propria, mixed but primarily mononuclear inflammatory population; edema, blunting, vascular congestion can be present.
1	2	ACR, mild	Altered mucosal architecture (e.g., mild blunting of villi), edema, vascular congestion; increased crypt epithelial cell apoptosis (six or more apoptotic bodies per 10 crypts); increased inflammatory infiltrate in lamina propria, mixed but primarily mononuclear inflammatory population with blastic and activated lymphocytes.
2	3	ACR, moderate	Features of grade 1 as well as multiple markedly increased crypt epithelial cell apoptoses (six or more apoptotic bodies per 10 crypts), accompanied by foci of "confluent apoptosis"; whole gland necrosis, and/or crypt abscess; extensively increased inflammatory infiltrate in lamina propria, mixed but primarily mononuclear inflammatory population with blastic and activated lymphocytes; edema, vascular congestion, and blunting of villi of higher degree of grade 1.
3	4	ACR, severe	Extensive morphological distortion and crypt damage with apoptosis, gland destruction, and associated mucosal ulceration; marked diffuse inflammatory infiltrate with blastic and activated lymphocytes, eosinophils, and neutrophils; granulation tissue and/or fibropurulent exudate with mucosal sloughing (exfoliative rejection).

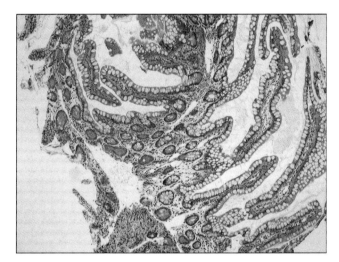

FIGURE 8.12: *No evidence of acute rejection (original magnification 200×, H&E): biopsy of a small bowel allograft seven days after transplantation and following induction with CAMPATH-1 immunosuppression therapy. There is no evidence of any significant alterations associated with acute rejection. Overall, the hematopoietic cell composition is less than seen with other immunosuppressive therapy.*

a. No Evidence of Acute Rejection, Grade 0

This grade is applied when there is histomorphology that is indistinguishable from normal bowel or if the bowel represents histological alterations that are definitely separate from those due to ACR (Figure 8.12).

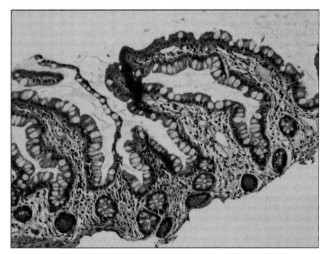

FIGURE 8.13: *Indeterminate for acute rejection (original magnification 100×, H&E): there is an increased inflammatory infiltrate within the interstitium that is composed of lymphocytes, eosinophils, immunoblasts, some plasma cells, and occasional neutrophils along with mild blunting of villi.*

b. Indeterminate for Acute Rejection, Grade IND

This grade can be seen at any stage including the early or resolving stages of ACR where there is a minor amount of epithelial cell injury or destruction but yet there is an increased inflammatory infiltrate within the interstitium that is composed of lymphocytes, eosinophils, immunoblasts, some plasma cells, and occasional neutrophils (Figures 8.13 and 8.14). The proportions of these cell types

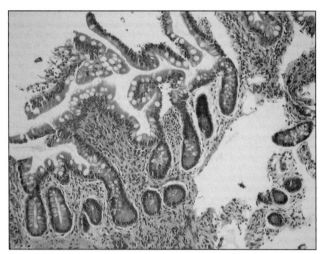

FIGURE 8.14: *Indeterminate for acute rejection (original magnification 200×, H&E): patient several months after transplantation who had clinical evidence of acute rejection. Morphology was suggestive of an ensuing acute rejection and there was early deposition of collagen in the lamina propria.*

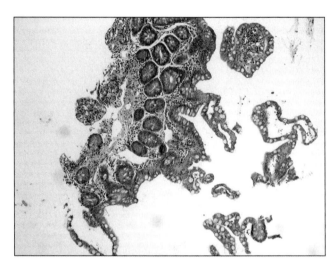

FIGURE 8.16: *ACR, mild (original magnification 40×, H&E): mild blunting of villi and mild intensity of inflammatory infiltrate are present.*

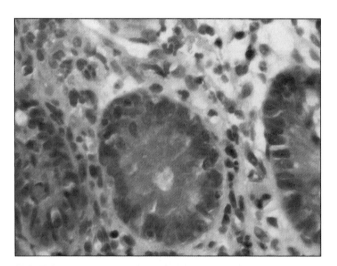

FIGURE 8.15: *Indeterminate for acute rejection (original magnification 400×, H&E): example of eosinophil-rich process.*

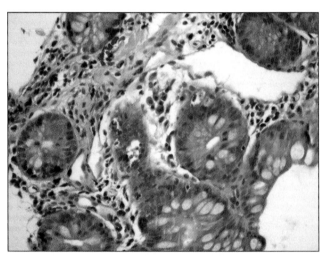

FIGURE 8.17: *ACR, mild (original magnification 200×, H&E): mixed inflammatory infiltrate and several apoptotic bodies are seen in crypts (less than six apoptotic bodies in ten crypts).*

varies (e.g., there may be an eosinophil-rich infiltrate) (Figure 8.15) but the intensity is clearly increased above normal and can be diffuse or localized. The intensity of the infiltrate may change according to the time after transplantation. Edema, blunting, and vascular congestion are occasionally present but these features are not necessary for the diagnosis. Crypts are infiltrated by the lymphocytes or eosinophils (cryptitis) and apoptotic bodies are present in the epithelial lining. However, the number of apoptotic bodies does not reach the level designated for grade 1 (mild) ACR.

c. ACR, Mild, Grade 1

The International Grading Scheme utilizes six apoptotic bodies or above per ten crypts as the cutoff for mild

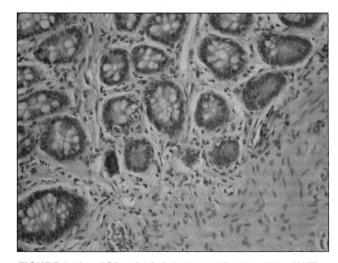

FIGURE 8.18: *ACR, mild (original magnification 400×, H&E): example of crypt epithelial cell apoptosis.*

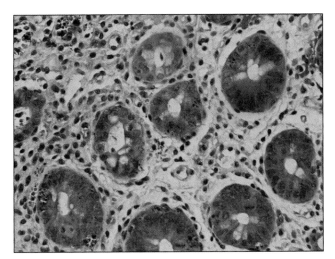

FIGURE 8.19: *ACR, mild (original magnification 200×, H&E): mixed inflammatory infiltrate marked edema and several apoptotic bodies are seen in crypts (less than six apoptotic bodies in ten crypts).*

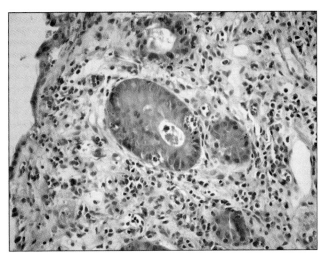

FIGURE 8.21: *ACR, moderate (original magnification 400×, H&E): multiple apoptotic bodies in crypt (more than six apoptotic bodies per ten crypts) with some "confluent apoptosis" seen. Nature of inflammatory infiltrate is mixed but predominantly mononuclear inflammatory population, including blastic or activated lymphocytes.*

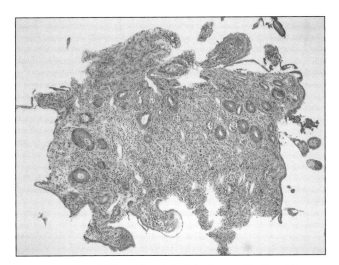

FIGURE 8.20: *ACR, moderate (original magnification 40×, H&E): significant mucosal alterations, blunting of villi, and vascular congestion are present with the higher degree than with grade 1 rejection. Moderate inflammatory infiltrate in lamina propria with focal edema and decreased number of crypts are also seen.*

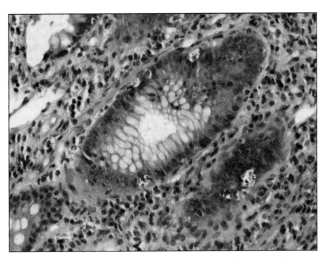

FIGURE 8.22: *ACR, moderate (original magnification 400×, H&E): example of multiple "confluent apoptosis" in crypts. Inflammatory infiltrate in lamina propria is dense in intensity and predominantly mononuclear inflammatory population with eosinophil component.*

ACR. There is typically edema, congestion, and altered architecture such as blunting of villi. In ACR, mild (grade 1), the crypt cell injury, inflammation, and all the other changes listed above are present but at higher levels than grade IND, including the level of apoptosis (Figures 8.16–8.19). The infiltrate is often diffusely distributed, mild to moderate in intensity, and tends to extend deeper within the submucosa and can involve muscle. These features are variable since the character and intensity of the infiltrate may change according to the time after transplantation. There may also be regen-

erative features such as mucin loss, epithelial cell nuclear enlargement, and hyperchromasia. Vascular congestion and endothelialitis are often present concomitantly with this and higher forms of ACR.

d. ACR, Moderate, Grade 2

In ACR, moderate (grade 2), there are the features of mild ACR but with heightened crypt cell injury including multiple apoptotic bodies in single crypts that are sometimes confluent (Figures 8.20–8.26). In some instances, there

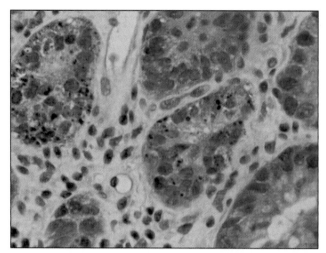

FIGURE 8.23: ACR, moderate (original magnification 400×, H&E): extended crypt cell injury with multiple apoptotic bodies.

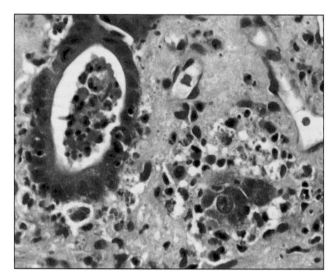

FIGURE 8.25: ACR, moderate (original magnification 100×, H&E).

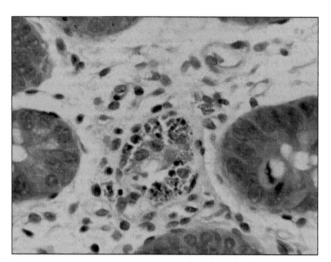

FIGURE 8.24: ACR, moderate (original magnification 400×, H&E): example of whole gland necrosis with multiple crypt epithelial cell apoptosis.

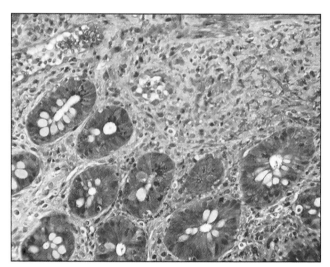

FIGURE 8.26: ACR, moderate (original magnification 400×, H&E): example of ACR, moderate with superimposed chronic rejection. Mucosal atrophy, loss of crypts, and increase of fibrosis in submucosal layer and lamina propria are seen. Multiple apoptotic bodies in crypts with focal "confluent apoptosis" are present.

may be whole gland necrosis and crypt abscesses can be evident (Figure 8.24). The inflammatory infiltrate in the lamina propria and submucosa is typically more intense than with mild ACR with the nature of the infiltrate being typically mixed but being predominantly a mononuclear inflammatory cell population, including blastic or activated lymphocytes and mucosal architectural alteration tends to be significant. The intensity of the infiltrate is often moderate to severe and is less affected by the time after transplantation. Edema, blunting of villi and vascular congestion tend to be more extensive with the higher degree than with grade 1 rejection.

e. ACR, Severe, Grade 3

ACR, severe (grade 3) is a not uncommon and potentially devastating form of ACR. There is pervasive crypt cell

injury and apoptosis, gland destruction, and related mucosal ulceration (Figures 8.27–8.30). The level of crypt epithelial apoptosis is variable; in fact, there may be an unimpressive level of apoptosis among the surviving crypts. There is a marked diffuse inflammatory infiltrate with blastic or activated lymphocytes, eosinophils, and neutrophils. Extended severe rejection typically results in complete loss of the bowel morphological architecture, and there may be predominantly granulation tissue and/ or fibropurulent (pseudomembranous) exudate, with mucosal sloughing. The endoscopist often finds the tissue friable and thus fragments of tissue with significant architectural alterations are obtained. Mucosal ulceration in the absence of active crypt cell injury should not be classified

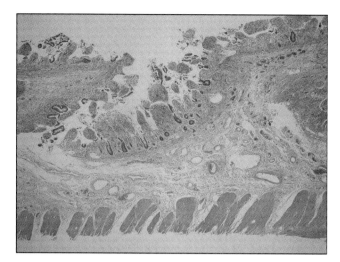

FIGURE 8.27: *ACR, severe (original magnification 40×, H&E): Extensive morphological distortions with marked diffuse inflammatory infiltrate are present. Severe blunting of villi with epithelial cell dropout is seen.*

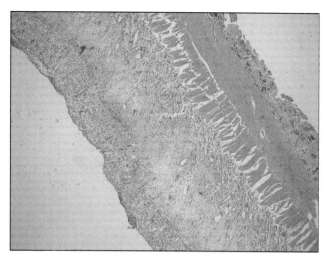

FIGURE 8.29: *ACR, severe (original magnification 40×, H&E): extensive loss of mucosa and crypts and replacement by granulation tissue consistent with severe "exfoliative rejection."*

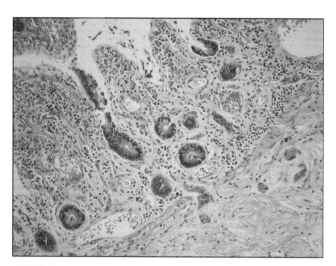

FIGURE 8.28: *ACR, severe (original magnification 100×, H&E): severe mucosal atrophy, loss of crypts, vascular congestion, and extravasation is accompanied by marked diffuse inflammatory infiltrate with blastic and activated lymphocytes, eosinophils, and occasional neutrophils. The level of apoptosis among the surviving crypts is not so impressive.*

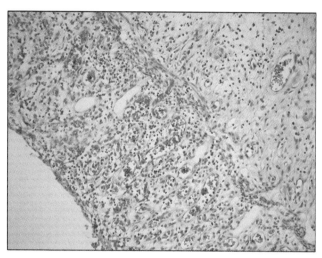

FIGURE 8.30: *ACR, severe (original magnification 200×, H&E): mucosal architecture is extensively distorted and replaced by granulation tissue. The evaluation of crypt epithelial cell apoptosis is difficult because of complete loss of crypts. Dense inflammatory infiltrate is seen which consists of mixed but predominantly mononuclear cell population with blastic and activated lymphocytes, eosinophils, and neutrophils.*

as grade 3 ACR but rather "consistent with ACR, severe" since ischemic and infectious processes can also lead to mucosal necrosis. This most extensive form of severe rejection with essentially only necrotic tissue has also been called "*exfoliative rejection*" (68,69). It is very useful with this grade of rejection to have tissue obtained from areas that grossly appear less involved. Animal models of intestinal transplantation most often demonstrate features of acute severe rejection (Figure 8.31).

Within the small bowel, certain regions appear to be more susceptible to ACR; in particular, the ileum displays ACR more frequently and often more intensely than biop-

sies obtained simultaneously from duodenum or jejunum (70). This typically correlates with endoscopic findings.

ACR can lead to intestinal graft loss as well as severe infectious complications as a consequence of the heavy immunosuppression to treat ACR; *bacterial translocation* can result from mucosal barrier impairment (71–73). Intestinal epithelial cells, intercellular tight junctions, and basement membranes play an important role in maintaining the barrier function of mucosa in intestinal graft. Alterations of intercellular tight junction structure have been reported during ACR which, along with epithelial cell injury, may be a cause of bacterial translocation (71).

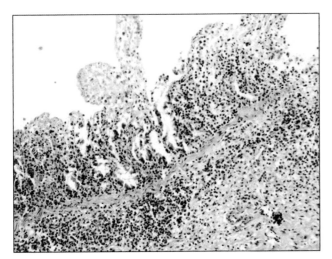

FIGURE 8.31: ACR in porcine intestinal allograft (original magnification 40×, H&E): extensive loss of mucosa and crypts and replacement by granulation tissue consistent with severe "exfoliative rejection."

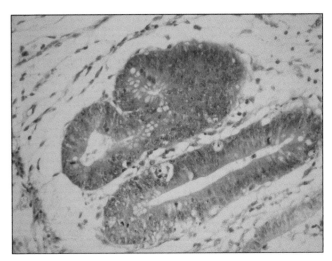

FIGURE 8.33: ACR in colonic allograft (original magnification 400×, H&E): multiple apoptotic bodies in crypt with "confluent apoptosis" are present.

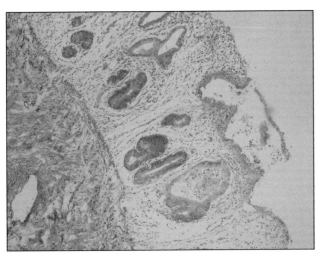

FIGURE 8.32: ACR in colonic allograft (original magnification 100×, H&E): example of ACR, moderate in colonic allograft. Extensive architectural distortion with marked edema and increased number of apoptotic bodies in crypt is seen.

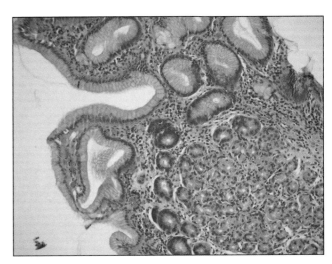

FIGURE 8.34: ACR in gastric allograft (original magnification 100×, H&E): example of ACR, mild in gastric allograft. Mild architectural disarray and significant increase of inflammatory infiltrate are present. Mild vascular congestion and extravasation are also seen.

iv. ACR in Colon and Stomach

ACR in colon allograft shows very similar changes (Figures 8.32 and 8.33) as seen with small intestine although experience with this organ is much less than with small bowel. The colon displays the same pattern and composition of the inflammatory cell infiltrate and there is a linear increase in the form of epithelial cell injury in crypts similar to small bowel. Surface architecture is more difficult to assess than in small bowel but there is often goblet cell loss and attenuation of the thickness of the surface epithelial cells. No grading system has been devised and at this point; we employ the same criteria in colon as we use in small intestine. There

is often native colon present in multivisceral transplant patients so that biopsying native and allograft simultaneously can be useful to the pathologist in distinguishing alloreactive versus other inflammatory processes.

In the stomach, there can be ACR in all regions of this organ (Figures 8.34 and 8.35). It is important to distinguish ACR in the stomach from other inflammatory processes such as various forms of chronic gastritis and infectious processes. As with small bowel and colon allografts, epithelial injury in the form of apoptosis and reactive changes are necessary components in order to identify ACR. In general, the degree of inflammation during acute rejection in the stomach is reduced compared to

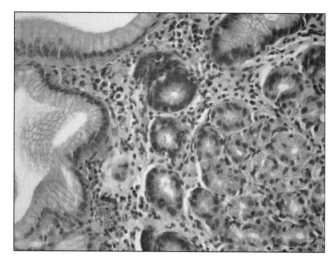

FIGURE 8.35: *ACR in gastric allograft (original magnification 400×, H&E): several crypt epithelial cell apoptotic bodies and mixed inflammatory infiltrate with microvascular congestion is present.*

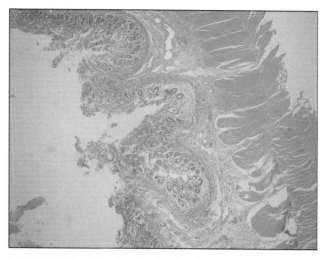

FIGURE 8.36: *Chronic rejection (original magnification 40×, H&E): example of explanted case of chronic rejection. Severe fibrosis in the lamina propria and submucosa with loss of crypts is present.*

TABLE 8.6 Characteristics of ACR in Gastric Allograft

Grade	Description	Histopathological Findings
0	No evidence of acute rejection	Absent to very minimal inflammatory infiltrate, normal cytology and architecture (glandular structures arranged back to back).
IND	Indeterminate for acute rejection	Scattered mixed inflammatory infiltrate, edema, or focal congestion; normal architecture; normal cytology; and no increased apoptotic bodies.
1	ACR, mild	Increased inflammation and apoptotic bodies, mild cytological atypia, and mild architectural disarray.
2	ACR, moderate	Prominent mixed inflammatory infiltrate, increased cytological atypia, vacuolization of parietal cells, erosion or ulceration of the surface epithelium, major architectural disarray, and increased or confluent apoptotic bodies.
3	ACR, severe	Significant distortion of the architecture with subtotal destruction of the gland and gastric pits, accompanied by ulceration.

intestine; thus, the pathologist should be cognizant that corresponding grades of acute rejection in stomach do not demonstrate the same level of inflammation and epithelial injury as in small bowel. For example, mild acute

rejection in stomach has a lower amount of inflammation and crypt apoptosis than seen in the small intestine (74). We have seen many exceptions where gastric rejection is solitary or exceeds the grades of rejection in other regions of the small bowel or colon. One useful approach to evaluating stomach allograft pathology is to score individual morphological features using a grading scheme that generates a numerical score to provide different levels of ACR (Table 8.6) (64).

V. CHRONIC REJECTION

As graft survival steadily improves in small bowel transplantation, there has been an increasing incidence of chronic allograft enteropathy (CAE) and it is becoming one of the principal causes of late graft loss in ITx and MVTx (75–77). As with other solid organ allografts, this entity is likely the result of several immune and nonimmune factors (see chapter 1). Clinical symptoms for CAE are nonspecific (e.g., protein losing enteropathy) but endoscopic information such as flattening can be very useful in correlating the pathological findings. Explanted bowels with chronic rejection (Figure 8.36) grossly show a transmural diffusely distributed thickening with an irregular flattened mucosal surface and occasional ulcerations. Serosal adhesions are abundant and generally the organ bloc is severely matted together. The pathognomonic lesion of bowel chronic rejection is similar to other transplanted organs, namely medium and large arteries with concentric intimal thickening with fibrous changes, medial hypertrophy of smooth muscle cells interspersed with foam cells, and adventitial fibrosis (Figures 8.37–8.41). Occasional thrombi in the arterial vessels at various stages can be sometimes seen along with

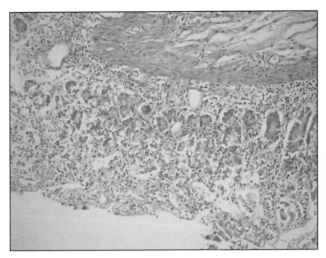

FIGURE 8.37: *Chronic rejection (original magnification 200×, H&E): marked architectural distortion and glandular atrophy are present.*

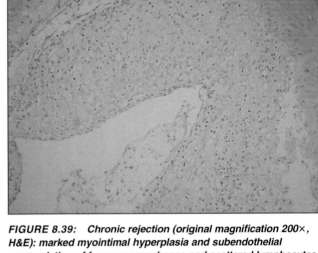

FIGURE 8.39: *Chronic rejection (original magnification 200×, H&E): marked myointimal hyperplasia and subendothelial accumulation of foamy macrophages and scattered lymphocytes are seen in obliterateive arteriopathy in large-sized vessel.*

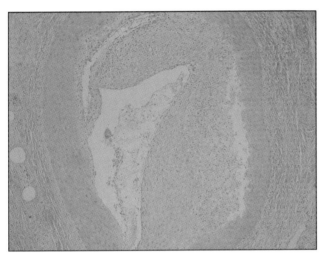

FIGURE 8.38: *Chronic rejection (original magnification 100×, H&E): Obliterative arteriopathy in a branch of superior mesenteric artery. Marked myointimal hyperplasia and subendothelial accumulation of foamy macrophages are present.*

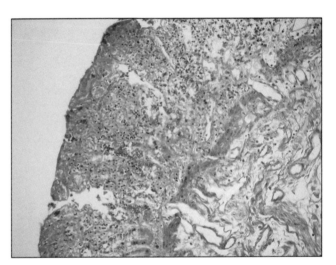

FIGURE 8.40: *Chronic rejection (original magnification 200×, trichrome stain): trichrome stain shows marked fibrosis in submucosa and lamina propria.*

occasional chronic inflammatory cells within the intimal space; the latter can be distinguished from the vigorous, fibrinous, and acutely destructive lesions of severe AVR. The mucosa shows a significant alteration in the architecture with variable fibrosis that extends into the submucosal and muscular layers, crypt loss, crypt separation, villous blunting, mucosal atrophy, and small arterial branches with evidence of transplant arteriopathy. Within the deeper layers there can be ganglion cell destruction and hyperplasia and the serosa is markedly thickened with extensive fibrinoid material. Chronic inflammatory cell infiltrates are irregularly distributed and there may be ulceration and superimposed acute rejection.

Mucosal biopsies of small bowel are typically limiting in being able to demonstrate the large vessel changes of chronic rejection since these arteries are not usually present in endoscopic biopsies. Despite this, mucosal biopsies from bowel with CAE can be very helpful in identifying the mucosal chronic injury (e.g., fibrosis, crypt loss and distortion, altered architecture) and thus with the clinical and endoscopic history provide a reasonable suspicion for chronic rejection. Multiple samples are encouraged since there is fluctuation in the degree of changes with this form of rejection. We have developed a scoring system for the mucosal biopsy evaluation of chronic rejection (Table 8.7) that incorporates semiquantitative assessment of several features seen with this entity. To date, immunohistochemical analysis of chronic rejection in GI allografts has not provided any increased level of specificity in the identification or prognostication of this serious complication.

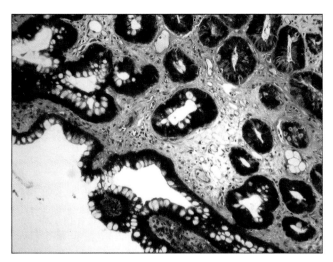

FIGURE 8.41: *Chronic rejection (original magnification 200×, trichrome stain): biopsy sample from small intestinal allograft showing moderate mucosal fibrosis and distortion of the epithelial architecture by the connective tissue deposition.*

TABLE 8.7 Semiquantitative Grading Schema for Mucosal Fibrosis

Grade	Description	Histopathological Findings
0	No fibrosis	No significant number of collagen fibers
1	Minimal fibrosis	Very few although readily visible collagen fibers
2	Mild fibrosis	Few collagen fibers arranged in bundle with preservation of the glandular architecture
3	Moderate fibrosis	Fibrous tissue in the lamina propria with decreased number of glands
4	Severe fibrosis	Areas devoid of glands and replaced by fibrous tissue

VI. INFECTIONS

Among the serious adverse effects associated with immunosuppression includes the appearance of opportunistic infections in the host. Patients with Itx and MVTx are subjected to extensive immunosuppression and often develop systemic infectious complications as well as infections that can often involve the GI allograft in the form of *infectious gastritis, enteritis or colitis* (note: the changes associated with infectious gastritis and colitis are similar to ones present in native tissue, and beyond the scope of this

chapter. *Infectious enteritis* will be addressed in this chapter since it is very common in bowel transplantation and can cause significant challenges in its identification from ACR in the small bowel). In bowel transplants, there are a number of pathogens that can emerge, potentially compromising graft function and placing the host at risk of death if the infection is not appropriately identified and treated. Many of these infectious agents can cause infectious enteritis with clinical symptoms mimicking acute rejection (e.g., diarrhea, fever) and that must be distinguished by culture and/or biopsy appearance since their treatment (e.g., decreasing immunosuppression) is typically opposite than what is initiated for rejection. The pathologist should be aware that there can be concomitant acute rejection during any of these infectious causes of enteritis. The incidence of infectious enteritis in small bowel transplant patients can be significant in our experience with the most common pathogens being viruses. A number of viruses can involve the bowel allograft (78) and are recognizable by characteristic morphological changes and confirmed by immunohistochemical, culture, or molecular techniques. Among these viruses are rotavirus, adenovirus, calicivirus (human calicivirus: HuCV), CMV, herpes simplex virus (HSV), and EBV. As in native bowel, the presence of these viruses is accompanied by an enteritis that is composed of a mixed acute and chronic inflammatory cell infiltrate with some epithelial damage and often disorderly cell proliferation and cytological changes. Necrosis may be focally present in more severe cases. Concomitant acute rejection may be present and in fact some of these viruses may show some changes that can be attributable to acute rejection; thus, it remains important that the transplant pathologist consider the patient's clinical history and microbiology results when looking at the slides. Molecular identification of these agents from tissue is emerging as an important adjunct to identifying infectious enteritis.

i. Rotavirus

Rotavirus is a common complication in the general pediatric population and likewise can complicate bowel transplant patients. There is little information as to the specific histopathological alterations that this virus displays in the small intestine since a great majority of the cases are diagnosed by the use of a rapid microbiology assay (78). Some experimental studies have shown superficial hyperplastic changes in the epithelium; our experience shows that in addition to this change, there can be a mixed inflammatory infiltrate near the surface, with occasional neutrophils and cell debris. The deeper crypts are not typically affected and do not show the epithelial injury ascribed to acute rejection. As with all other infectious enteritis causes, there can be coexistence of acute rejection and rotaviral infections.

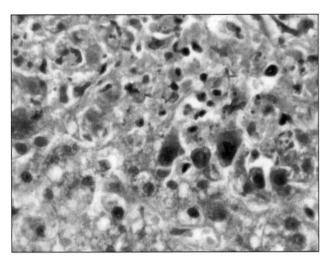

FIGURE 8.42: *Adenovirus enteritis (original magnification 400×, H&E): adenovirus inclusion bodies in small bowel allograft.*

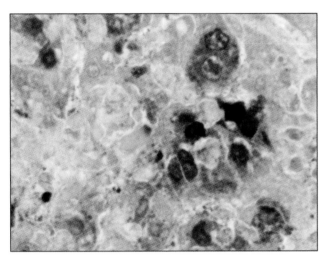

FIGURE 8.43: *Adenovirus enteritis (original magnification 400×, immunohistochemistry): immunostain demonstrating adenovirus positive cells.*

ii. Adenovirus

Adenovirus infection can be a challenging and dangerous infection for bowel transplant patients. We and others have previously reported infection with this virus during intestinal transplantation (79–81). Many of the histopathological changes that present with adenovirus infection can also be evident in acute rejection (Figures 8.42 and 8.43), namely crypt cell apoptosis and a mixed chronic inflammatory cell infiltrate with disarray of the surface epithelial cells associated with the presence of enlarged, often hyperchromatic cells. In addition, there can be eosinophilic nuclear inclusions as well as "smudge cells" with enlarged basophilic nuclei and proliferation of surface enterocytes. Immunostains and viral PCR assays (of tissue) for this virus are very useful and almost essential to help identify the presence of this pathogen; electron micro-

scopy, while helpful, involves a labor intensive effort that can be negative depending upon the location of the sampling. It is sometimes confusing to distinguish adenovirus enteritis from ACR because the histopathological features of both processes share some overlapping features. However, exact and rapid diagnosis of adenovirus enteritis is quite important because without proper treatment the clinical condition of patients tend to deteriorate quickly.

iii. Calicivirus

Calicivirus (HuCV) is a common cause of mild gastroenteritis in the general population (82). There are two groups of pathogenic HuCV: Norwalk-like virus and Sapporo virus. HuCV is usually detected by RT-PCR in fecal specimens (82). Clinical manifestations of this virus infection in small intestinal transplant recipients are mainly prolonged high-volume diarrhea (83,84). The information of histopathological alterations in the small intestinal transplant setting is quite limited, but several characteristic features have been reported (83,84); blunting and flattening of villi, mixed lymphoplasmacytic infiltrate with a small number of neutrophils in lamina propria, disarray and reactive changes of the superficial epithelium with loss of cellular polarity, increased apoptosis in the superficial epithelium and in the crypts, as well as in macrophages in the superficial portion of the lamina propria.

iv. Cytomegalovirus

Human CMV infection is common in small intestinal transplant recipients (78). Clinical manifestations of CMV enteritis include diarrhea, epigastric pain, and abdominal discomfort (85). Multiple erosions and superficial ulcers are found commonly in stomach and less often in small intestine by endoscopic examination (86). Microscopically, a chronic inflammatory infiltrate, composed of lymphocytes and histiocytes, with neutrophils is observed in the lamina propria in various severities (Figures 8.44 and 8.45). Characteristic large CMV-infected cells are observed which exhibit eosinophilic intranuclear inclusions surrounded by a clear halo and thickened nuclear membrane. Intranuclear inclusions are seen in endothelial, stromal, smooth muscle, and less often epithelial cells (85). The number of intranuclear inclusions varies in each case. Isolated intranuclear inclusions are sometimes hidden in dense chronic inflammatory infiltrates and hard to identify. Immunohistochemical staining for CMV and PCR assay of tissues for CMV are helpful to confirm the diagnosis of CMV enteritis (78,85].

v. Herpes Simplex Virus

Although HSV infection is commonly seen in immunocompromised patients, such as transplant recipients, patients with malignancy and AIDS, with most frequent sites of involvement being oral cavity, esophagus, perianum,

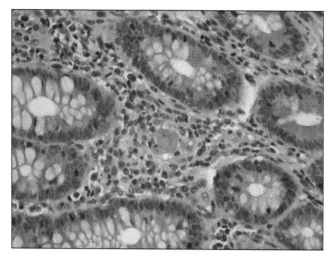

FIGURE 8.44: *CMV enteritis (original magnification 200×, H&E): CMV inclusion bodies in small bowel allograft.*

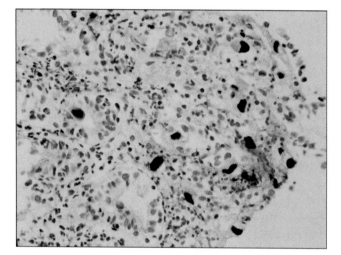

FIGURE 8.45: *CMV enteritis. (original magnification 400×, Immunohistochemistry): Immunostain demonstrating CMV: positive cell in bowel allograft.*

and rectum, HSV enteritis is relatively rare in small intestinal transplant recipients (87). In endoscopic examination, mucosal erythema and friability, aphthous and necrotic ulcers, and inflammatory pseudopolypoid lesions are commonly observed. Microscopically, there are nonspecific inflammatory changes, primarily composed of lymphoplasmacytic component with scattered eosinophils, in lamina propria (Figure 8.46). The presence of eosinophilic intranuclear inclusion and multinucleation of epithelial cells indicates HSV enteritis. Culturing of the biopsy sample is useful to confirm the diagnosis of HSV enteritis (87).

Typically, CMV and EBV disease including PTLD (discussed below) have been a common occurrence after ITx (1,2,4,7). By contrast, the incidence of CMV and EBV *acute* infection is low in our patient population as is the incidence of graft loss from these viruses or the development of PTLD (88,89). We attribute this to an aggressive protocol that involves both prophylactic and preemptive therapies directed against these viruses (90).

At times there may be some bacterial overgrowth in bowel allografts (as compared to the density of the normal flora) and the pathologist should communicate this information. Among potentially important bacterial infections in bowel allografts are *atypical mycobacteria* that can cause significant graft dysfunction (91). We have also observed several fungal and parasitic pathogens, including *Candida* and *cryptosporidium* (Figures 8.47 and 8.48) that are in the GI tract and which can involve the allograft (92).

VII. RECURRENT DISEASE AND OTHER ENTITIES

Although rare, there are occasionally patients whose original systemic or intestinal disease has the potential to recur in the bowel allograft. For example, patients with inflammatory bowel disease (e.g., Crohn's) may show reinvolvement of the bowel and this may be evident in

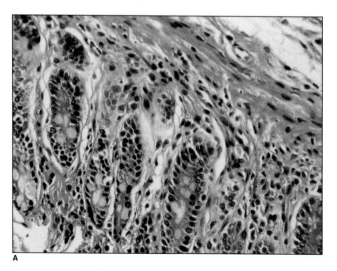

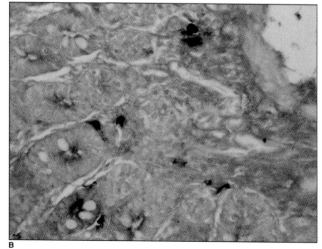

FIGURE 8.46: *Herpes simplex enteritis (HSV) (A: original magnification 200×, H&E): HSV inclusion bodies in small bowel allograft. (B: original magnification 200×, immunohistochemistry): immunostain demonstrating HSV positive cell in small bowel allograft.*

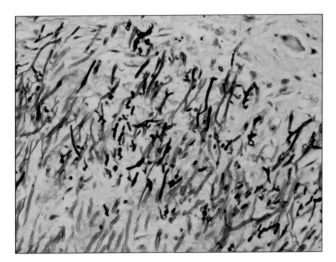

FIGURE 8.47: *Candida (original magnification 200×, H&E): candidal yeast forms in small bowel allograft.*

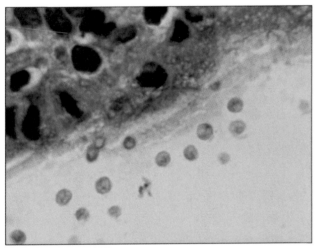

FIGURE 8.48: *Cryptosporidium (original magnification 400×, H&E): cryptosporidial organisms along mucosa of small bowel allograft.*

the mucosal biopsies (93–95). Recently, intestinal and multivisceral transplantation has been performed on patients with catastrophic intra-abdominal neoplastic diseases regardless of the nature of neoplastic disease, benign or malignant (96). Following surgical resection of those neoplasms, there may be tumor recurrence after transplantation. The recurrences of those neoplasms are usually intra-abdominal but may also occur outside the GI tract or extra peritoneal space; it is rare to find these tumors in the endoscopical biopsies.

Persistent ulcers (Figure 8.49) are a frequent problem in the later course of some Itx and MVTx patients. We have found that they can involve graft, native GI tissue, or both. In this regard, it appears that PTLD is the most common cause of these ulcers with positive EBV staining and molecular T/B antigen receptor rearrangement studies being crucial in helping to identify the underlying cause (97) Other causes of persistent ulcers include smoldering acute rejection, infections and some cases that remain of undetermined etiology.

In our experience, the most common etiologies of inflammation in the intestinal allograft are due to an alloimmune reaction between recipient and donor and active/chronic infectious process, each with characteristic morphological and immunohistochemical alterations. However, numerous miscellaneous inflammatory conditions can affect the small intestinal allograft as with native small intestine. *Active enteritis of undetermined etiology* is sometimes observed in the small intestinal mucosa taken by protocol surveillance or by clinical indication. Histopathological findings are characterized by acute inflammation, for example, polymorphic neutrophil infiltration, in lamina propria and/or surface epithelium with focal ulceration and crypt abscess, occurring on a background of chronic inflammation (Figures 8.50 and 8.51). The histopathological assessment of this active enteritis in small intestinal allograft

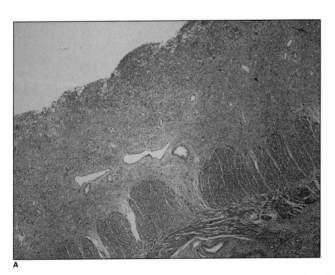

A

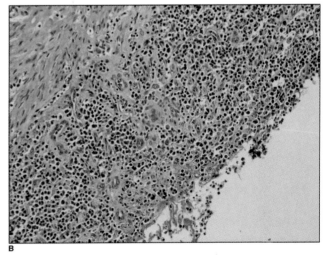

B

FIGURE 8.49: *Intestinal ulcers (A: original magnification 40×, B: original magnification 200×, H&E): persistent ulcer in small bowel allograft.*

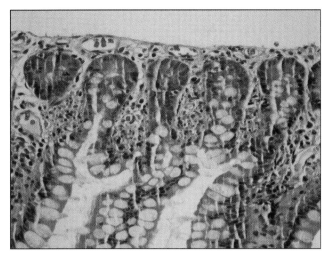

FIGURE 8.50: *Active enteritis in intestinal allograft (original magnification 100×, H&E).*

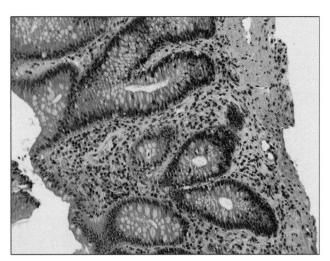

FIGURE 8.52: *Regenerative changes in intestinal allograft (original magnification 100×, H&E): changes similar to regenerative changes seen in native bowel that include branching, hyperplastic glands with reduced inflammation.*

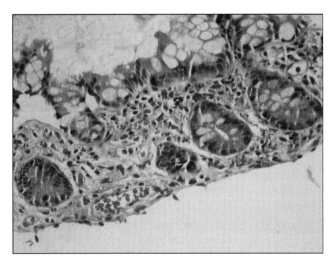

FIGURE 8.51: *Active enteritis in intestinal allograft (original magnification 100×, H&E).*

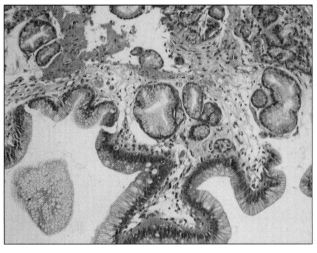

FIGURE 8.53: *Regenerative changes in intestinal allograft (original magnification 200×, H&E): changes similar to regenerative changes seen in native bowel that include branching, hyperplastic glands with reduced inflammation. Metaplastic changes are also present.*

has not been well documented because of a lack of uniformity and definition. However, several potential pathogenic mechanisms of this entity are envisioned, considering the possible counterpart in native small intestine, such as *pouchitis* in an ileal reservoir (98), "*backwash ileitis*" in ulcerative colitis (99), and *indeterminate enteritis/colitis* (100): these include stasis, changes in the bacterial flora of the intestinal mucosa, mucosal ischemia, mucosal prolapse, mucolysis, and mucosal pathology as a result of a lack of small intestinal or colonic nutrients. Moreover, a recent report suggested that Crohn's disease–associated polymorphism in the NOD2 gene, which was considered to play an important role in the maintenance of innate immunity in intestinal mucosa, were observed more frequently in intestinal recipients, and were associated with increased inflammatory infiltrate in intestinal mucosa and lower graft survival (101). Future investigation of alteration and reconstruction of innate immunity in association with inflammation in transplanted intestinal mucosa will enhance the understanding of pathophysiology in intestinal transplantation.

Regenerative changes are often evident in bowel allograft biopsies because of healing from protracted acute rejection or infectious enteritis, or after ischemic injury. The bowel allograft displays changes similar to regenerative changes seen in native bowel that include branching, hyperplastic glands with reduced inflammation (Figure 8.52), and metaplastic changes (Figure 8.53).

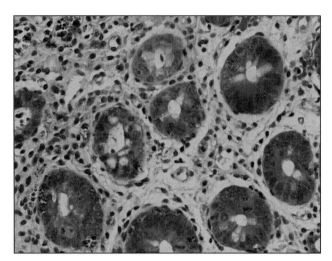

FIGURE 8.54: GVHD in native colon of patient with small intestinal allograft (original magnification 200×, H&E).

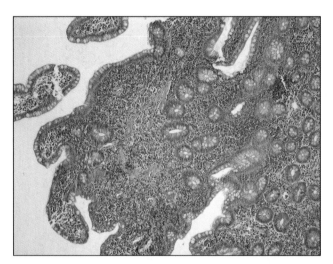

FIGURE 8.55: PTLD (original magnification 40×, H&E): example of possible early PTLD. Moderate lymphoplasmacytic infiltrate with indeterminate for acute rejection is present.

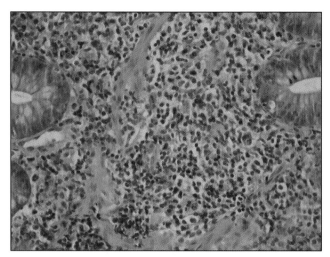

FIGURE 8.56: PTLD (original magnification 400×, H&E): example of possible early PTLD. Moderate lymphoplasmacytic infiltrate with indeterminate for acute rejection is present. Inflammatory infiltrate mainly consists of lymphoplasmacytic population along with eosinophil component. Gene rearrangement studies for T- and B-cell antigen receptors of this specimen suggested no B-cell rearrangement.

allograft or native), in order to diagnose GVHD. It is very important to share the clinical information of patients and obtained tissue samples with endoscopists.

VIII. POST-TRANSPLANT LYMPHOPROLIFERATIVE DISEASE

An additional consequence of the intense immunosuppression needed in small bowel transplantation is the increased incidence of several types of spontaneous neoplasms and development of direct organ toxicity by the immunosuppressive agent. These latter entities are typically manifested by involvement in organs other than small bowel and have been extensively reviewed (98,99). However, the development of PTLD is a frequent and critical complication in ITx and MVTx that often does demonstrate involvement of the allograft and hence must be recognized. PTLD can be present in a notable proportion of small bowel transplant recipients with the risk increasing as the time post-transplant increases. The majority (80 percent) of PTLD is associated with EBV infection that can cause polyclonal or monoclonal B-cell proliferation and, rarely, T-cell proliferation. The etiology of EBV-negative PTLD is not known but tends to occur later than EBV-positive PTLD. A majority of the PTLD in bowel allografts is of host origin. In calcineurin inhibitor–based immunosuppressive regimens (as used at our transplant center), PTLD tends to involve lymph nodes and the GI tract, as well as bone marrow, liver, and lungs.

There are a variety of morphological possibilities with PTLD in the bowel that range from plasmacytic hyperplasia (PH) (early lesion) to polymorphic PTLD

As with other types of organ transplantation, *graft-versus-host disease* (GVHD) can occur after intestinal transplantation (1,2,4,7,12). The GVHD occurring in Itx or MVTx patients can show the characteristic involvement seen in other patients with GVHD, including skin, GI tract and other systems (see chapter 9). Generally, there remains some part of *native* GI tract, such as native colon or rectum, in recipients after intestinal transplantation, which can be involved by GVHD. Histopathological features of GVHD in GI tract are very similar to those of ACR (Figure 8.54); increased crypt epithelial cell apoptosis and inflammatory infiltrate with a tendency for fewer apoptotic bodies and more intense inflammatory infiltrate in GVHD than in ACR (details described in other chapters) (12). Pathologists need to be aware of the clinical history and origin of the tissue sample (whether from

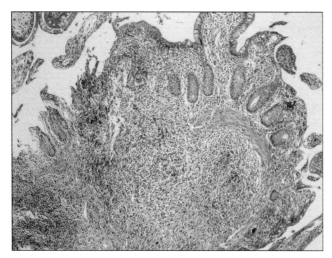

FIGURE 8.57: *PTLD (original magnification 40×, H&E). Expansile mild lymphoplasmacytic infiltrate with indeterminate for acute rejection.*

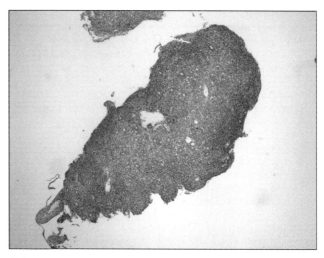

FIGURE 8.59: *PTLD (original magnification 40×, H&E). Example of malignant lymphoma (PTLD), large B-cell type.*

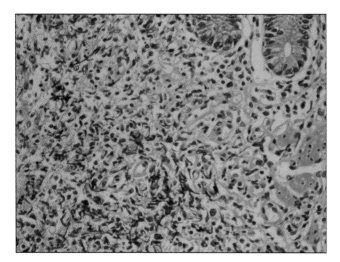

FIGURE 8.58: *PTLD (original magnification 400×, H&E): example of PTLD. Expansile mild lymphoplasmacytic infiltrate with indeterminate for acute rejection. In situ hybridization for EBV was negative. Gene rearrangement studies for T- and B-cell antigen receptors of this specimen suggested a B-cell monoclonal population.*

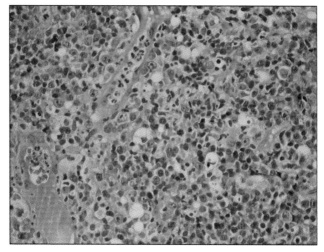

FIGURE 8.60: *PTLD (original magnification 400×, H&E): Example of malignant lymphoma (PTLD), large B-cell type. Mucosal ulceration, marked architectural distortion, and dense lymphoplasmacytic infiltrate is seen. Gene rearrangement studies for T- and B-cell antigen receptors of this specimen suggested B-cell monoclonal population.*

(Figures 8.55–8.58) and ultimately (if unsuccessfully treated) to monomorphic PTLD (Figures 8.59 and 8.60; Table 8.8) (see Chapter 10). PH (also called lymphoplasmacytic infiltrate) is a frequent observation in bowel allograft biopsies and should be considered as a separate diagnosis by the pathologist. The plasma cells and lymphocytes comprise the majority of the infiltrate present and extend throughout the tissue. Epithelial structures may be distorted and encroached upon by the infiltrate. The pathologist should attempt to characterize the intensity of the PH as mild, moderate, or severe and should be compared to previous biopsies. EBV staining by EBER and immunostaining for the presence and relative composition of B and T cells within the infiltrate is useful in evaluating possible PTLD (Figure 8.61). We also routinely utilize gene rearrangement studies for T- and B-cell antigen receptors from the paraffin block for an assessment of potential monoclonality. As the PTLD progresses, there can be effacement of the tissue with an infiltrate composed of plasma cells, intermediate-sized lymphoid cells, and immunoblasts (polymorphic PTLD, Figures 8.55 and 8.56). Monomorphic PTLDs can be of either T- or B-cell origin, and bear sufficient atypia and monomorphism as so to be recognized as neoplastic (Figures 8.57 and 8.58). These PTLD lymphomas are further

TABLE 8.8 Morphological Categories of PTLD

"Early" lesions: PH and infectious mononucleosis-like PTLD
Lymphoid proliferations that differ from typical reactive hyperplasia in having a diffuse proliferation of plasma cells and immunoblasts, but do not completely efface the architecture of the tissue.

Polymorphic PTLD
Destructive lesions composed of immunoblasts, plasma cells, and intermediate-sized lymphoid cells that efface the architecture of lymph nodes or form destructive extranodal masses.

Monomorphic PTLD
Monomorphic B-cell PTLD
Sufficient architectural and cytological atypia to be diagnosed as lymphoma on morphological grounds, and expression of B-cell antigens. Nodal architectural effacement and/or invasive tumoral growth in extranodal sites with confluent sheets of transformed cells.

Monomorphic T-cell PTLD
Sufficient atypia and monomorphism to be recognized as neoplastic, and should be classified according to the classification of T-cell neoplasms.

Hodgkin's lymphoma and Hodgkin's lymphoma–like PTLD
Since Reed-Sternberg–like cells may be seen in polymorphic PTLD, the diagnosis of Hodgkin's lymphoma should be based on both classical morphological and immunophenotypic features.

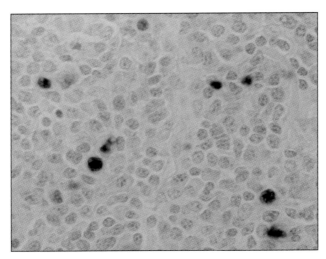

FIGURE 8.61: *PTLD (original magnification 100×, H&E): in situ hybridization for EBV shows mild number of positive cells.*

classified according to their architectural and cytological features in fashion identical to lymphomas occurring in native tissue. The types of PTLD lymphomas that have developed span the spectrum of most B- and T-cell neoplasms (Figures 8.59 and 8.60).

IX. SUMMARY

Small intestinal transplantation has become a viable treatment option for patients with GI failure and potential life-threatening complications due to parenteral nutrition. The surgical outcome has improved dramatically within the past decade, especially related to short-term patient and graft survival. In part, this improvement is related to an advancement of surgical techniques, improved and more selective immunosuppressive agents, and a better understanding of the underlying nature of pathologic injury after transplantation. Unfortunately, pathological entities such as acute rejection, chronic rejection, infectious enteritis, and PTLD still remain as challenging obstacles. Since the gold standard to diagnose those entities is histopathological evaluation, transplant pathologists have been assigned with a critical role within the bowel transplant team. Pathologists are required to comprehend and incorporate the clinical information of patients (e.g. age, primary disease, type of transplantation, post-transplant time, clinical symptoms, and history) with the morphological changes of tissue samples (e.g., native organ or graft, jejunum or ileum, endoscopical findings) in order to generate the most specific diagnosis in timely fashion to the treating physicians. Ultimately, the pathologist has the challenging responsibility of making an association between the pathological findings with the pathophysiological mechanisms of graft injury in order to offer a practical assessment of the probable clinical outcome.

REFERENCES

1. Grant, D., Abu-Elmagd, K., Reyes, J., Tzakis, A., Langnas, A., Fishbein, T., Goulet, O., and Farmer, D. 2003 report of the intestine transplant registry: a new era has dawned. *Ann Surg,* **241** (2005), 607–13.
2. Abu-Elmagd, K.M. Intestinal transplantation for short bowel syndrome and gastrointestinal failure: current consensus, rewarding outcomes, and practical guidelines. *Gastroenterology,* **130** (2006), S132–7.

3. Bakker, H., Bozzetti, F., Staun, M., Leon-Sanz, M., Hebuterne, X., Pertkiewicz, M., Shaffer, J., and Thul, P. Home parenteral nutrition in adults: a european multicentre survey in 1997. ESPEN-Home Artificial Nutrition Working Group. *Clin Nutr*, **18** (1999), 135–40.

4. Kato, T., Gaynor, J. J., Selvaggi, G., Mittal, N., Thompson, J., McLaughlin, G. E., Nishida, S., Moon, J., Levi, D., Madariaga, J., Ruiz, P., and Tzakis, A. Intestinal transplantation in children: a summary of clinical outcomes and prognostic factors in 108 patients from a single center. *J Gastrointest Surg*, **9** (2005), 75–89; discussion 89.

5. Liptak, P., and Ivanyi, B. Primer: Histopathology of calcineurin-inhibitor toxicity in renal allografts. *Nat Clin Pract Nephrol*, **2** (2006), 398–404.

6. Ruiz, P., Kato, T., and Tzakis, A. Current status of transplantation of the small intestine. *Transplantation*, **83** (2007), 1–6.

7. Tzakis, A. G., Kato, T., Levi, D.M., Defaria, W., Selvaggi, G., Weppler, D., Nishida, S., Moon, J., Madariaga, J. R., David, A. I., Gaynor, J. J., Thompson, J., Hernandez, E., Martinez, E., Cantwell, G. P., Augenstein, J. S., Gyamfi, A., Pretto, E. A., Dowdy, L., Tryphonopoulos, P., and Ruiz, P. 100 multivisceral transplants at a single center. *Ann Surg*, **242** (2005), 480–90; discussion 491–3.

8. Intestinal Transplant Registry; http://www.intestinaltransplant.org/

9. Grant, D., Zhong, R., Hurlbut, D., Garcia, B., Chen, H. F., Lamont, D., Wang, P. Z., Stiller, C., and Duff, J. A comparison of heterotopic and orthotopic intestinal transplantation in rats. *Transplantation*, **51** (1991), 948–54.

10. Ruiz, P., Bagni, A., Brown, R., Cortina, G., Harpaz, N., Magid, M. S., and Reyes, J. Histological criteria for the identification of acute cellular rejection in human small bowel allografts: results of the pathology workshop at the VIII International Small Bowel Transplant Symposium. *Transplant Proc*, **36** (2004), 335–7.

11. Wu, T., Abu-Elmagd, K., Bond, G., Nalesnik, M. A., Randhawa, P., and Demetris, A. J. A schema for histologic grading of small intestine allograft acute rejection. *Transplantation*, **75** (2003), 1241–8.

12. Lee, R. G., Nakamura, K., Tsamandas, A. C., Abu-Elmagd, K., Furukawa, H., Hutson, W. R., Reyes, J., Tabasco-Minguillan, J. S., Todo, S., and Demetris, A. J. Pathology of human intestinal transplantation. *Gastroenterology*, **110** (1996), 1820–34.

13. Schaefer, N., Tahara, K., Schmidt, J., Wehner, S., Kalff, J. C., Abu-Elmagd, K., Hirner, A., and Turler, A. Resident macrophages are involved in intestinal transplantation-associated inflammation and motoric dysfunction of the graft muscularis. *Am J Transplant*, **7** (2007), 1062–70.

14. Mallick, I. H., Yang, W., Winslet, M. C., and Seifalian, A. M. Ischemia-reperfusion injury of the intestine and protective strategies against injury. *Dig Dis Sci*, **49** (2004), 1359–77.

15. Tullius, S. G., Heemann, U., Hancock, W. W., Azuma, H., and Tilney, N. L. Long-term kidney isografts develop functional and morphologic changes that mimic those of chronic allograft rejection. *Ann Surg*, **220** (1994), 425–32; discussion 432–5.

16. Herrero-Fresneda, I., Torras, J., Cruzado, J. M., Condom, E., Vidal, A., Riera, M., Lloberas, N., Alsina, J., and Grinyo, J.M. Do alloreactivity and prolonged cold ischemia cause different elementary lesions in chronic allograft nephropathy? *Am J Pathol*, **162** (2003), 127–37.

17. Clavien, P. A., Harvey, P. R., and Strasberg, S. M. Preservation and reperfusion injuries in liver allografts. An overview and synthesis of current studies. *Transplantation*, **53** (1992), 957–78.

18. Dragun, D., Hoff, U., Park, J. K., Qun, Y., Schneider, W., Luft, F. C., and Haller, H. Prolonged cold preservation augments vascular injury independent of renal transplant immunogenicity and function. *Kidney Int*, **60** (2001), 1173–81.

19. Howard, T. K., Klintmalm, G. B., Cofer, J. B., Husberg, B. S., Goldstein, R. M., and Gonwa, T. A. The influence of preservation injury on rejection in the hepatic transplant recipient. *Transplantation*, **49** (1990), 103–7.

20. Quaedackers, J. S., Beuk, R. J., Bennet, L., Charlton, A., oude Egbrink, M. G., Gunn, A. J., and Heineman, E. An evaluation of methods for grading histologic injury following ischemia/reperfusion of the small bowel. *Transplant Proc*, **32** (2000), 1307–10.

21. Pillai, S. B., Luquette, M. H., Nowicki, P. T., and Besner, G. E. Segmental intestinal ischemia: an improved method of producing small bowel injury. *J Invest Surg*, **11** (1998), 123–8.

22. Martinez, O. M., and Rosen, H. R. Basic concepts in transplant immunology. *Liver Transpl*, **11** (2005), 370–81.

23. Briscoe, D. M., and Sayegh, M. H. A rendezvous before rejection: where do T cells meet transplant antigens? *Nat Med*, **8** (2002), 220–2.

24. He, G., Hart, J., Kim, O. S., Szot, G. L., Siegel, C. T., Thistlethwaite, J. R., and Newell, K. A. The role of CD8 and CD4 T cells in intestinal allograft rejection: a comparison of monoclonal antibody-treated and knockout mice. *Transplantation*, **67** (1999), 131–7.

25. Kellersmann, R., Ulrichs, K., Kellersmann, A., and Thiede, A. Intragraft distribution of lymphocytes expressing beta7 integrins after small bowel transplantation in mice. *Transpl Immunol*, **13** (2004), 249–58.

26. Bartlett, A. S., Ramadas, R., Furness, S., Gane, E., and McCall, J. L. The natural history of acute histologic rejection without biochemical graft dysfunction in orthotopic liver transplantation: a systematic review. *Liver Transpl*, **8** (2002), 1147–53.

27. Tippner, C., Nashan, B., Hoshino, K., Schmidt-Sandte, E., Akimaru, K., Boker, K. H., and Schlitt, H. J. Clinical and subclinical acute rejection early after liver transplantation: contributing factors and relevance for the long-term course. *Transplantation*, **72** (2001), 1122–8.

28. Nankivell, B. J., and Chapman, J. R. The significance of subclinical rejection and the value of protocol biopsies. *Am J Transplant*, **6** (2006), 2006–12.

29. Moreso, F., Ibernon, M., Goma, M., Carrera, M., Fulladosa, X., Hueso, M., Gil-Vernet, S., Cruzado, J. M., Torras, J., Grinyo, J. M., and Seron, D. Subclinical rejection associated with chronic allograft nephropathy in protocol biopsies as a risk factor for late graft loss. *Am J Transplant*, **6** (2006), 747–52.

30. Bohmig, G. A., Regele, H., and Horl, W. H. Protocol biopsies after kidney transplantation. *Transpl Int*, **18** (2005), 131–9.

31. Nankivell, B. J., Borrows, R. J., Fung, C. L., O'Connell, P. J., Allen, R. D., and Chapman, J. R. Natural history, risk factors, and impact of subclinical rejection in kidney transplantation. *Transplantation*, **78** (2004), 242–9.

32. Kee, T. Y., Chapman, J. R., O'Connell, P. J., Fung, C. L., Allen, R.D., Kable, K., Vitalone, M. J., and Nankivell, B. J. Treatment of subclinical rejection diagnosed by protocol biopsy of kidney transplants. *Transplantation*, **82** (2006), 36–42.

33. Takahashi, H., Kato, T., Selvaggi, G., Nishida, S., Gaynor, J J., Delacruz, V., Moon, JI., Levi, DM., Tzakis, AG., Ruiz, P. Subclinical rejection in the initial postoperative period in small intestinal transplantation: a negative influence on graft survival. *Transplantation*, **84(6)** (2007), 689–96.

34. Tilg, H., Vogel, W., Aulitzky, W. E., Schonitzer, D., Margreiter, R., Dietze, O., Judmaier, G., Wachter, H., and Huber, C. Neopterin excretion after liver transplantation and its value in differential diagnosis of complications. *Transplantation*, **48** (1989), 594–9.

35. Rodriguez-Iturbe, B. Cellular adhesion molecules in transplantation. *Transplant Proc*, **28** (1996), 3285–9.

36. Corti, B., Altimari, A., Gabusi, E., Pinna, A. D., Gruppioni, E., Lauro, A., Pirini, M. G., Fiorentino, M., Ridolfi, L., Grigioni, W. F., and Grigioni, A. D. Two years' experience of acute rejection monitoring of intestinal transplant recipients by real-time PCR assessment of granzyme B and perforin up-regulation: considerations on diagnostic accuracy. *Transplant Proc*, **38** (2006), 1726–7.

37. Han, D., Xu, X., Baidal, D., Leith, J., Ricordi, C., Alejandro, R., and Kenyon, N. S. Assessment of cytotoxic lymphocyte gene expression in the peripheral blood of human islet allograft recipients: elevation precedes clinical evidence of rejection. *Diabetes*, **53** (2004), 2281–90.

38. Windmueller, H. G., and Spaeth, A. E. Source and fate of circulating citrulline. *Am J Physiol*, **241** (1981), E473–80.

39. Wu, G. Intestinal mucosal amino acid catabolism. *J Nutr*, **128** (1998), 1249–52.

40. David, A. I., Gaynor, J. J., Zis, P.P., Conanan, L., Goldsmith, L., Esquenazi, V., Selvaggi, G., Weppler, D., Nishida, S., Moon, J., Madariaga, J. R., Ruiz, P., Kato, T., Levi, D. M., Kleiner, G., Tryphonopoulos, P., and Tzakis, A. G. An association of lower serum citrulline levels within 30 days of acute rejection in patients following small intestine transplantation. *Transplant Proc*, **38** (2006), 1731–2.

41. Gondolesi, G., Ghirardo, S., Raymond, K., Hoppenhauer, L., Surillo, D., Rumbo, C., Fishbein, T., Sansaricq, C., and Sauter, B. The value of plasma citrulline to predict mucosal injury in intestinal allografts. *Am J Transplant*, **6** (2006), 2786–90.

42. Nadalin, S., Biglarnia, A. R., Testa, G., Koppara, T. R., Schaffer, R., Johnson, C., Toetsch, M., Broelsch, C. E., and Malago, M. Role and significance of plasma citrulline in the early phase after small bowel transplantation in pigs. *Transpl Int*, **20** (2007), 425–31.

43. Kiyochi, H., Kellersmann, R., Blomer, A., Garcia, B. M., Zhang, Z., Zhong, R., and Grant, D. R. Rat-to-mouse small bowel xenotransplantation: a novel model for studying acute vascular and hyperacute xenograft rejection and xenogenic cell migration. *Xenotransplantation*, **6** (1999), 28–35.

44. Halloran, P. F., Wadgymar, A., Ritchie, S., Falk, J., Solez, K., and Srinivasa, N. S. The significance of the anti-class I antibody response. I. Clinical and pathologic features of anti-class I-mediated rejection. *Transplantation*, **49** (1990), 85–91.

45. Terasaki, P. I., and Cai, J. Humoral theory of transplantation: further evidence. *Curr Opin Immunol*, **17** (2005), 541–5.

46. Paul, L. C., Davidoff, A., Benediktsson, H., and Issekutz, T.B. The efficacy of LFA-1 and VLA-4 antibody treatment in rat vascularized cardiac allograft rejection. *Transplantation*, **55** (1993), 1196–9.

47. Hancock, W. W., Gao, W., Shemmeri, N., Shen, X. D., Gao, F., Busuttil, R. W., Zhai, Y., and Kupiec-Weglinski, J. W. Immunopathogenesis of accelerated allograft rejection in sensitized recipients: humoral and nonhumoral mechanisms. *Transplantation*, **73** (2002), 1392–7.

48. Kato, T., Mizutani, K., Terasaki, P., Quintini, C., Selvaggi, G., Thompson, J., Ruiz, P., and Tzakis, A. Association of emergence of HLA antibody and acute rejection in intestinal transplant recipients: a possible evidence of acute humoral sensitization. *Transplant Proc*, **38** (2006), 1735–7.

49. Terasaki, P. I. Humoral theory of transplantation. *Am J Transplant*, **3** (2003), 665–73.

50. Fujisaki, S., Murase, N., Demetris, A. J., Tanabe, M., Todo, S., and Starzl, T. E. Effects of preformed antibodies induced by whole blood transfusion on small bowel transplantation. *Transplant Proc*, **26** (1994), 1528–9.

51. Ruiz, P., Suarez, M., Nishida, S., de la Cruz, V., Nicolas, M., Weppler, D., Khaled, A., Bejarano, P., Kato, T., Mittal, N., Icardi, M., and Tzakis, A. Sclerosing mesenteritis in small bowel transplantation: possible manifestation of acute vascular rejection. *Transplant Proc*, **35** (2003), 3057–60.

52. Terasaki, P. I. Clinical Transplants 2006 (Los Angeles, CA: UCLA Immunogenetics Center 2007).

53. Ruiz, P., Garcia, M., Pappas, P., Berney, T., Esquenazi, V., Kato, T., Mittal, N., Weppler, D., Levi, D., Nishida, S., Nery, J., Miller, J., and Tzakis, A. Mucosal vascular alterations in isolated small-bowel allografts: relationship to humoral sensitization. *Am J Transplant*, **3** (2003), 43–9.

54. Colvin, R. B. Antibody-mediated renal allograft rejection: diagnosis and pathogenesis. *J Am Soc Nephrol*, **18** (2007), 1046–56.

55. Guo, W. H., Tian, L., Chan, K. L., Dallman, M., and Tam, P. K. Role of CD4+ and CD8+ T cells in early and late acute rejection of small bowel allograft. *J Pediatr Surg*, **36** (2001), 352–6.

56. Buonocore, S., Surquin, M., Le Moine, A., Abramowicz, D., Flamand, V., and Goldman, M. Amplification of T-cell responses by neutrophils: relevance to allograft immunity. *Immunol Lett*, **94** (2004), 163–6.

57. Ogura, Y., Martinez, O. M., Villanueva, J. C., Tait, J. F., Strauss, H. W., Higgins, J. P., Tanaka, K., Esquivel, C. O., Blankenberg, F. G., Krams, S. M. Apoptosis and allograft rejection in the absence of CD8+ T cells. *Transplantation*, **71** (2001), 1827–34.

58. Krams, S. M., Hayashi, M., Fox, C. K., Villanueva, J. C., Whitmer, K. J., Burns, W., Esquivel, C. O., Martinez, O. M. CD8+ cells are not necessary for allograft rejection or the induction of apoptosis in an experimental model of small intestinal transplantation. *J Immunol*, **160** (1998), 3673–80.

59. Corti, B., Altimari, A., Gabusi, E., Pinna, A. D., Gruppioni, E., Lauro, A., Pirini, M. G., Fiorentino, M., Ridolfi, L., Grigioni, W. F., Grigioni, A. D. Two years' experience of acute rejection monitoring of intestinal transplant recipients by real-time PCR assessment of granzyme B and perforin up-regulation: considerations on diagnostic accuracy. *Transplant Proc*, **38** (2006), 1726–7.

60. D'Errico, A., Corti, B., Pinna, A. D., Altimari, A., Gruppioni, E., Gabusi, E., Fiorentino, M., Bagni, A., Grigioni, W. F. Granzyme B and perforin as predictive markers for acute rejection in human intestinal transplantation. *Transplant Proc*, **35** (2003), 3061–5.

61. Veale, J. L., Liang, L. W., Zhang, Q., Gjertson, D. W., Du, Z., Bloomquist, E. W., Jia, J., Qian, L., Wilkinson, A. H., Danovitch, G. M., Pham, P. T., Rosenthal, J. T., Lassman, C. R., Braun, J., Reed, E. F., Gritsch, H. A. Noninvasive diagnosis of cellular and antibody-mediated rejection by perforin and granzyme B in renal allografts. *Hum Immunol*, **67** (2006), 777–86.

62. Stewart, S., Winters, G. L., Fishbein, M. C., Tazelaar, H. D., Kobashigawa, J., Abrams, J., Andersen, C. B., Angelini, A., Berry, G. J., Burke, M. M., Demetris, A. J., Hammond, E., Itescu, S., Marboe, C. C., McManus, B., Reed, E. F., Reinsmoen, N. L., Rodriguez, E. R., Rose, A. G., Rose, M., Suciu-Focia, N., Zeevi, A., and Billingham, M. E. Revision of the 1990 working formulation for the standardization of nomenclature in the diagnosis of heart rejection. *J Heart Lung Transplant*, **24** (2005), 1710–20.

63. Solez, K., Colvin, R. B., Racusen, L. C., Sis, B., Halloran, P. F., Birk, P. E., Campbell, P. M., Cascalho, M., Collins, A. B., Demetris, A. J., Drachenberg, C. B., Gibson, I. W., Grimm, P. C., Haas, M., Lerut, E., Liapis, H., Mannon, R. B., Marcus, P. B., Mengel, M., Mihatsch, M. J., Nankivell, B. J., Nickeleit, V., Papadimitriou, J. C., Platt, J. L., Randhawa, P., Roberts, I., Salinas-Madriga, L., Salomon, D. R., Seron, D., Sheaff, M., et al. Banff '05 Meeting Report: differential diagnosis of chronic allograft injury and elimination of chronic allograft nephropathy ('CAN'). *Am J Transplant*, **7** (2007), 518–26.

64. Garcia, M., Delacruz, V., Ortiz, R., Bagni, A., Weppler, D., Kato, T., Tzakis, A., and Ruiz, P. Acute cellular rejection grading scheme for human gastric allografts. *Hum Pathol*, **35** (2004), 343–9.

65. Nishida, S., Levi, D. M., Moon, J. I., Madariaga, J. R., Kato, T., Selvaggi, G., Tryphonopoulos, P., DeFaria, W., Santiago, S., Gaynor, J., Weppler, D., Martinez, E., Ruiz, P., and Tzakis, A. G. Intestinal transplantation with alemtuzumab (Campath-1H) induction for adult patients. *Transplant Proc*, **38** (2006), 1747–9.

66. Garcia, M., Weppler, D., Mittal, N., Nishida, S., Kato, T., Tzakis, A., and Ruiz, P. Campath-1H immunosuppressive therapy reduces incidence and intensity of acute rejection in intestinal and multivisceral transplantation. *Transplant Proc*, **36** (2004), 323–4.

67. Tzakis, A. G., Kato, T., Nishida, S., Levi, D. M., Tryphonopoulos, P., Madariaga, J. R., De Faria, W., Nery, J. R., Regev, A., Vianna, R., Miller, J., Esquenazi, V., Weppler, D., and Ruiz, P. Alemtuzumab (Campath-1H) combined with tacrolimus in intestinal and multivisceral transplantation. *Transplantation*, **75** (2003), 1512–7.

68. Ishii, T., Mazariegos, G. V., Bueno, J., Ohwada, S., and Reyes, J. Exfoliative rejection after intestinal transplantation in children. *Pediatr Transplant*, **7** (2003), 185–91.

69. Kato, T., Ruiz, P., and Tzakis, A. Exfoliative bowel rejection – a dangerous loss of integrity. *Pediatr Transplant*, **8** (2004), 426–7.

70. Sigurdsson, L., Reyes, J., Todo, S., Putnam, P. E., and Kocoshis, S. A. Anatomic variability of rejection in intestinal allografts after pediatric intestinal transplantation. *J Pediatr Gastroenterol Nutr*, **27** (1998), 403–6.

71. Wang, M., Li, Q., Wang, J., Li, Y., Zhu, W., Li, N., Li, J. Intestinal tight junction in allograft after small bowel transplantation. *Transplant Proc*, **39** (2007), 289–91.

72. Zou, Y., Hernandez, F., Burgos, E., Martinez, L., Gonzalez-Reyes, S., Fernandez-Dumont, V., Lopez, G., Romero, M., Lopez-Santamaria, M., Tovar, J. A. Bacterial translocation in acute rejection after small bowel transplantation in rats. *Pediatr Surg Int*, **21** (2005), 208–11.

73. Cicalese, L., Sileri, P., Green, M., Abu-Elmagd, K., Kocoshis, S., Reyes, J. Bacterial translocation in clinical intestinal transplantation. *Transplantation*, **71** (2001), 1414–7.

74. Takahashi, H., Selvaggi, G., Nishida, S., Weppler, D., Levi, D., Kato, T., Tzakis, A., and Ruiz, P. Organ-specific differences in acute rejection intensity in a multivisceral transplant. *Transplantation*, **81** (2006), 297–9.

75. Takahashi, H., Delacruz, V., Sarwar, S., Selvaggi, G., Moon, J., Nishida, S., Weppler, D., Levi, D., Kato, T., Tzakis, A., and Ruiz, P. Contemporaneous chronic rejection of multiple allografts with principal pancreatic involvement in modified multivisceral transplantation. *Pediatr Transplant*, **11** (2007), 448–52.

76. Ma, H., Wang, J., Wang, J., Li, Y., and Li, J. Features of chronic allograft rejection on rat small intestine transplantation. *Pediatr Transplant*, **11** (2007), 165–72.

77. Parizhskaya, M., Redondo, C., Demetris, A., Jaffe, R., Reyes, J., Ruppert, K., Martin, L., and Abu-Elmagd, K. Chronic rejection of small bowel grafts: pediatric and adult study of risk factors and morphologic progression. *Pediatr Dev Pathol*, **6** (2003), 240–50.

78. Ziring, D., Tran, R., Edelstein, S., McDiarmid, S. V., Gajjar, N., Cortina, G., Vargas, J., Renz, J. F., Cherry, J. D., Krogstad, P., Miller, M., Busuttil, R. W., and Farmer, D. G. Infectious enteritis after intestinal transplantation: incidence, timing, and outcome. *Transplantation*, **79** (2005), 702–9.

79. Parizhskaya, M., Walpusk, J., Mazariegos, G., and Jaffe, R. Enteric adenovirus infection in pediatric small bowel transplant recipients. *Pediatr Dev Pathol*, **4** (2001), 122–8.

80. Pinchoff, R. J., Kaufman, S. S., Magid, M. S., Erdman, D. D., Gondolesi, G. E., Mendelson, M. H., Tane, K., Jenkins, S. G., Fishbein, T. M., and Herold, B. C.

Adenovirus infection in pediatric small bowel transplantation recipients. *Transplantation*, **76** (2003), 183–9.

81. Berho, M., Torroella, M., Viciana, A., Weppler, D., Thompson, J., Nery, J., Tzakis, A., and Ruiz, P. Adenovirus enterocolitis in human small bowel transplants. *Pediatr Transplant*, **2** (1998), 277–82.

82. Fankhauser, R. L., Monroe, S. S., Noel, J. S., Humphrey, C. D., Bresee, J. S., Parashar, U. D., Ando, T., and Glass, R. I. Epidemiologic and molecular trends of "Norwalk-like viruses" associated with outbreaks of gastroenteritis in the United States. *J Infect Dis*, **186** (2002), 1–7.

83. Morotti, R. A., Kaufman, S. S., Fishbein, T. M., Chatterjee, N. K., Fuschino, M. E., Morse, D. L., and Magid, M. S. Calicivirus infection in pediatric small intestine transplant recipients: pathological considerations. *Hum Pathol*, **35** (2004), 1236–40.

84. Kaufman, S. S., Chatterjee, N. K., Fuschino, M. E., Magid, M. S., Gordon, R. E., Morse, D. L., Herold, B. C., LeLeiko, N. S., Tschernia, A., Florman, S. S., Gondolesi, G. E., and Fishbein, T. M. Calicivirus enteritis in an intestinal transplant recipient. *Am J Transplant*, **3** (2003), 764–8.

85. Maiorana, A., Baccarini, P., Foroni, M., Bellini, N., and Giusti, F. Human cytomegalovirus infection of the gastrointestinal tract in apparently immunocompetent patients. *Hum Pathol*, **34** (2003), 1331–6.

86. Xiao, S. Y., and Hart, J. Marked gastric foveolar hyperplasia associated with active cytomegalovirus infection. *Am J Gastroenterol*, **96** (2001), 223–6.

87. Delis, S., Kato, T., Ruiz, P., Mittal, N., Babinski, L., and Tzakis, A. Herpes simplex colitis in a child with combined liver and small bowel transplant. *Pediatr Transplant*, **5** (2001), 374–7.

88. Sarkar, S., Selvaggi, G., Mittal, N., Cenk Acar, B., Weppler, D., Kato, T., Tzakis, A., and Ruiz, P. Gastrointestinal tract ulcers in pediatric intestinal transplantation patients: etiology and management. *Pediatr Transplant*, **10** (2006), 162–7.

89. Quintini, C., Kato, T., Gaynor, J. J., Ueno, T., Selvaggi, G., Gordon, P., McLaughlin, G., Tompson, J., Ruiz, P., and Tzakis, A. Analysis of risk factors for the development of posttransplant lymphoproliferative disorder among 119 children who received primary intestinal transplants at a single center. *Transplant Proc*, **38** (2006), 1755–8.

90. Berney, T., Delis, S., Kato, T., Nishida, S., Mittal, N. K., Madariaga, J., Levi, D., Nery, J. R., Cirocco, R. E., Gelman, B., Ruiz, P., and Tzakis, A. G. Successful treatment of posttransplant lymphoproliferative disease with prolonged rituximab treatment in intestinal transplant recipients. *Transplantation*, **74** (2002), 1000–6.

91. Kato, T., Dowdy, L., Weppler, D., Ruiz, P., Thompson, J., Raskin, J., and Tzakis, A. Non-tuberculous mycobacterial associated enterocolitis in intestinal transplantation. *Transplant Proc*, **30** (1998), 2537–8.

92. Delis, S. G., Tector, J., Kato, T., Mittal, N., Weppler, D., Levi, D., Ruiz, P., Nishida, S., Nery, J. R., and Tzakis, A. G. Diagnosis and treatment of cryptosporidium infection in intestinal transplant recipients. *Transplant Proc*, **34** (2002), 951–2.

93. Harpaz, N., Schiano, T., Ruf, A. E., Shukla, D., Tao, Y., Fishbein, T. M., Sauter, B. V., and Gondolesi, G. E. Early and frequent histological recurrence of Crohn's disease in small intestinal allografts. *Transplantation*, **80** (2005), 1667–70.

94. Glas, J., Folwaczny, M., Folwaczny, C., and Torok, H. P. Crohn's disease recurrence in small bowel transplant. *Am J Gastroenterol*, **99** (2004), 2067.

95. Sustento-Reodica, N., Ruiz, P., Rogers, A., Viciana, A. L., Conn, H. O., and Tzakis, A. G. Recurrent Crohn's disease in transplanted bowe *Lancet*, **349** (1997), 688–91.

96. Moon, J. I., Selvaggi, G., Nishida, S., Levi, D. M., Kato, T., Ruiz, P., Bejarano, P., Madariaga, J. R., and Tzakis, A. G. Intestinal transplantation for the treatment of neoplastic disease. *J Surg Oncol*, **92** (2005), 284–91.

97. Selvaggi, G., Sarkar, S., Mittal, N., Weppler, D., Kato, T., Tryphonopoulos, P., Tzakis, A. and P. Ruiz. Etiology and management of alimentary tract ulcers in pediatric intestinal transplantation patients. *Transplant Proc*, **38** (2006), 1768–1769.

98. Desilva, H. J., Kettlewell, M., Mortensen, N., et al. Acute-inflammation in ileal pouches (pouchitis). *Eur J Gastro Hepatol*, **3**(4) (1991), 343–9.

99. Villanacci, V., and Bassotti, G. Histological aspects of the terminal ileum: a windows on coeliac disease too? *Diges Liv Dis*, **38**(11) (2006), 820–2.

100. Martland, G. T., and Shepherd, N. A. Indeterminate colitis: definition, diagnosis, implications and a plea for nosological sanity. *Histopathology*, **50** (2007), 83–96.

101. Fishbein, T., Novitskiy, G., Mishra, L., Matsumoto, C., Kaufman, S., Goyal, S., Shetty, K., Johnson, L., Lu, A., Wang, A., Hu, F., Kallakury, B., Lough, D., and M. Zasloff. Nod 2 expressing bone marrow derived cells appear to regulate epithelial innate immunity of the transplanted human small intestine. *Gut* **57** (2008), 323–330.

102. Ruiz, P., Soares, M. F., Garcia, M., Nicolas, M., Kato, T., Mittal, N., Nishida, S., Levi, D., Selvaggi, G., Madariaga, J., and Tzakis, A. Lymphoplasmacytic hyperplasia (possibly pre-PTLD) has varied expression and appearance in intestinal transplant recipients receiving Campath immunosuppression. *Transplant Proc*, **36** (2004), 386–387.

103. Finn, L., Reyes, J., Bueno, J., and Yunis, E. Epstein-Barr virus infections in children after transplantation of the small intestine. *Am J Surg Pathol*, **22** (1998), 299–309.

CHAPTER 9

Pathology of Hematopoietic Stem Cell Transplantation

Gary Kleiner, M.D., Ph.D.

Michael Kritzer-Cheren, B.S.

Phillip Ruiz, M.D., Ph.D.

I. INTRODUCTION

The field of stem cell transplantation is growing and evolving with increased success as compared to when it was first initiated. Despite this accomplishment, pathological processes involving hematopoietic stem cell transplants (HSCT) often occur and may be present early or late in the course of treatment. Early on, the conditioning regimens may create pathology and toxicities associated with the treatments themselves. Soon after, as the new hematopoietic cell system develops, immunologically based pathologies such as graft rejection or graft-versus-host disease (GVHD) may occur. In addition, long-term sequelae from extended immunosuppressive therapies results in increased susceptibility to various and life-threatening infections (1).

Our current understanding concerning HSCT in humans is based on pioneering work of clinical scientists and animal models. As expected, the first clinical trials were unsuccessful and in 1957, only one transient successful graft was seen (2). Despite their failure, an important tenet was established from these experiments. Bone marrow transplants could be infused in large amount without adverse effects so long as it was anticoagulated properly and infused as a cellular suspension.

Three important discoveries occurred in 1959; the *first* being two acute lymphoblast leukemia (ALL) patients who each received marrow infusions from their respective identical twin. This is referred to as a *syngeneic graft*. Prior to the infusion, they received a dose of total body irradiation (TBI) (3). The recovery of each patient, both clinically and hematologically, was observed within two weeks. This illustrated the fact that a matched bone marrow graft is capable of protecting against the normally lethal aplasia associated with irradiation. Unfortunately, the leukemia recurred in both of these patients within months following reconstitution, indicating chemotherapy was also required in addition to irradiation. After his studies of syngeneic mice, Barnes et al. (4) suggested a cure could be by a reaction of the graft against the leukemia; this illustrated the potential importance of using an allogeneic graft. A *second finding* in 1959 demonstrated that allogeneic grafts could reconstitute a patients' bone marrow. However, this was displayed prior to major histocompatibility complex (MHC) matching and the result was probably due to the reconstitution by the patients' original marrow (5). The *third finding* in that year reported a treatment of a patient with ALL by first performing TBI and then infusing the same patient's marrow (i.e., *autologous*), stored from a previous remission (6). At first the patient went into remission but then subsequently died because of leukemic cells in the stored marrow. Eventually, more promising experiments based on newly acquired knowledge of the *MHC* (human MHC = HLA) occurred, and investigators began to look to siblings as marrow donors (7). The continued success of HSCT therapy with other diseases such as aplastic anemia legitimized it as a viable treatment option and brought it into the modern day era where it remains as a mainstay in the treatment of a variety of hematological disorders and malignancies.

II. AUTOLOGOUS CELL TRANSPLANTS

Autologous HSCT reemerged in the 1980s (8) as a treatment for lymphomas that responded poorly to other therapies. The benefits for autologous transplants are threefold. They do not require a donor, which is of particular importance because of a frequent lack of suitable allogeneic donors. Secondly, autologous transplants have a lower transplant-related mortality due to the reduced incidence of GVHD and the faster recovery and reconstitution than allogeneic transplants. Finally, these procedures can be carried out in the community sector because of the ease of collection and preparation of this type of transplant. Peripheral blood can be taken by leukapheresis after a regimen of growth factors such as granulocyte and granulocyte macrophage colony stimulating factors. The resulting stem cell product displaying large quantities of hematopoietic progenitors could be collected and infused for quicker reconstitution (9–11).

III. ALLOGENEIC CELL TRANSPLANTS

Successful unrelated HLA-matched donor transplant engraftments were documented as early as 1973 (12,13). However, the vast amount of polymorphisms in the MHC creates a limited pool of possible donors. This heralded the coordination of many national and international organizations to create registries designed to increase the chances a HLA-matched donor could be found. By 1996, there were over three million HLA-typed people listed to help patients in need of a transplant (14). *Bone Marrow Donors Worldwide* is a worldwide collaborator of all the registries from individual countries. The largest to date is the *United States National Marrow Donor Program*, currently with over three million registered donors itself (15). The advent of these registries created to supply for unrelated allogeneic transplant resulted in an increase in these procedures. In 1985, less than 10 percent of transplants were unrelated allogeneic donors; by 1995, the number had risen to 25 percent.

Recent research has illustrated the possibility of umbilical cord blood (UCB), which can be used as a source for allogeneically matched donor stem cells. UCB is typically discarded at birth and has been shown to be a significant source of stem cells that may be used in transplants for bone marrow reconstitution (16). An advantage of UCB is that the blood is already stored and can therefore be easily accessed when needed. There is no screening of live donors needed and no harvesting of bone marrow through that painful procedure.

IV. GRAFT-VERSUS-LEUKEMIA (GVL)

Barnes et al. (4) originally proposed in an experimental murine leukemia model that engrafted bone marrow against leukemia could be protective to the host by cellular interaction with the leukemia. This phenomenon was later confirmed when it was shown that patients with GVHD after a transplant for leukemia had a lower risk of recurrence (17). In addition, a recipient of bone marrow syngeneically showed higher incidence of leukemia recurrence than matched HLA from siblings (18). Subsequently, GVL could be induced by the addition of *immunomodulatory cytokines* such as interleukin-2 (IL-2). IL-2 activates T cells and natural killer (NK) cells, both of which are thought to play a significant role in GVL. Studies in vitro showed that IL-2 induced GVL in peripheral blood lymphocytes post-transplantation (19,20). Mackinnon et al. then proceeded to illustrate that donor leukocytes with a T-cell count as low as 1×10^7 per kilogram could result in donor chimerism with potent GVL effects, even without clinical signs of GVHD (21). Current studies are determining the effects of low-dose donor lymphocyte infusions following transplants to reduce relapse in patients with CML.

V. PRETRANSPLANTATION EVALUATION

HSCT is a multifaceted and intricate procedure that requires physicians to be knowledgeable of a constellation of complex signs and symptoms from potential complications. In preparation for transplant, patients undergo a systematic *ablation* of their existing bone marrow. These regimens are given to patients eligible for transplant (Table 9.1), whose illnesses include solid and blood borne malignancies, immunodeficiency diseases, and metabolic and non-malignant hematological disorders (i.e., sickle cell disease, thalassemia major). The chemically or radiation-induced ablation renders the patient *immunodeficient*, predisposing the subject to a myriad of complications such as infection and de novo malignancies. Different primary disorders may require special approaches and conditioning regimens in preparation for HSCT (22). For example, the myelodysplastic syndromes refractory anemia and refractory anemia with excess blasts require careful analysis for

TABLE 9.1 Conditions Treated by Hematopoietic Stem Cell Transplantation

Condition	Malignant	Nonmalignant
Acute lymphoblastic leukemia	√	
Acute myelogenous leukemia	√	
Aplastic anemia		√
Chronic myelogenous leukemia	√	
Hodgkin's disease	√	
Multiple myeloma	√	
Myelodysplasia		√*
Non-Hodgkin's lymphoma	√	
Paroxysmal nocturnal hemoglobinuria		√
Radiation poisoning		√
Chronic lymphocytic leukemia	√	
AL amyloidosis		√
Essential thrombocytosis		√
Polycythemia vera		√
Adrenoleukodystrophy		√
Amegakaryocytic thrombocytopenia		√
Sickle cell disease		√
Griscelli syndrome type II		√
Hurler syndrome		√
Kostmann syndrome		√
Krabbe disease		√
Metachromatic leukodystrophy		√
Thalassemia		√
Hemophagocytic lymphohistiocytosis		√
Wiskott-Aldrich syndrome		√
Neuroblastoma	√	
Some inborn errors of metabolism		√

* Predisposes for malignancy.

distinctive preparation regimens. In addition to the limited amount of time aplastic anemic patients have to receive a transplant, they also must not receive extensive quantities of blood transfusions prior to allogeneic transplantation to avoid sensitization and graft rejection (23). Patients presenting with chronic myeloid leukemia, acute myelofibrosis, myelodysplastic syndromes, and metastatic disease must have bone marrow biopsies taken for baseline determination of changes such as myelofibrosis. Liver biopsies may need to be taken for evaluation of hepatic integrity and determine the risk of developing veno-occlusive disorder early post-transplant. Additionally, active hepatitis and cirrhosis prior to transplant must be determined because of the possibility of severe toxicity that can develop from the conditioning regimens.

VI. POST-TRANSPLANT CHANGES

Early after transplant, patients may display evidence of marked injury to the bone marrow, with most marrow elements destroyed except for plasma cells, and the accumulation of fat and iron-rich macrophages. Bone marrow morphology in the early transplantation period (days one to twenty-eight) include aplasia/hypocellularity with extensive necrosis, debris, fat necrosis, stromal edema, and phagocytic macrophages (Figure 9.1). *Bone marrow regeneration* is evident seven to ten days after HSCT, with small, nonparatrabecular colonies of uniform immature cells; erythroid and myeloid cells precede megakaryocytic regeneration. Bone marrow cellularity reaches about 50 percent of normal levels by day 21 and by day 28 there should be engraftment of all cell lineages and a normocellular appearance. At first, lymphoid cell numbers are low and remain diffusely spread in the recipient. Platelet cells are typically the last cell type to regain adequate titers. Relapse of primary disease is unlikely to occur prior to 100 days after transplantation, unless the recipient displays a persistence of bone marrow tumor cells within days 7–21. Cytogenetics, restriction length polymorphism analysis, and Y chromosome DNA detection are techniques that aid in the *prediction of relapse status versus chimeric*

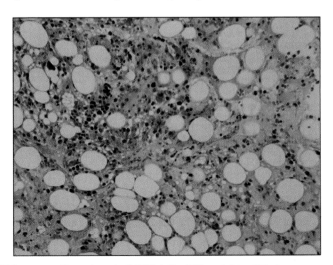

FIGURE 9.1: *Bone marrow regeneration fourteen days after HSCT (hematoxylin and eosin [H&E], left – 200×; right – 400×).*

establishment (24). Secondary tumors, excluding post-transplant lymphoproliferative disease, will typically present late following transplantation (25). If no regeneration is evident after four weeks, the hematopoietic stem cells have failed to engraft.

To combat infection in HSCT patients, *T-cell immunity* must be intact. If T-cell immunity is not regained following a HSCT, then the transplant is considered to have failed (26–32). Temporary antigen-specificity is observed in patients who receive peripheral blood stem cells (PBSC) as well as bone marrow. (*Note*: there are 1–1.5 logs more T cells in peripheral blood than in the bone marrow.) There are fewer complications and infections following a transplant performed with additional PBSC. These antigen-specific T cells protect the recipient short term; however, long-term immunity needs a continual production of new antigen-specific T cells.

Unlike T-cell immunity, *antibody formation* is found early after a HSCT (33). Circulating antibody levels to various antigens increase when either the donor or the recipient has an immunization prior to transplant. The maximum amount of antibody achieved is seen when both the donor and the recipient are immunized prior to transplant (34–40). Without immunization, there is no maintenance of antibody production after one year after transplantation. There is also a temporary transfer of donor-derived salivary immunoglobulin A (IgA) after transplantation (41). Residual B lymphocytes and plasma cells are nondividing cells and are therefore frequently seen in patients undergoing cytoablative regimens (40). Increased antibody titer post HSCT can be seen likely due to immunocompetent donor B lymphocytes, antigen-primed donor antigen-presenting cells (APCs), and also immune donor T lymphocytes. Immediately after transplant, patients are given intravenous immunoglobulin (IVIg), especially in patients not displaying this antibody titer increase (42). Few patients are completely void of humoral cellular responses after HSCT.

T cells following an HSCT can either be derived from mature T lymphocytes in the bone marrow inoculum or result from the transplanted hematopoietic stem cells that were transplanted. Patients who receive unmanipulated (not depleted of T cells) autologous bone marrow reach a lymphocyte count of 500/µl faster than patients who receive untreated histoincompatible transplants (fifteen days compared to twenty-seven to thirty) (43,44). The delay seen in allogeneic transplants is secondary to GVHD prophylactic drug treatments (45). While it takes between six and eight weeks for autologous HSCT recipients to reconstitute their T cells, it takes allogeneic recipients about twelve weeks following transplantation. The onset of acute GVHD has no effect on the reconstitution of T cells. The next step is for the T cells to become either helper or cytotoxic, observed by the addition of either CD4 or CD8 cell surface molecules, respectively (43,45–48). Cyto-

toxic T cells recover their appropriate amount by four months after transplantation, while helper T-cells titers remain low for at least six months. Recovery of T-cell function is represented by a proliferative response to antigenic stimulation (toxins, viral antigens) or nonspecific stimuli (PHA or anti-CD3 antibodies). Patients receiving non-T-cell–depleted bone marrow transplants display functionality within two months (45).

Following a bone marrow transplant the first cell type to repopulate is the *NK cell* (49). This typically occurs within the first month after transplantation (50). The appearance of NK cells effectively alters the phenotypic ratio of helper to cytotoxic T cells (50). The reconstitution of helper T cells decreases naturally with age, resulting from a decrease in thymic tissue (51,52). The number of these T cells is inversely correlated with the age of the transplant patient, which makes it more difficult for older transplant patients to reach normal T-cell capacity. Studies have shown that initial increases in T cells after transplantation occur via proliferation of mature donor T cells from the graft (51,53). Production of CD4 T cells is severely compromised in adult patients due to the lack of thymic tissue.

B lymphocytes reach normal levels within two months after transplantation and this is independent of T-cell depletion prior to transplant (50,54). B-cell reconstitution follows that same maturation as ontogeny, shown by post-HSCT immunoglobulin variable heavy chain to be similar to those fetal immunoglobulin (55). B cells following transplant have increased frequency of expression of CD5, indicating a greater propensity for autoimmunity. There are persistent secretory IgA synthesis defects for six months after HSCT, which necessitates administration of IVIg (54). It may take up to nine months for their IgG levels to normalize, twelve months for IgM, and two to three years for IgA. If a patient suffers from chronic GVHD, their IgM and IgG levels may be elevated beginning at six to nine months following transplantation.

In patients not victim to chronic GVHD, partial immune reconstitution is observed by one year. Patients should receive immunization to diphtheria, pertussis, tetanus, and pneumococcus and the vaccines should illicit an immune response. Live attenuate vaccines such as measles, mumps, rubella, and oral polio should be avoided until at least year 2 after transplantation. Patients with chronic GVHD will not become immunocompetent until the GVHD is resolved.

VII. ENGRAFTMENT AND REJECTION

Animal models have shown that the *rejection* of a HSCT graft in a recipient is mediated by NK cells and T cells (56). NK cells are associable with the innate immune system and initiate rejection relatively immediately; they do not need the immunological priming that T cells require.

Experiments in rodents have shown that NK precursors are sensitive to radiation, and therefore, pre-transplant regimens of cyclophosphamide or split-dose irradiation are ways to eliminate this arm of rejection. In humans, the exact mechanism of rejection is unknown, but T lymphocytes have been strongly implicated. Interestingly, rejection still occurs in experimental hosts lacking perforin, granzyme B, and/or Fas ligand (57–59). Recipient-derived lymphocytes with anti-donor HLA-specific cytotoxicity have been observed in patients following a graft rejection after a T-cell–depleted HLA-mismatched bone marrow transplant.

Graft rejection in humans is ultimately fatal in most cases. There is very little chance for spontaneous reconstitution with host hematopoietic cells and the chemotherapy regimen is too difficult to withstand another transplant. The *diagnosis* of graft rejection is complicated—there is a failure of engraftment initially and pancytopenia (the latter that can be associated with other causes). The major suggestion of graft rejection is elevated host T cells, indicating a cell-mediated immune response. The probability of rejection depends on many factors, but particularly, the *HLA compatibility* of the donor cells to the recipient. An HLA-identical transplant has a failure to graft reconstitution of about 2 percent, with a slight 1 percent chance of graft rejection. When the donor is HLA haploidentical, the chances of graft failure is 3–15 percent (60), which can vary by the degree of HLA disparities. If there is one disparity with HLA-A, -B, or -DR, the risk is 5 percent, while two or three disparities raise that chance to 15 percent. *Alloimmunization by antibodies* induced by prior transfusions can also cause graft rejection. This can be detected by finding cytotoxic antibodies to donor T or B cells.

There are at least *three* different ways hematopoietic grafts fail: the *first* occurs when there is a failure to achieve an absolute neutrophil count of 500 per µl for three consecutive days any time after transplantation; the *second* occurs when initial engraftment develops into a pancytopenia and bone marrow aplasia; *third* occurs when there is late graft failure with or without the reconstitution of the recipient's own bone marrow (61,62). These three pathways have been observed in patients that were HLA-identical, -nonidentical, and closely matched unrelated donors (MUDs).

When lymphocytes are taken from recipients of HLA-identical marrow at the time of graft failure, they do not display any cytotoxicity toward the donor peripheral blood. In contrast, the pathogenesis in graft failure may be a result of specifically inhibiting donor bone marrow colony forming units in vitro (63,64) and then after in vitro expansion, their ability to lyse the donor-derived peripheral blood cells (65). The lysis of the donor-derived peripheral blood cells is thought to arise as a result of minor histocompatibility antigens.

VIII. COMPLICATIONS

Infection is a common and dangerous complication associated with HSCT. Rapid and specific diagnosis and treatment is essential to ensure the survival of patients after transplantation. Patients receiving bone marrow transplants require regular blood sampling and additional infusions of many blood products, intravenous antibiotics, and nutritional support, all provided by needles through ports, thereby serving as potential routes for infection. The considerable immunosuppression occurring weeks to months after HSCT significantly predisposes the recipient to infection. Allogeneic transplants have extended immunosuppression durations, compared to syngeneic or autologous. GVHD results in even more immunosuppression as a means to treat the disease. Many normally nonpathogenic organisms that are typically part of normal flora grow to invasive and detrimental quantities with destructive consequences. These organisms are mostly, but not exclusively, bacteria such as coagulase-negative staphylococcus, many viruses (specifically cytomegalovirus [CMV]), and fungi such as *Candida* (Figure 9.2) and *Aspergillus*; protozoa such as *Pneumocystis carinii* have been indicated as well (66–68). Conditioning regimens ablate a patient's virus-specific immunity, and because GVHD treatment and prophylaxis render a patient immunocompromised, latent viruses reactivate and reemerge, especially herpes and adenoviruses, causing pain and disease (69–71). Accurate diagnosis is of utmost importance for proper treatment. For example, severe abdominal pain may be thought of as a complication from gastrointestinal (GI) GVHD, when it could easily be adenoviral hepatitis or a member of the herpes virus family (Figures 9.3 and 9.4) in the same way that hematuria and costovertebral tenderness can be adenoviral nephritis. (70). Prophylaxis with antivirals has shown to greatly reduce the incidence of CMV and HSV infections. Patients who underwent transplant but have not yet reconstituted their marrow are at severe risk for fatal respiratory virus infections when there is significant prevalence in the community (68).

i. GI and Hepatic Complications

There has been significant improvement regarding the severity of GI complications; still, the incidence remains high. Infection, mainly viral, cause much of the intestinal and hepatic pathologies associated with HSCT (Figures 9.3 and 9.4). The advent of antiviral therapies has reduced the incidence of herpes simplex virus, as well as CMV infections; however, these cases still occur. There are many pretransplant contraindications, which range from viral hepatitis to tumors.

Cytoreductive pretransplant therapies lower platelet counts significantly and this can cause an increased incidence of bleeding in patients with GI ulcers. Any indication of pain should be investigated with endoscopy to be

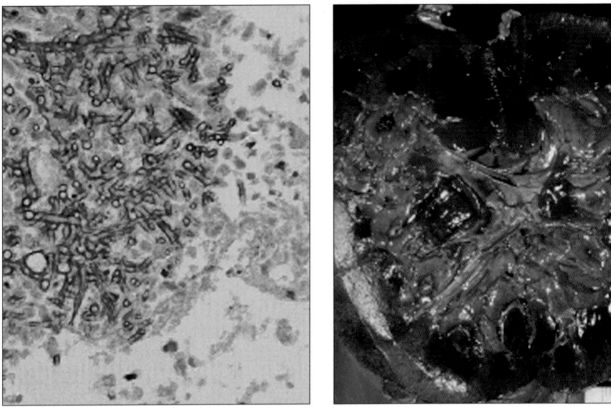

FIGURE 9.2: *Disseminated Candida in transplant patient showing renal involvement (right) with photomicrograph (left) displaying hyphal forms (periodic acid Schiff, 400×).*

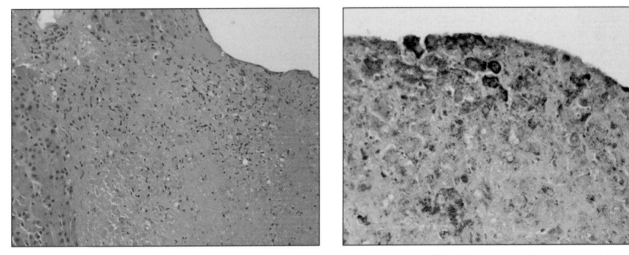

FIGURE 9.3: *Native liver showing focal necrosis with viral cytopathic changes (left – H&E, 200×) and positive immunostain to HSV (right – 200 ×, immunohistochemistry [IHC] to HSV).*

certain of their absence or for treatment prior to transplant. If duodenal or gastric ulcers are present as a result of *Helicobacter pylori* infection, treatment can eliminate this organism and should be done prior to HSCT (72). It is necessary to allow all ulcers to heal, especially those of idiopathic ulcerative colitis or Crohn's disease.

Parasitic infection can be fatal in immunocompromised patients following HSCT, particularly *Entamoeba histolytica* and *Strongyloides* (73). In addition, *Giardia lamblia, E. histolytica,* and *Cryptosporidium* can cause significant diarrhea (74–76). Stool should be checked for *Giardia* antigens, and serum should be checked for antibodies to *E. histolytica* (77).

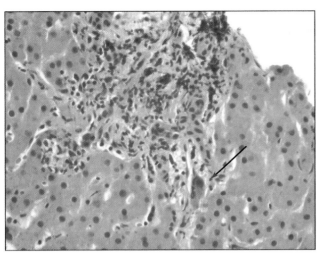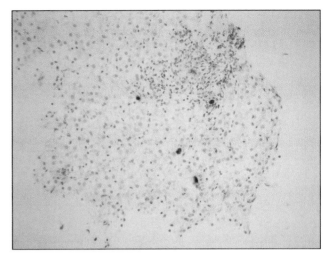

FIGURE 9.4: *Native liver showing inflammation with CMV-like viral cytopathic changes (left – H&E, 400×) and positive immunostain to CMV (right – 200 ×, IHC to CMV).*

Patients with tender hepatomegaly may have a fungal infection or a tumor in their liver. Without the presence of tumors elsewhere in the patient, a search for *fungi* and subsequent treatment systemically should commence (78,79). *Candida* is most likely to be the pathogen but infections may result from numerous fungi species, including *Scopulariopsis, Trichosporon, Pseudallescheria, Coniothyrium, Fusarium, Mucor, Absidia,* and *Dactylaria* (80,81). Fungal infections of the liver tend to present with fever, tender hepatomegaly, and increased serum levels of alkaline phosphatase (78,82). Fungal infections rarely infiltrate the vasculature, so there is little veno-occlusive changes resulting from these infections (82); however, there have been cases of bile duct obstruction by *Candida* (83,84).

Patients presenting with clostridium infections should be treated prior to transplant, whereas with the transplant associated granulocytopenia, typhlitis may develop from *Clostridium septicum* (85). It is necessary to treat perianal infections prior to transplant because tissue necrosis and septicemia may result (86,87). Latent mycobacterium may activate when a patient becomes immunocompromised resulting in hepatic infection (88). Bacillus Calmette-Guerin infections may become disseminated and infect the bone marrow, liver, or spleen (88,89).

There are many *viruses* that create GI and hepatic complications following HSCT. These include HSV (Figure 9.3), CMV (Figure 9.4), varicella-zoster virus (VZV), adenoviruses, echoviruses, hepatitis B, and hepatitis C. A liver biopsy must be taken to see if a patient that acquires HSV after HSCT has liver involvement. The biopsy will have foci of necrosis, surrounded by an area of hepatocytes filled with lightly basophilic intranuclear inclusions (Figure 9.3). Other techniques such as immunohistochemistry or in situ hybridization can determine between HSV types 1 and 2 (90). Computed tomography scans of the abdomen may reveal multiple necrotic lesions

that look like pyogenic abscess; however, the causative agent is difficult to determine (91). Large doses of antiviral acyclovir should be administered to avoid acute hepatitis, which may be deadly if not treated (92).

Infections with VZV are extremely common, with as many as 50 percent of HSCT patients acquiring it (93–96). It is typically seen within eighteen months, mainly presenting within four to seven months after transplantation (97). Infections are typically *disseminated* and occur more frequently in GVHD patients, probably attributed to the extended period of an immunocompromised state. Liver biopsy will reveal necrosis, variable lobular inflammatory cellular infiltrate, and multinucleated giant cells filled with intranuclear inclusions (90).

CMV infections are rare because of prophylactic antiviral regimens. If infection does occur, however, it will be disseminated and the liver will be involved. Even with liver infection, CMV rarely causes hepatic dysfunction (98–100). When examined histologically, there are scattered microabscesses, intranuclear and intracytoplasmic inclusions, as well as bile duct abnormalities (98) (Figure 9.4). These infections are difficult to distinguish between others like it. Determination of a CMV infection can be made with PCR with a sample from the liver biopsy (100,101). CMV can cause enteritis and may contribute to biliary obstruction in cases where ampulla of Vater is involved (102,103).

Complications arising from *adenovirus* in immunocompromised patients are vast, including hemorrhagic enterocolitis, interstitial pneumonitis, myocarditis, hemorrhagic cystitis and nephritis, meningoencephalitis, and fulminant hepatitis (70,104). Liver biopsy is the best determinant of adenovirus infection of the liver. It will appear to have discrete foci of coagulative necrosis surrounded by hepatocytes that have intranuclear inclusions, if the samples are stained (105). Confirmation can come from PCR of stool samples (106).

While there have been no cases of *echovirus* infection in patients after HSCT; immunocompromised patients can develop chronic meningoencephalitis (107). Additionally, echovirus was isolated from the liver of an infant with bone marrow hypoplasia (108) as well as a causative agent in adult hepatitis (109); this implies a possible echoviral hepatitis in patients after post-HSCT.

Hepatitis B (HBV) virus infection in immunosuppressed patients can be detrimental if not fatal. There are three possible ways of becoming infected with HBV. One is an activation from a latent infection, another is a pretransplant infection that progresses as the patient recovers from the transplant, and thirdly, if the transplant donor is infected, the recipient will unfortunately acquire the virus (110). Liver biopsy can reveal a fibrosing cholestatic hepatitis with elevated levels of hepatitis B surface antigen and the associated core antigen in many of the hepatocytes (111) (Figure 9.5). HBV infections can lead to acute hepatitis and liver failure (112), and therefore, levels of viral DNA in the patients' serum should be monitored to avoid this. When levels of HBV DNA are detected, antiviral therapy must be administered and continued throughout recovery. When a patient becomes stable and there is no immunosuppression, a mild liver disease is likely to persist (113).

There are two ways to acquire hepatitis C virus (HCV) after transplantation; there may be progression of a pre-transplant infection or the recipient may be exposed to HCV or HCV-infected blood products, including the transplant itself (114,115). HCV mainly causes chronic viral hepatitis and may lead to cirrhosis (116).

Hepatic veno-occlusive disease (VOD) or sinusoidal obstruction syndrome (SOS) is the most common complication following HSCT, occurring in to 50 percent of patients. Hepatic VOD refers to occlusive lesions in the tiny hepatic venules and endothelium-lined pores that connect the sinusoids to those venules (117). This is a result of the cytotoxic preparations and subsequent treatment associated with the transplant. There is often no venous involvement and the disease is initiated by changes in the hepatic sinusoids. The most common cause of SOS in North America and Western Europe is the myeloablative regimen in preparation for HSCT (Table 9.2). The clinical signs of this syndrome typically develop within few weeks and are jaundice, painful hepatomegaly, and fluid retention especially ascites, all due to liver failure (118). Diagnosis is best determined with a liver biopsy, followed by trichrome staining. Inspection of the biopsy will reveal venular luminal narrowing resulting from subendothelial erythrocytes trapped within the extracellular matrix.

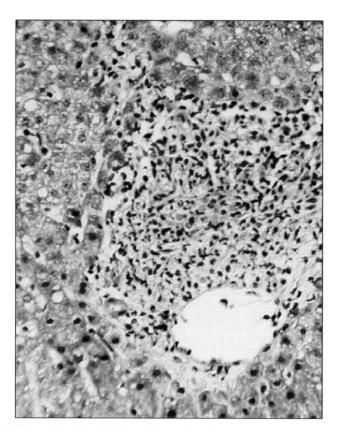
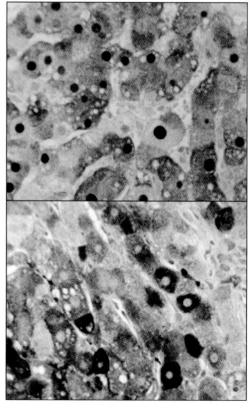

FIGURE 9.5: *Hepatitis B in liver. Left – photomicrograph showing chronic hepatitis with parenchymal injury (H, 200×); immunohistochemical stains confirming hepatitis B infection (upper right—IHC to hepatitis B core antigen, 400×; lower right—IHC to hepatitis B surface antigen, 400×).*

TABLE 9.2 Causes of VOD or SOS

Myeloablative regimens for HSCT
Busulfan/cyclophosphamide/total body irradiation, busulfan/
cyclophosphamide, cyclophosphamide/total body irradiation,
busulfan/melphalan/thiotepa
Gemtuzumab-ozogamicin
Actinomycin D
Pyrrolizidine alkaloids
Dacarbazine
Alkaloids from the plant species *Crotalaria, Heliotropium, Senecio, Symphytum*
6-Thioguanine

There may also be hepatocyte necrosis, embolization of hepatocytes into the portal or terminal hepatic venules, and sinusoidal dilation, filled with red blood cells (Figure 9.6). This is followed by complete obliteration of these venules, a thickening of the outer layer of the hepatic venules, called phlebosclerosis, along with fibrosis of the sinusoids adjacent to the terminal hepatic venules, the third zone of the acinus (119,120). The final event is the accumulation of factor VIII in the VOD lesions, followed by deposits of collagen and extracellular matrix proteins (121). The only treatment for this constellation of symptoms is supportive.

Iron overload is seen both acutely, when patients are transplanted for thalassemia or aplastic anemia, and chronically, when patients suffer from hemosiderosis. Patients undergoing HSCT for hematological malignancies may present with a 25 percent increase in iron, designating a grade 3 or 4 siderosis (122). Chelation prior to

transplant has significant increase in survival rates in patients with thalassemia (123). Studies have shown that either excess iron in the liver or circulating free iron is associated with regimen toxicity and early post-transplant fatalities (124–126). With this in mind, it is possible to postpone iron quantification until after patient recovery, unless there is indicated liver injury.

Long-term survivors of HSCT for hematological malignancies have a 90 percent prevalence of iron overload (127,128); this is thought to be related to the multiple red blood cell transfusions and dyserythropoiesis. Ferritin levels should be measured as it provides the best indicator of iron stores in tissues in patients without complication, while patients with viral infections or GVHD should also have liver biopsies (129). It is thought that persistent hepatic dysfunction in post-HSCT patients is due to lipid peroxidation of membranes by free radicals and intracellular accumulations of iron (130–134). Patients receiving HSCT for thalassemia or hematological malignancies may also suffer from portal fibrosis, cirrhosis, and hepatocellular carcinoma with hemosiderosis; however, these patients are typically coinfected with HCV and this tends to increase the pathologies associated with iron overload (135,136). Additionally, free iron is a growth requirement for many opportunistic bacterial infections, particularly *Listeria monocytogenes*, mucormycosis, *Yersinia enterocolitica*, and noncholera *Vibrio* species, observed especially in immunocompromised patients (137–140). So, every patient should be evaluated for iron overload, especially when displaying abnormal liver function tests.

Malignancies may recur within the first post-transplant year in many patients. This may be determined by elevated

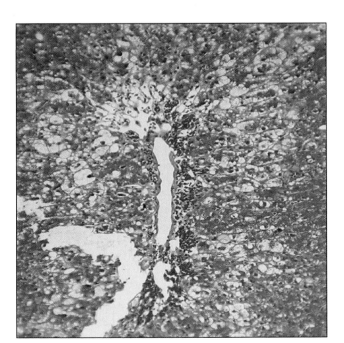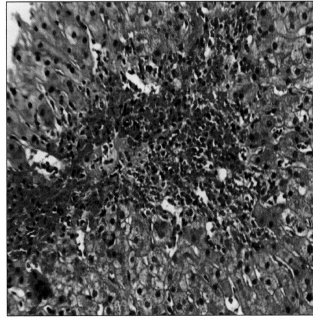

FIGURE 9.6: *Mild (left—H&E, 200×) and severe (right—H&E, 400×) centrilobular hemorrhage in hepatic VOD.*

liver enzymes, hepatomegaly, or imaging study abnormalities and should by recognized and taken into consideration following bone marrow transplantation. EBV-associated lymphoproliferative disorder is frequently seen in patients recovering from allogeneic HSCT, with up to 25 percent incidence in HLA-mismatched, T-cell–depleted transplants, while extremely rare after autologous transplants (25,141,142). There is liver involvement in about 50 percent of these patients, indicated by elevated alkaline phosphatase levels in the blood, as well as hepatosplenomegaly. Biopsies display portal inflammatory cellular infiltrate with plasma cells, lymphocytes and immunoblasts (25). Diagnostic confirmation is made by immunohistological staining for EBV-associated markers (143).

Gross GI bleeding including hematemesis, melena, or rectal bleeding occurs in less than 10 percent of patients post-HSCT within the first 100 days (144,145); however, other minor bleeding consequences occur as a result of low platelet counts. The most common cause of severe bleeding is from diffuse small intestinal ulceration from acute GVHD. Mucosal trauma of the stomach from vomiting leads to "coffee-ground" emesis (146). Intramural esophageal hematomas from Mallory-Weiss tears at the gastroesophageal junction in combination with low platelets counts are a large source of severe bleeding (145). Nausea and vomiting lasting longer than sixty days may be from GVHD or from infection from HSV and CMV causing esophagitis (146–149). These bleeds typically resolve themselves when platelet counts rise above 60,000/μl.

ii. Gallbladder and Biliary Complications

After HSCT, it is common for biliary sludge to develop within one to four days after transplantation (150,151). Risk is increased in patients who fasted for extended periods while on total parenteral nutrition were administered ceftriaxone or narcotics, and possibly from the endothelial injury resulting from the conditioning regimen or GVHD (152). Most patients recover and the sludge resolves, however some patients may acquire a biliary obstruction (103). Biliary sludge has been indicated as a cause of acute "acalculous" cholecystitis, acute pancreatitis, and acute bacterial cholangitis and may also obscure the gallbladder from sight when performing scintigraphy (150,153–156). It may also exacerbate the symptoms of hepatic GVHD, because there is a correlation to its resolution with an improvement of symptoms (157).

Acute cholecystitis is rarely observed in HSCT patients (150) but when seen, it is not associated with a presentation of gall stones (i.e., acalculous cholecystitis) (158,159). It may represent a recurrence of leukemia with a gallbladder involvement (160), from biliary sludge production, or from an infection, either CMV or fungal (161,162).

iii. Pulmonary Complications

The lungs are particularly susceptible to disease resulting from hematopoietic stem cell transplantation. Complications include chemical toxicity, damage from irradiation, tumor metastasis, and given its function, it is particularly susceptible to infection. Many organisms are capable of infecting a patient and causing *pneumonia*, typically implicated pathogens are respiratory syncytial virus (RSV), mycobacteria, streptococcus pneumonia; patients recovering from HSCT may be infected with other organisms, most notably *Legionella, Mycoplasma, Chlamydia, Cryptosporidia, Campylobacter, Toxoplasma* spp., and human herpes virus (HHV)-6, -7, and -8 (66,163). It is estimated that 35 percent of allogeneic HSCT patients treated for leukemia have developed nonbacterial pneumonia (Figure 9.7), a clinical syndrome referred to as *interstitial pneumonia* (IP) (69). This syndrome is typically acute and severe, a sharp contrast to the chronic pneumonia usually associated with IP in non-transplanted patients. Improved prophylaxis, such as antivirals, antibiotics, and antimycotics, has notably reduced the overall prevalence. About one-third of the IPs are labeled idiopathic, with no known origin of disease. These cases probably result from many factors, including the chemical and irradiative pretransplant conditioning regimens (164–167). Acute GVHD increases the risk for this idiopathic interstitial pneumonia (IIP) (164,168). IIP has not been shown to be a consequence of allogeneic HSCT; however, it has been shown in mice to develop when there is a presentation of GVHD after irradiation (169). HHV-6 has been implicated as well (170).

Pulmonary veno-occlusive disorder has been observed in several instances following chemotherapy and it may be associated with hepatic VOD and IP (166,171,172). Clinical identification of this complication is important

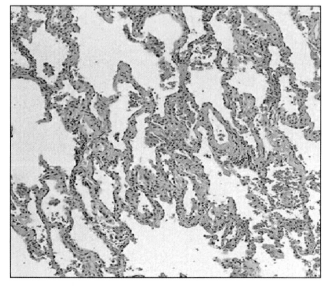

FIGURE 9.7: *Mild interstitial inflammation in open lung biopsy, representative of interstitial pneumonia (H&E, 200×).*

since early detection and treatment with high doses of steroids has improved outcomes (173).

iv. Neurological Complications

Neurological complications have been observed in all phases of an HSCT, including the conditioning regimen, the post-transplant pancytopenia, and the immunosuppressed or GVHD phases (174–177). The adverse neurological effects can be divided into five groups: infectious, cerebrovascular, metabolic, toxic, and immune mediated. These complications can occur within different phases of HSCT and with varying severity. Toxic complications can occur during all three phases, secondary to administered chemotherapies. The infectious, metabolic and cerebrovascular complications mainly manifest during the latter two phases. *Infections* such as bacterial meningitis arise during the pancytopenic phase when patients are leukopenic. When a patient has GVHD, other complications can manifest, including fungal abscesses, meningoencephalitis, and septic or mycotic embolisms. Overall patient survival with neurological complications has increased significantly over the past ten years, mainly as a result of better treatment of infection (178). Patients with neurological infection present with altered mental status, delirium, and depressed sensorium, mostly without meningeal signs or obvious lateralizing neurological signs. Cerebrospinal fluid from a lumbar puncture should be used to aid in diagnosis of infectious organisms. Meningeal infection tends to disrupt the blood-brain barrier and hydrophilic drugs such as chloramphenicol, trimethoprim, and sulfonamides. Typically, the organisms responsible for central nervous system (CNS) infection in allogeneic transplants are *Listeria monocytogenes*, which occurs within the first four months after transplantation (179,180), and long-term survivors may acquire a meningitis from *Streptococcus pneumoniae* (180,181). Autologous transplants have only two cases described, *L. monocytogenes* and one case of *Stomatococcus mucilaginous* (180). Additionally, one fatal case of *Mycobacterium tuberculosis* CNS infection has been seen; this organism in the CNS is rare, present only in 0.47 percent of allogeneic transplants and 0.25 percent of autologous transplants (177,182). Toxoplasmosis is occasionally observed early after transplant (183,184). Many viral infections have been seen, as described before, and incidence can be decreased with prophylactic antiviral regimens.

Cerebrovascular accidents such as intracranial bleeds and ischemic stroke can occur, and are typically fatal. In autopsies of 105 HSCT patients, 13 percent had subarachnoid hemorrhages, 10 percent subdural hematomas, and 5 percent intraparenchymal hematomas (185). Computed tomography is preferred to magnetic resonance imaging (MRI) to determine an acute bleed since MRI only shows bleeds after methemoglobin has formed, which

takes approximately twelve hours (185). Neurosurgical intervention is necessary to remove any hematomas. Patients with intraparenchymal bleeds can show signs of hemiparesis or other cerebral hemisphere deficit, followed by depression of sensorium and then a brain stem transtentorial herniation may occur. Cerebellar hemorrhages are difficult to distinguish before they evolve to paresis and then coma. Patients have a 44 percent risk of developing a subdural hematoma, and this complication occurs more frequently after autologous transplantation (177). The removal of cerebrospinal fluid by lumbar puncture allows room for the hematoma to heal and relieves symptoms associated with the increase in pressure.

Ischemic strokes may arise due to embolisms from endocarditis or thrombus. Thrombotic thrombocytopenic purpura (TTP) has been seen after allogeneic transplant, and may cause seizures or other neurological signs associated with focal disruption of blood flow (186). A hypercoagulable state is observed in many patients as a result of endothelial damage from the conditioning chemotherapy (187,188). This may cause a nonbacterial thrombotic endocarditis, which is prone to embolism and causing ischemic stroke (189).

The *metabolic complications* that occur during the pancytopenic phase include gram-negative sepsis, sedative-hypnotic drug reactions, and hepatic encephalopathy of VOD. The GVHD phase manifests hypoxic encephalopathy of IP, hepatic encephalopathy of GVHD, and uremic encephalopathy. Metabolic encephalopathy following HSCT is most commonly associated with gram-negative sepsis or after sedative-hypnotic drug treatment. Hypoxic encephalopathy, which may cause permanent neurological damage, can result from IP or hypoxemia following hemolytic-uremic syndrome, which is hallmarked by the lysis of erythrocytes. GVHD may cause hepatic encephalopathy from GVHD liver involvement or from the fulminant hepatic failure of hepatic VOD.

Toxic complications are the result of chemotherapies administered throughout transplantation treatment. Encephalopathies may result during the conditioning phase from drugs such as BCNU, busulfan, mechlorethamine, and ifosfamide. Neuropathies may result from treatment with VP-16, cisplatin, and paclitaxel. Cisplatin neurotoxicity, steroid toxicity, and leukoencephalopathies may occur during the pancytopenia or GVHD phases, while thalidomide neuropathy can occur during the GVHD phase. Finally, during the GVHD phase, *immune-mediated complications* can arise, most commonly, polymyositis, myasthenia gravis, and demyelinating polyneuropathy.

v. Hemolytic Complications

Major ABO compatibility issues: Hemolytic anemia (HA) and thrombotic microangiopathic syndromes are potential immune-mediated complications after HSCT. Most HA cases result from alloimmune reactions against noncompatible ABO antigens, while autoimmune HA (AIHA) has also been seen following allogeneic HSCT. Patients receiving HSCT from unrelated donors or that develop chronic extensive GVHD are at heightened risk of AIHA (190). ABO incompatibilities are present in 23–30 percent of all HSCTs. This is because donor-recipient ABO incompatibility is not a contraindication for a HSCT. With allogeneic transplantation, there have been no evidence to illustrate that ABO mismatched donors increase transplant associated GVHD, graft rejection, or overall survival (191,192). However, the risks for several immunological complications remain high. There can be *severe hemolytic reactions* immediately or a delayed response due to erythropoiesis after reconstitution. Red blood cells are removed by buffy-coat removal prior to transplantation to eliminate possible adverse immunological effects (193–195). Isohemagglutinins are produced by lymphocytes and can cause hemolysis immediately if present in the marrow infusion or later if produced by the donor lymphocytes (192,196–199). Isohemagglutinins can be removed by plasma exchange, plasma immunoadsorption, or whole blood immunoadsorption performed three to four days prior to infusion, reducing the isohemagglutinin titers to 1:16 or less (200). Using donor typed–fresh frozen plasma to get A and B antigens is another technique for the in vitro adsorption and removal of these antigens (201). There is about a 10 percent chance of adverse reaction after these procedures, and is shown to be higher if patients have high isohemagglutinin titers prior to transplant and are given GVHD prophylaxis with cyclosporine or prednisone (202). If the erythrocyte depletion is incomplete, it may result in hemolytic anemia. It is preferred to have a smaller amount of stem cells transplanted than a larger amount because there is the possibility of contamination by erythrocytes. There has been evidence that shows an increase likelihood of graft failure in recipients of MUD marrow (203). Hemolysis can occur several weeks after transplant in patients where donor-derived RBCs appear in circulation and immune reactions are mounted against them. This occurs when residual host lymphocytes respond to donor-derived RBCs (192,196–199).

Minor ABO mismatch occurs in 15–20 percent of HLA-matched donor-recipient transplants. As with major ABO incompatibility, *immediate hemolysis* may occur because of isohemagglutinins infused with the transplant or delayed as a result of their production later by donor lymphocytes. Immediate reactions have not been shown to be lethal, but delayed reactions have serious complications that may result in organ failure or death (192). Patients with GVHD prophylaxis are at an increased risk (196,204). Bystander blood group O has been affected by hemolysis as a result of minor ABO incompatibility. The occurrence rate is higher in patients receiving peripheral blood transplants (205). Two methods to reduce the risk of minor

ABO complications for both immediate and delayed hemolytic reactions is the *removal of plasma* from donor reactions and a pre-HSCT dilution of the recipient's erythrocytes with blood type O erythrocytes (204).

While an Rh factor mismatch has not been shown to adversely affect engraftment, overall survival, or GVHD (192,206,207), mismatched Rh can result in a positive antiglobulin test (192), with described cases of severe delayed alloimmune hemolytic reactions (208). Pancytopenia in all three cell lines was seen in one patient (209). There is also a 10–15 percent chance of hemolysis from minor Rh mismatches (196). This is thought to result from a primary antibody response mediated by the infused donor lymphocytes. It is recommended to prophylactically infuse Rh-negative blood or anti-Rh immunoglobulin to reduce the risk (207,209). When a patient is Rh-factor negative and the donor is Rh-factor positive, Rh-negative blood products should be administered. When the patient is Rh-factor positive and the donor is Rh-factor negative, Rh-negative blood products should be administered as well.

The mechanism of AIHA is not fully understood but is thought to be multifactorial (190). Only a few cases of true AIHA following allogeneic and autologous transplants have been observed. This complication is a result of antigen processing by the new marrow, which begins to recognize "self" most likely after a viral infection. B-cell dysfunction as a result of T-cell dysfunction leads to the production of autoantibodies. It may result from regulatory T-cell dysfunction (210). This hypothesis is supported by the autoimmune thrombocytopenia seen in GVHD (211,212). Seven cases have been described in a 236-patient study that underwent a T-cell–depleted allogeneic HSCT. Additionally, four patients with Evans syndrome developed this as well (213,214). It is therefore thought that the immunosuppressive effect of T-cell depletion that leads to this B-cell dysfunction may be a contributing factor.

Many complications may result from thrombotic microangiopathies, including a hemolytic syndrome and visceral injury (Figure 9.8). Consequence of chemotherapy prior to and after transplantation, the endothelial vascular lining is compromised and therefore prone to thrombus development. There is complete or partial obstruction of many small arterioles and capillaries by microthrombi formed from activated platelets that become overlaid with endothelial cell proliferation. Mid-sized vessels may also be occluded (Figure 9.8). Implicated chemicals are cyclophosphamide, nitrosoureas, and platinum-based compounds; also GVHD prophylactic agents, cytokines from acute GVHD, CMV, and fungal infections (215–221). Finally, *Bartonella*-like inclusions have been found in RBCs following HSCT with thrombotic microangiopathy (222).

Elevated levels of thrombomodulin, P-selectin (GMP-140), and tissue plasminogen activating factor are observed

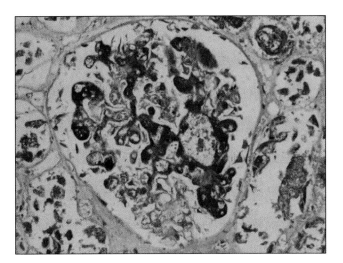

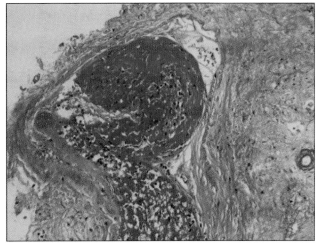

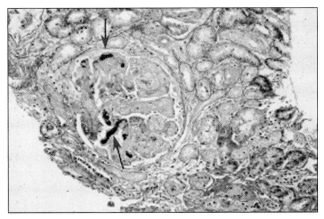

FIGURE 9.8: *Renal biopsy of patient with thrombotic glomerulopathy (upper left—glomerulus with thrombi and necrosis, H&E, 400×) and microangiopathy (right—arterial thrombus, H&E, 200×). (lower) Glomerulus showing fibrin thrombi in capillary loops (arrows) (PTAH stain, 400×).*

in patients with TTP or HUS (223). The three- to six-month delay observed between the cellular injury from chemotherapy and radiation and the onset of clinical symptoms may be a result from the formation of autoantibodies to endothelial cells or platelet glycoprotein IV (CD36) or other endothelial antigens (224). Additional support for this hypothesis is the presence of elevated plasma levels of IL-1 and -6, soluble IL-2 receptor, and tumor necrosis factor (TNF) (225). Animal models have shown that accumulation of von Willebrand factor (vWF) instigates the formation of microthrombi (226); animal models, however, displayed thrombi in vessels supporting the liver and spleen, while humans with TTP or HUS typically have pathology associated with the brain and kidney (227) (Figure 9.8). Human plasma samples display a correlation to these findings by having a notable amount of vWF multimers (ULvWF for "unusually large") representing accumulations of this clotting factor with higher affinity for platelets, particularly in high-flow arterioles. Additionally, the amount of monomeric vWF is decreased in the plasma of the same patients (228,229).

vi. Oral Cavity Complications

The oral cavity and its' mucosa are susceptible to many infections, both invasive and opportunistic. It is also damaged by chemotherapies administered pretransplant. Continual assessment is of utmost importance in the prevention of disease. The oral cavity is a gateway to the bloodstream and therefore has considerable influence on the outcome of patients after bone marrow transplantation. Simple and routine *oral hygiene* has significant impact on patient survival. Prior to transplant, a patient should be in the best possible oral health. Unknown underlying oral disease can manifest terrible outcomes after chemotherapy. Dental decay, perio- and endodontal diseases are typical causes of infection and complication; these should be identified and treated prior to transplant.

Oropharyngeal mucositis is the most common and worrisome outcome from the oral toxicity of the HSCT therapy. Its detriment varies from benign or absent to significant bleeding and pain. The extent of damage is related to the conditioning regimen and the type of HSCT the patient receives. The transplant contribution to the

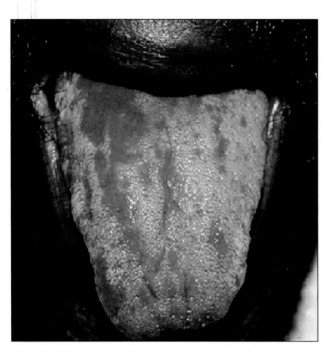

FIGURE 9.9: *Oral candidiasis in a transplant patient.*

damage is determined by the extent of mismatch with the donor (230). About five to ten days after myeloablative chemotherapy, oral manifestations arise (230). At first, the nonkeratinized oral mucosa atrophies and there is erythema. This typically progresses to ulceration and becomes more severe as time passes, at its worst by day 11 (231). Mechanistically, there is radiation- or chemotherapy-induced injury to basal epithelial cells among other cells in the mucosa resulting in cell death or injury. Endothelial cells, fibroblasts, and epithelial cells participate in upregulation of genes that modulate the damage response, while lymphocytes and macrophages secrete proinflammatory cytokines that potentiate further tissue injury (231). The inflammatory cycle accelerates with damage to *epithelial stem cells*. The latter injury results in thinned epithelium and an initiation of ulceration. Bacteria in the oral cavity colonize the ulcer, where their presence in the connective tissue induces cytokine release. The inflammatory infiltrate during the ulcerative stage consists of a mixture of macrophages, lymphocytes, plasma cells, and mast cells.

The *oral regions* most affected are the lateral and ventral parts of the tongue and the mucosa of the labia and bucca, typically healing over the following two weeks (232). These affects are worsened by salivary gland dysfunction (xerostomia) associated with chemotherapy, which removes the lubricating and antimicrobial effects of saliva and the reactivation of latent viruses such as HSV, VSV, and CMV that create sores that become ports of entry for other organisms (233–235). Opportunistic infections include *Pseudomonas aeruginosa*, *Neisseria* species,

Escherichia coli, streptococcus and staphylococcus species. Candidiasis is the most common fungal infection to the oral mucosa (Figure 9.9), with *C. albicans* being the most pathogenic.

The lateral and ventrolateral portions of the tongue may develop painless exophytic soft tissue masses that resemble polyps and can range from millimeters to several centimeters in length with a height up to 1.5 cm. They are typically overlaid by mucosa, but sometimes may become covered by a pseudomembranous fibrin exudate and histological examination shows granulomatous tissue (236,237).

IX. GRAFT-VERSUS-HOST DISEASE

GVHD is the occurrence of an immunologically mediated and injurious set of reactions by the transplanted cells that are genetically disparate to their host; it is a unique phenomenon that has been described as the age of bone marrow and solid organ transplantation has emerged. In 1955, Barnes and Loutit first described GVHD in mice (238). In 1966, Billingham (239) proposed three conditions required for the development of GVHD as follows 1) the graft must contain immunologically competent cells, 2) the host must possess important transplant alloantigens that are lacking in the donor graft so that the host appears foreign to the graft, and 3) the host itself must be incapable of mounting an effective immunologic reaction to the graft.

GVHD occurs when the recipient is recognized as foreign by the graft and consequently subject to rejection. The response is initiated by the *donor T cells*, which recognize the recipients' alloantigens and deems them foreign (240–242). There is a constellation of events that trigger this response. Donor CD8+ cytotoxic T cells recognize the mismatched MHC class I on host cells and subsequently become activated, while donor CD4+ helper T cells are activated when there is mismatched MHC class II presenting polymorphic peptides as minor histocompatibility complexes (MiHC) (i.e., direct presentation). In addition, there is a vigorous activation of donor T cells by the host APCs (i.e., indirect presentation) that remain after the pretransplant regimen (241,243,244). If the donor APC indirectly expresses alloantigens, then donor T cells are easily activated and subsequently attack the host.

GVHD is an exaggeration of normal cellular and humoral responses to injury, resulting in detrimental inflammation that is often fatal. Lymphocytes transplanted into a donor are responding to foreign antigens in recipients of bone marrow transplants that are due to chemotherapy regimens are in a *proinflammatory* state (Figure 9.10). Recipient endothelial and epithelial cells secrete and overexpress immunomodulatory factors that include adhesion molecules, cytokines, and cell surface

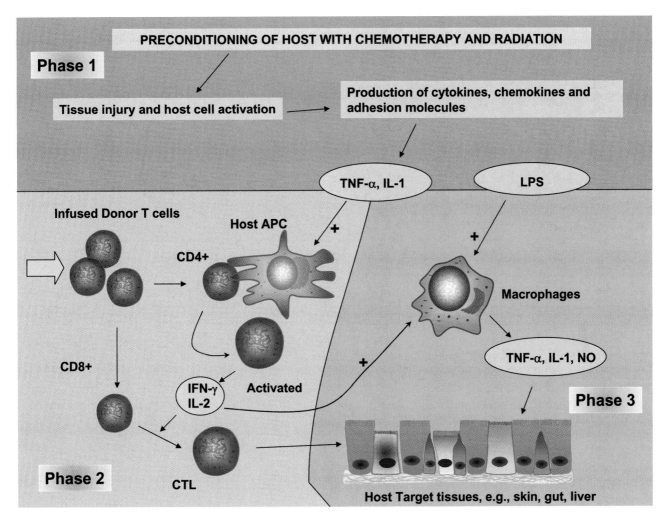

FIGURE 9.10: Phases of acute GVHD.

recognition molecules. Thus, the pathophysiology is two-fold: donor cells respond to foreign material and proliferate only after being introduced to an environment primed for this destruction. One may consider the response parallel to a person's immune response to viral infection, or that of gram-negative bacteria.

Certain organs are *more susceptible* to the effects of GVHD, mainly because of their elevated exposure to proinflammatory endotoxin and other bacterial products that trigger and amplify cellular responses. These include the skin, gut, and liver. Other organs such as the heart and kidneys can be rejected by cellular processes when placed into a recipient, but are rarely, if ever, the targets for GVHD. The *lungs* are not classic targets of GVHD; however, there is some controversy as to whether or not they are susceptible. The lungs are constantly introduced to foreign and inflammatory producing material and as a result have large numbers of APCs such as macrophages and dendritic cells that have been shown to enhance GVHD (245–247). In both experimental and clinical scenarios, *acute GVHD* describes a syndrome consisting of

dermatitis, enteritis, and hepatitis occurring within the first 100 days, but typically within thirty to forty days, following HSCT. *Chronic GVHD* usually develops after 100 days and describes an autoimmune syndrome consisting of impairment of multiple organs or organ systems.

There are three distinct phases associated with acute GVHD (Figure 9.10). The *first phase* is initiated in response to stressors resulting in tissue damage, these include previous infection, underlying illness, and also the transplant-conditioning regimen. With HSCT, the proinflammatory environment is the product of the extremely toxic conditioning regimen given prior to the bone marrow infusion. Various tissues, especially intestinal mucosa and the liver, are damaged and display proinflammatory changes. This process attracts and retains white blood cells in these tissues. The activated tissues secrete inflammatory cytokines such as TNF-αa and IL-1 (241,248). They also secrete growth factors such as granulocyte-macrophage colony stimulating factor, transforming growth factor alpha (249,250), and many others as well (251). These cytokines may upregulate cellular adhesion molecules (252) and

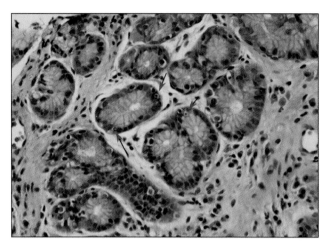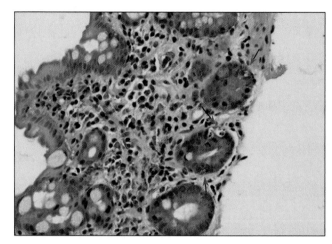

FIGURE 9.11: *Grade 1 acute GVHD involving ileum (left, H&E, 400×) and stomach (right, H&E, 400×).*

MHC antigens (253–257), thus increasing T-cell responses and contributing to GVHD.

The *second phase* occurs after antigen is presented and donor T cells become activated. The process begins with antigen presentation by APCs on their MHC molecules. T cells recognize MHC or MiHC with synthesis of cytokines such as IL-2, IL-12, interferon gamma (IFN-γ), and their respective receptors (Figure 9.10). Both IL-2 and IFN-γ have been implicated in GVHD's pathophysiology. Th1 cells are thought to increase GVHD effects, while Th2 do not (258). In addition to T cells, NK cells, and other cell types are recruited for clonal expansion and differentiation. All this occurs in as little as twenty-four hours, and will commence within five days (259,260). Cell surface molecule expression is changed to facilitate the cellular migration to carry out those functions (261).

Phase three begins when, in response to Th1 cytokines, cytotoxic T cells, and NK cells specifically target and injure cells through Fas-FasL and perforin-granzyme B systems; through the release of additional cytokines, the reaction is perpetuated by recruiting additional macrophages, granulocytes and NK cells (Figure 9.10). In addition, macrophages may become stimulated directly when lipopolysaccharide (LPS) from intestinal bacteria crossing damaged gut epithelia, thereby activating this response through a different pathway, resulting in the same pathology. NK cells do not recognize HLAs but are recruited by secreted factors released by the T cells (262,263).

Mononuclear phagocytic cells that have been primed by Th1 cells during the second phase of GVHD now receive a second signal that increases their release of inflammatory cytokines TNF-α and IL-1. This may be stimulated by the bacterial endotoxin (LPS), which stimulates gut-associated lymphocytes and macrophages (264). LPS that reaches the skin may stimulate a similar reaction via keratinocytes, dermal fibroblasts, and macrophages (249–251). TNF-α causes tissue damage by initiating necrosis of target tissues

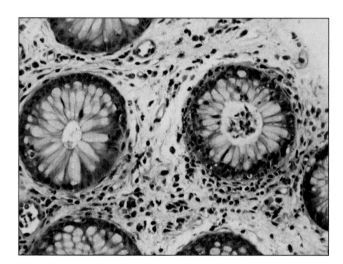

FIGURE 9.12: *Grade 2 GVHD in ileum (H&E, 400×).*

or by inducing apoptosis. *Apoptosis* is particularly critical in the gut (265) (Figures 9.11 and 9.12), skin (266,267), and endothelium (268) following an allogeneic HSCT. Activated macrophages proceed to release large amounts of nitric oxide (NO), this can cause significant immunosuppression (269–271). These processes amplify and synergize each other to produce massive inflammatory responses, typically resulting in GVHD (272).

There are *three established pathways* that contribute to GVHD effectors: 1) the perforin-granzyme B pathway, 2) the Fas-FasL pathway, and 3) the direct cytokine-mediated injury pathway. There is certainly overlap between these pathways, and an understanding is crucial to the prevention and treatment of GVHD (273).

Viral infections are more frequently associated with GVHD and are known to trigger and exacerbate this process. CMV, HSV, and possibly HHV-6 have been described as suspects (99,274,275). The hypothesis is that viral antigens presented by cells on MHC class I complexes may function as a MiHC and stimulate a T-cell response.

TABLE 9.3 Grading of Acute GVHD

Organ	Grade	Description
Skin	+1	Maculopapular rash over <25% of body area
	+2	Maculopapular rash over 25–50% of body area
	+3	Generalized erythroderma
	+4	Generalized erythroderma with bullous formation and often with desquamation
Hepatic	+1	Bilirubin 2.0–3.0 mg/dl; SGOT 150–750 IU
	+2	Bilirubin 3.1–6.0 mg/dl
	+3	Bilirubin 6.1–15.0 mg/dl
	+4	Bilirubin >15.0 mg/dl
GI	+1	Diarrhea >30 ml/kg or >500 ml/day
	+2	Diarrhea >60 ml/kg or >1,000 ml/day
	+3	Diarrhea >90 ml/kg or >1500 ml/day
	+4	Diarrhea >90 ml/kg or >2,000 ml/day; or severe abdominal pain with or without ileus

The *clinical presentation* is often a triad of dermatitis, hepatitis, and gastroenteritis although symptoms may occur alone or in different combinations. Skin: maculopapular rash may present with the onset occurring five to forty-seven days after transplantation. Pruritis involving the palms and soles may precede the rash. In the early stage, the rash is confined to the nape of the neck, shoulder, palms, or soles. It may be confluent and involve the entire surface of the body. In severe cases, bullous lesions similar to third degree burns may develop. Liver: the liver is the second most common organ involved. GVHD first manifests as elevated liver transaminase levels. Cholestatic jaundice is common, but hepatic failure with encephalopathy is unusual. Hepatic and GI involvement may manifest with or following skin involvement. GI: GVHD results in profuse diarrhea; intestinal bleeding; and cramping, abdominal pain, and paralytic ileus. Common symptoms of upper GI involvement are anorexia, nausea and vomiting.

Grading: Acute GVHD is graded in five steps from 0–IV based on involvement of the skin, liver, and GI tract. Grade 0 indicates no clinical evidence of disease. Grades I–IV are graded functionally. Grade I indicates rash on less than 50 percent of skin, and no gut or liver involvement. Grade II indicates rash covering more than 50 percent of cells, bilirubin 2–3 mg/dl, diarrhea 10–15 ml/kg/day, or persistent nausea. Grade III or IV indicates generalized erythroderma with bullous formation, bilirubin greater than 3 mg/dl, or diarrhea more than 16 ml/kg/day (Table 9.3).

Histologically, the skin (Figure 9.13) (also see chapter 2) demonstrates epidermal basal vacuolization, followed by epidermal basal cell apoptotic death with lymphoid infiltration. Eosinophilic bodies may be observed with increased severity. Bullous formation with epidermal separation and necrosis is observed in later stages. T cells are the primary infiltrating population (Figure 9.14) and there is marked increased expression of class II MHC molecules

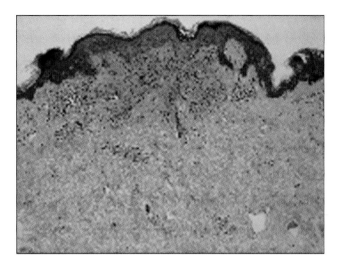

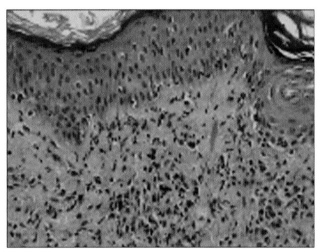

FIGURE 9.13: *Skin with GVHD changes including subepidermal infiltrate and focal epidermal injury and inflammatory cell infiltration (top, H&E, 100×; bottom, H&E, 400×).*

(Figure 9.14). Liver tissue undergoing acute GVHD can demonstrate damage to more than 50 percent of bile ducts with vacuolated cytoplasm, with duct cell nuclear pleomorphism and necrosis of individual cells (apoptosis). There is a lymphocytic infiltrate of portal tracts with endothelialitis along with ballooning degeneration of hepatocytes and/or acidophil bodies (Figure 9.15). GI biopsy specimens show diffuse edema and mucosal swelling followed by variable crypt apoptosis, a mixed chronic and predominantly lymphoplasmacytic infiltrate, and possibly crypt dropout. The acquisition of serial biopsies is useful in determining a diagnosis of GVHD (276).

An accurate diagnosis of GVHD is critical to the treatment and its grading typically predicts the clinical course and outcome (277). There are a variety of possible diagnoses associated with the intestinal involvement when patients present with anorexia and vomiting; these include peptic ulceration, GVHD, and mycotic or viral infection (146,278). Biopsy and upper GI endoscopy may not elucidate

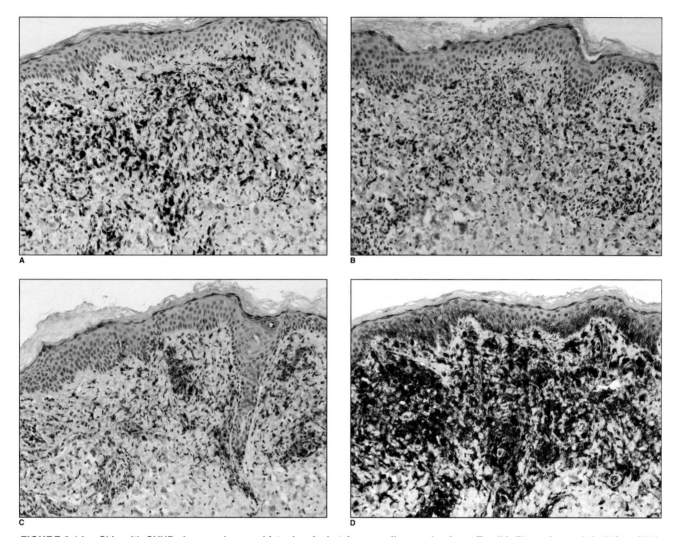

FIGURE 9.14: *Skin with GVHD changes. Immunohistochemical stains revealing predominant T-cell infiltrate (upper left, IHC to CD3), with slight CD8+ T cell (upper right, IHC to CD8) predominance compared to CD4+ cells (lower left, IHC to CD4). HLA-DR expression is markedly upregulated on the infiltrating cells and some of the epidermal structure (lower right, IHC to HLA-DR). All pictures at 200×.*

the diagnosis properly. Liver biopsy may not reveal abnormal pathology, making diagnosis difficult (279). It is of utmost importance that physicians recognize the constellation of symptoms and reach a proper diagnosis.

Chronic GVHD has a pathogenetic mechanism unlike that of acute GVHD and has been approached as an *autoimmune disease* (280). The T cells in chronic GVHD are considered autoreactive because they recognize MHC class II molecule determinants, instead of recognizing the polymorphic major and/or MiHC. Reactive T cells in acute GVHD are specific for host alloantigens (281,282). There is evidence of anti-cytoskeletal, antinuclear, anti–double–stranded DNA, antinucleolar, and anti–smooth muscle autoantibodies in patients with chronic GVHD with a prevalence ranging from 11 to 62 percent (283,284). Cytokine profiles of chronic GVHD often show elevated levels of IL-4 or IFN-γ, and no IL-2 – this combination of cytokines may be potentiating the production of collagen by fibroblasts. The autoreactive T cells appear

to arising from a dysfunctional thymus, which may have been damaged by a bout of acute GVHD, by the conditioning regimen, or even by the age-related involution of the organ. Syngeneic GVHD may also have autoreactive T cells underlying its pathology.

Chronic GVHD occurs in approximately one-third of HLA-identical sibling HSCT patients, 49 percent of HLA-identical related HSCT patients, and 64 percent of MUD transplant patients surviving over 150 days after transplantation (285). It has been estimated to have a prevalence of up to 80 percent in unrelated HLA-nonidentical, one-antigen matched transplant patients.

The *pattern of organ involvement* observed in chronic GVHD differs from acute GVHD. Chronic GVHD can cause damage to the liver, gut, and skin, such as in acute GVHD; however, it is *also* known to involve the eyes, lungs, oral, and neuromuscular systems.

Liver function tests and biopsies are used to determine the degree of pathology associated with chronic GVHD.

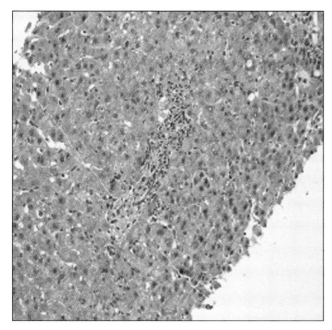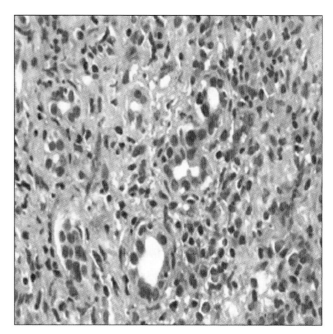

FIGURE 9.15: *Liver undergoing acute GVHD (left, 100×, H&E) (right, 200×, H&E).*

Cholestatic alterations are seen in chronic GVHD, typically absent from acute GVHD (286,287) with rare cases having development of portal hypertension, cirrhosis, and even death from liver failure (288). The differential diagnosis is broad and complex, including infection (either viral or mycotic), adverse drug reactions, gallstones, and also neoplastic disease (287). The liver shows a portal mononuclear infiltrate with damage to the bile ducts and eventually ductopenia, changes that can be seen in the absence of clinical manifestations.

Unlike acute GVHD, *GI involvement* is less likely with chronic GVHD and if present may be esophageal injury. Symptoms can be misleading, including dysphagia, pain, and weight loss (289). Poor acid clearance and motility issues ranging from aperistalsis to high-amplitude contractions are seen. Fortunately, a distinguishing factor of chronic GVHD from pathology associated with systemic sclerosis is that nerve fibers and silver stains of the myenteric plexus are normal in patients with chronic GVHD, in contrast to patients suffering from scleroderma (289,290). GI findings of crypt destruction, lymphoplasmacytic infiltrate with single cell dropout, and fibrosis of lamina propria can be seen.

Skin: It is possible that patients may lose hair and nails as a consequence of chronic GVHD, and their return is indicative of disease improvement. It is rare to see patients manifest vesicles, bullae, or bullous pemphigoid lesions; however, these pathologies have been reported (291). More likely to appear on the chest and abdominal skin are guttate lesions, resembling shiny indurated areas; these lesions may appear localized to areas of pressure-point trauma, previous irradiation or current irradiation, other injury, or herpes-zoster infection (292–294). The develop-

ment of skin abnormalities may vary largely among patients and a time frame is not indicated with these pathologies. Solar exposure may increase the likeliness of manifesting skin abnormalities. Erythema, hyperkeratosis, and desquamation may develop rapidly after exposure to the sun. Erythemic lesions may resemble lupus erythematosus but can be differentiated by observation of sun-exposed areas solely containing these lesions. Other abnormalities have insidious onsets and may present with patches of hyper- and hypopigmented skin, reticular mottling, perifollicular papules, and papulosquamous plaques. Also, less observed is total leukoderma (295). Physicians must take care not to wrongly assume these lesions to be the result of trimethoprim-sulfamethoxazole. Skin biopsies are useful in making this distinction. Also, patients receiving allogeneic HSCT for aplastic amenia may develop dyskeratosis and this distinction should be made as well (296,297). Skin biopsy specimens can demonstrate epithelial acanthosis, dyskeratosis, and hyperkeratosis with mononuclear infiltrate at the dermal-epidermal junction and in adnexal structures. This inflammatory process can evolve to dermal fibrosis and epidermal atrophy.

Keratoconjuntivitis sicca may represent an ocular manifestation and could present with symptoms of irritation, burning, pain, and photophobia (298). Schirmer's test can help evaluate tear function. If punctate keratopathy occurs, it may range from a minimal stippling to massive erosion. It is important to carefully evaluate the eyes for ocular sicca, and even without presentation of symptoms, patients should be started on supplementary artificial tears and if severe, lacrimal puncti ligation is recommended to preserve ocular lubrication. More commonly, cataracts develop post-HSCT (299,300).

Pulmonary pathology typically manifests as a broncho-dilator-resistant obstructive disease (301,302). Lung biopsy illustrates lesions characteristic of obliterative bronchitis. It has been shown that prophylaxis with methotrexate actually increased the incidence of obliterative bronchitis (301). The incidence of late obstructive airway disease is markedly increased in patients with chronic GVHD or inpatients with hypogammaglobulinemia, which is a deficiency in an IgG subclass (303,304). When pulmonary pathology presents, a patient typically displays an increased three-year mortality rate, compared to patients with chronic GVHD who do not develop this complication (305). Double lung transplants can be performed and have been with success (306). Still, the debate is out on whether these lung complications are a direct result of chronic GVHD (307).

After 100 days following transplantation, when chronic GVHD typically manifests, the patient may experience oral dryness accompanied by an extreme sensitivity to acidic or spicy foods (308–310). HSCT patients have demonstrated a correlation of chronic GVHD with oral atrophy, erythema, and lichenoid lesions of the buccal and labial mucosa (309). A mononuclear infiltrate is seen in the salivary glands on lip biopsy. Oral candidiasis is frequently confused with signs of lichen planus-like lesions of chronic GVHD. Additionally, HSV can cause painful lesions in a patient with chronic GVHD and therefore viral cultures should be taken to diagnose and appropriately treat these patients.

There is a lack of evidence to directly associate chronic GVHD to neurological symptoms and disease (311). Typically, post-transplant metabolic and infectious diseases are capable of causing neurological disease, and one case of cerebral involvement has been observed (312). The immunosuppressive regimen patients receive has been shown to create a peripheral neuropathy (313). The autoimmunity resulting from chronic GVHD has been linked to myasthenia gravis, and patients receiving cholinesterase inhibitors have responded well (311,314,315). Another possibility is the development of polymyositis, where symptoms were typically relieved with corticosteroid treatment (286,316).

Some women experiencing chronic GVHD have manifested *vaginal symptoms* (317). Initially thought to be a result of the irradiation from the conditioning regimen, a study of allogeneic HSCT female patients was able to distinguish the pathologies (318). Renal consequences of chronic GVHD are more difficult to correlate (319–321). Autoimmune-like thrombocytopenia and anemia (212,322), hypogammaglobulinemi,a and factor VIII deficiency have been observed (323,324).

Patients receiving long-term corticosteroid treatment are at a increased risk of developing cataracts, avascular necrosis, and osteoporosis (300,325–327). Also with steroid therapy, growth may be arrested in children when chronic GVHD presents severely and typically resolves upon termination of such therapies (328).

Additional clinical manifestations associated with chronic GVHD include progressive systemic sclerosis, systemic lupus erythematosus, lichen planus, Sjogren syndrome, eosinophilic fasciitis, rheumatoid arthritis, and primary biliary cirrhosis (286,287,329–331). The range of disorders and complications resulting from chronic GVHD is changing over the years as a consequence of earlier diagnosis and the implementation of immunosuppressive therapy (286).

Chronic GVHD has two stages: 1) *limited* chronic GVHD presents with localized skin involvement, hepatic dysfunction, or both and 2) *extensive* chronic GVHD presents with the following: generalized skin involvement, or localized skin involvement and/or hepatic dysfunction caused by chronic GVHD plus liver histological finding showing chronic aggressive hepatitis, bridging necrosis, or cirrhosis. Eye involvement may be diagnosed by the Schirmer test (<5 mm wetting), involvement of minor salivary glands or oral mucosa demonstrated by buccal/labial biopsy, and involvement of any other target organ.

The diagnosis of GVHD is established by clinical judgment, imaging studies, laboratory workup, and biopsy results (332).

- Anemia and thrombocytopenia are observed early in acute GVHD or in chronic GVHD.

- Eosinophilia and Howell-Jolly bodies are observed on peripheral smear in chronic GVHD.

- In hepatic involvement, elevation of transaminases is observed early and followed by an increase in bilirubin and finally, cholestatic picture with increased alkaline phosphatase and glucose tolerance.

Although biopsy is not performed routinely, it can be very helpful to distinguish changes of GVHD from drug toxicity in skin and liver.

REFERENCES

1. Muller-Hermelink, H.K., Sale, G.E. 1983. [Pathologic findings in bone marrow transplantation]. *Verh Dtsch Ges Pathol*, 67: 335–61.
2. Thomas, E.D., Lochte, H.L., Jr., Lu, W.C., Ferrebee, J.W. 1957. Intravenous infusion of bone marrow in patients receiving radiation and chemotherapy. *N Engl J Med*, 257: 491–6.
3. Thomas, E.D., Lochte, H.L., Jr., Cannon, J.H., Sahler, O.D., Ferrebee, J.W. 1959. Supralethal whole body irradiation and isologous marrow transplantation in man. *J Clin Invest*, 38: 1709–16.
4. Barnes, D.W., Corp, M.J., Loutit, J.F., Neal, F.E. 1956. Treatment of murine leukaemia with X rays and homologous bone marrow; preliminary communication. *Br Med J*, 2: 626–7.

5. Andrews, G.A. 1962. Criticality accidents in Vinca, Yugoslavia, and Oak Ridge, Tennessee. Comparison of radiation injuries and results of therapy. *JAMA, 179*: 191–7.

6. Mc, G.J., Jr., Russell, P.S., Atkins, L., Webster, E.W. 1959. Treatment of terminal leukemic relapse by total-body irradiation and intravenous infusion of stored autologous bone marrow obtained during remission. *N Engl J Med, 260*: 675–83.

7. Thomas, E.D., Bryant, J.I., Buckner, C.D., Clift, R.A., Fefer, A., Fialkow, P.J., Funk, D.D., Neiman, P.E., Rudolph, R.H., Slichter, S.J. et al. 1971. Allogeneic marrow grafting using HL-A matched donor-recipient sibling pairs. *Trans Assoc Am Physicians, 84*: 248–61.

8. Appelbaum, F.R., Herzig, G.P., Ziegler, J.L., Graw, R.G., Levine, A.S., Deisseroth, A.B. 1978. Successful engraftment of cryopreserved autologous bone marrow in patients with malignant lymphoma. *Blood, 52*: 85–95.

9. Reiffers, J., Bernard, P., David, B., Vezon, G., Sarrat, A., Marit, G., Moulinier, J., Broustet, A. 1986. Successful autologous transplantation with peripheral blood hemopoietic cells in a patient with acute leukemia. *Exp Hematol, 14*: 312–15.

10. Kessinger, A., Armitage, J.O., Landmark, J.D., Weisenburger, D.D. 1986. Reconstitution of human hematopoietic function with autologous cryopreserved circulating stem cells. *Exp Hematol, 14*: 192–6.

11. Korbling, M., Dorken, B., Ho, A.D., Pezzutto, A., Hunstein, W., Fliedner, T.M. 1986. Autologous transplantation of blood-derived hemopoietic stem cells after myeloablative therapy in a patient with Burkitt's lymphoma. *Blood, 67*: 529–32.

12. Speck, B., Zwaan, F.E., van Rood, J.J., Eernisse, J.G. 1973. Allogeneic bone marrow transplantation in a patient with aplastic anemia using a phenotypically HL-A-identifcal unrelated donor. *Transplantation, 16*: 24–8.

13. Hansen, J.A., Clift, R.A., Thomas, E.D., Buckner, C.D., Storb, R., Giblett, E.R. 1980. Transplantation of marrow from an unrelated donor to a patient with acute leukemia. *N Engl J Med, 303*: 565–7.

14. Oudshoorn, M., van Leeuwen, A., vd Zanden, H.G., van Rood, J.J. 1994. Bone Marrow Donors Worldwide: a successful exercise in international cooperation. *Bone Marrow Transplant, 14*: 3–8.

15. Stroncek, D., Bartsch, G., Perkins, H.A., Randall, B.L., Hansen, J.A., McCullough, J. 1993. The National Marrow Donor Program. *Transfusion, 33*: 567–77.

16. Kurtzberg, J., Laughlin, M., Graham, M.L., Smith, C., Olson, J.F., Halperin, E.C., Ciocci, G., Carrier, C., Stevens, C.E., Rubinstein, P. 1996. Placental blood as a source of hematopoietic stem cells for transplantation into unrelated recipients. *N Engl J Med, 335*: 157–66.

17. Weiden, P.L., Flournoy, N., Thomas, E.D., Prentice, R., Fefer, A., Buckner, C.D., Storb, R. 1979. Antileukemic effect of graft-versus-host disease in human recipients of allogeneic-marrow grafts. *N Engl J Med, 300*: 1068–73.

18. Fefer, A., Sullivan, K.M., Weiden, P., Buckner, C.D., Schoch, G., Storb, R., Thomas, E.D. 1987. Graft versus leukemia effect in man: the relapse rate of acute leukemia is lower after allogeneic than after syngeneic marrow transplantation. *Prog Clin Biol Res, 244*: 401–8.

19. Hauch, M., Gazzola, M.V., Small, T., Bordignon, C., Barnett, L., Cunningham, I., Castro-Malaspinia, H., O'Reilly, R.J., Keever, C.A. 1990. Anti-leukemia potential of interleukin-2 activated natural killer cells after bone marrow transplantation for chronic myelogenous leukemia. *Blood, 75*: 2250–62.

20. Mackinnon, S., Hows, J.M., Goldman, J.M. 1990. Induction of in vitro graft-versus-leukemia activity following bone marrow transplantation for chronic myeloid leukemia. *Blood, 76*: 2037–45.

21. Mackinnon, S., Papadopoulos, E.B., Carabasi, M.H., Reich, L., Collins, N.H., Boulad, F., Castro-Malaspina, H., Childs, B.H., Gillio, A.P., Kernan, N.A. et al. 1995. Adoptive immunotherapy evaluating escalating doses of donor leukocytes for relapse of chronic myeloid leukemia after bone marrow transplantation: separation of graft-versus-leukemia responses from graft-versus-host disease. *Blood, 86*: 1261–8.

22. Sale, G.E., Buckner, C.D. 1988. Pathology of bone marrow in transplant recipients. *Hematol Oncol Clin North Am, 2*: 735–56.

23. Sievers, E.L., Lange, B.J., Buckley, J.D., Smith, F.O., Wells, D.A., Daigneault-Creech, C.A., Shults, K.E., Bernstein, I.D., Loken, M.R. 1996. Prediction of relapse of pediatric acute myeloid leukemia by use of multidimensional flow cytometry. *J Natl Cancer Inst, 88*: 1483–8.

24. Radich, J.P., Gehly, G., Gooley, T., Bryant, E., Clift, R.A., Collins, S., Edmands, S., Kirk, J., Lee, A., Kessler, P. et al. 1995. Polymerase chain reaction detection of the BCR-ABL fusion transcript after allogeneic marrow transplantation for chronic myeloid leukemia: results and implications in 346 patients. *Blood, 85*: 2632–8.

25. Zutter, M.M., Martin, P.J., Sale, G.E., Shulman, H.M., Fisher, L., Thomas, E.D., Durnam, D.M. 1988. Epstein-Barr virus lymphoproliferation after bone marrow transplantation. *Blood, 72*: 520–9.

26. Meyers, J.D., Flournoy, N., Thomas, E.D. 1980. Cytomegalovirus infection and specific cell-mediated immunity after marrow transplant. *J Infect Dis, 142*: 816–24.

27. Meyers, J.D., Flournoy, N., Thomas, E.D. 1980. Cell-mediated immunity to varicella-zoster virus after allogeneic marrow transplant. *J Infect Dis, 141*: 479–87.

28. Meyers, J.D., Flournoy, N., Thomas, E.D. 1980. Infection with herpes simplex virus and cell-mediated immunity after marrow transplant. *J Infect Dis, 142*: 338–46.

29. Wade, J.C., Day, L.M., Crowley, J.J., Meyers, J.D. 1984. Recurrent infection with herpes simplex virus after marrow transplantation: role of the specific immune response and acyclovir treatment. *J Infect Dis, 149*: 750–6.

30. Quinnan, G.V., Jr., Kirmani, N., Esber, E., Saral, R., Manischewitz, J.F., Rogers, J.L., Rook, A.H., Santos, G.W., Burns, W.H. 1981. HLA-restricted cytotoxic T lymphocyte and nonthymic cytotoxic lymphocyte responses to cytomegalovirus infection of bone marrow transplant recipients. *J Immunol, 126*: 2036–41.

31. Ljungman, P., Wilczek, H., Gahrton, G., Gustavsson, A., Lundgren, G., Lonnqvist, B., Ringden, O., Wahren, B. 1986. Long-term acyclovir prophylaxis in bone marrow transplant recipients and lymphocyte proliferation responses

to herpes virus antigens in vitro. *Bone Marrow Transplantat, 1*: 185–92.

32. Gratama, J.W., Verdonck, L.F., van der Linden, J.A., van Heugten, J.G., Kreeft, H.A., D'Amaro, J., Zwaan, F.E., de Gast, G.C. 1986. Cellular immunity to vaccinations and herpesvirus infections after bone marrow transplantation. *Transplantation, 41*: 719–24.

33. Ottinger, H.D., Beelen, D.W., Scheulen, B., Schaefer, U.W., Grosse-Wilde, H. 1996. Improved immune reconstitution after allotransplantation of peripheral blood stem cells instead of bone marrow. *Blood, 88*: 2775–9.

34. Lum, L.G., Munn, N.A., Schanfield, M.S., Storb, R. 1986. The detection of specific antibody formation to recall antigens after human bone marrow transplantation. *Blood, 67*: 582–7.

35. Shiobara, S., Lum, L.G., Witherspoon, R.P., Storb, R. 1986. Antigen-specific antibody responses of lymphocytes to tetanus toxoid after human marrow transplantation. *Transplantation, 41*: 587–92.

36. Lum, L.G., Seigneuret, M.C., Storb, R. 1986. The transfer of antigen-specific humoral immunity from marrow donors to marrow recipients. *J Clin Immunol, 6*: 389–96.

37. Lum, L.G. 1987. The kinetics of immune reconstitution after human marrow transplantation. *Blood, 69*: 369–80.

38. Wimperis, J.Z., Brenner, M.K., Prentice, H.G., Reittie, J.E., Karayiannis, P., Griffiths, P.D., Hoffbrand, A.V. 1986. Transfer of a functioning humoral immune system in transplantation of T-lymphocyte-depleted bone marrow. *Lancet, 1*: 339–43.

39. Wahren, B., Gahrton, G., Linde, A., Ljungman, P., Lonnqvist, B., Ringden, O., Sundqvist, V.A. 1984. Transfer and persistence of viral antibody-producing cells in bone marrow transplantation. *J Infect Dis, 150*: 358–65.

40. Witherspoon, R.P., Schanfield, M.S., Storb, R., Thomas, E.D., Giblett, E.R. 1978. Immunoglobulin production of donor origin after marrow transplantation for acute leukemia or aplastic anemia. *Transplantation, 26*: 407–8.

41. Chaushu, S., Chaushu, G., Garfunkel, A., Slavin, S., Or, R., Yefenof, E. 1994. Salivary immunoglobulins in recipients of bone marrow grafts. II. Transient secretion of donor-derived salivary IgA following transplantation of T cell-depleted bone marrow. *Bone Marrow Transplant, 14*: 925–8.

42. Sullivan, K.M., Kopecky, K.J., Jocom, J., Fisher, L., Buckner, C.D., Meyers, J.D., Counts, G.W., Bowden, R.A., Peterson, F.B., Witherspoon, R.P. et al. 1990. Immunomodulatory and antimicrobial efficacy of intravenous immunoglobulin in bone marrow transplantation. *N Engl J Med, 323*: 705–12.

43. Atkinson, K. 1990. Reconstruction of the haemopoietic and immune systems after marrow transplantation. *Bone Marrow Transplant, 5*: 209–26.

44. Linch, D.C., Knott, L.J., Thomas, R.M., Harper, P., Goldstone, A.H., Davis, E.G., Levinski, R.J. 1983. T cell regeneration after allogeneic and autologous bone marrow transplantation. *Br J Haematol, 53*: 451–8.

45. Keever, C.A., Small, T.N., Flomenberg, N., Heller, G., Pekle, K., Black, P., Pecora, A., Gillio, A., Kernan, N.A., O'Reilly, R.J. 1989. Immune reconstitution following bone marrow transplantation: comparison of recipients of T-cell depleted marrow with recipients of conventional marrow grafts. *Blood, 73*: 1340–50.

46. Friedrich, W., O'Reilly, R.J., Koziner, B., Gebhard, D.F., Jr., Good, R.A., Evans, R.L. 1982. T-lymphocyte reconstitution in recipients of bone marrow transplants with and without GVHD: imbalances of T-cell subpopulations having unique regulatory and cognitive functions. *Blood, 59*: 696–701.

47. Forman, S.J., Nocker, P., Gallagher, M., Zaia, J., Wright, C., Bolen, J., Mills, B., Hecht, T. 1982. Pattern of T cell reconstitution following allogeneic bone marrow transplantation for acute hematological malignancy. *Transplantation, 34*: 96–8.

48. Atkinson, K. 1986. T cell subpopulations defined by monoclonal antibodies after HLA-identical sibling marrow transplantation. II. Activated and functional subsets of helper-inducer and cytotoxic-suppressor subpopulations defined by two-colour fluorescence flow cytometry. *Bone Marrow Transplant, 1*: 121–32.

49. Keever, C.A., Welte, K., Small, T., Levick, J., Sullivan, M., Hauch, M., Evans, R.L., O'Reilly, R.J. 1987. Interleukin 2-activated killer cells in patients following transplants of soybean lectin-separated and E rosette-depleted bone marrow. *Blood, 70*: 1893–903.

50. Ault, K.A., Antin, J.H., Ginsburg, D., Orkin, S.H., Rappeport, J.M., Keohan, M.L., Martin, P., Smith, B.R. 1985. Phenotype of recovering lymphoid cell populations after marrow transplantation. *J Exp Med, 161*: 1483–502.

51. Storek, J., Witherspoon, R.P., Storb, R. 1995. T cell reconstitution after bone marrow transplantation into adult patients does not resemble T cell development in early life. *Bone Marrow Transplant, 16*: 413–25.

52. Weinberg, K., Annett, G., Kashyap, A., Lenarsky, C., Forman, S.J., Parkman, R. 1995. The effect of thymic function on immunocompetence following bone marrow transplantation. *Biol Blood Marrow Transplant, 1*: 18–23.

53. Vavassori, M., Maccario, R., Moretta, A., Comoli, P., Wack, A., Locatelli, F., Lanzavecchia, A., Maserati, E., Dellabona, P., Casorati, G. et al. 1996. Restricted TCR repertoire and long-term persistence of donor-derived antigen-experienced CD4+ T cells in allogeneic bone marrow transplantation recipients. *J Immunol, 157*: 5739–47.

54. Noel, D.R., Witherspoon, R.P., Storb, R., Atkinson, K., Doney, K., Mickelson, E.M., Ochs, H.D., Warren, R.P., Weiden, P.L., Thomas, E.D. 1978. Does graft-versus-host disease influence the tempo of immunologic recovery after allogeneic human marrow transplantation? An observation on 56 long-term survivors. *Blood, 51*: 1087–105.

55. Storek, J., King, L., Ferrara, S., Marcelo, D., Saxon, A., Braun, J. 1994. Abundance of a restricted fetal B cell repertoire in marrow transplant recipients. *Bone Marrow Transplant, 14*: 783–90.

56. Murphy, W.J., Kumar, V., Bennett, M. 1987. Acute rejection of murine bone marrow allografts by natural killer cells and T cells. Differences in kinetics and target antigens recognized. *J Exp Med, 166*: 1499–509.

57. Baker, M.B., Podack, E.R., Levy, R.B. 1995. Perforin- and Fas-mediated cytotoxic pathways are not required for

allogeneic resistance to bone marrow grafts in mice. *Biol Blood Marrow Transplant*, *1*: 69–73.

58. Aguila, H.L., Weissman, I.L. 1996. Hematopoietic stem cells are not direct cytotoxic targets of natural killer cells. *Blood*, *87*: 1225–31.

59. Graubert, T.A., Russell, J.H., Ley, T.J. 1996. The role of granzyme B in murine models of acute graft-versus-host disease and graft rejection. *Blood*, *87*: 1232–7.

60. Anasetti, C., Amos, D., Beatty, P.G., Appelbaum, F.R., Bensinger, W., Buckner, C.D., Clift, R., Doney, K., Martin, P.J., Mickelson, E. et al. 1989. Effect of HLA compatibility on engraftment of bone marrow transplants in patients with leukemia or lymphoma. *N Engl J Med*, *320*: 197–204.

61. Kernan, N.A., Flomenberg, N., Dupont, B., O'Reilly, R.J. 1987. Graft rejection in recipients of T-cell-depleted HLA-nonidentical marrow transplants for leukemia. Identification of host-derived antidonor allocytotoxic T lymphocytes. *Transplantation*, *43*: 842–7.

62. Kernan, N.A., Bordignon, C., Heller, G., Cunningham, I., Castro-Malaspina, H., Shank, B., Flomenberg, N., Burns, J., Yang, S.Y., Black, P. et al. 1989. Graft failure after T-cell-depleted human leukocyte antigen identical marrow transplants for leukemia: I. Analysis of risk factors and results of secondary transplants. *Blood*, *74*: 2227–36.

63. Bordignon, C., Keever, C.A., Small, T.N., Flomenberg, N., Dupont, B., O'Reilly, R.J., Kernan, N.A. 1989. Graft failure after T-cell-depleted human leukocyte antigen identical marrow transplants for leukemia: II. In vitro analyses of host effector mechanisms. *Blood*, *74*: 2237–43.

64. Bunjes, D., Heit, W., Arnold, R., Schmeiser, T., Wiesneth, M., Carbonell, F., Porzsolt, F., Raghavachar, A., Heimpel, H. 1987. Evidence for the involvement of host-derived OKT8-positive T cells in the rejection of T-depleted, HLA-identical bone marrow grafts. *Transplantation*, *43*: 501–5.

65. Marijt, W.A., Kernan, N.A., Diaz-Barrientos, T., Veenhof, W.F., O'Reilly, R.J., Willemze, R., Falkenburg, J.H. 1995. Multiple minor histocompatibility antigen-specific cytotoxic T lymphocyte clones can be generated during graft rejection after HLA-identical bone marrow transplantation. *Bone Marrow Transplant*, *16*: 125–32.

66. Slavin, M.A., Meyers, J.D., Remington, J.S., Hackman, R.C. 1994. Toxoplasma gondii infection in marrow transplant recipients: a 20 year experience. *Bone Marrow Transplant*, *13*: 549–57.

67. van Burik, J.A., Hackman, R.C., Nadeem, S.Q., Hiemenz, J.W., White, M.H., Flowers, M.E., Bowden, R.A. 1997. Nocardiosis after bone marrow transplantation: a retrospective study. *Clin Infect Dis*, *24*: 1154–60.

68. Harrington, R.D., Hooton, T.M., Hackman, R.C., Storch, G.A., Osborne, B., Gleaves, C.A., Benson, A., Meyers, J.D. 1992. An outbreak of respiratory syncytial virus in a bone marrow transplant center. *J Infect Dis*, *165*: 987–93.

69. Meyers, J.D., Flournoy, N., Thomas, E.D. 1982. Nonbacterial pneumonia after allogeneic marrow transplantation: a review of ten years' experience. *Rev Infect Dis*, *4*: 1119–32.

70. Shields, A.F., Hackman, R.C., Fife, K.H., Corey, L., Meyers, J.D. 1985. Adenovirus infections in patients undergoing bone-marrow transplantation. *N Engl J Med*, *312*: 529–33.

71. Ruutu, P., Ruutu, T., Volin, L., Tukiainen, P., Ukkonen, P., Hovi, T. 1990. Cytomegalovirus is frequently isolated in bronchoalveolar lavage fluid of bone marrow transplant recipients without pneumonia. *Ann Intern Med*, *112*: 913–16.

72. Walsh, J.H., Peterson, W.L. 1995. The treatment of Helicobacter pylori infection in the management of peptic ulcer disease. *N Engl J Med*, *333*: 984–91.

73. Walzer, P.D., Milder, J.E., Banwell, J.G., Kilgore, G., Klein, M., Parker, R. 1982. Epidemiologic features of Strongyloides stercoralis infection in an endemic area of the United States. *Am J Trop Med Hyg*, *31*: 313–19.

74. Bromiker, R., Korman, S.H., Or, R., Hardan, I., Naparstek, E., Cohen, P., Ben-Shahar, M., Engelhard, D. 1989. Severe giardiasis in two patients undergoing bone marrow transplantation. *Bone Marrow Transplant*, *4*: 701–3.

75. Bavaro, P., Di Girolamo, G., Di Bartolomeo, P., Angrilli, F., Olioso, P., Papalinetti, G., Del Vecchio, A., Torlontano, G. 1994. Amebiasis after bone marrow transplantation. *Bone Marrow Transplant*, *13*: 213–14.

76. Collier, A.C., Miller, R.A., Meyers, J.D. 1984. Cryptosporidiosis after marrow transplantation: person-to-person transmission and treatment with spiramycin. *Ann Intern Med*, *101*: 205–6.

77. Long, E.G., Christie, J.D. 1995. The diagnosis of old and new gastrointestinal parasites. *Clin Lab Med*, *15*: 307–31.

78. Thaler, M., Pastakia, B., Shawker, T.H., O'Leary, T., Pizzo, P.A. 1988. Hepatic candidiasis in cancer patients: the evolving picture of the syndrome. *Ann Intern Med*, *108*: 88–100.

79. Bjerke, J.W., Meyers, J.D., Bowden, R.A. 1994. Hepatosplenic candidiasis—a contraindication to marrow transplantation? *Blood*, *84*: 2811–14.

80. Rossetti, F., Brawner, D.L., Bowden, R., Meyer, W.G., Schoch, H.G., Fisher, L., Myerson, D., Hackman, R.C., Shulman, H.M., Sale, G.E. et al. 1995. Fungal liver infection in marrow transplant recipients: prevalence at autopsy, predisposing factors, and clinical features. *Clin Infect Dis*, *20*: 801–11.

81. Jantunen, E., Ruutu, P., Niskanen, L., Volin, L., Parkkali, T., Koukila-Kahkola, P., Ruutu, T. 1997. Incidence and risk factors for invasive fungal infections in allogeneic BMT recipients. *Bone Marrow Transplant*, *19*: 801–8.

82. Lewis, J.H., Patel, H.R., Zimmerman, H.J. 1982. The spectrum of hepatic candidiasis. *Hepatology (Baltimore, MD)*, *2*: 479–87.

83. Magnussen, C.R., Olson, J.P., Ona, F.V., Graziani, A.J. 1979. Candida fungus balls in the common bile duct. Unusual manifestation of disseminated candidiasis. *Arch Intern Med*, *139*: 821–2.

84. Marcucci, R.A., Whitely, H., Armstrong, D. 1978. Common bile duct obstruction secondary to infection with Candida. *J Clin Microbiol*, *7*: 490–2.

85. McFarland, L.V., Mulligan, M.E., Kwok, R.Y., Stamm, W.E. 1989. Nosocomial acquisition of Clostridium difficile infection. *N Engl J Med*, *320*: 204–10.

86. Hiatt, J.R., Kuchenbecker, S.L., Winston, D.J. 1986. Perineal gangrene in the patient with granulocytopenia: the importance of early diverting colostomy. *Surgery*, *100*: 912–5.

87. Cohen, J.S., Paz, I.B., O'Donnell, M.R., Ellenhorn, J.D. 1996. Treatment of perianal infection following bone marrow transplantation. *Dis Colon Rect*, *39*: 981–5.

88. Navari, R.M., Sullivan, K.M., Springmeyer, S.C., Siegel, M.S., Meyers, J.D., Buckner, C.D., Sanders, J.E., Stewart, P.S., Clift, R.A., Fefer, A. et al. 1983. Mycobacterial infections in marrow transplant patients. *Transplantation*, *36*: 509–13.

89. Skinner, R., Appleton, A.L., Sprott, M.S., Barer, M.R., Magee, J.G., Darbyshire, P.J., Abinun, M., Cant, A.J. 1996. Disseminated BCG infection in severe combined immunodeficiency presenting with severe anaemia and associated with gross hypersplenism after bone marrow transplantation. *Bone Marrow Transplant*, *17*: 877–80.

90. Nikkels, A.F., Delvenne, P., Sadzot-Delvaux, C., Debrus, S., Piette, J., Rentier, B., Lipcsei, G., Quatresooz, P., Pierard, G.E. 1996. Distribution of varicella zoster virus and herpes simplex virus in disseminated fatal infections. *J Clin Pathol*, *49*: 243–8.

91. Wolfsen, H.C., Bolen, J.W., Bowen, J.L., Fenster, L.F. 1993. Fulminant herpes hepatitis mimicking hepatic abscesses. *J Clin Gastroenterol*, *16*: 61–4.

92. Hayashi, M., Takeyama, K., Takayama, J., Ohira, M., Tobinai, K., Shimoyama, M. 1991. Severe herpes simplex virus hepatitis following autologous bone marrow transplantation: successful treatment with high dose intravenous acyclovir. *Jpn J Clin Oncol*, *21*: 372–6.

93. Locksley, R.M., Flournoy, N., Sullivan, K.M., Meyers, J.D. 1985. Infection with varicella-zoster virus after marrow transplantation. *J Infect Dis*, *152*: 1172–81.

94. Atkinson, K., Meyers, J.D., Storb, R., Prentice, R.L., Thomas, E.D. 1980. Varicella-zoster virus infection after marrow transplantation for aplastic anemia or leukemia. *Transplantation*, *29*: 47–50.

95. Ljungman, P., Lonnqvist, B., Gahrton, G., Ringden, O., Sundqvist, V.A., Wahren, B. 1986. Clinical and subclinical reactivations of varicella-zoster virus in immunocompromised patients. *J Infect Dis*, *153*: 840–7.

96. Schuchter, L.M., Wingard, J.R., Piantadosi, S., Burns, W.H., Santos, G.W., Saral, R. 1989. Herpes zoster infection after autologous bone marrow transplantation. *Blood*, *74*: 1424–7.

97. Han, C.S., Miller, W., Haake, R., Weisdorf, D. 1994. Varicella zoster infection after bone marrow transplantation: incidence, risk factors and complications. *Bone Marrow Transplant*, *13*: 277–83.

98. Snover, D.C., Hutton, S., Balfour, H.H., Jr., Bloomer, J.R. 1987. Cytomegalovirus infection of the liver in transplant recipients. *J Clin Gastroenterol*, *9*: 659–65.

99. Meyers, J.D., Flournoy, N., Thomas, E.D. 1986. Risk factors for cytomegalovirus infection after human marrow transplantation. *J Infect Dis*, *153*: 478–88.

100. Einsele, H., Waller, H.D., Weber, P., Frickhofen, N., Dette, S., Horny, H.P., Roos, A., Roos, H., Hebart, H., Schmidt, H. et al. 1994. Cytomegalovirus in liver biopsies of marrow transplant recipients: detection methods, clinical, histological and immunohistological features. *Med Microbiol and Immunol*, *183*: 205–16.

101. Evans, M.J., Edwards-Spring, Y., Myers, J., Wendt, A., Povinelli, D., Amsterdam, D., Rittenhouse-Diakun, K., Armstrong, D., Murray, B.M., Greenberg, S.J. et al. 1997. Polymerase chain reaction assays for the detection of cytomegalovirus in organ and bone marrow transplant recipients. *Immunol Invest*, *26*: 209–29.

102. Cheung, A.N., Ng, I.O. 1993. Cytomegalovirus infection of the gastrointestinal tract in non-AIDS patients. *Am J Gastroenterol*, *88*: 1882–6.

103. Murakami, C.S., Louie, W., Chan, G.S., O'Donnell, M., David, D., Forman, S.J., McDonald, G.B. 1999. Biliary obstruction in hematopoietic cell transplant recipients: an uncommon diagnosis with specific causes. *Bone Marrow Transplant*, *23*: 921–7.

104. Blanke, C., Clark, C., Broun, E.R., Tricot, G., Cunningham, I., Cornetta, K., Hedderman, A., Hromas, R. 1995. Evolving pathogens in allogeneic bone marrow transplantation: increased fatal adenoviral infections. *Am J Med*, *99*: 326–8.

105. Niemann, T.H., Trigg, M.E., Winick, N., Penick, G.D. 1993. Disseminated adenoviral infection presenting as acute pancreatitis. *Human pathology*, *24*: 1145–8.

106. Allard, A., Girones, R., Juto, P., Wadell, G. 1991. Polymerase chain reaction for detection of adenoviruses in stool samples. *Journal of clinical microbiology*, *29*: 2683.

107. Cree, B.C., Bernardini, G.L., Hays, A.P., Lowe, G. 2003. A fatal case of coxsackievirus B4 meningoencephalitis. *Arch Neurol*, *60*: 107–12.

108. Ho-Yen, D.O., Hardie, R., McClure, J., Cunningham, N.E., Bell, E.J. 1989. Fatal outcome of echovirus 7 infection. *Scand J Infect Dis*, *21*: 459–61.

109. Schleissner, L.A., Portnoy, B. 1968. Hepatitis and pneumonia associated with ECHO virus, type 9, infection in two adult siblings. *Ann Intern Med*, *68*: 1315–9.

110. Webster, A., Brenner, M.K., Prentice, H.G., Griffiths, P.D. 1989. Fatal hepatitis B reactivation after autologous bone marrow transplantation. *Bone Marrow Transplant*, *4*: 207–8.

111. McIvor, C., Morton, J., Bryant, A., Cooksley, W.G., Durrant, S., Walker, N. 1994. Fatal reactivation of precore mutant hepatitis B virus associated with fibrosing cholestatic hepatitis after bone marrow transplantation. *Ann Intern Med*, *121*: 274–5.

112. Mertens, T., Kock, J., Hampl, W., Schlicht, H.J., Tillmann, H.L., Oldhafer, K.J., Manns, M.P., Arnold, R. 1996. Reactivated fulminant hepatitis B virus replication after bone marrow transplantation: clinical course and possible treatment with ganciclovir. *J Hepatol*, *25*: 968–71.

113. Reed, E.C., Myerson, D., Corey, L., Meyers, J.D. 1991. Allogeneic marrow transplantation in patients positive for hepatitis B surface antigen. *Blood*, *77*: 195–200.

114. Shuhart, M.C., Myerson, D., Childs, B.H., Fingeroth, J.D., Perry, J.J., Snyder, D.S., Spurgeon, C.L., Bevan, C.A., McDonald, G.B. 1994. Marrow transplantation from hepatitis C virus seropositive donors: transmission rate and clinical course. *Blood*, *84*: 3229–35.

115. Shuhart, M.C., Myerson, D., Spurgeon, C.L., Bevan, C.A., Sayers, M.H., McDonald, G.B. 1996. Hepatitis C virus (HCV) infection in bone marrow transplant patients after

transfusions from anti-HCV-positive blood donors. *Bone Marrow Transplant, 17*: 601–6.

116. Strasser, S.I., Sullivan, K.M., Myerson, D., Spurgeon, C.L., Storer, B., Schoch, H.G., Murakami, C.S., McDonald, G.B. 1999. Cirrhosis of the liver in long-term marrow transplant survivors. *Blood, 93*: 3259–66.

117. Shulman, H.M., McDonald, G.B., Matthews, D., Doney, K.C., Kopecky, K.J., Gauvreau, J.M., Thomas, E.D. 1980. An analysis of hepatic venocclusive disease and centrilobular hepatic degeneration following bone marrow transplantation. *Gastroenterology, 79*: 1178–91.

118. McDonald, G.B., Sharma, P., Matthews, D.E., Shulman, H.M., Thomas, E.D. 1984. Venocclusive disease of the liver after bone marrow transplantation: diagnosis, incidence, and predisposing factors. *Hepatology (Baltimore, Md, 4*: 116–22.

119. McDonald, G.B., Shulman, H.M., Wolford, J.L., Spencer, G.D. 1987. Liver disease after human marrow transplantation. *Semin Liver Dis, 7*: 210–29.

120. Shulman, H.M., Hinterberger, W. 1992. Hepatic veno-occlusive disease – liver toxicity syndrome after bone marrow transplantation. *Bone Marrow Transplant, 10*: 197–214.

121. Shulman, H.M., Gown, A.M., Nugent, D.J. 1987. Hepatic veno-occlusive disease after bone marrow transplantation. Immunohistochemical identification of the material within occluded central venules. *Am J Pathol, 127*: 549–58.

122. Scheimberg, I.B., Pollock, D.J., Collins, P.W., Doran, H.M., Newland, A.C., van der Walt, J.D. 1995. Pathology of the liver in leukaemia and lymphoma. A study of 110 autopsies. *Histopathology, 26*: 311–21.

123. Lucarelli, G., Galimberti, M., Polchi, P., Angelucci, E., Baronciani, D., Giardini, C., Andreani, M., Agostinelli, F., Albertini, F., Clift, R.A. 1993. Marrow transplantation in patients with thalassemia responsive to iron chelation therapy. *N Engl J Med, 329*: 840–4.

124. Walters, M.C., Sullivan, K.M., O'Reilly, R.J., Boulad, F., Brockstein, J., Blume, K., Amylon, M., Johnson, F.L., Klemperer, M., Graham-Pole, J. et al. 1994. Bone marrow transplantation for thalassemia. The USA experience. *The Am J Pediatr Hematol Oncol, 16*: 11–7.

125. Foerder, C.A., Tobin, A.A., McDonald, G.B., Zager, R.A. 1992. Bleomycin-detectable iron in plasma of bone-marrow transplant patients–its correlation with liver injury. *Transplantation, 54*: 1120–3.

126. Chapko, M.K., Syrjala, K.L., Schilter, L., Cummings, C., Sullivan, K.M. 1989. Chemoradiotherapy toxicity during bone marrow transplantation: time course and variation in pain and nausea. *Bone Marrow Transplant, 4*: 181–6.

127. McKay, P.J., Murphy, J.A., Cameron, S., Burnett, A.K., Campbell, M., Tansey, P., Franklin, I.M. 1996. Iron overload and liver dysfunction after allogeneic or autologous bone marrow transplantation. *Bone Marrow Transplant, 17*: 63–6.

128. Iqbal, M., Creger, R.J., Fox, R.M., Cooper, B.W., Jacobs, G., Stellato, T.A., Lazarus, H.M. 1996. Laparoscopic liver biopsy to evaluate hepatic dysfunction in patients with hematologic malignancies: a useful tool to effect changes in management. *Bone Marrow Transplant, 17*: 655–62.

129. Jensen, P.D., Jensen, F.T., Christensen, T., Ellegaard, J. 1995. Evaluation of transfusional iron overload before and during iron chelation by magnetic resonance imaging of the liver and determination of serum ferritin in adult non-thalassaemic patients. *Br J Haematol, 89*: 880–9.

130. Mahendra, P., Hood, I.M., Bass, G., Patterson, P., Marcus, R.E. 1996. Severe hemosiderosis post allogenic bone marrow transplantation. *Hematol Oncol, 14*: 33–5.

131. Harrison, P., Neilson, J.R., Marwah, S.S., Madden, L., Bareford, D., Milligan, D.W. 1996. Role of non-transferrin bound iron in iron overload and liver dysfunction in long term survivors of acute leukaemia and bone marrow transplantation. *J Clin Pathol, 49*: 853–6.

132. Cross, C.E., Halliwell, B., Borish, E.T., Pryor, W.A., Ames, B.N., Saul, R.L., McCord, J.M., Harman, D. 1987. Oxygen radicals and human disease. *Ann Intern Med, 107*: 526–45.

133. Lesnefsky, E.J. 1994. Tissue iron overload and mechanisms of iron-catalyzed oxidative injury. *Adv Exp Med Biol, 366*: 129–46.

134. Stal, P. 1995. Iron as a hepatotoxin. *Dig Dis, 13*: 205–22.

135. Angelucci, E., Baronciani, D., Lucarelli, G., Giardini, C., Galimberti, M., Polchi, P., Martinelli, F., Baldassarri, M., Muretto, P. 1993. Liver iron overload and liver fibrosis in thalassemia. *Bone Marrow Transplant, 12 Suppl 1*: 29–31.

136. Schafer, A.I., Cheron, R.G., Dluhy, R., Cooper, B., Gleason, R.E., Soeldner, J.S., Bunn, H.F. 1981. Clinical consequences of acquired transfusional iron overload in adults. *N Engl J Med, 304*: 319–24.

137. Blei, F., Puder, D.R. 1993. Yersinia enterocolitica bacteremia in a chronically transfused patient with sickle cell anemia. Case report and review of the literature. *Am J Pediatr Hematol Oncol, 15*: 430–4.

138. Bullen, J.J., Spalding, P.B., Ward, C.G., Gutteridge, J.M. 1991. Hemochromatosis, iron and septicemia caused by Vibrio vulnificus. *Arch Intern Med, 151*: 1606–9.

139. Gaziev, D., Baronciani, D., Galimberti, M., Polchi, P., Angelucci, E., Giardini, C., Muretto, P., Perugini, S., Riggio, S., Ghirlanda, S. et al. 1996. Mucormycosis after bone marrow transplantation: report of four cases in thalassemia and review of the literature. *Bone Marrow Transplant, 17*: 409–14.

140. Lee, A.C., Ha, S.Y., Yuen, K.Y., Lau, Y.L. 1995. Listeria septicemia complicating bone marrow transplantation for Diamond-Blackfan syndrome. *Pediatr Hematol Oncol, 12*: 295–9.

141. Chao, N.J., Berry, G.J., Advani, R., Horning, S.J., Weiss, L.M., Blume, K.G. 1993. Epstein-Barr virus-associated lymphoproliferative disorder following autologous bone marrow transplantation for non-Hodgkin's lymphoma. *Transplantation, 55*: 1425–8.

142. Shapiro, R.S., McClain, K., Frizzera, G., Gajl-Peczalska, K.J., Kersey, J.H., Blazar, B.R., Arthur, D.C., Patton, D.F., Greenberg, J.S., Burke, B. et al. 1988. Epstein-Barr virus associated B cell lymphoproliferative disorders following bone marrow transplantation. *Blood, 71*: 1234–43.

143. O'Reilly, R.J., Lacerda, J.F., Lucas, K.G., Rosenfield, N.S., Small, T.N., Papadopoulos, E.B. 1996. Adoptive cell therapy with donor lymphocytes for EBV-associated lymphomas developing after allogeneic marrow transplants. *Important Adv Oncol*: 149–66.

144. Kaur, S., Cooper, G., Fakult, S., Lazarus, H.M. 1996. Incidence and outcome of overt gastrointestinal bleeding in patients undergoing bone marrow transplantation. *Dig Dis Sci, 41*: 598–603.

145. Schwartz, J.M., Wolford, J.L., Thornquist, M.D., Hockenbery, D.M., Murakami, C.S., Drennan, F., Hinds, M., Strasser, S.I., Lopez-Cubero, S.O., Brar, H.S. et al. 2001. Severe gastrointestinal bleeding after hematopoietic cell transplantation, 1987–1997: incidence, causes, and outcome. *Am J Gastroenterol, 96*: 385–93.

146. Spencer, G.D., Hackman, R.C., McDonald, G.B., Amos, D.E., Cunningham, B.A., Meyers, J.D., Thomas, E.D. 1986. A prospective study of unexplained nausea and vomiting after marrow transplantation. *Transplantation, 42*: 602–7.

147. Weisdorf, D.J., Snover, D.C., Haake, R., Miller, W.J., McGlave, P.B., Blazar, B., Ramsay, N.K., Kersey, J.H., Filipovich, A. 1990. Acute upper gastrointestinal graft-versus-host disease: clinical significance and response to immunosuppressive therapy. *Blood, 76*: 624–9.

148. Reed, E.C., Wolford, J.L., Kopecky, K.J., Lilleby, K.E., Dandliker, P.S., Todaro, J.L., McDonald, G.B., Meyers, J.D. 1990. Ganciclovir for the treatment of cytomegalovirus gastroenteritis in bone marrow transplant patients. A randomized, placebo-controlled trial. *Ann Intern Med, 112*: 505–10.

149. Wu, D., Hockenberry, D.M., Brentnall, T.A., Baehr, P.H., Ponec, R.J., Kuver, R., Tzung, S.P., Todaro, J.L., McDonald, G.B. 1998. Persistent nausea and anorexia after marrow transplantation: a prospective study of 78 patients. *Transplantation, 66*: 1319–24.

150. Jacobson, A.F., Teefey, S.A., Lee, S.P., Hollister, M.S., Higano, C.A., Bianco, J.A. 1993. Frequent occurrence of new hepatobiliary abnormalities after bone marrow transplantation: results of a prospective study using scintigraphy and sonography. *Am J Gastroenterol, 88*: 1044–9.

151. Teefey, S.A., Hollister, M.S., Lee, S.P., Jacobson, A.F., Higano, C.S., Bianco, J.A., Colacurcio, C.J. 1994. Gallbladder sludge formation after bone marrow transplant: sonographic observations. *Abdomin Imaging, 19*: 57–60.

152. Messing, B., Bories, C., Kunstlinger, F., Bernier, J.J. 1983. Does total parenteral nutrition induce gallbladder sludge formation and lithiasis? *Gastroenterology, 84*: 1012–9.

153. Grier, J.F., Cohen, S.W., Grafton, W.D., Gholson, C.F. 1994. Acute suppurative cholangitis associated with choledochal sludge. *Am J Gastroenterol, 89*: 617–9.

154. Ko, C.W., Gooley, T., Schoch, H.G., Myerson, D., Hackman, R.C., Shulman, H.M., Sale, G.E., Lee, S.P., McDonald, G.B. 1997. Acute pancreatitis in marrow transplant patients: prevalence at autopsy and risk factor analysis. *Bone Marrow Transplant, 20*: 1081–6.

155. Lee, S.P., Nicholls, J.F., Park, H.Z. 1992. Biliary sludge as a cause of acute pancreatitis. *N Engl J Med, 326*: 589–93.

156. Ohara, N., Schaefer, J. 1990. Clinical significance of biliary sludge. *J Clin Gastroenterol, 12*: 291–4.

157. Frick, M.P., Snover, D.C., Feinberg, S.B., Salomonowitz, E., Crass, J.R., Ramsay, N.K. 1984. Sonography of the gallbladder in bone marrow transplant patients. *Am J Gastroenterol, 79*: 122–7.

158. Pitkaranta, P., Haapiainen, R., Taavitsainen, M., Elonen, E. 1991. Acalculous cholecystitis after bone marrow transplantation in adults with acute leukaemia. Case report. *Eur J Surg Acta Chirurgica, 157*: 361–4.

159. Jardines, L.A., O'Donnell, M.R., Johnson, D.L., Terz, J.J., Forman, S.J. 1993. Acalculous cholecystitis in bone marrow transplant patients. *Cancer, 71*: 354–8.

160. Hurley, R., Weisdorf, D.J., Jessurun, J., Vercellotti, G.M., Miller, W.J. 1992. Relapse of acute leukemia presenting as acute cholecystitis following bone marrow transplantation. *Bone Marrow Transplant, 10*: 387–9.

161. Bigio, E.H., Haque, A.K. 1989. Disseminated cytomegalovirus infection presenting with acalculous cholecystitis and acute pancreatitis. *Arch Pathol Lab Med, 113*: 1287–9.

162. Valainis, G.T., Sachitano, R.A., Pankey, G.A. 1987. Cholecystitis due to Torulopsis glabrata. *J Infect Dis, 156*: 244–5.

163. Harrington, R.D., Woolfrey, A.E., Bowden, R., McDowell, M.G., Hackman, R.C. 1996. Legionellosis in a bone marrow transplant center. *Bone Marrow Transplant, 18*: 361–8.

164. Clark, J.G., Hansen, J.A., Hertz, M.I., Parkman, R., Jensen, L., Peavy, H.H. 1993. NHLBI workshop summary. Idiopathic pneumonia syndrome after bone marrow transplantation. *Am Rev Respir Dis, 147*: 1601–6.

165. Kantrow, S.P., Hackman, R.C., Boeckh, M., Myerson, D., Crawford, S.W. 1997. Idiopathic pneumonia syndrome: changing spectrum of lung injury after marrow transplantation. *Transplantation, 63*: 1079–86.

166. Wingard, J.R., Mellits, E.D., Jones, R.J., Beschorner, W.E., Sostrin, M.B., Burns, W.H., Santos, G.W., Saral, R. 1989. Association of hepatic veno-occlusive disease with interstitial pneumonitis in bone marrow transplant recipients. *Bone Marrow Transplant, 4*: 685–9.

167. Applebaum, F.R., Meyers, J.D., Fefer, A., Fluornoy, N., Cheever, M.A., Greenberg, P.D., Hackman, R., Thomas, E.D. 1982. Nonbacterial nonfungal pneumonia following marrow transplantation in 100 identical twins. *Transplantation, 33*: 265–8.

168. Crawford, S.W., Longton, G., Storb, R. 1993. Acute graft-versus-host disease and the risks for idiopathic pneumonia after marrow transplantation for severe aplastic anemia. *Bone Marrow Transplant, 12*: 225–31.

169. Lehnert, S., Rybka, W.B., Seemayer, T.A. 1986. Amplification of the graft-versus-host reaction by partial body irradiation. *Transplantation, 41*: 675–9.

170. Cone, R.W., Hackman, R.C., Huang, M.L., Bowden, R.A., Meyers, J.D., Metcalf, M., Zeh, J., Ashley, R., Corey, L. 1993. Human herpesvirus 6 in lung tissue from patients with pneumonitis after bone marrow transplantation. *N Engl J Med, 329*: 156–61.

171. Lombard, C.M., Churg, A., Winokur, S. 1987. Pulmonary veno-occlusive disease following therapy for malignant neoplasms. *Chest, 92*: 871–6.

172. Troussard, X., Bernaudin, J.F., Cordonnier, C., Fleury, J., Payen, D., Briere, J., Vernant, J.P. 1984. Pulmonary veno-occlusive disease after bone marrow transplantation. *Thorax, 39*: 956–7.

173. Hackman, R.C., Madtes, D.K., Petersen, F.B., Clark, J.G. 1989. Pulmonary venoocclusive disease following bone marrow transplantation. *Transplantation*, 47: 989–92.

174. Wiznitzer, M., Packer, R.J., August, C.S., Burkey, E.D. 1984. Neurological complications of bone marrow transplantation in childhood. *Ann Neurol*, 16: 569–76.

175. Patchell, R.A., White, C.L., 3rd, Clark, A.W., Beschorner, W.E., Santos, G.W. 1985. Neurologic complications of bone marrow transplantation. *Neurology*, 35: 300–6.

176. Davis, D.G., Patchell, R.A. 1988. Neurologic complications of bone marrow transplantation. *Neurol Clin*, 6: 377–87.

177. Graus, F., Saiz, A., Sierra, J., Arbaiza, D., Rovira, M., Carreras, E., Tolosa, E., Rozman, C. 1996. Neurologic complications of autologous and allogeneic bone marrow transplantation in patients with leukemia: a comparative study. *Neurology*, 46: 1004–9.

178. Wingard, J.R. 1990. Advances in the management of infectious complications after bone marrow transplantation. *Bone Marrow Transplant*, 6: 371–83.

179. Long, S.G., Leyland, M.J., Milligan, D.W. 1993. Listeria meningitis after bone marrow transplantation. *Bone Marrow Transplant*, 12: 537–9.

180. Abraham, J., Bilgrami, S., Dorsky, D., Edwards, R.L., Feingold, J., Hill, D.R., Tutschka, P.J. 1997. Stomatococcus mucilaginosus meningitis in a patient with multiple myeloma following autologous stem cell transplantation. *Bone Marrow Transplant*, 19: 639–41.

181. D'Antonio, D., Di Bartolomeo, P., Iacone, A., Olioso, P., Di Girolamo, G., Angrilli, F., Papalinetti, G., Fioritoni, G., Betti, S., Torlontano, G. 1992. Meningitis due to penicillin-resistant Streptococcus pneumoniae in patients with chronic graft-versus-host disease. *Bone Marrow Transplant*, 9: 299–300.

182. Roy, V., Weisdorf, D. 1997. Mycobacterial infections following bone marrow transplantation: a 20 year retrospective review. *Bone Marrow Transplant*, 19: 467–70.

183. Lowenberg, B., van Gijn, J., Prins, E., Polderman, A.M. 1983. Fatal cerebral toxoplasmosis in a bone marrow transplant recipient with leukemia. *Transplantation*, 35: 30–4.

184. Jehn, U., Fink, M., Gundlach, P., Schwab, W.D., Bise, K., Deckstein, W.D., Wilske, B. 1984. Lethal cardiac and cerebral toxoplasmosis in a patient with acute myeloid leukemia after successful allogeneic bone marrow transplantation. *Transplantation*, 38: 430–3.

185. Mohrmann, R.L., Mah, V., Vinters, H.V. 1990. Neuropathologic findings after bone marrow transplantation: an autopsy study. *Hum Pathol*, 21: 630–9.

186. Tschuchnigg, M., Bradstock, K.F., Koutts, J., Stewart, J., Enno, A., Seldon, M. 1990. A case of thrombotic thrombocytopenic purpura following allogeneic bone marrow transplantation. *Bone Marrow Transplant*, 5: 61–3.

187. Patchell, R.A., White, C.L., 3rd, Clark, A.W., Beschorner, W.E., Santos, G.W. 1985. Nonbacterial thrombotic endocarditis in bone marrow transplant patients. *Cancer*, 55: 631–5.

188. Jerman, M.R., Fick, R.B., Jr. 1986. Nonbacterial thrombotic endocarditis associated with bone marrow transplantation. *Chest*, 90: 919–22.

189. Doll, D.C., Ringenberg, Q.S., Yarbro, J.W. 1986. Vascular toxicity associated with antineoplastic agents. *J Clin Oncol*, 4: 1405–17.

190. Sanz, J., Arriaga, F., Montesinos, P., Orti, G., Lorenzo, I., Cantero, S., Puig, N., Moscardo, F., de la Rubia, J., Sanz, G. et al. 2007. Autoimmune hemolytic anemia following allogeneic hematopoietic stem cell transplantation in adult patients. *Bone Marrow Transplant*, 39: 555–61.

191. Buckner, C.D., Clift, R.A., Sanders, J.E., Williams, B., Gray, M., Storb, R., Thomas, E.D. 1978. ABO-incompatible marrow transplants. *Transplantation*, 26: 233–8.

192. Lasky, L.C., Warkentin, P.I., Kersey, J.H., Ramsay, N.K., McGlave, P.B., McCullough, J. 1983. Hemotherapy in patients undergoing blood group incompatible bone marrow transplantation. *Transfusion*, 23: 277–85.

193. Dinsmore, R.E., Reich, L.M., Kapoor, N., Gulati, S., Kirkpatrick, D., Flomenberg, N., O'Reilly, R.J. 1983. ABH incompatible bone marrow transplantation: removal of erythrocytes by starch sedimentation. *Br J Haematol*, 54: 441–9.

194. Ho, W.G., Champlin, R.E., Feig, S.A., Gale, R.P. 1984. Transplantation of ABH incompatible bone marrow: gravity sedimentation of donor marrow. *Br J Haematol*, 57: 155–62.

195. Warkentin, P.I., Hilden, J.M., Kersey, J.H., Ramsay, N.K., McCullough, J. 1985. Transplantation of major ABO-incompatible bone marrow depleted of red cells by hydroxyethyl starch. *Vox Sang*, 48: 89–104.

196. Hows, J., Beddow, K., Gordon-Smith, E., Branch, D.R., Spruce, W., Sniecinski, I., Krance, R.A., Petz, L.D. 1986. Donor-derived red blood cell antibodies and immune hemolysis after allogeneic bone marrow transplantation. *Blood*, 67: 177–81.

197. Haas, R.J., Rieber, P., Helmig, M., Strobel, E., Belohradsky, B.H., Heim, M.U. 1986. Acquired immune haemolysis by anti A 1 antibody following bone marrow transplantation. *Blut*, 53: 401–4.

198. Robertson, V.M., Henslee, P.J., Jennings, C.D., Hill, M.G., Thompson, J.T., Dickson, L.G. 1987. Early appearance of anti-A isohemagglutinin after allogeneic, ABO minor incompatible, T cell depleted bone marrow transplant. *Transplant Proc*, 19: 4612–7.

199. Hazlehurst, G.R., Brenner, M.K., Wimperis, J.Z., Knowles, S.M., Prentice, H.G. 1986. Haemolysis after T-cell depleted bone marrow transplantation involving minor ABO incompatibility. *Scand J Haematol*, 37: 1–3.

200. Bensinger, W.I., Buckner, C.D., Thomas, E.D., Clift, R.A. 1982. ABO-incompatible marrow transplants. *Transplantation*, 33: 427–9.

201. Webb, I.J., Soiffer, R.J., Andersen, J.W., Cohen, C.A., Freeman, A., Sugrue, M., Ritz, J., Anderson, K.C. 1997. In vivo adsorption of isohemagglutinins with fresh frozen plasma in major ABO-incompatible bone marrow transplantation. *Biol Blood Marrow Transplant*, 3: 267–72.

202. Sniecinski, I.J., Oien, L., Petz, L.D., Blume, K.G. 1988. Immunohematologic consequences of major ABO-mismatched bone marrow transplantation. *Transplantation*, 45: 530–4.

203. Bensinger, W.I. 1992. Supportive care in marrow transplantation. *Curr Opin Oncol*, 4: 614–23.

204. Gajewski, J.L., Petz, L.D., Calhoun, L., O'Rourke, S., Landaw, E.M., Lyddane, N.R., Hunt, L.A., Schiller, G.J., Ho, W.G., Champlin, R.E. 1992. Hemolysis of transfused group O red blood cells in minor ABO-incompatible

unrelated-donor bone marrow transplants in patients receiving cyclosporine without posttransplant methotrexate. *Blood*, 79: 3076–85.

205. Oziel-Taieb, S., Faucher-Barbey, C., Chabannon, C., Ladaique, P., Saux, P., Gouin, F., Gastaut, J.A., Maraninchi, D., Blaise, D. 1997. Early and fatal immune haemolysis after so-called 'minor' ABO-incompatible peripheral blood stem cell allotransplantation. *Bone Marrow Transplant*, 19: 1155–6.

206. Niethammer, D., Bienzle, U., Rodt, H., Goldmann, S.F., Korbling, M., Flad, H.D., Netzel, B., Haas, R.J., Fischer, K., Poschmann, A. et al. 1980. Rhesus incompatibility and aplastic anemia as the consequence of split chimerism after bone-marrow transplantation for severe combined immunodeficiency. *Thymus*, 2: 75–82.

207. Rigal, D., Monestier, M., Meyer, F., Tremisi, P.J., Vu Van, H., Fiere, D., Jouvenceaux, A. 1985. Transplant of rhesus-positive bone marrow in a rhesus-negative woman having anti-rhesus D alloantibodies. *Acta Haematol*, 73: 153–6.

208. Girelli, G., Arcese, W., Bianchi, A., Mauro, F.R., Malagnino, F., Adorno, G., Iurlo, A., Perrone, M.P., Papa, G. 1986. Hemolysis in Rh-negative female recipient after Rh-incompatible bone marrow transplantation for chronic myeloid leukemia. *Haematologica*, 71: 46–9.

209. Falkenburg, J.H., Schaafsma, M.R., Jansen, J., Brand, A., Goselink, H.M., Zwaan, F.E., Eernisse, J.G. 1985. Recovery of hematopoiesis after blood-group-incompatible bone marrow transplantation with red-blood-cell-depleted grafts. *Transplantation*, 39: 514–20.

210. Klumpp, T.R., Caligiuri, M.A., Rabinowe, S.N., Soiffer, R.J., Murray, C., Ritz, J. 1990. Autoimmune pancytopenia following allogeneic bone marrow transplantation. *Bone Marrow Transplant*, 6: 445–7.

211. Bierling, P., Cordonnier, C., Fromont, P., Rodet, M., Tanzer, J., Vernant, J.P., Bracq, C., Duedari, N. 1985. Acquired autoimmune thrombocytopenia after allogeneic bone marrow transplantation. *Br J Haematol*, 59: 643–6.

212. Anasetti, C., Rybka, W., Sullivan, K.M., Banaji, M., Slichter, S.J. 1989. Graft-v-host disease is associated with autoimmune-like thrombocytopenia. *Blood*, 73: 1054–8.

213. Drobyski, W.R., Potluri, J., Sauer, D., Gottschall, J.L. 1996. Autoimmune hemolytic anemia following T cell-depleted allogeneic bone marrow transplantation. *Bone Marrow Transplant*, 17: 1093–9.

214. Keung, Y.K., Cobos, E., Bolanos-Meade, J., Issarachai, S., Brideau, A., Morgan, D. 1997. Evans syndrome after autologous bone marrow transplant for recurrent Hodgkin's disease. *Bone Marrow Transplant*, 20: 1099–101.

215. Chappell, M.E., Keeling, D.M., Prentice, H.G., Sweny, P. 1988. Haemolytic uraemic syndrome after bone marrow transplantation: an adverse effect of total body irradiation? *Bone Marrow Transplant*, 3: 339–47.

216. Guinan, E.C., Tarbell, N.J., Niemeyer, C.M., Sallan, S.E., Weinstein, H.J. 1988. Intravascular hemolysis and renal insufficiency after bone marrow transplantation. *Blood*, 72: 451–5.

217. Rabinowe, S.N., Soiffer, R.J., Tarbell, N.J., Neuberg, D., Freedman, A.S., Seifter, J., Blake, K.W., Gribben, J.G., Anderson, K.C., Takvorian, T. et al. 1991. Hemolytic-uremic

218. syndrome following bone marrow transplantation in adults for hematologic malignancies. *Blood*, 77: 1837–44.

218. Juckett, M., Perry, E.H., Daniels, B.S., Weisdorf, D.J. 1991. Hemolytic uremic syndrome following bone marrow transplantation. *Bone Marrow Transplant*, 7: 405–9.

219. Spruce, W.E., Forman, S.J., Blume, K.G., Bearman, R.M., Bixby, H., Ching, A., Drinkard, J., San Marco, A. 1982. Hemolytic uremic syndrome after bone marrow transplantation. *Acta Haematol*, 67: 206–10.

220. Pettitt, A.R., Clark, R.E. 1994. Thrombotic microangiopathy following bone marrow transplantation. *Bone Marrow Transplant*, 14: 495–504.

221. van der Lelie, H., Baars, J.W., Rodenhuis, S., van Dijk, M.A., de Glas-Vos, C.W., Thomas, B.L., van Oers, R.H., von dem Borne, A.E. 1995. Hemolytic uremic syndrome after high dose chemotherapy with autologous stem cell support. *Cancer*, 76: 2338–42.

222. Tarantolo, S.R., Landmark, J.D., Iwen, P.C., Kessinger, A., Chan, W.C., Hinrichs, S.H. 1997. Bartonella-like erythrocyte inclusions in thrombotic thrombocytopenic purpura. *Lancet*, 350: 1602.

223. Chong, B.H., Murray, B., Berndt, M.C., Dunlop, L.C., Brighton, T., Chesterman, C.N. 1994. Plasma P-selectin is increased in thrombotic consumptive platelet disorders. *Blood*, 83: 1535–41.

224. Tandon, N.N., Rock, G., Jamieson, G.A. 1994. Anti-CD36 antibodies in thrombotic thrombocytopenic purpura. *Br J Haematol*, 88: 816–25.

225. Wada, H., Kaneko, T., Ohiwa, M., Tanigawa, M., Tamaki, S., Minami, N., Takahashi, H., Deguchi, K., Nakano, T., Shirakawa, S. 1992. Plasma cytokine levels in thrombotic thrombocytopenic purpura. *Am J Hematol*, 40: 167–70.

226. Asada, Y., Sumiyoshi, A., Hayashi, T., Suzumiya, J., Kaketani, K. 1985. Immunohistochemistry of vascular lesion in thrombotic thrombocytopenic purpura, with special reference to factor VIII related antigen. *Thromb Res*, 38: 469–79.

227. Sanders, W.E., Jr., Reddick, R.L., Nichols, T.C., Brinkhous, K.M., Read, M.S. 1995. Thrombotic thrombocytopenia induced in dogs and pigs. The role of plasma and platelet vWF in animal models of thrombotic thrombocytopenic purpura. *Arterioscler Thromb Vasc Biol*, 15: 793–800.

228. Zeigler, Z.R., Rosenfeld, C.S., Andrews, D.F., 3rd, Nemunaitis, J., Raymond, J.M., Shadduck, R.K., Kramer, R.E., Gryn, J.F., Rintels, P.B., Besa, E.C. et al. 1996. Plasma von Willebrand Factor Antigen (vWF:AG) and thrombomodulin (TM) levels in Adult Thrombotic Thrombocytopenic Purpura/Hemolytic Uremic Syndromes (TTP/HUS) and bone marrow transplant-associated thrombotic microangiopathy (BMT-TM). *Am J Hematol*, 53: 213–20.

229. Moake, J.L. 1997. Studies on the pathophysiology of thrombotic thrombocytopenic purpura. *Semin Hematol*, 34: 83–9.

230. Schubert, M.M., Williams, B.E., Lloid, M.E., Donaldson, G., Chapko, M.K. 1992. Clinical assessment scale for the rating of oral mucosal changes associated with bone marrow transplantation. Development of an oral mucositis index. *Cancer*, 69: 2469–77.

231. Sonis, S.T. 2004. The pathobiology of mucositis. *Nat Rev Cancer*, 4: 277–84.

232. Walter, E.A., Bowden, R.A. 1995. Infection in the bone marrow transplant recipient. *Infect Dis Clin N Am*, 9: 823–47.

233. Schubert, M.M., Izutsu, K.T. 1987. Iatrogenic causes of salivary gland dysfunction. *J Dent Res*, 66 Spec No: 680–8.

234. Schubert, M.M. 1991. Oral manifestations of viral infections in immunocompromised patients. *Curr Opin Dent*, 1: 384–97.

235. Schubert, M.M., Epstein, J.B., Lloid, M.E., Cooney, E. 1993. Oral infections due to cytomegalovirus in immunocompromised patients. *J Oral Pathol Med*, 22: 268–73.

236. Woo, S.B., Allen, C.M., Orden, A., Porter, D., Antin, J.H. 1996. Non-gingival soft tissue growths after allogeneic marrow transplantation. *Bone Marrow Transplant*, 17: 1127–32.

237. Sonis, S.T., Woods, P.D., White, B.A. 1990. Oral complications of cancer therapies. Pretreatment oral assessment. *NCI Monogr*: 29–32.

238. Barnes, D.W.H., Loutit, J.F. 1955. The radiation recovery factor—preservation by the Polge-Smith-Parkes technique. *J Natl Cancer Inst*, 15: 901–5.

239. Billingham, R.E. 1966. The biology of graft-versus-host reactions. *Harvey Lectures*, 62: 21–78.

240. Holler, E. 2007. Progress in acute graft versus host disease. *Curr Opin Hematol*, 14: 625–31.

241. Shlomchik, W.D. 2007. Graft-versus-host disease. *Nat Rev Immunol*, 7: 340–52.

242. Sun, Y., Tawara, I., Toubai, T., Reddy, P. 2007. Pathophysiology of acute graft-versus-host disease: recent advances. *Translational Res J Lab Clin Med*, 150: 197–214.

243. Steinmuller, D., Shelby, J. 1980. Lymphoid target cell replacement and refractoriness to graft-versus-host disease. *Transplantation*, 30: 313–4.

244. Kosaka, H., Surh, C.D., Sprent, J. 1992. Stimulation of mature unprimed CD8+ T cells by semiprofessional antigen-presenting cells in vivo. *J Exp Med*, 176: 1291–302.

245. Antin, J.H., Ferrara, J.L. 1992. Cytokine dysregulation and acute graft-versus-host disease. *Blood*, 80: 2964–8.

246. Jadus, M.R., Wepsic, H.T. 1992. The role of cytokines in graft-versus-host reactions and disease. *Bone Marrow Transplant*, 10: 1–14.

247. Krenger, W., Ferrara, J.L. 1996. Dysregulation of cytokines during graft-versus-host disease. *J Hematother*, 5: 3–14.

248. Xun, C.Q., Thompson, J.S., Jennings, C.D., Brown, S.A., Widmer, M.B. 1994. Effect of total body irradiation, busulfan-cyclophosphamide, or cyclophosphamide conditioning on inflammatory cytokine release and development of acute and chronic graft-versus-host disease in H-2-incompatible transplanted SCID mice. *Blood*, 83: 2360–7.

249. Luger, T.A., Schwarz, T. 1990. Evidence for an epidermal cytokine network. *J Invest Dermatol*, 95: 100S–4S.

250. McKenzie, R.C., Sauder, D.N. 1990. The role of keratinocyte cytokines in inflammation and immunity. *J Invest Dermatol*, 95: 105S–7S.

251. Kupper, T.S. 1990. Immune and inflammatory processes in cutaneous tissues. Mechanisms and speculations. *J Clin Invest*, 86: 1783–9.

252. Norton, J., Sloane, J.P. 1991. ICAM-1 expression on epidermal keratinocytes in cutaneous graft-versus-host disease. *Transplantation*, 51: 1203–6.

253. Cavender, D.E., Haskard, D.O., Joseph, B., Ziff, M. 1986. Interleukin 1 increases the binding of human B and T lymphocytes to endothelial cell monolayers. *J Immunol*, 136: 203–7.

254. Chang, R.J., Lee, S.H. 1986. Effects of interferon-gamma and tumor necrosis factor-alpha on the expression of an Ia antigen on a murine macrophage cell line. *J Immunol*, 137: 2853–6.

255. Leeuwenberg, J.F., Van Damme, J., Meager, T., Jeunhomme, T.M., Buurman, W.A. 1988. Effects of tumor necrosis factor on the interferon-gamma-induced major histocompatibility complex class II antigen expression by human endothelial cells. *Eur J Immunol*, 18: 1469–72.

256. Pober, J.S., Gimbrone, M.A., Jr., Lapierre, L.A., Mendrick, D.L., Fiers, W., Rothlein, R., Springer, T.A. 1986. Overlapping patterns of activation of human endothelial cells by interleukin 1, tumor necrosis factor, and immune interferon. *J Immunol*, 137: 1893–6.

257. Thornhill, M.H., Wellicome, S.M., Mahiouz, D.L., Lanchbury, J.S., Kyan-Aung, U., Haskard, D.O. 1991. Tumor necrosis factor combines with IL-4 or IFN-gamma to selectively enhance endothelial cell adhesiveness for T cells. The contribution of vascular cell adhesion molecule-1-dependent and -independent binding mechanisms. *J Immunol*, 146: 592–8.

258. Allen, R.D., Staley, T.A., Sidman, C.L. 1993. Differential cytokine expression in acute and chronic murine graft-versus-host-disease. *Eur J Immunol*, 23: 333–7.

259. Mosmann, T.R., Cherwinski, H., Bond, M.W., Giedlin, M.A., Coffman, R.L. 1986. Two types of murine helper T cell clone. I. Definition according to profiles of lymphokine activities and secreted proteins. *J Immunol*, 136: 2348–57.

260. Sad, S., Marcotte, R., Mosmann, T.R. 1995. Cytokine-induced differentiation of precursor mouse CD8+ T cells into cytotoxic CD8+ T cells secreting Th1 or Th2 cytokines. *Immunity*, 2: 271–9.

261. Hemler, M.E. 1988. Adhesive protein receptors on hematopoietic cells. *Immunol Today*, 9: 109–13.

262. Gisselbrecht, C., Maraninchi, D., Pico, J.L., Milpied, N., Coiffier, B., Divine, M., Tiberghien, P., Bosly, A., Tilly, H., Boulat, O. et al. 1994. Interleukin-2 treatment in lymphoma: a phase II multicenter study. *Blood*, 83: 2081–5.

263. Meloni, G., Foa, R., Vignetti, M., Guarini, A., Fenu, S., Tosti, S., Tos, A.G., Mandelli, F. 1994. Interleukin-2 may induce prolonged remissions in advanced acute myelogenous leukemia. *Blood*, 84: 2158–63.

264. Nestel, F.P., Price, K.S., Seemayer, T.A., Lapp, W.S. 1992. Macrophage priming and lipopolysaccharide-triggered release of tumor necrosis factor alpha during graft-versus-host disease. *J Exp Med*, 175: 405–13.

265. Suzuki, M., Suzuki, Y., Ikeda, H., Koike, M., Nomura, M., Tamura, J., Sato, S., Hotta, Y., Itoh, G. 1994. Apoptosis of murine large intestine in acute graft-versus-host disease after allogeneic bone marrow transplantation across minor histocompatibility barriers. *Transplantation*, 57: 1284–7.

266. Langley, R.G., Walsh, N., Nevill, T., Thomas, L., Rowden, G. 1996. Apoptosis is the mode of keratinocyte death in

cutaneous graft-versus-host disease. *J Am Acad Dermatol*, *35*: 187–90.

267. Gilliam, A.C., Whitaker-Menezes, D., Korngold, R., Murphy, G.F. 1996. Apoptosis is the predominant form of epithelial target cell injury in acute experimental graft-versus-host disease. *J Invest Dermatol*, *107*: 377–83.

268. Lindner, H., Holler, E., Ertl, B., Multhoff, G., Schreglmann, M., Klauke, I., Schultz-Hector, S., Eissner, G. 1997. Peripheral blood mononuclear cells induce programmed cell death in human endothelial cells and may prevent repair: role of cytokines. *Blood*, *89*: 1931–8.

269. Falzarano, G., Krenger, W., Snyder, K.M., Delmonte, J., Jr., Karandikar, M., Ferrara, J.L. 1996. Suppression of B-cell proliferation to lipopolysaccharide is mediated through induction of the nitric oxide pathway by tumor necrosis factor-alpha in mice with acute graft-versus-host disease. *Blood*, *87*: 2853–60.

270. Langrehr, J.M., Murase, N., Markus, P.M., Cai, X., Neuhaus, P., Schraut, W., Simmons, R.L., Hoffman, R.A. 1992. Nitric oxide production in host-versus-graft and graft-versus-host reactions in the rat. *J Clin Invest*, *90*: 679–83.

271. Krenger, W., Falzarano, G., Delmonte, J., Jr., Snyder, K.M., Byon, J.C., Ferrara, J.L. 1996. Interferon-gamma suppresses T-cell proliferation to mitogen via the nitric oxide pathway during experimental acute graft-versus-host disease. *Blood*, *88*: 1113–21.

272. Hakim, F.T., Sharrow, S.O., Payne, S., Shearer, G.M. 1991. Repopulation of host lymphohematopoietic systems by donor cells during graft-versus-host reaction in unirradiated adult F1 mice injected with parental lymphocytes. *J Immunol*, *146*: 2108–15.

273. Duke, R.C., Persechini, P.M., Chang, S., Liu, C.C., Cohen, J.J., Young, J.D. 1989. Purified perforin induces target cell lysis but not DNA fragmentation. *J Exp Med*, *170*: 1451–6.

274. Gratama, J.W., Sinnige, L.G., Weijers, T.F., Zwaan, F.E., van Heugten, J.G., Stijnen, T., D'Amaro, J., The, T.H., Hekker, A.C., de Gast, G.C. 1987. Marrow donor immunity to herpes simplex virus: association with acute graft-versus-host disease. *Exp Hematol*, *15*: 735–40.

275. Appleton, A.L., Sviland, L., Peiris, J.S., Taylor, C.E., Wilkes, J., Green, M.A., Pearson, A.D., Kelly, P.J., Malcolm, A.J., Proctor, S.J. et al. 1995. Human herpes virus-6 infection in marrow graft recipients: role in pathogenesis of graft-versus-host disease. Newcastle upon Tyne Bone Marrow Transport Group. *Bone Marrow Transplant*, *16*: 777–82.

276. Vogelsang, G.B., Hess, A.D., Santos, G.W. 1988. Acute graft-versus-host disease: clinical characteristics in the cyclosporine era. *Medicine (Baltimore)*, *67*: 163–74.

277. Storb, R., Prentice, R.L., Buckner, C.D., Clift, R.A., Appelbaum, F., Deeg, J., Doney, K., Hansen, J.A., Mason, M., Sanders, J.E. et al. 1983. Graft-versus-host disease and survival in patients with aplastic anemia treated by marrow grafts from HLA-identical siblings. Beneficial effect of a protective environment. *N Engl J Med*, *308*: 302–7.

278. Roy, J., Snover, D., Weisdorf, S., Mulvahill, A., Filipovich, A., Weisdorf, D. 1991. Simultaneous upper and lower endoscopic biopsy in the diagnosis of intestinal graft-versus-host disease. *Transplantation*, *51*: 642–6.

279. Shulman, H.M., Sharma, P., Amos, D., Fenster, L.F., McDonald, G.B. 1988. A coded histologic study of hepatic graft-versus-host disease after human bone marrow transplantation. *Hepatology (Baltimore, MD)*, *8*: 463–70.

280. Parkman, R. 1986. Clonal analysis of murine graft-vs-host disease. I. Phenotypic and functional analysis of T lymphocyte clones. *J Immunol*, *136*: 3543–8.

281. Hess, A.D., Horwitz, L., Beschorner, W.E., Santos, G.W. 1985. Development of graft-vs.-host disease-like syndrome in cyclosporine-treated rats after syngeneic bone marrow transplantation. I. Development of cytotoxic T lymphocytes with apparent polyclonal anti-Ia specificity, including autoreactivity. *J Exp Med*, *161*: 718–30.

282. Hess, A.D., Bright, E.C., Thoburn, C., Vogelsang, G.B., Jones, R.J., Kennedy, M.J. 1997. Specificity of effector T lymphocytes in autologous graft-versus-host disease: role of the major histocompatibility complex class II invariant chain peptide. *Blood*, *89*: 2203–9.

283. Dighiero, G., Intrator, L., Cordonnier, C., Tortevoye, P., Vernant, J.P. 1987. High levels of anti-cytoskeleton autoantibodies are frequently associated with chronic GVHD. *Br J Haematol*, *67*: 301–5.

284. Kier, P., Penner, E., Bakos, S., Kalhs, P., Lechner, K., Volc-Platzer, B., Wesierska-Gadek, J., Sauermann, G., Gadner, H., Emminger-Schmidmeier, W. et al. 1990. Autoantibodies in chronic GVHD: high prevalence of antinucleolar antibodies. *Bone Marrow Transplant*, *6*: 93–6.

285. Sullivan, K.M., Agura, E., Anasetti, C., Appelbaum, F., Badger, C., Bearman, S., Erickson, K., Flowers, M., Hansen, J., Loughran, T. et al. 1991. Chronic graft-versus-host disease and other late complications of bone marrow transplantation. *Semin Hematol*, *28*: 250–9.

286. Sullivan, K.M., Shulman, H.M., Storb, R., Weiden, P.L., Witherspoon, R.P., McDonald, G.B., Schubert, M.M., Atkinson, K., Thomas, E.D. 1981. Chronic graft-versus-host disease in 52 patients: adverse natural course and successful treatment with combination immunosuppression. *Blood*, *57*: 267–76.

287. Epstein, O., Thomas, H.C., Sherlock, S. 1980. Primary biliary cirrhosis is a dry gland syndrome with features of chronic graft-versus-host disease. *Lancet*, *1*: 1166–8.

288. Yau, J.C., Zander, A.R., Srigley, J.R., Verm, R.A., Stroehlein, J.R., Korinek, J.K., Vellekoop, L., Dicke, K.A. 1986. Chronic graft-versus-host disease complicated by micronodular cirrhosis and esophageal varices. *Transplantation*, *41*: 129–30.

289. McDonald, G.B., Sullivan, K.M., Schuffler, M.D., Shulman, H.M., Thomas, E.D. 1981. Esophageal abnormalities in chronic graft-versus-host disease in humans. *Gastroenterology*, *80*: 914–21.

290. McDonald, G.B., Sullivan, K.M., Plumley, T.F. 1984. Radiographic features of esophageal involvement in chronic graft-vs.-host disease. *AJR Am J Roentgenol*, *142*: 501–6.

291. Ueda, M., Mori, T., Shiobara, S., Harada, M., Yoshida, T., Matsuda, T., Hattori, K., Mizoguchi, H., Sullivan, K.M., Witherspoon, R.P. 1986. Development of bullous pemphigoid after allogeneic bone marrow transplantation. Report of a case. *Transplantation*, *42*: 320–2.

292. Fenyk, J.R., Jr., Smith, C.M., Warkentin, P.I., Krivit, W., Goltz, R.W., Neely, J.E., Nesbit, M.E., Ramsay, N.K.,

Coccia, P.F., Kersey, J.H. 1978. Sclerodermatous graft-versus-host disease limited to an area of measles exanthem. *Lancet*, *1*: 472–3.

293. Socie, G., Gluckman, E., Cosset, J.M., Devergie, A., Girinski, T., Esperou, H., Dutreix, J. 1989. Unusual localization of cutaneous chronic graft-versus-host disease in the radiation fields in four cases. *Bone Marrow Transplant*, *4*: 133–5.

294. Freemer, C.S., Farmer, E.R., Corio, R.L., Altomonte, V.L., Wagner, J.E., Vogelsang, G.B., Santos, G.W. 1994. Lichenoid chronic graft-vs-host disease occurring in a dermatomal distribution. *Arch Dermatol*, *130*: 70–2.

295. Nagler, A., Goldenhersh, M.A., Levi-Schaffer, F., Bystryn, J.C., Klaus, S.N. 1996. Total leucoderma: a rare manifestation of cutaneous chronic graft-versus-host disease. *Br J Dermatol*, *134*: 780–3.

296. Ling, N.S., Fenske, N.A., Julius, R.L., Espinoza, C.G., Drake, L.A. 1985. Dyskeratosis congenita in a girl simulating chronic graft-vs-host disease. *Arch Dermatol*, *121*: 1424–8.

297. Ivker, R.A., Woosley, J., Resnick, S.D. 1993. Dyskeratosis congenita or chronic graft-versus-host disease? A diagnostic dilemma in a child eight years after bone marrow transplantation for aplastic anemia. *Pediatr Dermatol*, *10*: 362–5.

298. Tichelli, A., Duell, T., Weiss, M., Socie, G., Ljungman, P., Cohen, A., van Lint, M., Gratwohl, A., Kolb, H.J. 1996. Late-onset keratoconjunctivitis sicca syndrome after bone marrow transplantation: incidence and risk factors. European Group or Blood and Marrow Transplantation (EBMT) Working Party on Late Effects. *Bone Marrow Transplant*, *17*: 1105–11.

299. Deeg, H.J., Flournoy, N., Sullivan, K.M., Sheehan, K., Buckner, C.D., Sanders, J.E., Storb, R., Witherspoon, R.P., Thomas, E.D. 1984. Cataracts after total body irradiation and marrow transplantation: a sparing effect of dose fractionation. *Int J Radiat Oncol Biol Phys*, *10*: 957–64.

300. Benyunes, M.C., Sullivan, K.M., Deeg, H.J., Mori, M., Meyer, W., Fisher, L., Bensinger, R., Jack, M.K., Hicks, J., Witherspoon, R. et al. 1995. Cataracts after bone marrow transplantation: long-term follow-up of adults treated with fractionated total body irradiation. *Int J Radiat Oncol Biol Phys*, *32*: 661–70.

301. Clark, J.G., Schwartz, D.A., Flournoy, N., Sullivan, K.M., Crawford, S.W., Thomas, E.D. 1987. Risk factors for airflow obstruction in recipients of bone marrow transplants. *Ann Intern Med*, *107*: 648–56.

302. Sullivan, K.M., Shulman, H.M. 1989. Chronic graftversus-host disease, obliterative bronchiolitis, and graftversus-leukemia effect: case histories. *Transplant Proc*, *21*: 51–62.

303. Holland, H.K., Wingard, J.R., Beschorner, W.E., Saral, R., Santos, G.W. 1988. Bronchiolitis obliterans in bone marrow transplantation and its relationship to chronic graft-v-host disease and low serum IgG. *Blood*, *72*: 621–7.

304. Sullivan, K.M. 1989. Intravenous immune globulin prophylaxis in recipients of a marrow transplant. *J Allergy Clin Immunol*, *84*: 632–8; discussion 638–9.

305. Clark, J.G., Crawford, S.W., Madtes, D.K., Sullivan, K.M. 1989. Obstructive lung disease after allogeneic marrow transplantation. Clinical presentation and course. *Ann Intern Med*, *111*: 368–76.

306. Boas, S.R., Noyes, B.E., Kurland, G., Armitage, J., Orenstein, D. 1994. Pediatric lung transplantation for graftversus-host disease following bone marrow transplantation. *Chest*, *105*: 1584–6.

307. Schwarer, A.P., Hughes, J.M., Trotman-Dickenson, B., Krausz, T., Goldman, J.M. 1992. A chronic pulmonary syndrome associated with graft-versus-host disease after allogeneic marrow transplantation. *Transplantation*, *54*: 1002–8.

308. Lawley, T.J., Peck, G.L., Moutsopoulos, H.M., Gratwohl, A.A., Deisseroth, A.B. 1977. Scleroderma, Sjogren-like syndrome, and chronic graft-versus-host disease. *Ann Intern Med*, *87*: 707–9.

309. Schubert, M.M., Sullivan, K.M., Morton, T.H., Izutsu, K.T., Peterson, D.E., Flournoy, N., Truelove, E.L., Sale, G.E., Buckner, C.D., Storb, R. et al. 1984. Oral manifestations of chronic graft-v-host disease. *Arch Intern Med*, *144*: 1591–5.

310. Schubert, M.M., Sullivan, K.M. 1990. Recognition, incidence, and management of oral graft-versus-host disease. *NCI Monogr*: 135–43.

311. Nelson, K.R., McQuillen, M.P. 1988. Neurologic complications of graft-versus-host disease. *Neurol Clin*, *6*: 389–403.

312. Marosi, C., Budka, H., Grimm, G., Zeitlhofer, J., Sluga, E., Brunner, C., Schneeweiss, B., Volc, B., Bettelheim, P., Panzer, S. et al. 1990. Fatal encephalitis in a patient with chronic graft-versus-host disease. *Bone Marrow Transplant*, *6*: 53–7.

313. Greenspan, A., Deeg, H.J., Cottler-Fox, M., Sirdofski, M., Spitzer, T.R., Kattah, J. 1990. Incapacitating peripheral neuropathy as a manifestation of chronic graft-versus-host disease. *Bone Marrow Transplant*, *5*: 349–52.

314. Smith, C.I., Aarli, J.A., Biberfeld, P., Bolme, P., Christensson, B., Gahrton, G., Hammarstrom, L., Lefvert, A.K., Lonnqvist, B., Matell, G. et al. 1983. Myasthenia gravis after bone-marrow transplantation. Evidence for a donor origin. *N Engl J Med*, *309*: 1565–8.

315. Bolger, G.B., Sullivan, K.M., Spence, A.M., Appelbaum, F.R., Johnston, R., Sanders, J.E., Deeg, H.J., Witherspoon, R.P., Doney, K.C., Nims, J. et al. 1986. Myasthenia gravis after allogeneic bone marrow transplantation: relationship to chronic graft-versus-host disease. *Neurology*, *36*: 1087–91.

316. Parker, P., Chao, N.J., Ben-Ezra, J., Slatkin, N., Openshaw, H., Niland, J.C., Linker, C.A., Greffe, B.S., Kashyap, A., Molina, A. et al. 1996. Polymyositis as a manifestation of chronic graft-versus-host disease. *Medicine (Baltimore)*, *75*: 279–85.

317. Corson, S.L., Sullivan, K., Batzer, F., August, C., Storb, R., Thomas, E.D. 1982. Gynecologic manifestations of chronic graft-versus-host disease. *Obstet Gynecol*, *60*: 488–92.

318. Schubert, M.A., Sullivan, K.M., Schubert, M.M., Nims, J., Hansen, M., Sanders, J.E., O'Quigley, J., Witherspoon, R.P., Buckner, C.D., Storb, R. et al. 1990. Gynecological abnormalities following allogeneic bone marrow transplantation. *Bone Marrow Transplant*, *5*: 425–30.

319. Gomez-Garcia, P., Herrera-Arroyo, C., Torres-Gomez, A., Gomez-Carrasco, J., Aljama-Garcia, P., Lopez-Rubio, F., Martinez-Guibelalde, F., Fornes-Torres, G., Rojas-Contreras, R. 1988. Renal involvement in chronic graft-

versus-host disease: a report of two cases. *Bone Marrow Transplant*, 3: 357–62.

320. Miralbell, R., Bieri, S., Mermillod, B., Helg, C., Sancho, G., Pastoors, B., Keller, A., Kurtz, J.M., Chapuis, B. 1996. Renal toxicity after allogeneic bone marrow transplantation: the combined effects of total-body irradiation and graft-versus-host disease. *J Clin Oncol*, 14: 579–85.

321. Peralvo, J., Bacigalupo, A., Pittaluga, P.A., Occhini, D., Van Lint, M.T., Frassoni, F., Nardelli, E., Transino, A., Pantarotto, M., Marmout, A.M. 1987. Poor graft function associated with graft-versus-host disease after allogeneic marrow transplantation. *Bone Marrow Transplant*, 2: 279–85.

322. Godder, K., Pati, A.R., Abhyankar, S.H., Lamb, L.S., Armstrong, W., Henslee-Downey, P.J. 1997. De novo chronic graft-versus-host disease presenting as hemolytic anemia following partially mismatched related donor bone marrow transplant. *Bone Marrow Transplant*, 19: 813–7.

323. Siadak, M.F., Kopecky, K., Sullivan, K.M. 1994. Reduction in transplant-related complications in patients given intravenous immuno globulin after allogeneic marrow transplantation. *Clin Exp Immunol*, 97 Suppl 1: 53–7.

324. Seidler, C.W., Mills, L.E., Flowers, M.E., Sullivan, K.M. 1994. Spontaneous factor VIII inhibitor occurring in association with chronic graft-versus-host disease. *Am J Hematol*, 45: 240–3.

325. Socie, G., Selimi, F., Sedel, L., Frija, J., Devergie, A., Esperou Bourdeau, H., Ribaud, P., Gluckman, E. 1994. Avascular necrosis of bone after allogeneic bone marrow transplantation: clinical findings, incidence and risk factors. *Br J Haematol*, 86: 624–8.

326. Stern, J.M., Chesnut, C.H., 3rd, Bruemmer, B., Sullivan, K.M., Lenssen, P.S., Aker, S.N., Sanders, J. 1996. Bone density loss during treatment of chronic GVHD. *Bone Marrow Transplant*, 17: 395–400.

327. Fink, J.C., Leisenring, W.M., Sullivan, K.M., Sherrard, D.J., Weiss, N.S. 1998. Avascular necrosis following bone marrow transplantation: a case-control study. *Bone*, 22: 67–71.

328. Sanders, J.E. 1991. Long-term effects of bone marrow transplantation. *Pediatrician*, 18: 76–81.

329. Graze, P.R., Gale, R.P. 1979. Chronic graft versus host disease: a syndrome of disordered immunity. *Am J Med*, 66: 611–20.

330. Furst, D.E., Clements, P.J., Graze, P., Gale, R., Roberts, N. 1979. A syndrome resembling progressive systemic sclerosis after bone marrow transplantation. A model for scleroderma? *Arthritis Rheum*, 22: 904–10.

331. Shulman, H.M., Sullivan, K.M., Weiden, P.L., McDonald, G.B., Striker, G.E., Sale, G.E., Hackman, R., Tsoi, M.S., Storb, R., Thomas, E.D. 1980. Chronic graft-versus-host syndrome in man. A long-term clinicopathologic study of 20 Seattle patients. *Am J Med*, 69: 204–17.

332. Kim, S.T., Jung, C.W., Lee, J., Kwon, J.M., Oh, S.Y., Park, B.B., Lee, H.R., Kim, H.J., Kim, K., Kim, W.S. et al. 2007. New clinical grading system for chronic GVHD predicts duration of systemic immunosuppressive treatment and GVHD-specific and overall survival. *Bone Marrow Transplant*, 39: 711–16.

CHAPTER 10

Pathology and Pathogenesis of Post-Transplant Lymphoproliferative Disorders

Lawrence Tsao, M.D.

Eric D. Hsi, M.D.

Izidore S. Lossos, M.D.

I. INTRODUCTION

Post-transplant lymphoproliferative disorders (PTLDs) represent a major complication of organ transplantation and account for severe morbidity and mortality among transplant patients. In recent years, the prevalence of PTLDs has markedly increased. The reasons are multifactorial and include expanded indications and diversity of transplanted organs, increased number of performed transplantations, more potent immunosuppressive regimens, and improved long-term survival after transplantation. First described in 1968 by Doak et al. (1) in a renal transplant recipient, PTLDs comprise a spectrum of diseases characterized by lymphoid proliferation ranging from *Epstein-Barr virus* (EBV)–driven polyclonal benign lymphoid hyperplasia to highly aggressive monomorphic proliferations, which may be indistinguishable from aggressive types of lymphoma, such as diffuse large B-cell lymphoma (DLBCL) (2). Most PTLDs are thought to arise as a result of iatro-genic immunosuppression after transplantation, leading to decreased immunosurveillance by EBV-specific T cells, which in turn may lead to uncontrolled proliferation of EBV-infected B cells. However, PTLDs are not exclusively associated with EBV infection and EBV-negative cases are also encountered, especially after many years of immuno-supression (3,4). PTLDs differ in their pathogenesis and clinical characteristics from lymphoproliferative disorders that occur in immunocompetent individuals. Despite advances in our understanding of PTLD pathogenesis, improved diagnostic tools and earlier diagnosis, and expanded therapeutic options, these disorders are still associated with a high rate of graft loss and a mortality of more than 50 percent at one year following diagnosis (5–7).

II. INCIDENCE AND PREDISPOSING FACTORS

Patients who have received solid organ transplants have a 20- to 120-fold higher incidence of non-Hodgkin's

TABLE 10.1 Incidence of PTLD in Specific Organ Transplants

Organ	Incidence (%)
Kidney	0.4–2
Liver	1–3.5
Heart	3.4–5
Lung	7.9
Multivisceral	11–20
Bone marrow	1

TABLE 10.2 Risk Factors for PTLD

Transplant Organ	Risk Factors
Solid organ	Type of organ transplant
	Degree and type of immunosuppressive regimens
	EBV serostatus of the recipient at the time of transplant
	Development of primary EBV infection after transplantation
	Recipients' age at the time of the transplant (pediatric age-group)
Bone marrow transplant	Mismatched bone marrow transplant
	T-cell depletion of the graft
	Use of monoclonal anti-CD3 antibodies

lymphoma (NHL) (8–10). The incidence of PTLD after organ transplantation correlates with the type of organ transplanted and is probably related to the intensity of associated immunosuppressive therapy (Table 10.1). In renal transplantation, the risk for PTLD was found to be about forty times greater than in the general population, with an incidence in adults ranging between 0.4 and 2 percent (11–15). Caillard et al. (14) investigated the incidence and risk of PTLD in a prospective French nationwide cohort of adult kidney transplant recipients. The PTLD incidence in the first post-transplant year was 0.46 percent and the cumulative five-year incidence was around 1.2 percent. Analysis of the U.S. Renal Data System showed a cumulative PTLD incidence of 1.4 percent in the three years following kidney transplantation. A similar incidence of 1.2 percent was reported in pediatric recipients of renal transplants (16). The incidence of PTLD was found to be between 3.4 and 5 percent in heart transplant recipients, 7.9 percent in lung transplant recipients, between 1 and 3.5 percent in liver transplant recipients, and between 11 and 20 percent in primary intestinal transplants (Table 10.1) (7,8,17–24). In all types of transplants, the incidence of PTLD is highest in the first year, with largest risk at around six months, followed by continuous fall in risk for this complication. However, even after many years after transplantation, the risk for PTLD always remains higher than in the general population. The incidence of PTLD after first year following transplant is approximately 0.04 percent per year in renal and 0.30 percent in cardiac recipients (8–10). The lifetime increased risk for PTLD accounts for the increased number of PTLD patients encountered with longer survival of transplant recipients. The incidence of PTLD after allogeneic bone marrow transplantation (BMT) is typically low, with a cumulative incidence of 1 percent at ten years based on the analysis of 18,014 BMT recipients reported to the International Bone Marrow Transplant Registry (IBMTR) (25). This incidence rate is comparable to the 0.5–1.8 percent incidence reported from single institutions (26,27). In the IBMTR cohort, the incidence was highest in the first five months after transplantation, followed by a steep decline in the incidence between six and twelve months after transplant (25). Although a significantly increased risk of PTLD continues among longer term BMT survivors, the rate is greatly diminished and is mark-

edly lower compared to the survivors of solid organ transplants. The differences in the long-term PTLD risks between BMT and solid organ recipients is likely due to the fact that immunosuppression therapies are usually discontinued at approximately one year after BMT but are maintained lifelong in most solid organ recipients.

The risk for developing PTLD is influenced by several factors, including type of organ transplant, (7,8,17–23) the degree and type of immunosuppressive regimens used, (15,16,25) EBV serostatus of the recipient, (28) the development of primary EBV infection after transplantation, and recipients' age at the time of the transplant (pediatric age group) (29) (Table 10.2). The incidence of PTLD has consistently been higher in nonrenal than in renal transplants possibly because of the greater intensity of immunosuppression in vital organ recipients. Patients receiving liver and heart transplants are commonly maintained on higher levels of cyclosporine A than kidney transplant recipients. The role of higher cyclosporine A levels or doses as potential risk factor for PTLD was suggested in some studies (30) but was not confirmed in others (15). Further, as newer immunosuppressive agents improved the rates of graft survival over the past decades, many centers have noticed an accompanying rise in the number of cases of PTLD. A marked rise in the prevalence of PTLD was reported with the use of tacrolimus in pediatric renal and liver transplant recipients versus those receiving cyclosporine A (31,32). Various anti-T-cell antibodies used for induction or rejection treatment were also implicated as risk factors for PTLD. Swinnen et al. (33) reported an increased prevalence of PTLD (more than fourfold) in cardiac transplant recipients receiving more than 75-mg cumulative dose of OKT3. Walker et al. (34) reported that the use of OKT3 independently increased the risk of PTLD five- to sixfold in a multivariate analysis. Other studies also demonstrated an increased risk of post–solid organ transplant PTLD in recipients of OKT3 or antithymocyte globulin (15,23,25). However, not all studies were able to confirm these observations (16). Caillard et al. (15)

reported that treatment with antimetabolites (mycophenolate nofetil and azathioprine) was associated with a lower risk of PTLD in renal recipients. The effect of mammalian target of rapamycin (mTOR) inhibitors (sirolimus, everolimus) on PTLD development is not clear yet. However, these drugs might theoretically be associated with a lower risk since constitutive activation of mTOR signaling pathway was observed in PTLD (35) and these inhibitors displayed an inhibitory effect on PTLD-derived cells in both in vitro and in vivo animal models (36,37). Overall, currently available data suggest that the *total amount of immunosuppression*, including induction and rejection therapy, represents an important risk factor for PTLD following solid organ transplant. The precise role of specific immunosuppressive agents in PTLD risk is less clear since most of the currently available data stem from single institution reports or retrospective analysis of transplant registries. Unequivocal proof of specific association between risk of PTLD and specific single immunosuppressive agents is ideally obtained only from prospective randomized trials.

Pretransplant EBV seronegativity is a major risk factor for PTLD. In one report, the risk of PTLD in EBV-seronegative recipients was estimated to be seventy-six times higher than in seropositive recipients (28). The higher risk of EBV seronegativity among pediatric patients may account for increased risk for PTLD in this age-group. Virtually all seronegative recipients seroconvert shortly after transplantation and the incidence of EBV-associated PTLD is highest during the first year after transplantation.

Another virus associated with PTLD is *herpes type-8* (HHV-8) detected in all the cases of post-transplant primary effusion lymphoma (38). Whether cytomegalovirus and hepatitis virus infections are also associated with increased risk of PTLD is debatable (14,15,39,40).

III. PATHOLOGICAL FEATURES AND CLASSIFICATION

The classification of PTLD is currently based on the World Health Organization (WHO) system for classifying hematopoietic neoplasms (2). The key morphological, immunophenotypic, and molecular characteristics of each type of PTLD are listed in Table 10.3. The WHO divides PTLD into four major categories: early lesions, polymorphic PTLD, monomorphic PTLD, and Hodgkin's lymphoma (HL) and HL-like PTLD. Early lesions, polymorphic PTLD, and monomorphic PTLD represent a pathological spectrum that can be observed synchronously within a single specimen or from multiple specimens from a single patient. Patients may also manifest with different types of lesions at different times and progress from one type (e.g., early lesion) to another (e.g., monomorphic PTLD).

i. Early Lesions

Florid follicular hyperplasia may be seen in lymph nodes from transplant patients and some regard this as the earliest precursor of PTLD. The WHO, however, currently recognizes two subtypes of early lesions: plasmacytic hyperplasia (PH) and infectious mononucleosis-like (IM-like) PTLD. The common defining morphological characteristic of early lesions is some degree of architectural preservation of the involved tissue. PH (Figure 10.1) is a lesion characterized by numerous plasma cells with rare immunoblasts. The plasma cells are mature and atypical cytological features are absent. Binucleated plasma cells may be seen in reactive conditions and are not considered atypical. Cytoplasmic inclusions (Russell bodies) may be seen but Dutcher bodies are generally absent and, when present, should raise suspicion of a monotypic process. IM-like lesions (Figure 10.2) resemble typical IM with florid follicular hyperplasia and marked paracortical expansion by a mixed T-cell and plasma cell infiltrate and a prominent immunoblastic proliferation. Some early lesions may show overlapping features between PH and IM-like lesions.

Immunophenotyping of early lesions is of limited diagnostic utility, as it will confirm the morphological impression of variable mixtures of B cells, T cells, and plasma cells with polytypic light chain expression. Immunoblasts will frequently show evidence of EBV infection using in situ hybridzation for EBV-encoded RNA (EBER) or EBV latent membrane protein (LMP)-1 immunohistochemical stain. Other EBV-associated nuclear antigens are not reliably expressed (41).

Analysis of *IGH* and episomal EBV genome will frequently yield polyclonal or oligoclonal patterns. Occasionally, a minor clone is seen but is of no clinical significance. Clonal cytogenetic changes are rare in early lesions but have been reported (42,43). They are usually only present in a small number of metaphases when present.

ii. Polymorphic Lesions

Polymorphic PTLDs (Figure 10.3) are characterized by a mixed infiltrate consisting of immunoblasts, plasma cells, and intermediately sized lymphocytes. In contrast to early lesions, polymorphic PTLD is characterized by loss of the underlying architecture of the involved tissue due to the lymphoid proliferation. However, in contrast to monomorphic PTLD, polymorphic PTLD shows a full spectrum of B cells from small- to intermediate-sized lymphocytes to immunoblasts and mature plasma cells. Cytological atypia, areas of necrosis, and numerous mitotic figures are all acceptable in the spectrum of polymorphic PTLD. In the past, these features of "malignancy" were used to distinguish "polymorphic lymphoma" from "polymorphic hyperplasia." (44) However, subdividing

TABLE 10.3 WHO classification[2] of PTLD

Subtype	Morphology	Immunophenotype	Molecular	EBV status
Early Lesion	Preservation of the underlying architecture	Mixture of B-, T-, and plasma cells	IgH: polyclonal or oligoclonal EBV: polyclonal or oligoclonal	(+), virtually all
IM like	Increased numbers of immunoblasts	CD30+ immunoblasts will be present	See *Early lesion*	(+), virtually all Immunoblasts EBER+
Plasma cell hyperplasia	Large aggregates and sheets of plasma cells	Kappa and lambda show polytypic plasma cells	See *Early lesion*	(+), majority occasionally can be (−)
Polymorphic	Some degree of effacement of underlying architecture with a spectrum of lymphoid cells ranging from small lymphocytes to intermediate to immunoblasts	B-cell markers may highlight the spectrum of B-cells present CD30 will highlight immunoblasts	IgH: clonal EBV: clonal	(+), majority variable numbers of EBER+ cells
Monomorphic	Effacement of underlying architecture with cytologic atypia sufficient for a lymphoma	Varies with lineage	Varies with lineage	Varies with lineage
B cell	Majority will resemble diffuse large B-cell lymphoma A subset may resemble Burkitt lymphoma	Positive for B-cell markers, but can show abnormal phenotype (i.e. aberrant expression or loss of antigens) Burkitt immunophenotype (CD20+, CD10+, CD43+, BCL-6+, BCL-2−, Ki-67: ~100%)	IgH: clonal EBV: clonal	(+), majority large numbers EBER+ cells
T/NK cell	Varies with type	Varies with type (WHO T-cell lymphomas) Pan-T-cell antigens should be evaluated for aberrant loss	**T cell:** TCR: clonal **NK cell:** TCR: germline EBV: clonal (if present)	(−), majority of T cell (+), virtually all NK cell
Plasma cell myeloma Plasmacytoma	Sheets of plasma cells Must be differentiated for early lesion	Positive for plasma cell markers Kappa and lambda show monotypic plasma cells	IgH: clonal EBV: clonal (if present)	Variable
HL and HL like	RS cells in the classic HL mileu	**HL:** Classic HL immunophenotype (CD30+, CD15+, CD45−, CD20−/+, CD3−, weak PAX-5) **HL like:** Aberrant immunophenotype (i.e. CD20+)	IgH: varies EBV: clonal (if present)	(+), majority RS-cells EBER+
MALT-type PTLD	Lymphoid infiltrate of small, mature-appearing lymphocytes expanding underlying mucosa and submucosa Lymphocytes show slightly irregular nuclei with moderate amounts of pale cytoplasm	Similar to MALT-type lymphomas is immunocompetent patients (CD20+, CD5−, CD10−, CD43+/−)	IgH: clonal	(−), majority *H. pylori* associated

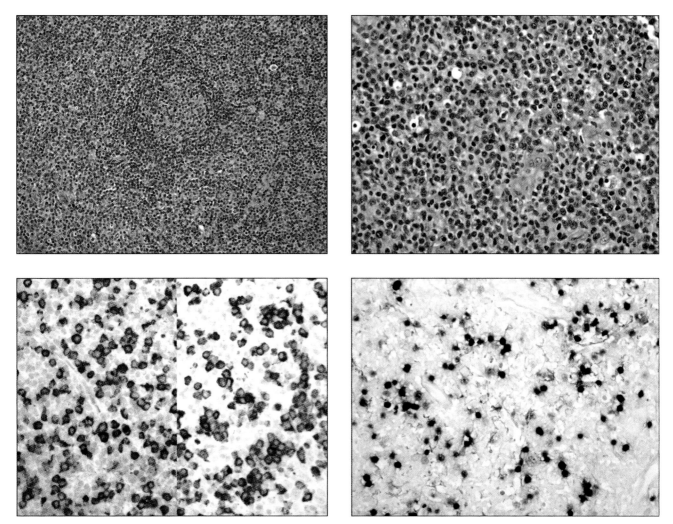

FIGURE 10.1: *Early-lesion PTLD, plasma cell hyperplasia is seen in the tonsil of a patient after solid organ transplantation. The overall architecture is preserved with small residual follicles surrounded by a marked expansion of the paracortical area (upper left, hematoxylin and eosin [H&E] 200×). The paracortical expansion consists of numerous plasma cells and plasmacytoid cells (upper right, H&E 400×). These plasma cells show polytypic expression of kappa and lambda light chains (lower left, immunohistochemistry [IHC] 200×, kappa right panel and lambda left panel). EBER in situ hybridization highlights numerous EBV-infected cells, the majority most likely representing B cells (lower right, EBER ISH 200×).*

polymorphic PTLD into such morphological types does not reliably predict clinical behavior and is not necessary in the WHO classification (45).

Immunophenotyping of polymorphic PTLD will show variable mixtures of B and T cells. Analysis of surface or cytoplasmic immunoglobulin expression is useful for identifying monotypic B-cell populations. However, B cells may show polytypic immunoglobulin expression in polymorphic PTLD. The majority of polymorphic PTLD will show EBV latency II and III patterns, expressing EBER and EBV LMP-1 with variable expression of EBNA-2 and other viral antigens (41). Although immunophenotyping may appear polytypic, molecular analysis of *IGH* or episomal EBV genome will virtually always show a clonal pattern (45). Clonal cytogenetic changes may be present.

iii. Monomorphic Lesions

Monomorphic PTLDs are divided according to B- or T-cell lineage and further subclassified according to the WHO classification of lymphomas in the nontransplant population (2). B-cell monomorphic PTLDs are by far the most common type. They are characterized by architectural and cytological atypia sufficient to be classified as a lymphoma based on morphological features (2). In general, monomorphic PTLDs show invasion and architectural effacement by large aggregates and confluent sheets of transformed cells with large nuclei with prominent nucleoli. The neoplastic cells can show marked pleomorphism or plasmacytoid/plasma cell differentiation. These cases of monomorphic PTLD generally are not diagnostically problematic. However, occasional cases of PTLD may span the spectrum of polymorphic PTLD and

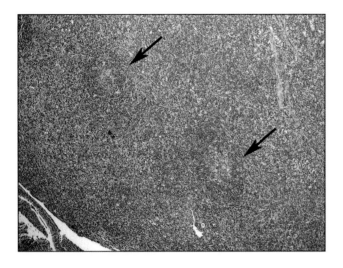

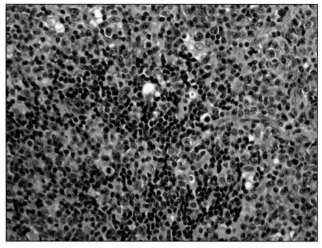

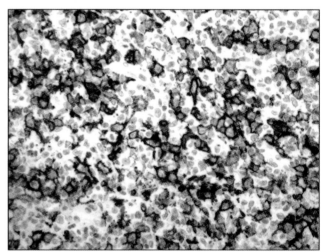

FIGURE 10.2: Early-lesion PTLD, infectious mononucleosis like, is seen in a patient after solid organ transplantation. The overall architecture is preserved with two small residual follicles (arrows) surrounded by a marked paracortical expansion (upper left, H&E 40×). The paracortical expansion consists of a mixture of small lymphocytes with scattered large transformed cells and rare plasma cells (upper right, H&E 400×). CD20 highlights only the scattered large transformed cells (lower right, IHC 400×). The majority of small lymphoid cells are actually residual paracortical T cells. EBV is present by EBER in situ hybridization (not shown).

monomorphic PTLD. These cases are difficult to classify within a single category but are best considered monomorphic lesions.

1. Monomorphic B-Cell PTLD

The majority of the B-cell PTLD will resemble DLBCL [in nontransplant patients (Figure 10.4)]. Sheets of large, transformed lymphoma cells are present. Morphological variants include immunoblastic, centroblastic, and less commonly anaplastic morphology. Immunoblastic cells are large with single central prominent nucleolus and abundant cytoplasm. Centroblasts have vesicular chromatin with multiple small nucleoli. Anaplastic B-cell PTLDs have numerous pleomorphic and highly atypical multilobulated or multinucleated cells. As with DLBCL, these morphological variants do not appear to have any clinical significance.

Cases resembling Burkitt lymphoma (BL) or atypical BL have been reported and have the morphological, phenotypic, and molecular genetic features of BL. Cytologically, the cells are intermediate in size (similar size to a histocyte nucleus). Numerous mitotic figures are present and a starry-sky pattern is present due to many interspersed tingible body macrophages. Diagnosis of BL should be confirmed with appropriate immunophenotypic and cytogenetic studies.

Immunophenotypically, monomorphic B-cell PTLDs demonstrate monotypic surface immunoglobulin expression. Occasionally, it may be absent, which is an abnormal finding that should prompt investigation of monoclonality at the genetic level. The majority of B-cell PTLDs show presence of EBV infection within the transformed cells, with variable latency patterns (46). Virtually, all cases show a clonal pattern of *IGH* rearrangement and, if present,

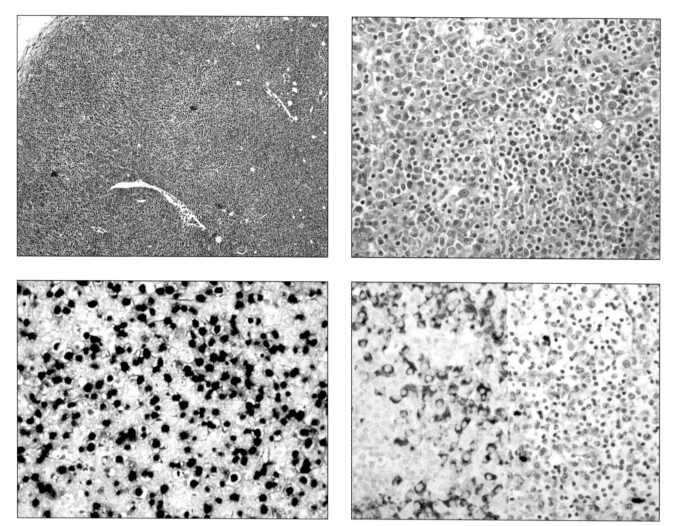

FIGURE 10.3: *Polymorphic PTLD is seen in the lymph node of a patient after solid organ transplantation. The normal lymph node architecture is replaced by a diffuse proliferation (upper left, H&E 40×) of mixed plasma cells and lymphocytes. The lymphocytes are predominantly small in size but show a spectrum including scattered large transformed immunoblasts (upper right, H&E 200×). EBER in situ hybridization highlights numerous EBV-infected cells (lower left, EBER ISH 200×). In addition, the plasma cells show kappa light chain restriction (left panel) with only rare plasma cells expressing lambda light chain (right panel) (lower right, IHC 200×).*

episomal EBV genomes. Cytogenetic evaluation will show clonal karyotypic abnormalities, which can include trisomies 9 and/or 11 and abnormalities of 8q24.1, 3q27, and 14q32.

Rare cases of B-cell PTLD are morphologically and immunophenotypically identical to plasma cell neoplasms (Figure 10.5) (47,48). Plasma cell myeloma and plasmacytoma-like PTLD can also be EBV associated in about 50 percent of the cases reported (47,48). Clinically, these can present as rare extramedullary plasmacytic neoplasms similar to plasmacytomas or plasma cell myeloma. Plasma cell PTLDs need to be differentiated from PH, a nondestructive early lesion, and DLBCL with marked plasmacytic differentiation, a monomorphic PTLD. Due to the rarity of plasma cell PTLDs, it is currently unclear if plasma cell directed, B cell directed, or both are the most effective therapy. The evaluation for

urine and serum M-components, serum immunoglobulin levels, and lytic bone lesions, although not always conclusive, can be helpful in the diagnosis of plasma cell myeloma PTLD (48). Immunophenotypic evaluation of B-cell PTLD should include B-cell and plasma cell associated antigens.

2. Monomorphic T-Cell PTLD

Monomorphic T-cell PTLDs (T-PTLDs) are uncommon and are classified according to the WHO classification. Many histological types of T-cell lymphomas have been reported in the post-transplantation setting. These include peripheral T-cell lymphoma unspecified; cutaneous T-cell lymphoma; subcutaneous panniculitis-like, anaplastic large cell lymphoma (both ALK− and ALK+); hepatosplenic T-cell lymphoma; and adult T-cell leukemia; and

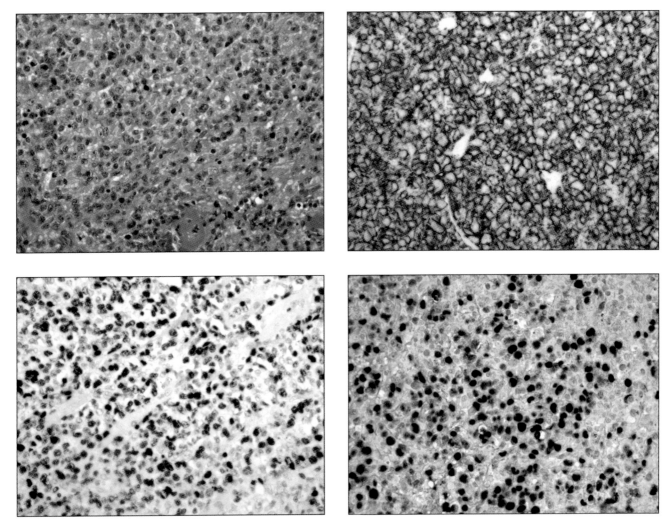

FIGURE 10.4: *Monomorphic PTLD, DLBCL, is seen in a patient after solid organ transplantation. There is a diffuse proliferation of large transformed lymphoid cells with irregular nuclei, vesiculated chromatin, multiple prominent nucleoli, and scant cytoplasm (upper left, H&E 400×). These large transformed lymphoid cells show uniform expression of CD20 confirming a B-cell lineage (upper right, IHC 400×). Ki-67, a proliferation marker, shows a high proliferation index but not approaching 100 percent (lower left, IHC 400×). EBV is present by EBER in situ hybridization in numerous transformed neoplastic cells (lower right, ISH 400×).*

angioimmunoblastic T-cell lymphoma. These PTLDs usually occur late after transplantation and are often EBV negative. Thus, one may wonder whether they represent incidental occurrences in immunocompromised individuals. However, since some cases respond to reduction in immunosuppression, it seems likely that most consider them within the spectrum of PTLD. Examples of T-PTLDs are shown in Figures 10.6 and 10.7.

Immunophenotyping is essential for diagnosis and subtyping of T-PTLDs. Depending on the subtype, the immunophenotype will vary. Evaluation of pan-T-cell antigens, although not always conclusive, is useful for demonstrating any aberrant losses of expression. The expression of CD4 or CD8 is variable and generally follows what is known for particular T-cell lymphomas in the nontransplant setting. Evaluation of alpha-beta and gamma-delta T-cell receptors (TCRs) can also show

expression of either receptor type. Markers of immaturity (CD1a, TdT, CD34) can be seen in cases of precursor T-lymphoblastic lymphoma. CD30 expression can be present and although characteristic of anaplastic large cell lymphoma, it is not a specific marker. CD56 and cytotoxic markers are variably expressed by T-PTLD. Most (60–80 percent) T-PTLDs *lack* EBV; however, a minor subset may be EBV positive (49). Molecular analysis of the *TCR* gene should show a clonal pattern. Analysis of episomal EBV genome is usually not indicated but will show a clonal pattern when EBV is present.

3. *Monomorphic NK PTLD*

Only rare NK cell PTLDs have been reported corresponding to aggressive NK cell leukemia/lymphoma (12,13) and nasal type PTLD. They have the characteristic

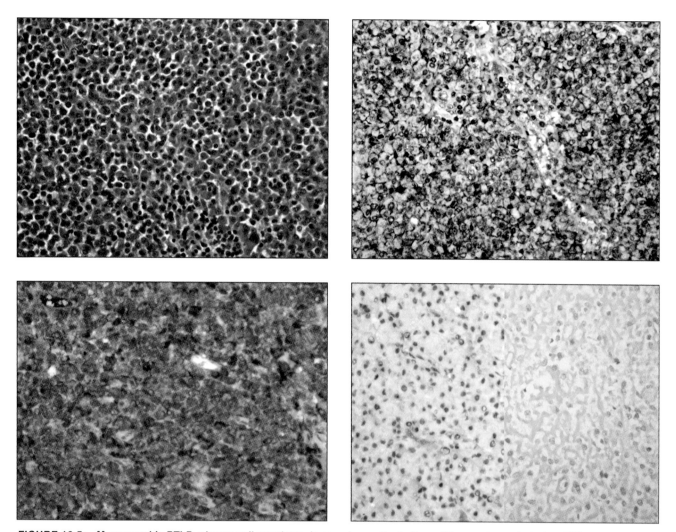

FIGURE 10.5: *Monomorphic PTLD, plasma cell neoplasm, is seen in a patient after solid organ transplantation. Diffuse sheets of plasma cells are present and scattered plasma cells have enlarged nuclei with distinct nucleoli (upper left, H&E 400×). Membranous expression of CD138 is consistent with plasma cells (upper right, IHC 400×). The plasma cells are kappa light chain restricted with almost all plasma cells expressing kappa light chain (lower left, IHC 400×). No plasma cells are seen expressing lambda light chain (lower right, left panel, IHC 400×). No evidence of EBV is identified by EBER in situ hybridization (lower right, right panel, EBER ISH 400×).*

morphological features of the lymphomas occurring in non-immunocompromised patients.

True NK cell PTLDs will express CD56 and cytotoxic markers but must lack surface CD3. Variable expression of pan-T-cell antigens, CD2 and CD7, can be seen. Unlike T-PTLDs, the vast majority (80–90 percent) of true NK cell PTLDs shows EBV infection with clonal episomal EBV genome (50). Along with the appropriate NK cell phenotype, molecular analysis of *TCR* must show a germline pattern to be diagnosed as true NK cell PTLDs.

4. *Hodgkins Lymphoma (HL) and HL-Like Lesion*

HL and HL-like PTLD is a rare category of PTLD classified independently from other monomorphic PTLDs, comprising 1–2 percent of all PTLDs (Figure 10.8). These cases usually arise late in transplantation and frequently show evidence of EBV infection. While classified together currently, there is evidence that these may be distinct from one another (14,15). HL-like PTLD have a heterogeneous, polymorphic lymphocytic background with scattered Reed-Sternberg (RS)–like cells scattered within the infiltrate and may resemble the mixed cellularity or lymphocyte depleted type of HL. The rare HL as a PTLD may have a more uniform small lymphocytic background with eosinophils and more marked pleomorphism of the RS cells compared to HL-like PTLDs.

Immunophenotypic studies reveal further differences. The RS-like cells of HL-like PTLDs strongly express CD20 and CD45RB (unlike true RS cells of HL). Although CD30 is uniformly expressed, CD15 is absent in HL-like PTLDs. HL-PTLDs have the more typical

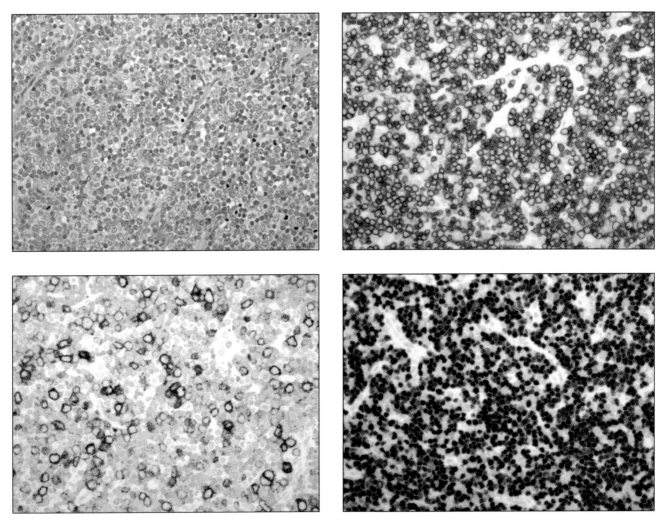

FIGURE 10.6: *Monomorphic PTLD, precursor T-cell acute lymphoblastic lymphoma, is seen arising in a patient after cardiac transplant. An involved lymph node shows a diffuse proliferation of medium-sized lymphoid cells with irregular cleaved nuclei, fine blastic chromatin pattern, small indistinct nucleoli, and scant cytoplasm (upper left, H&E 200×). CD3 expression is present in these lymphoid cells (upper right, IHC 200×). Surface expression of CD3 is confirmed by flow cytometric analysis confirming a T-cell lineage (not shown). The majority of these lymphoid cells show a loss of pan-T-cell antigen, CD7 (lower left, IHC 200×). TdT, a marker of immaturity expressed by acute lymphoblastic leukemias/lymphomas, is seen in the majority of the neoplastic lymphoid cells (lower right, IHC 200×).*

phenotype (CD20 weak+/−, CD15+, CD30+, CD45RB−). EBER ISH also reveals with both the large RS-like cells and the small lymphocytes positive in HL-like PTLD, whereas only the RS cells are positive on HL-PTLD. Thus, HL-like PTLDs may best be considered related to B-cell PTLDs and managed as such. Some have been reported to regress with reduction in immunosuppression, while others have progressed (51). At the molecular level, IGH rearrangement from DNA extracted from whole tissue section (rather than single or groups of RS cells) has been demonstrated in many cases of HL-like PTLD (51).

Distinction of an HL-like PTLD from polymorphic B-cell PTLD is problematic. RS-like cells can be seen in polymorphic PTLD; however, they are generally seen only sparsely scattered in the infiltrate of a polymorphic PTLD in a background of heterogeneous B lymphocytes. In HL-like PTLD, the RS-like cells are frequent.

5. Low-Grade B-Cell Lymphoproliferative Disorders

The current WHO classification does not recognize low-grade B-cell lymphoproliferative disorders as PTLD; however, they do occur. Extranodal marginal zone B-cell lymphomas of mucosa-associated lymphoid tissue (MALT) type occurring as PTLDs morphologically and immunophenotypically resemble their counterparts in immunocompetent patients (Figure 10.9) (52,53). A dense lymphoid infiltrate is present that destroys normal elements of the primary extranodal site. The cells are

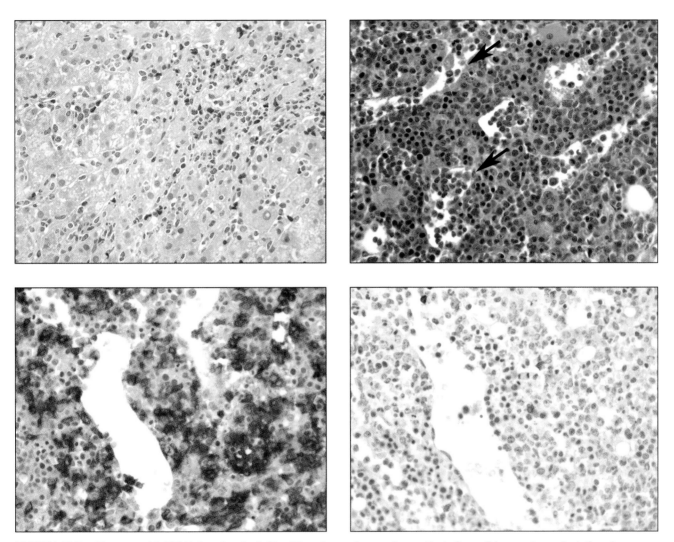

FIGURE 10.7: *Monomorphic PTLD, hepatosplenic T-cell lymphoma, is seen in a patient after solid organ transplantation. An intrasinusoidal lymphoid infiltrate is seen in the liver consisting of predominantly medium-sized lymphocytes with round to irregular nuclei, small but distinct nucleoli, and scant cytoplasm (upper left, H&E 400×). An infiltrate of similar lymphoid cells is also seen in the spleen within sinusoidal spaces (arrows) (upper right, H&E 400×). These lymphocytes express the pan-T-cell antigens CD2, CD3 (lower left, IHC 400×), and CD7, and are predominantly CD8+ T cells (not shown). Aberrant loss of the pan-T-cell antigen, CD5, is seen (lower right, IHC 400×). No evidence of EBV is detected by EBER in situ hybridization (not shown).*

small with round to slightly irregular nuclei. Cytoplasm is lightly eosinophilic and moderate in amount. Some degree of plasmacytic maturation can be seen, with some cases showing a prominent plasma cell component that may be monotypic. Immunophenotyping shows a pattern similar to MALT lymphoma in nonimmunocompromised patients (CD20+, CD5, CD10−, sIG−). These MALT lymphomas do not show evidence of EBV but are frequently associated with *Helicobacter* organisms, especially in gastric sites (52). Molecular analysis of *IGH* will show a clonal pattern (53). Other low-grade B-cell lymphoproliferative disorders reported after transplantation include hairy cell leukemia (54). This is extremely rare. Clinically, morphologically, and immunophenotypically, these cases are identical to those seen

in the nontransplant setting and may represent coincidental events.

IV. MOLECULAR PATHOGENESIS

PTLD is a clinically, pathologically, and biologically heterogeneous disease. Similar to other types of cancer, the pathogenesis of PTLD represents a multistep process that involves accumulation of multiple genetic and molecular lesions leading to the selection of a malignant clone. However, unlike lymphomas in immunocompetent hosts, *viral-induced* cell proliferation and immunosuppression of the host significantly contribute to the pathogenesis of PTLD. The differences in cellular derivation of PTLD, EBV infection, and aberrations common to other malignancies

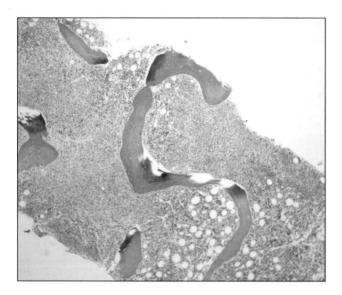

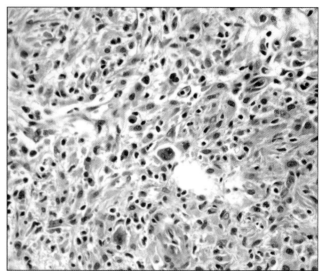

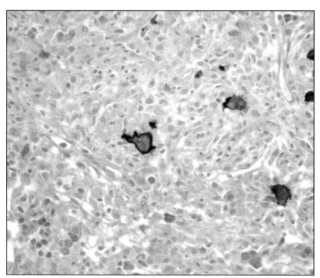

FIGURE 10.8:   *HL PTLD is seen in a patient presenting with cytopenias after renal transplantation. Bone marrow biopsy shows a diffuse fibrotic replacement of normal hematopoietic elements with only patchy residual hematopoeisis (upper left, H&E 40×). There is a mixed inflammatory infiltrate consisting of lymphocytes, eosinophils, neutrophils, and scattered histiocytes with rare large atypical cells showing multilobated nuclei, prominent eosinophilic macronucleoli, and moderate cytoplasm. Rare RS cells are identified (upper right, H&E 200×). These RS cells and variants express CD30 (red, cytoplasmic) and show weak expression of PAX-5 (brown, nuclear) (lower left, IHC 200×). These cells show the characteristic phenotype for classical Hodgkin lymphoma: CD45−, CD20−, CD30+, and CD15+ (not shown).*

such as gene amplifications, deletions, and mutations, all contribute to the complex process of the molecular pathogenesis of PTLD. Although marked advances in our understanding of the pathobiology of this disease have been made, many pathogenetic mechanisms and biological features of PTLD remain largely unknown.

i. Cellular Derivation of PTLD

The majority of PTLD are of B-cell origin. B-cell lymphomas arise from normal lymphocytes at different stages of B-cell differentiation. Comparison of the biological features and surface markers of a given type of lymphoma to

different maturation stages of normal lymphocytes can suggest the stage of B-cell ontogeny at which malignant transformation occurred. Analysis of immunoglobulin V-region mutations can provide important information regarding the ontogenetic stage of various B-cell populations (55). Moreover, analysis of V-gene mutations in B-cell lymphomas has helped to trace the developmental stage at which malignant transformation and clonal selection have taken place and assign these cells to their corresponding normal counterparts (55–59). The presence of somatic mutations in the variable (V) region of immunoglobulin (*Ig*) genes is commonly used as a marker of germinal center (GC) transit since normal pregerminal center

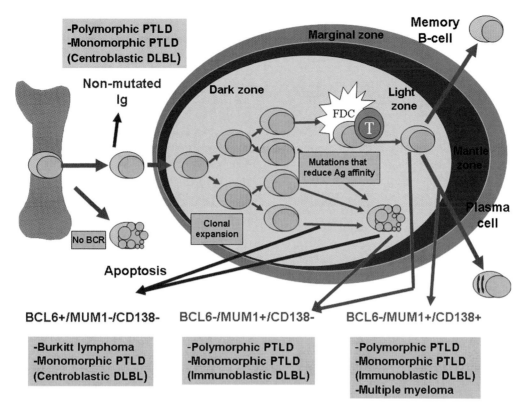

FIGURE 10.9: *Schematic representation of cellular origin of PTLD subtypes.*

lymphocytes harbor unmutated *Ig* genes. Furthermore, the presence of intraclonal heterogeneity in *Ig* gene mutations is regarded as a marker of ongoing somatic mutations that occur almost exclusively in the GC and thus is used as a marker of GC origin. In addition, the biased use of Ig variable heavy (V_H) genes and analysis of the rate and distribution of silent and replacement mutations in the complementarity-determining and framework regions (CDR and FR, respectively) may point to the contribution of antigen selection process to lymphoma pathogenesis (60).

Analysis of *Ig* heavy and light chains rearrangements has revealed that the majority of PTLD tumors harbor mutated *Ig* genes, suggesting that they arise from GC-experienced cells (61). Analysis of intraclonal heterogeneity in *Ig* gene mutations have demonstrated the presence of ongoing mutations in 48 percent of cases belonging to the monomorphic centroblastic DLBCL and BL subtypes (61). No intraclonal heterogeneity was detected in the remaining 62 percent of PTLD, including all the polymorphic PTLD, immunoblastic DLBCL, and some centroblastic DLBCL (61). These findings suggested that based on *Ig* analysis, most PTLD tumors, including all the polymorphic PTLD and immunoblastic DLBCL subtypes are of post-GC origin, while the majority of PTLD of the centroblastic DLBCL variant are of GC origin.

The distribution of IgV_H families used by PTLD reflects the complexity of the rearranged IgV_H repertoire of mature B cells, with the V_H3 family used most commonly (61). Molecular studies have revealed the presence of functional rearrangements in 80 percent of PTLD cases, while in 20 percent the tumors carried crippling mutations precluding expression of functional B-cell receptor (BCR) Ig (61,62). Further immunohistochemical studies showed detectable expression of Ig light chains in only about 50 percent of cases, thus suggesting that about 50 percent of PTLD derive from B cells that have lost the ability to express functional BCR (62). Since the expression of functional BCR is necessary for B-cell survival, PTLDs lacking BCR are hypothesized to acquire the ability to escape apoptotic death in the absence of antigen stimulation, as was previously also observed in Hodgkin's disease (HD) tumors (63). EBV infection is one possible explanation for the potential rescue from the cell death induced by loss of antigen stimulation (64).

Among the PTLD tumors that express functional BCR, 60 percent select mutations to maintain intact FR structure and only 30 percent select mutations to increase antigen binding affinity (62). Overall, these observations suggest that BCR stimulation does not play a major role in pathogenesis of many PTLD tumors.

Further analysis combining *Ig* mutational status with immunohistochemical phenotypic characterization based on BCL6 (GC marker), MUM1 (late GC and post-GC), and CD138 (post-GC, terminal differentiation) has allowed subclassification of PTLD into four ontogenic subtypes (61): (1) 25 percent of polymorphic PTLD and 10 percent of DLBCL carry unmutated *IgV* genes, thus denoting a pre-GC origin; (2) 25 percent of DLBCL, mainly of centroblastic morphology, and 100 percent BL carry ongoing *IgV* mutations and BCL6+/MUM1−/CD138− phenotype denoting an origin from GC centroblasts; (3) 65 percent of polymorphic PTLD and 30 percent of DLBCL, mainly with immunoblastic features, do not exhibit *Ig* intraclonal heterogeneity and carry the BCL6−/MUM1+/CD138− suggesting origin from B cells that have concluded the GC reaction but have not yet undergone terminal differentiation; (4) 35 percent of polymorphic PTLD and some of the immunoblastic DLBCL, commonly with plasmacytic differentiation, that also do not exhibit *Ig* intraclonal heterogeneity but carry the BCL6−/MUM1+/CD138+ phenotype reminiscent of post-GC and preterminally differentiated B cells. All the latter tumors are EBV positive and express LMP-1 antigen.

ii. Viral Infection in PTLD

Oncogenic viruses implicated in PTLD pathogenesis include EBV and human herpesvirus-8 (HHV-8) (28,38,65–67). EBV infects about 60–80 percent of PTLD, including almost 100 percent of early PTLD occurring within the first year after transplantation and 80–100 percent post-transplant HD (4,68). EBV infection is usually monoclonal in monomorphic PTLD, suggesting that the virus has been present in the tumor precursor cells at the early phases of clonal selection and expansion. In contrast, lesions consisting of polyclonal or multiclonal B-cell proliferations contain multiple EBV clones. In most cases, the infected cells have a latency type III pattern; however, cases with a latency pattern II, as seen in HD, or type I pattern, as seen in BL, are reported (46,69,70). In some cases, evidence of lytic activity has been reported (70,71). It has been postulated, that the immunosuppression-induced decrease in EBV-specific cytotoxic T cells allows uncontrolled virus proliferation, as manifested by increase in EBV viral load that frequently precedes the PTLD (72). Latent genes of EBV have transforming activity and may even rescue from apoptosis B lacking surface immunoglobulin BCR. Although the precise mechanism of transformation is presently unknown, it has been shown that EBV proteins LMP-1 and LMP-2A may activate intracellular signaling pathways, mimicking CD40 and BCR signals leading to activation of NFkB – an important survival mediator (73). Treatment of EBV-positive PTLD with autologous EBV-specific cytotoxic T cells was reported to reduce the viral load and lead to tumor size reduction (74).

Although EBV infection is detected in a majority of PTLD cases, documentation of intratumoral EBV is not required for tissue diagnosis of PTLD. Further, approx-

imately 15–30 percent of PTLD do not demonstrate evidence of EBV infection (3,4,75). EBV-negative cases are more likely to be of monomorphic type than EBV-positive cases and are more likely to occur later after transplantation. Leblond et al (4). reported a series of eleven patients who developed EBV-negative PTLD. In EBV-negative group, the PTLD was diagnosed at a median time of sixty months after transplantation, with the earliest tumor arising at six months. In contrast, EBV-positive tumors were diagnosed at a median of six months after transplantation, with the earliest arising one month after transplantation. EBV negativity, more common in adult PTLD patients, was reported to be an adverse prognostic factor. Certain types of PTLD are more likely to be EBV negative, such as those of multiple myeloma type. Only about one third of T-PTLD is EBV positive (49,76). In the EBV-negative tumors, the mechanism of transformation and the signals rescuing B cells with crippled *Ig* gene mutation from spontaneous apoptosis are presently unknown.

iii. Genetic Alterations

Several genetic alterations in oncogenes or tumor suppressor genes have been found in PTLDs. These include *MYC*, *BCL6*, *NRAS*, and *TP53* (77–79). Chromosomal translocations involving *MYC* and mutations in *MYC*, *BCL6*, *NRAS*, and *TP53* have been described (77–79). Alterations in *MYC*, *NRAS*, and *TP53* are uncommon and seen only in monomorphic (immunoblastic lymphoma histology) or multiple myeloma types of PTLDs and are never present in polymorphic lesions (79). Rearrangement (translocation) of *BCL6* is very uncommon in PTLD as opposed to DLBCL in immunocompetent patients. However, *BCL6* mutations are common (approximately 50 percent), and have been associated with shorter survival and nonresponsiveness to reduced immunosuppression (77). Rearrangements of *MYC* have also been associated with more aggressive disease and poor outcome (42). Microsatellite instability has been described in a higher proportion of PTLDs than in NHL from immunocompetent hosts, corresponding to the high degree of genetic instability in PTLDs (80).

Recently, epigenetic alterations have been examined. In particular, hypermethylation of O6-methylguanine-DNA methyltransferase (*MGMT*), a DNA repair gene, has been found in 60 percent of monomorphic PTLD. MGMT inactivation has been shown to be lymphomagenic in knockout mice and may promote genetic instability with acquisition of *TP53* and *RAS* mutations (81,82). Other genes identified as abnormally methylated include death-associated protein kinase (*DAPK1*), a proapoptotic molecule, and *TP73*, a putative tumor suppressor gene related to *TP53* (81). Much work remains to be done and new tools such as array-based comparative genomic hybridization studies have identified other abnormalities

(83). However, the exact role of these abnormalities in the development of PTLD remains largely unknown.

iv. Pathological Evaluation—What Needs to Be Done?

Practically speaking, excisional biopsies of masses or enlarged lymph nodes are essential because one of the characteristics differentiating features between early lesions and polymorphic and monomorphic PTLD relies on the ability to document preservation of underlying architecture. Extranodal disease is common, with particular predisposition to allografted organ, gastrointestinal tract, liver, lung, and central nervous system. If endoscopic or needle biopsies are used, several biopsies or passes are advised to obtain adequate tissue for ancillary studies.

When multiple sites of involvement are present, sampling of several lesions should be considered since early, polymorphic, and monomorphic lesions can be *synchronously* present in different sites. In addition, since synchronous lesions may actually represent different clonal proliferations, separate workup at the genetic level (i.e., molecular analysis of *IGH* gene) may be of interest for follow-up purposes (84). In patients with allograft involvement where rejection enters into the clinical differential diagnosis, allograft biopsies can help differentiate rejection from PTLD. Assessment of EBV can be helpful since PTLDs are often positive, whereas EBV is absent in rejection. Overall, focusing the diagnostic evaluation based on organ dysfunction or presence of a mass lesion provides the highest yield for obtaining adequate tissue for diagnosis. Screening blood or bone marrow evaluations in patients suspected of PTLD are usually of low diagnostic yield.

Immunophenotyping PTLDs is essential because of the significant differences in prognosis and therapy between B-cell and NK/T-cell lymphomas. Evaluation for presence of EBV by immunohistochemical or molecular techniques is also essential because of the differences in prognosis between the EBV-positive and EBV-negative cases. EBER in situ hybridization is preferred given its presence in all latency patterns.

Although not absolutely required for diagnosis in the majority of cases, testing for *clonality* (usually by antigen receptor rearrangement studies) is also helpful for complete characterization and can be used for comparison to simultaneous or future PTLDs. A distinct clone at a later date would suggest a new independent PTLD, rather than a relapse. Cytogenetic studies, also not necessary, may similarly be helpful. Assessment of oncogene mutations or translocations, by molecular or cytogenetic techniques, is currently not routinely performed. Diagnostically, the type of PTLD, lineage of the PTLD (if a monomorphic lesion), clonal status, and EBV status should be clearly indicated in the pathology report.

REFERENCES

1. Doak PB, Montgomerie JZ, North JD, Smith F. Reticulum cell sarcoma after renal homotransplantation and azathioprine and prednisone therapy. Br Med J. 1968;4: 746–748.
2. Harris NL SS, Frizzera G, Knowles DM. Post-transplant lymphoproliferative disorders. In: Jaffe ES HN, Stein H, Vardiman JW, ed. World Health Organization Classification of Tumours. Lyon France: IARC Press; 2001:264–269.
3. Nelson BP, Nalesnik MA, Bahler DW, Locker J, Fung JJ, Swerdlow SH. Epstein-Barr virus-negative post-transplant lymphoproliferative disorders: a distinct entity? Am J Surg Pathol. 2000;24:375–385.
4. Leblond V, Davi F, Charlotte F, et al. Posttransplant lymphoproliferative disorders not associated with Epstein-Barr virus: a distinct entity? J Clin Oncol. 1998;16:2052–2059.
5. Martin-Gomez MA, Pena M, Cabello M, et al. Posttransplant lymphoproliferative disease: a series of 23 cases. Transplant Proc. 2006;38:2448–2450.
6. Faull RJ, Hollett P, McDonald SP. Lymphoproliferative disease after renal transplantation in Australia and New Zealand. Transplantation. 2005;80:193–197.
7. Opelz G, Dohler B. Lymphomas after solid organ transplantation: a collaborative transplant study report. Am J Transplant. 2004;4:222–230.
8. Opelz G, Henderson R. Incidence of non-Hodgkin lymphoma in kidney and heart transplant recipients. Lancet. 1993;342:1514–1516.
9. Opelz G. Collaborative Transplant Study—10-year report. Transplant Proc. 1992;24:2342–2355.
10. Opelz G. Are post-transplant lymphomas inevitable? Nephrol Dial Transplant. 1996;11:1952–1955.
11. Penn I. Cancers in renal transplant recipients. Adv Ren Replace Ther. 2000;7:147–156.
12. Penn I. Occurrence of cancers in immunosuppressed organ transplant recipients. Clin Transpl. 1998:147–158.
13. Kasiske BL, Snyder JJ, Gilbertson DT, Wang C. Cancer after kidney transplantation in the United States. Am J Transplant. 2004;4:905–913.
14. Caillard S, Lelong C, Pessione F, Moulin B. Post-transplant lymphoproliferative disorders occurring after renal transplantation in adults: report of 230 cases from the French Registry. Am J Transplant. 2006;6:2735–2742.
15. Caillard S, Dharnidharka V, Agodoa L, Bohen E, Abbott K. Posttransplant lymphoproliferative disorders after renal transplantation in the United States in era of modern immunosuppression. Transplantation. 2005;80:1233–1243.
16. Dharnidharka VR, Sullivan EK, Stablein DM, Tejani AH, Harmon WE. Risk factors for posttransplant lymphoproliferative disorder (PTLD) in pediatric kidney transplantation: a report of the North American Pediatric Renal Transplant Cooperative Study (NAPRTCS). Transplantation. 2001;71:1065–1068.
17. Armitage JM, Kormos RL, Stuart RS, et al. Posttransplant lymphoproliferative disease in thoracic organ transplant patients: ten years of cyclosporine-based immunosuppression. J Heart Lung Transplant. 1991;10:877–886; discussion 886–877.

18. Domingo-Domenech E, de Sanjose S, Gonzalez-Barca E, et al. Post-transplant lymphomas: a 20-year epidemiologic, clinical and pathologic study in a single center. Haematologica. 2001;86:715–721.

19. Nalesnik MA, Makowka L, Starzl TE. The diagnosis and treatment of posttransplant lymphoproliferative disorders. Curr Probl Surg. 1988;25:367–472.

20. Raymond E, Tricottet V, Samuel D, Reynes M, Bismuth H, Misset JL. Epstein-Barr virus-related localized hepatic lymphoproliferative disorders after liver transplantation. Cancer. 1995;76:1344–1351.

21. Chen JM, Barr ML, Chadburn A, et al. Management of lymphoproliferative disorders after cardiac transplantation. Ann Thorac Surg. 1993;56:527–538.

22. Reyes J, Green M, Bueno J, et al. Epstein Barr virus associated posttransplant lymphoproliferative disease after intestinal transplantation. Transplant Proc. 1996;28:2768–2769.

23. Quintini C, Kato T, Gaynor JJ, et al. Analysis of risk factors for the development of posttransplant lymphoproliperative disorder among 119 children who received primary intestinal transplants at a single center. Transplant Proc. 2006;38:1755–1758.

24. Webber SA, Naftel DC, Fricker FJ, et al. Lymphoproliferative disorders after paediatric heart transplantation: a multi-institutional study. Lancet. 2006;367:233–239.

25. Curtis RE, Travis LB, Rowlings PA, et al. Risk of lymphoproliferative disorders after bone marrow transplantation: a multi-institutional study. Blood. 1999;94:2208–2216.

26. Bhatia S, Ramsay NK, Steinbuch M, et al. Malignant neoplasms following bone marrow transplantation. Blood. 1996;87:3633–3639.

27. Zutter MM, Martin PJ, Sale GE, et al. Epstein-Barr virus lymphoproliferation after bone marrow transplantation. Blood. 1988;72:520–529.

28. Walker RC, Paya CV, Marshall WF, et al. Pretransplantation seronegative Epstein-Barr virus status is the primary risk factor for posttransplantation lymphoproliferative disorder in adult heart, lung, and other solid organ transplantations. J Heart Lung Transplant. 1995;14:214–221.

29. Ho M, Jaffe R, Miller G, et al. The frequency of Epstein-Barr virus infection and associated lymphoproliferative syndrome after transplantation and its manifestations in children. Transplantation. 1988;45:719–727.

30. Dantal J, Hourmant M, Cantarovich D, et al. Effect of long-term immunosuppression in kidney-graft recipients on cancer incidence: randomised comparison of two cyclosporin regimens. Lancet. 1998;351:623–628.

31. Sokal EM, Antunes H, Beguin C, et al. Early signs and risk factors for the increased incidence of Epstein-Barr virus-related posttransplant lymphoproliferative diseases in pediatric liver transplant recipients treated with tacrolimus. Transplantation. 1997;64:1438–1442.

32. Cox KL, Lawrence-Miyasaki LS, Garcia-Kennedy R, et al. An increased incidence of Epstein-Barr virus infection and lymphoproliferative disorder in young children on FK506 after liver transplantation. Transplantation. 1995;59:524–529.

33. Swinnen LJ, Costanzo-Nordin MR, Fisher SG, et al. Increased incidence of lymphoproliferative disorder after immunosuppression with the monoclonal antibody OKT3 in cardiac-transplant recipients. N Engl J Med. 1990;323:1723–1728.

34. Walker RC, Marshall WF, Strickler JG, et al. Pretransplantation assessment of the risk of lymphoproliferative disorder. Clin Infect Dis. 1995;20:1346–1353.

35. El-Salem M, Raghunath PN, Marzec M, et al. Constitutive activation of mTOR signaling pathway in post-transplant lymphoproliferative disorders. Lab Invest. 2007;87:29–39.

36. Majewski M, Korecka M, Joergensen J, et al. Immunosuppressive TOR kinase inhibitor everolimus (RAD) suppresses growth of cells derived from posttransplant lymphoproliferative disorder at allograft-protecting doses. Transplantation. 2003;75:1710–1717.

37. Nepomuceno RR, Balatoni CE, Natkunam Y, Snow AL, Krams SM, Martinez OM. Rapamycin inhibits the interleukin 10 signal transduction pathway and the growth of Epstein Barr virus B-cell lymphomas. Cancer Res. 2003;63:4472–4480.

38. Gaidano G, Carbone A. Primary effusion lymphoma: a liquid phase lymphoma of fluid-filled body cavities. Adv Cancer Res. 2001;80:115–146.

39. McLaughlin K, Wajstaub S, Marotta P, et al. Increased risk for posttransplant lymphoproliferative disease in recipients of liver transplants with hepatitis C. Liver Transpl. 2000;6:570–574.

40. Buda A, Caforio A, Calabrese F, et al. Lymphoproliferative disorders in heart transplant recipients: role of hepatitis C virus (HCV) and Epstein-Barr virus (EBV) infection. Transpl Int. 2000;13 Suppl. 1:S402–S405.

41. Shaknovich R, Basso K, Bhagat G, et al. Identification of rare Epstein-Barr virus infected memory B cells and plasma cells in non-monomorphic post-transplant lymphoproliferative disorders and the signature of viral signaling. Haematologica. 2006;91:1313–1320.

42. Djokic M, Le Beau MM, Swinnen LJ, et al. Post-transplant lymphoproliferative disorder subtypes correlate with different recurring chromosomal abnormalities. Genes Chromosomes Cancer. 2006;45:313–318.

43. Vakiani E, Nandula SV, Subramaniyam S, et al. Cytogenetic analysis of B-cell posttransplant lymphoproliferations validates the World Health Organization classification and suggests inclusion of florid follicular hyperplasia as a precursor lesion. Hum Pathol. 2007;38:315–325.

44. Frizzera G, Hanto DW, Gajl-Peczalska KJ, et al. Polymorphic diffuse B-cell hyperplasias and lymphomas in renal transplant recipients. Cancer Res. 1981;41:4262–4279.

45. Chadburn A, Chen JM, Hsu DT, et al. The morphologic and molecular genetic categories of posttransplantation lymphoproliferative disorders are clinically relevant. Cancer. 1998;82:1978–1987.

46. Rea D, Fourcade C, Leblond V, et al. Patterns of Epstein-Barr virus latent and replicative gene expression in Epstein-Barr virus B cell lymphoproliferative disorders after organ transplantation. Transplantation. 1994;58:317–324.

47. Caillard S, Agodoa LY, Bohen EM, Abbott KC. Myeloma, Hodgkin disease, and lymphoid leukemia after renal transplantation: characteristics, risk factors and prognosis. Transplantation. 2006;81:888–895.

48. Sun X, Peterson LC, Gong Y, Traynor AE, Nelson BP. Post-transplant plasma cell myeloma and polymorphic lymphoproliferative disorder with monoclonal serum protein occurring in solid organ transplant recipients. Mod Pathol. 2004;17:389–394.

49. Dockrell DH, Strickler JG, Paya CV. Epstein-Barr virus-induced T cell lymphoma in solid organ transplant recipients. Clin Infect Dis. 1998;26:180–182.

50. Tsao L, Draoua HY, Mansukhani M, Bhagat G, Alobeid B. EBV-associated, extranodal NK-cell lymphoma, nasal type of the breast, after heart transplantation. Mod Pathol. 2004;17:125–130.

51. Ranganathan S, Webber S, Ahuja S, Jaffe R. Hodgkin-like posttransplant lymphoproliferative disorder in children: does it differ from posttransplant Hodgkin lymphoma? Pediatr Dev Pathol. 2004;7:348–360.

52. Hsi ED, Singleton TP, Swinnen L, Dunphy CH, Alkan S. Mucosa-associated lymphoid tissue-type lymphomas occurring in post-transplantation patients. Am J Surg Pathol. 2000;24:100–106.

53. Wotherspoon AC, Diss TC, Pan L, Singh N, Whelan J, Isaacson PG. Low grade gastric B-cell lymphoma of mucosa associated lymphoid tissue in immunocompromised patients. Histopathology. 1996;28:129–134.

54. Tsao L, Chu KE, Bhagat G, Alobeid B. Development of hairy cell leukemia in a patient after cardiac transplantation. Leuk Lymphoma. 2006;47:361–363.

55. Lossos IS, Okada CY, Tibshirani R, et al. Molecular analysis of immunoglobulin genes in diffuse large B-cell lymphomas. Blood. 2000;95:1797–1803.

56. Stevenson F, Sahota S, Zhu D, et al. Insight into the origin and clonal history of B-cell tumors as revealed by analysis of immunoglobulin variable region genes. Immunol Rev. 1998;162:247–259.

57. Hamblin TJ, Davis Z, Gardiner A, Oscier DG, Stevenson FK. Unmutated Ig V(H) genes are associated with a more aggressive form of chronic lymphocytic leukemia. Blood. 1999;94:1848–1854.

58. Lossos IS. Molecular pathogenesis of diffuse large B-cell lymphoma. J Clin Oncol. 2005;23:6351–6357.

59. Lossos IS, Alizadeh AA, Eisen MB, et al. Ongoing immunoglobulin somatic mutation in germinal center B cell-like but not in activated B cell-like diffuse large cell lymphomas. Proc Natl Acad Sci U S A. 2000;97:10209–10213.

60. Amit AG, Mariuzza RA, Phillips SE, Poljak RJ. Three-dimensional structure of an antigen-antibody complex at 6 A resolution. Nature. 1985;313:156–158.

61. Capello D, Cerri M, Muti G, et al. Molecular histogenesis of posttransplantation lymphoproliferative disorders. Blood. 2003;102:3775–3785.

62. Capello D, Cerri M, Muti G, et al. Analysis of immunoglobulin heavy and light chain variable genes in post-transplant lymphoproliferative disorders. Hematol Oncol. 2006;24:212–219.

63. Kanzler H, Kuppers R, Hansmann ML, Rajewsky K. Hodgkin and Reed-Sternberg cells in Hodgkin's disease represent the outgrowth of a dominant tumor clone derived from (crippled) germinal center B cells. J Exp Med. 1996; 184:1495–1505.

64. Re D, Kuppers R, Diehl V. Molecular pathogenesis of Hodgkin's lymphoma. J Clin Oncol. 2005;23:6379–6386.

65. Paya CV, Fung JJ, Nalesnik MA, et al. Epstein-Barr virus-induced posttransplant lymphoproliferative disorders. ASTS/ASTP EBV-PTLD Task Force and The Mayo Clinic Organized International Consensus Development Meeting. Transplantation. 1999;68:1517–1525.

66. Cleary ML, Nalesnik MA, Shearer WT, Sklar J. Clonal analysis of transplant-associated lymphoproliferations based on the structure of the genomic termini of the Epstein-Barr virus. Blood. 1988;72:349–352.

67. Young L, Alfieri C, Hennessy K, et al. Expression of Epstein-Barr virus transformation-associated genes in tissues of patients with EBV lymphoproliferative disease. N Engl J Med. 1989;321:1080–1085.

68. Capello D, Rossi D, Gaidano G. Post-transplant lymphoproliferative disorders: molecular basis of disease histogenesis and pathogenesis. Hematol Oncol. 2005;23:61–67.

69. Delecluse HJ, Kremmer E, Rouault JP, Cour C, Bornkamm G, Berger F. The expression of Epstein-Barr virus latent proteins is related to the pathological features of post-transplant lymphoproliferative disorders. Am J Pathol. 1995;146:1113–1120.

70. Oudejans JJ, Jiwa M, van den Brule AJ, et al. Detection of heterogeneous Epstein-Barr virus gene expression patterns within individual post-transplantation lymphoproliferative disorders. Am J Pathol. 1995;147:923–933.

71. Montone KT, Hodinka RL, Salhany KE, Lavi E, Rostami A, Tomaszewski JE. Identification of Epstein-Barr virus lytic activity in post-transplantation lymphoproliferative disease. Mod Pathol. 1996;9:621–630.

72. Weinstock DM, Ambrossi GG, Brennan C, Kiehn TE, Jakubowski A. Preemptive diagnosis and treatment of Epstein-Barr virus-associated post transplant lymphoproliferative disorder after hematopoietic stem cell transplant: an approach in development. Bone Marrow Transplant. 2006; 37:539–546.

73. Kuppers R. B cells under influence: transformation of B cells by Epstein-Barr virus. Nat Rev Immunol. 2003;3:801–812.

74. Comoli P, Maccario R, Locatelli F, et al. Treatment of EBV-related post-renal transplant lymphoproliferative disease with a tailored regimen including EBV-specific T cells. Am J Transplant. 2005;5:1415–1422.

75. Ghobrial IM, Habermann TM, Maurer MJ, et al. Prognostic analysis for survival in adult solid organ transplant recipients with post-transplantation lymphoproliferative disorders. J Clin Oncol. 2005;23:7574–7582.

76. van Gorp J, Doornewaard H, Verdonck LF, Klopping C, Vos PF, van den Tweel JG. Posttransplant T-cell lymphoma. Report of three cases and a review of the literature. Cancer. 1994;73:3064–3072.

77. Cesarman E, Chadburn A, Liu YF, Migliazza A, Dalla-Favera R, Knowles DM. BCL-6 gene mutations in posttransplantation lymphoproliferative disorders predict response to therapy and clinical outcome. Blood. 1998;92:2294–2302.

78. Delecluse HJ, Rouault JP, Jeammot B, Kremmer E, Bastard C, Berger F. Bcl6/Laz3 rearrangements in post-transplant lymphoproliferative disorders. Br J Haematol. 1995;91:101–103.

79. Knowles DM, Cesarman E, Chadburn A, et al. Correlative morphologic and molecular genetic analysis demonstrates three distinct categories of posttransplantation lymphoproliferative disorders. Blood. 1995;85:552–565.

80. Duval A, Raphael M, Brennetot C, et al. The mutator pathway is a feature of immunodeficiency-related lymphomas. Proc Natl Acad Sci U S A. 2004;101:5002–5007.

81. Rossi D, Gaidano G, Gloghini A, et al. Frequent aberrant promoter hypermethylation of O6-methylguanine-DNA methyltransferase and death-associated protein kinase genes in immunodeficiency-related lymphomas. Br J Haematol. 2003;123:475–478.

82. Gerson SL. MGMT: its role in cancer aetiology and cancer therapeutics. Nat Rev Cancer. 2004;4:296–307.

83. Rinaldi A, Kwee I, Poretti G, et al. Comparative genome-wide profiling of post-transplant lymphoproliferative disorders and diffuse large B-cell lymphomas. Br J Haematol. 2006;134:27–36.

84. Chadburn A, Cesarman E, Liu YF, et al. Molecular genetic analysis demonstrates that multiple posttransplantation lymphoproliferative disorders occurring in one anatomic site in a single patient represent distinct primary lymphoid neoplasms. Cancer. 1995;75:2747–2756.

CHAPTER 11

Laboratory Medicine in Transplantation

Phillip Ruiz, M.D., Ph.D.

Manuel Carreno, M.D.

Robert Cirocco, M.D.

Rolando Garcia-Morales, M.D.

I. INTRODUCTION

In addition to the routine testing provided to all potential transplant candidates, the clinical laboratories afford highly specialized services that are essential for the clinical support of a transplant program. The histocompatibility laboratory is involved early in the transplant process through the precise genotypic screening of cadaveric and living-related donors as well as future transplant recipients. In addition, donors are also tested for a variety of infectious agents that could be potentially transmitted to allograft recipients. The immune status of recipients is constantly monitored for possible levels of immunological sensitization to specific donor histocompatibility antigens, whether in the form of antibodies (humoral sensitization) or as immune effector cells (cellular sensitization). Finally, a variety of standard histocompatibility and molecular-based tests are utilized after the transplant takes place that assist in the monitoring and delicate clinical maintenance that is required for the long-term successful transplant to take place.

II. THE HISTOCOMPATIBILITY LABORATORY

Histocompatibility testing of the donor and the recipient, as well as the evaluation and monitoring for anti-donor sensitization to human leukocyte antigens (HLA) is an essential and a critical responsibility of the histocompatibility laboratory. The major histocompatibility complex (MHC), in humans termed the HLA complex (1), is a 4-megabase (Mb) region on chromosome 6 (6p21.3) that is heavily filled with a variety of expressed genes (Figure 11.1). HLA class I and class II genes are the best known and characterized in the HLA complex, and these genes play a crucial role in host immune responses and possible susceptibility to several autoimmune diseases (2). In addition, HLA class III genes are essential to a variety of functions, some immunological in origin (3). Other additional HLA region genes are also essential to the innate and antigen-specific components (i.e., acquired immunity) of the immune system (4). There is extensive conservation of the human HLA region's genomic organization, gene sequence, and protein structure with the MHC of other mammals.

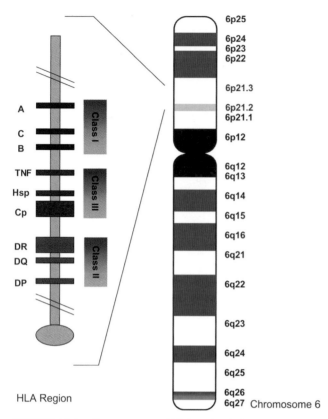

FIGURE 11.1: *Genome map of HLA region in human chromosome 6.*

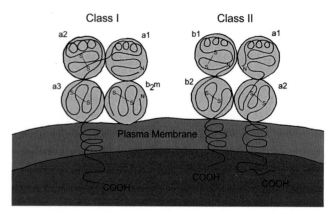

FIGURE 11.2: *Structure of class I and class II HLA proteins. This cartoon illustrates the structural similarities and differences between class I and class II molecules. Components of the figures are not drawn to scale.*

Interestingly, the proteins (Figure 11.2) that ultimately translate from these genes also unwittingly serve as powerful antigenic determinants that are the primary targets of allograft rejection (5); this makes the MHC molecules the most important barriers in allotransplantation within any species and in xenotransplantation. These proteins behave as antigens and can be expressed at different levels and/or restricted to select cellular types, so that a transplanted organ (e.g., liver) may not be as immunogenic as another (e.g., kidney) for a particular donor-recipient pair. Regardless, a high level of HLA antigen compatibility or matching between the donor and recipient tends to augment the chances for a successful transplant acceptance by the recipient due to a lower level of immune response to the donor, which looks more like self than non-self. In contrast, the opposite scenario is true when there is a significant level of *histoincompatibility* or mismatching. There is tremendous diversity in the number of HLA alleles or polymorphisms that arose through evolution presumably as a means to combat various infections and provide populations with heterogeneity and immune vigor. The combinations of ancestral alleles inherited by an individual is therefore the result of a natural selection process and ultimately phenotype frequencies for HLA class I and class II that vary among different populations. Unfortunately, due to the extensive genetic variability of the HLA genetic loci,

the great majority of human transplantation combinations for donors and recipients will have some degree of MHC incompatibility between each other. In general, cumulative mismatches at HLA, B, C, DR, and DQ are associated with poorer graft survival. Thus, it is incumbent for a transplant program to be able to identify these major and, in many cases, minor mismatched differences and try to arrive at the best acceptable combination possible for the potential transplant recipient.

The methodology used to determine HLA compatibility has evolved significantly since its first application in the early 1960s. Initial techniques only allowed discriminating among HLA identical and fully mismatched individuals; however the development of human T-cell clones and molecular genetic techniques has led to a detailed understanding of the phenotypic polymorphism and diversity of HLA antigens (6). HLA typing is still performed by serological and cellular assays in some centers. Since the mid-1980s, more sensitive and specific tools such as flow cytometry have been applied to pretransplant HLA typing and cross-matching (7,8). In addition, over the past two decades, a variety of highly sensitive and specific molecular-based assays have been developed for HLA typing. These include southern blotting (9), polymerase chain reaction (PCR) (10), restriction fragment length polymorphism analysis of PCR products (PCR-RFLP) (11), and the ultimate gold standard for DNA characterization, that is, nucleotide sequencing (12).

i. HLA Typing

Typing of the polymorphic HLA genes is used to determine the number of antigens in those genes that are similar (compatible) or different (incompatible) within potential donor/recipient pairs. Two sources can be used for testing: one source is from DNA, while the other is through the study of molecular products or gene expression of these antigens that can be detected on leukocyte cell surfaces. Lymphocytes can be obtained from peripheral blood, lymph node, and spleen. The two types of HLA antigens that are typed for are class I and class II. Class I is ubiquitously expressed on most nucleated cells, while class II molecules tend to be present on antigen-presenting cells (APCs) such as B cells, macrophages, and dendritic cells (13,14).

The most common class I antigens that are identified or typed are HLA-A, HLA-B, and HLA-C, while in class II it is HLA-DR, HLA-DRB1, HLA-DP, and HLA-DQ.

The *leukocyte typing assay* is a qualitative cytotoxicity procedure that identifies these HLA antigens based on their expression. The microlymphocytotoxicity assay uses lymphocytes as the target. Viable cells are easily extracted from peripheral blood, lymph nodes, spleen, and so forth. This *serological* assay measures cell death by the activation of complement (rabbit) in the presence of specific HLA antigen-antibody combinations. The antibody-antigen complement reaction is measured by viewing the test microscopically using phase-contrast illumination and a vital stain such as eosin Y, trypan blue, or propidium iodide. A lymphocyte suspension of at least 90 percent viability and purity is prepared from whole blood and adjusted to a cell concentration of $2–3 \times 10^6$ cells/ml. A purity and viability of greater than 90 percent is essential for optimum performance of leukocyte typing sera. Lymphocytes may be prepared according to a standard procedure, which is listed in the ASHI Laboratory Procedure Manual (15). Viable cells (those lacking the antigen), exclude the dye, and appear slightly brighter and smaller in size as compared to dead cells. The number of lysed lymphocytes compared with the total number of lymphocytes is quoted as a score value in each well.

Cross-reactivity of HLA antigens and antisera may cause the expression of "too many" antigens (i.e., more than two antigens per locus) for an individual's HLA phenotype. Also, cross-reactivity may cause erroneous identification of an antigen within a locus, which is actually "blank" or unidentified. These cases can be helped by testing cells using a less sensitive cytotoxicity technique and by performing sera absorptions.

Before antisera were available to identify distinct specificities of HLA, family members were typed against panels of unknown or partially known antisera, many which were multispecific. Segregation analysis was made by observing the patterns of reactivity these sera gave within a family. Retrospective typing of early families has shown that this method of genotyping was very accurate. It is still a useful method when families do not have clearly defined antigens, when typing panels do not contain the best reagent antisera, and when non-HLA or new HLA specificities are being sought in unknown or multispecific sera. So these patterns of reactivity of one or more antisera are sought, which are positive with one parent, negative with the other parent, and inherited reciprocally by the children. When antisera react against the same antigen on two parental haplotypes, or when the antisera is dual specific and reacts against two specificities, each on separate haplotypes, "sum patterns" are observed. When an antiserum or, specifically, groups of antisera do not fit the expected patterns, there are four possibilities: the wrong patterns are selected; there is an illegitimate, an adopted, or a step-child among the children; genetic recombination occurs; and/or the antiserum contains non-HLA factors or there is an error in reactivity.

1. Molecular Methods for HLA Typing

Molecular HLA typing can be accomplished at several levels of discrimination between alleles, with the categories being low, medium, and high resolution. *Low resolution* characterizes broad families of alleles that may have many members. *High-resolution* typing is an attempt to definitively identify the allele residing at a given locus for the recipient. *Medium resolution* lies between high and low, narrowing the choices to fewer subtypes than by low-resolution typing. Solid organ transplant programs can generally operate well with low-resolution typing; bone marrow programs need the support of high-resolution typing to promote long-term graft survival and minimize graft-versus-host disease. Earlier molecular methods used tests such as RFLP; however, these tests did not often provide the level of sensitivity needed for the high level of polymorphism present in the different HLA loci. With the advent of the PCR, amplification became available and this revolutionized DNA typing for HLA. Ultimately, the DNA sequence coding for the RNA that is translated into the protein sequence of the HLA antigen is the most reliable template for molecular HLA typing.

In molecular HLA typing, there are four general steps involved: 1) isolation of the genomic DNA from the nucleated cell; 2) PCR amplification of the region to be typed (short-arm chromosome 6); 3) analysis of the PCR product either by gel, hybridization on strip, or Luminex beads; and 4) interpretation of the results.

The isolation of genomic DNA is performed by using chaotropic salts, detergents, and proteolytic enzymes. These agents disrupt both the cellular and nuclear membrane releasing the super-coiled DNA. These agents also lyse and disrupt the histones that keep the DNA in a super helix. Ethanol is added to the mixture making the DNA sticky. The solution can be applied to a column, the DNA sticks to the column, and the cell waste is centrifuged or vacuumed away. This is followed by a high-salt/ethanol wash and a low-salt/ethanol wash. The purified DNA is eluted with an aqueous solution. Solutions must be basic since acid solutions or water will hydrolyze the DNA. Another method pellets the sticky DNA followed by the salt/ethanol washes. This method is more difficult due to the fact that one can take the pellet with the supernatant of the wash solutions and discard the DNA.

a. PCR Sequence–Specific Oligonucleotide Probes

A commonly used technique with molecular HLA typing is a process whereby there is amplification of DNA followed by probing with sequence-specific oligonucleotide probes (16). This approach identifies different alleles at a locus by probes recognizing the allele differences and binding to the complementary region of the amplified HLA region. Assays often have immobilized DNA strands as part of the procedure; there are multiple permutations of these assays such that there can be immobilization of the probe or the target. Dot blot (dots on a filter paper) assays have immobilized amplified product with application of labeled probes (17), while slot blot assays have the labeled probe added in a line over fixed product. There are assays where the probe is immobilized and the amplified target is labeled; these assays are referred to as a reverse dot blot or *reverse probe hybridization* (18). In the latter assay, probes can be bound to a strip or to beads. The method is as follows. As described above, the region of choice is PCR amplified with labeled primers to the entire region. If the patients' DNA sequence matches the informative probe, it binds to it permanently. If there is a one base mismatch, it will melt off at a certain temperature under low-salt conditions. The labeled probes are now visualized by using a reporter substrate to highlight the probes that are a match. The strip is scored by using a template guide and a computer algorithm that resolves the individual's typing. In another version, the beads are run thru a Luminex cytometer and positive beads are scored to resolve the individuals' HLA molecular typing. These assays can have a high throughput and may be able to evaluate large numbers of samples.

b. PCR Sequence–Specific Primer

Sequence-specific primer (SSP) or amplification refractory mutation system (ARMS) typing is the amplification of alleles at a locus using allele-specific primers (19). Within the primer pair, *one primer* is specific to an area conserved across many alleles, while the *second primer* is specific for a one-base pair difference (the 3′ end of the second primer is specific for a complementary base in the target – if the 3′ end of a primer binds to the target then the polymerase will extend the strand and there will be amplification) (Figure 11.3). The detection is usually via agarose gel product fractionation. Since there is an advantage in using multiple primer sets to type for many alleles at a locus or loci, companies have to design kits where there is optimization of the melting curves of the primers so that simultaneous thermal cycling of all reactions can take place in a single instrument. Some primer sets allow for high-resolution typing with this methodology. Testing using SSP and ARMS can yield low-, medium-, or high-resolution results,

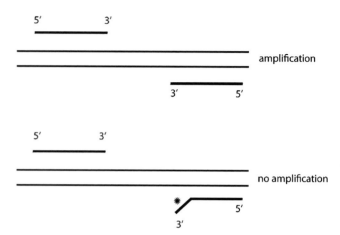

FIGURE 11.3: *Illustration of the principle for allele-specific PCR amplification. A completely matched primer will be more efficiently used in the PCR reaction than a primer with several mismatches, allowing the discrimination of alleles differing by a single base pair. Single base pair mismatches, denoted by *, should be placed in the extreme 3′-end of primers as the Taq polymerase lacks 3′ → 5′ proof-reading exonuclease activity.*

depending on the primer sets used. For example, this method could employ ninety-six different primer sets to resolve intermediate resolution of HLA-A, B, and DRB1 (Figure 11.4).

The pros of this technique are it is fast from two to three hours to get the typing. This is ideal for cadaveric typing since cold ischemia time is minimized resulting in better graft survival. The cons of this procedure are it takes large volumes of highly concentrated DNA and it is costly because it uses large quantities of the enzyme Taq polymerase. This methodology is robust and can be employed to do high-resolution allele-level typing. A final drawback is the freezer space necessary to store all the kits necessary to resolve all the alleles and the large amount of DNA required. SSP can also be used to determine the presence of infectious viral agents, such as HCV, HBV, and HIV.

Sequence-based typing (SBT) of MHC alleles is the current definitive high-resolution technique (20) and is necessary for unrelated bone marrow matching. There are several methods that can be employed to perform SBT. The first step in SBT is isolation of good quality DNA that allows for efficient primary PCR amplification. This is followed by *locus-specific* PCR amplification. Depending on which HLA locus is being typed there will be variation in the size of the primary amplicon. The amplicon will typically be a portion of exon 2 for class II and exons 1–5 for class I. Following stringent purification, the primary amplification product is then used as a *template* in forward and reverse sequencing reactions specifically designed for either exons of the class I alleles or the class II alleles. To emphasize, purification is necessary before the reaction products are sequenced. Capillary instruments are generally being used more frequently than traditional slab-gel instruments – this provides more automation and efficient

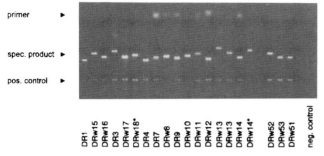

FIGURE 11.4: *Illustration of the relative sizes of the PCR products obtained in DR "low-resolution" PCR-SSP typing. The length of the allele- and group-specific PCR products ranges from 130 to 260 base pairs. Each PCR reaction includes the positive control primer pair C3 and C5, which gives rise to a 796-base pair fragment. PCR reaction mixtures containing primer pairs identifying allelic DRB1 variability corresponding to the serologically defined series DR1-DRw18 are size separated in the left seventeen lanes. An empty lane is followed by three lanes with the external positive control reactions assigning the DRB5*0101 to DRB*0301 (DRw52), the DRB4*0101 (DRw53), and the DRB5*0101 to DRB5*0202 (DRw51) group of alleles, and finally, the negative amplification control is separated from the external positive control lanes by an empty lane. * denotes that the primer mix will amplify alleles belonging to more than one serologically defined specificity.*

unattended laboratory operation. Thus, SBT can be a means of producing high-resolution typing with high throughput.

c. Chimerism Analysis *Single tandem repeats (STR) or variable nucleotide tandem repeats (VNTR)* (21,22) is a molecular method to determine chimerism, that is, the amount of donor cells in the recipient's total white blood cells. It is primarily employed to determine if bone marrow transplants are successful. Initially after the transplant, the recipient has 100 percent donor cells. The patient is followed to see if reemergence of the cancer or recipient cells occurs. The donor and recipient often possess the same HLA alleles. The twelve or so sets of primers look for noncoding DNA that will be different in these individuals. The method involves extracting the DNA and PCR multiplexing twelve different primer sets and will differentiate HLA-identical HLA siblings. The PCR-labeled amplicons are separated by capillary electrophoresis and read by a laser, and the amount of donor and recipient DNA is calculated as area under the curve. This method has a lower sensitivity from 1 to 5 percent of either donor or recipient.

Expression analysis is a molecular method that measures the amount of messenger RNA (mRNA) of a specific gene within an individual's blood or tissue. All cellular mRNA is isolated from the specimen and transcribed to complementary DNA (cDNA) by a reverse transcriptase and random decamer priming. The cDNA is run on a real-time PCR machine with a negative control and four recombi-

nant standards. The *amount* of mRNA is calculated from this standard curve. Certain genes have been implicated in rejection such as granzyme B and/or perforin. These molecules have been shown to be responsible for white cell lysis and/or rejection. FOX P-3 has been demonstrated to be a marker for T regulatory cells that are mediating suppression of rejection. When this type of analysis is performed, a housekeeping gene should be monitored to normalize the gene of interest's copy number.

ii. HLA Antibody Detection

Antibodies to HLA antigens are one of the primary immunological barriers to successful transplantation and can be produced after the primary transplant or can be preformed prior to a transplant (e.g., from a previous transplant, pregnancies, or transfusions). Alloantibodies to HLA can mediate hyperacute rejection, acute rejection, and most likely contribute to chronic rejection (23,24). The testing of patient's serum with donor cells or *cross-match* is likely the most important test performed by the histocompatibility laboratory since a negative test is required before the transplant can be performed (25). This test measures in large part the presence of preformed anti-HLA antibodies in the potential recipient with the donor being evaluated.

1. *Complement-Dependent Cytotoxicity (CDC) Cross-match*

The cytotoxic cross-match, also known as lymphocytotoxicity cross-match, is used to detect the presence of preformed allogeneic lymphocytotoxic antibodies specific to a potential donor or to detect self-autologous lymphocytotoxic antibodies (26). This technique is a routine test performed in many histocompatibility laboratories. One can perform this test with lymphocytes from peripheral blood (at room temperature), lymph nodes, or spleen samples (at 4°C). It is typically performed in microtiter plates and is based on the interaction of patient serum with donor strain lymphocytes followed by incubation with complement. The complement will fix to cells with bound antibody and cause cell lysis, which can be detected in a variety of ways.

The target cell used may be unseparated lymphocytes or lymphocyte populations enriched for T cells (used because they express class I HLA antigens) or B cells (used because they express both class I and class II antigens).

The antibody formed is usually specific for the immunizing antigen, although antibodies that cross-react with the primary antigen may also be formed. After immunization, the usual time lapse for antibody to be detected by cytotoxicity is between seven and fourteen days. In most cases, an IgM type of antibody circulating in the recipient blood may change in strength (or titer) and may change in specificity as that recipient receives different immunizations.

Historically, when cytotoxic antibodies were not detected, a cross-match was interpreted as negative with this test. However, there was still some graft loss in some of these "negative" cases. As a result, more sensitive indirect complement-dependent assays were developed, sometimes with a second wash step or reagent added to increase the sensitivity to find these detrimental antibodies.

The Amos test is a CDC procedure developed to eliminate anticomplementary factors that promote false-negative CDC cross-matches; this procedure removes unbound serum components from the lymphocyte suspension before the addition of complement, and it is used with T-cell and B-cell targets. Another test is called the extended CDC in which the incubation time is extended in order to increase sensitivity (27). The anti-human globulin (AHG)-CDC is a test in which an anti-human globulin is added to identify antibodies that do not fix complement in vitro and are expressed at low titers, including the cytotoxicity-negative adsorption-positive antibodies. In this assay, a complement-fixing AHG (i.e., goat anti-human light chain) is added after the serum incubation, but before the addition of complement. The AHG-CDC for B and T cells allows B cells and T cells to be used as targets.

2. Flow Cytometry Cross-match

Another test that has proven to be more sensitive than the ones described above is the flow cytometry cross-match (7,8). This method allows detecting reactive antibodies that do not fix complement although there are methods for the detection of complement fixation using this methodology (28). It is performed by incubation of patients' sera with donor lymphocytes from peripheral blood, lymph nodes, or spleen. After this incubation, the cells are stained with a fluorochrome-conjugated secondary antibody to immunoglobulin that is either monoclonal or polyclonal. After this step, the mononuclear cells are incubated with CD3 and CD19 monoclonal antibodies to identify T- and B-cell reactivity (anti-class I or class II reactivity, respectively). The flow cytometer provides more objective reading as compared to the more subjective approach of a technologist looking in a microscope to determine the positive or negative reaction.

Many laboratories perform the flow cytometry cross-match as well as the AHG-CDC tests. There have been different studies trying to identify the testing procedure to perform cross-matches; however, there is no a clear consensus delineating which one is the best because of significant variations in the methodology such as reagents, sera conditions, cell isolation, and numbers used as targets. Autologous antibodies like IgG and IgM can be interpreted as positive yet are not a contraindication to transplantation so there is a component of the reaction where autologous lymphocytes or platelets are exposed to sera and analyzed.

With these techniques, generally a negative end result will mean that the transplant can take place. A positive cross-match indicates a high risk to develop antibody-mediated rejection, and is a contraindication to transplantation unless the patient is subjected to a desensitization protocol and donor-specific antibodies reduced. However, not all positive cross-matches with CDC-based assays predict a graft rejection and not all negative cross-matches will predict graft survival (29).

Panel reactive antibody (PRA) is a test with patient sera that is routinely performed on patients waiting for transplants. This test can be performed with complement-based assays as described above or by flow cytometry–based or Luminex (or bead)–based assays (30,31). This test is a way of measuring *all* of the anti-HLA antibodies, to all specificities, including any prospective donor. Thus, a person's PRA can be anywhere from 0 to 99 percent and this number represents the percent of the population that the anti-HLA antibodies in the patient's serum reacts with. For example, if a patient has a PRA of 50 percent, then the antibodies in the patient would bind to the tissue types of 50 percent of the people in the population. Patients with antibodies to a large portion of the population means that obtaining a donor will be difficult since any prospective donor should not have the HLA antigens to which the antibodies are directed (32). Due to the serious problem with an inadequate number of donors in transplantation compared to the number of persons on waiting lists for organs, some centers have now employed desensitization techniques to reduce or eliminate PRA levels so that these individuals become more viable candidates.

The detection of PRAs by enzyme-linked immunosorbent assay (ELISA) is considered a helpful screening test that employs purified HLA antigens as target for the binding of the patient's antibody. In this case it helps to eliminate non-HLA–positive reactions and gives a percentage of the true positive ones. It is also capable of detecting non-complement–fixing HLA-specific antibody that sometimes could be missed. Other methods target only IgG antibody specificity (33).

Another useful method to identify HLA antibody specificities uses Luminex technology (31). This technique uses a panel of color-coded microbeads coated with HLA antigens detected by a laser-based analyzer that assigns HLA specificity and percentages. In this method, serum is incubated with the coated microbeads and the antigens bound are labeled with R-phycoerythrin-conjugated goat anti-human IgG, detected by a flow analyzer and assigning a percent PRA and its specificity.

The detection of the spectrum of HLA antibodies (i.e., PRA) by flow cytometry is also becoming more helpful in assigning percentages and specificities (34). This test has high sensitivity and can distinguish from IgG and IgM antibodies, as well as non-complement–fixing antibodies.

This test can also exclude non-HLA antigens that by other methods could be read as false positive; at the same time, it allows identification of class I from class II antibodies. To detect the percentage and specificity of HLA antibodies, the beads, previously incubated with serum, labeled with a fluorochrome, and run in a flow cytometer, would have a fluorescent channel shift as compared against the negative control. Eventually, HLA antibody specificities identified by PRA and antigen frequencies will be used by United Network for Organ Sharing to estimate PRA (35) and this will help determine whether there is potential allosensitization to the possible donor. There will be correlation of cross-match with the PRA data – this will be used as a *virtual cross-match* that will be used to accept or reject certain potential donor : recipient combinations.

III. THE CLINICAL IMMUNOLOGY AND GENERAL LABORATORIES

i. Drug Monitoring in Organ Transplantation

Monitoring of immunosuppressive drug levels is another task performed in the clinical transplant laboratory. Some of the standard immunosuppressive agents used in transplantation, particularly cyclosporine (CsA) and tacrolimus, have a very narrow therapeutic range and become ineffective at low concentrations and toxic at high concentrations (36). Continuous monitoring of the dosage and trough level of immune suppressive drugs in organ transplantation therefore is critical in the management of the recipient's immune response to the allograft (37–39). Among the adverse side effects of immunosuppressive drugs are toxicity, cancer, and infection and there is often an association between acute complications and the elevated levels present in the recipient. Likewise, suboptimal levels of these drugs can have an association with rejection episodes occurring in the host, although the utility of post-transplant monitoring of immunosuppressive drugs to prevent rejection episodes so far is not conclusive.

The optimal method to monitor these drugs has been a matter of debate (40). There is extensive metabolizing in the liver of these compounds and an accumulation of metabolites may contribute to their toxicity; therefore, determination of not only the parent drug but also of its metabolites is of clinical importance (41,42). High-pressure liquid chromatography is considered the gold standard method for monitoring levels of many drugs (43); however, this technique requires expensive instrumentation. Immunoassays utilizing monoclonal antibodies have also proved to be excellent alternatives for drug monitoring (44). It is of paramount importance that these techniques demonstrate accuracy, precision, sensitivity, and specificity since drug doses are taken at a specific time of the day and the sample should be taken before the next dose is due. These immunosuppressive drugs often target cell activation pathways to inhibit immune cell populations (45,46) and to a certain extent there may be synergistic effects between them. Some of the drugs (Figure 11.5) that are monitored by the lab are as follows:

Tacrolimus (FK506, Prograf): Tacrolimus inhibits the activation of T cells, and it appears that the active compound binds to the immunophilin, FKBP-12. A complex of tacrolimus-FKBP-12, calcium, calmodulin, and calcineurin is then formed and the phosphatase activity of calcineurin is inhibited (47). Thereafter, there is dephosphorylation and translocation of nuclear factor of activated T-cells (NF-AT), a nuclear component that initiates gene transcription and production of cytokines such as interleukin 2 (IL-2) and IFN-γ (Figure 11.6). With this action there is an inhibition of T-lymphocyte activation (i.e., immunosuppression). There are many side effects associated with tacrolimus since it can affect many organ systems including gastrointestinal, nervous, and renal, and their incidence is high; the effects are typically dose related (48). The principal adverse reactions are tremor, headache, diarrhea, hypertension, nausea, and abnormal renal function. In some cases, tacrolimus can be used to reverse acute rejection episodes using higher doses. It is usually

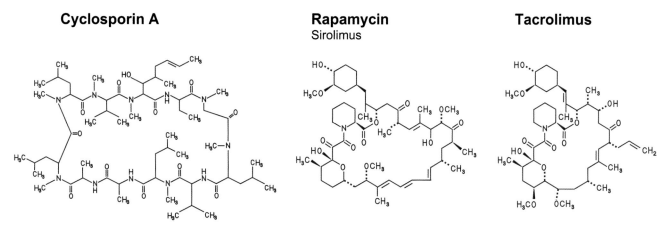

FIGURE 11.5: *Chemical structures of common immunosuppressant agents.*

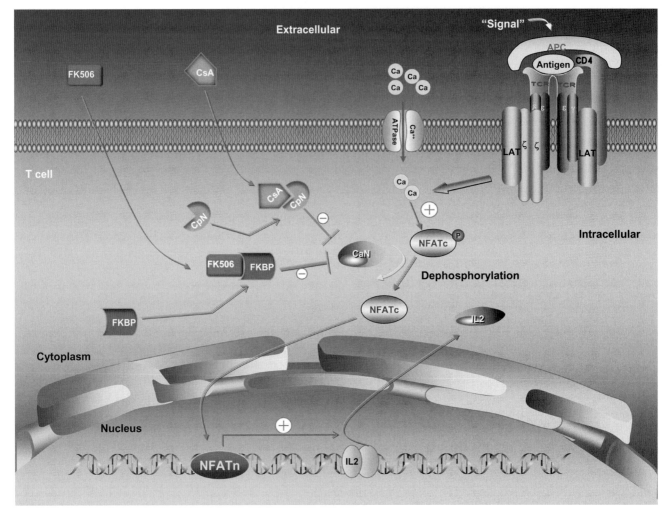

FIGURE 11.6: Pathways in lymphocytes affected by tacrolimus and CsA.

administered in the morning and the monitoring level is taken shortly before the morning dose. The optimal trough levels tend to be between 5 and 15 µg/l.

Cyclosporine (Neoral, CsA, Gengraf): It is another potent immunosuppressive agent and also a calcineurin inhibitor, blocking IL-2 production, which in turn down-regulates T-cell production and activation. CsA binds to its immunophilin, cyclophilin (CpN), forming a complex between CsA and CpN (Figure 11.6). The CsA-CpN complex binds and blocks calcineurin, blocking its phosphatase activity. As described above, calcineurin fails to dephosphorylate the cytoplasmic component of NF-AT and its transport to the nucleus. There is no promoter for the IL-2 gene, a lack of IL-2 production and no T-cell activation. Thus, although the predrugs CsA and FK506 bind to different target molecules, both drugs inhibit T-cell activation in the same fashion (Figure 11.6). The principal adverse reactions can be similar to tacrolimus and include renal dysfunction, tremor, hirsutism, hypertension, and gum hyperplasia. Renal CsA toxicity may be acute (e.g., glomer-

ular capillary thrombosis) (Figure 11.7) or chronic (49). The target level for CSA is 100–400 µg/l. As with tacrolimus, there are a variety of oral and intravenous formulations.

Sirolimus (Rapamune): Sirolimus is a macrocyclic lactone (Figure 11.5) produced by *Streptomyces hygroscopicus*, which in cells binds to the immunophilin, FKBP-12, forming a complex that binds to and inhibits the activation of the mammalian target of rapamycin (mTOR), a key regulatory kinase (Figure 11.8) (50). The sirolimus : FKBP-12 complex has no effect on calcineurin activity. The mTOR inhibition suppresses cytokine-driven T-cell proliferation, inhibiting the progression from the G_1 to the S phase of the cell cycle. It can be administered concomitantly with calcineurin inhibitors. Among the side effects of sirolimus are hypercholesterolemia, hyperlipemia, hypertension, rash, anemia, arthralgia, diarrhea, hypokalemia, and thrombocytopenia.

Mycophenylate mofetil (MMF, Cellcept): Mycophenolate (MPA) is an inhibitor of inosine monophosphate dehydrogenase, affecting the de novo pathway of guanosine

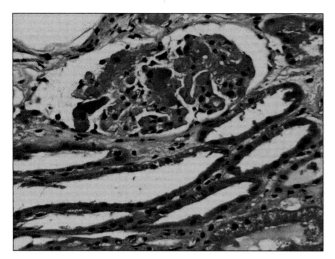

FIGURE 11.7: *Renal biopsy showing glomerular thrombosis and isometric vacuolization (toxic tubulopathy) secondary to CsA toxicity (hematoxylin and eosin, 400×).*

nucleotide synthesis without incorporation into DNA (Figure 11.9) (51). T cells and B cells are dependent on de novo synthesis of purines for their proliferation and have no salvage pathways; thus, MMF has potent cytostatic effects on lymphocytes. MPA also suppresses anti-

body formation by B lymphocytes. MPA prevents the glycosylation of lymphocyte and monocyte glycoproteins involved in adhesion to endothelial cells and thus affects immune cell recruitment into sites of graft rejection.

ii. Measurement of Graft Status and Host Immune Function

Due to the morbidity and risks sometimes associated with obtaining biopsies of allograft and native organs, there are ongoing attempts to monitor graft function and assess general immune status by the measurement of numerous molecules and the performance of functional and phenotypic cellular assays. In general, there has not been any one marker or assay that has been able to provide the specificity and detail regarding graft status as actual histological examination of the transplant tissue. However, many markers can now provide additional and valuable information for the clinician that enhances the decision-making process for treatment of graft dysfunction. Moreover, there are a variety of assays that help assess the immune functional status of the host and this may intuitively relate to whether there is an ongoing assault by the host immune response.

A variety of soluble substances are measured in the serum of transplant patients that reflect a static measurement of

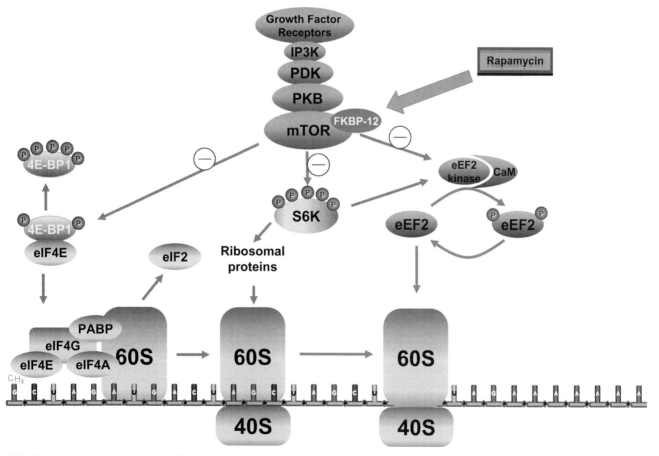

FIGURE 11.8: *Cellular pathway affected by rapamycin.*

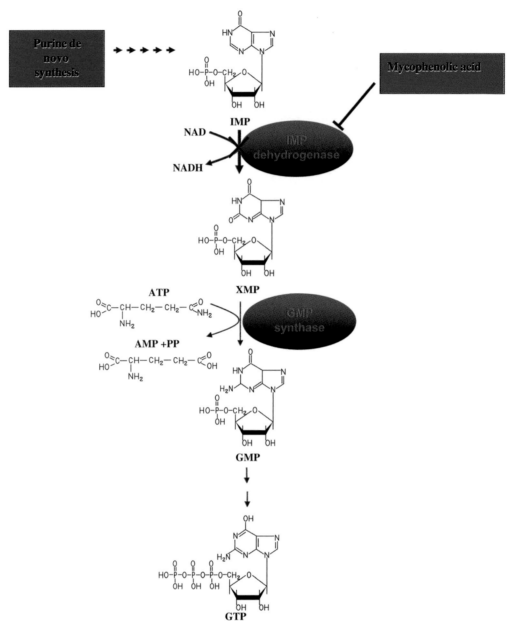

FIGURE 11.9: *Cellular pathway affected by mycophenolate.*

some pathway in the host that ultimately relates to organ function (e.g., creatinine for kidney; GGT, ALT, AST for liver; amylase for pancreas; citrulline for bowel) or some component of inflammation (e.g., cytokines, chemokines). The determination of substances such as soluble IL-2 receptor (52), neopterin (53), CD30 (54,55), cytokines (56,57), and adhesion molecules (58) tend to lack specificity and may be increased in infections and even in allograft injury related to causes other than rejection.

The search for soluble biomarkers in transplantation has been largely being performed via *genomic* and *proteomic* profile assessment from transplanted patients. The future of this work may yield an identification of one or more molecules that can be measured and possibly placed into

an algorithm that will yield precise information as to the status of the graft or what complications are present in the host. These biomarkers should have good sensitivity and specificity, be rapidly performed, and be cost effective. Initially, these markers could help predict rejection or immunological tolerance but ultimately they may provide a means to individualize immunosuppressive treatment and identify novel targets for new drug development.

1. Flow Cytometry in Organ Transplantation

Immune status monitoring by flow cytometry following organ transplantation has become a useful tool (59) to identify and monitor peripheral lymphocyte subpopulations that change in close relationship with the organ recipient's immune status during the principal complications (i.e., infections and rejections) in the post-transplant period. Multicolor flow cytometry is performed as a means of enumerating a variety of cell populations in the peripheral blood while simultaneously measuring their coexpression of many molecules that relate to activation status, maturation, and clonality. T lymphocytes are critical for the initiation and maintenance of allograft rejection, and cytofluorographic analysis of peripheral blood during rejection episodes reveals increases in CD4+ and CD8+ T lymphocytes expressing IL-2 receptors and/or HLA-DRw antigens, suggesting lymphocyte activation. Immunophenotyping can also evaluate the presence of regulatory cells that may be associated with immunological quiescence and that may be leading to operational tolerance (e.g., FoxP3+ cells) (60), the effects caused by immunosuppressive drugs, monoclonal and polyclonal antibodies (whether depleting or nondepleting), and the magnitude of cellular depletion (e.g., CD52+ subpopulations following Campath®/alemtuzumab therapy). Infectious and malignant processes (e.g., clonality studies of B cells in PTLD), and antibody-dependent injury (e.g., platelet antibody studies) can also be assessed by flow cytometry. The most commonly used monoclonal antibody panels used to stain cells postoperatively aim to characterize T cells and their subsets (CD2, CD3, CD4, CD8, TcR alpha/beta, CD7), B cells (CD19, CD20, CD22, kappa, lambda), natural killer (NK) cells (CD16/56), along with the coexpression of a variety of surface molecules (CD25, CD34, CD45, CD52, HLA-DRw, and CD138) (Figure 11.10); intracellular molecules (FoxP3, IFN-γ, IL-2, IL-4, and IL10) can also be evaluated (61–63).

2. Infectious Disease Screening

The presence of infectious agents remains as one of the principal causes of morbidity and mortality in following transplantation, understandably secondary to the profound immunosuppression these patients typically have to endure. Infectious disease serological screening is a stalwart component of the microbiology laboratory since it measures the presence of host antibody responses to bacterial, fungal, or viral antigens. There are a variety of means to measure antibodies in the clinical lab including solid-phase ELISA, nephelometry, and immunofixation techniques. Microbial antigens may also be detected with these methods. Among the limitations of serological assessment are that some individuals have a poor antibody response or the measurement may be within the time period between initial infection and seroconversion. In addition to screening patients in the post-transplant period, these methods can also be used to screen potential donors for infectious pathogens.

Molecular methods for the identification of infectious agents identify the presence of the actual pathogen DNA or RNA sequence and these methods have become an essential part of the microbiology laboratory. The PCR, which amplifies very few nucleic acid molecules to a detectable level, is used for detection and quantification. It is the method of choice for immunocompromised transplant patients. SSPs may be used for qualitative analysis and/or a labeled oligonucleotide probe to do quantitative analysis. In addition to being able to detect few molecules, this methodology is capable of rapid turnaround time (often two–four hours) to diagnosis. Several latent viruses such as Cytomegalovirus (CMV) and Epstein-Barr Virus (EBV) are monitored with these PCR quantitative methods (64). The presence of Human Immunodeficiency Virus (HIV), Hepatitis B Virus (HBV), Hepatitis C Virus (HCV), and polyomavirus (65) can be resolved without laborious and time-consuming culture methods.

The clinical laboratory also assists in the detection and monitoring of disease recurrence in allograft organs. Chronic HCV infection is a common cause of end-stage liver disease requiring liver transplantation. Although almost all patients who receive a liver allograft for HCV will have detectable HCV RNA levels after transplantation (66,67), there is a wide variation in the severity of the clinical course and histological response. In this regard, investigators have focused on the levels of HCV viremia and the different HCV genotypes (68). There are some laboratories that offer highly sophisticated PCR-based techniques to detect and quantitate HCV RNA and genotype the virus. HCV RNA levels performed monthly following transplantation are used in conjunction with surgical biopsies to evaluate the appropriateness of antiviral therapy.

3. Functional Immune Assessment

The evaluation of immune status in transplantation and other patients with immune-based disorders is a growing area of the clinical laboratory. Three general types of measurements are possible: in vivo, immune activity is measured within the patient; ex vivo, cells from the patient are put directly into an assay to measure activity; in vitro, cells, usually from peripheral blood mononuclear cells (PBMC), are cultured before activity assay. The source of cells is generally from PBMC. The assays described below use ex vivo or in vitro measurements. Among the primary issues with the studies of the immune function assays is the establishment of test standardization, communication pathways, and assessments of all events in anticipation of possible response during the different phases of the transplantation settings. Since many areas of the immune response can be measured, it is very important to correctly identify which phase is to be measured (e.g., assessment of naive, effector, or memory T-cell function; APC functions such as phagocytosis and antigen presentation; T-cell recognition and activation). These tests are typically multistep assays with complex readouts. Their high level of

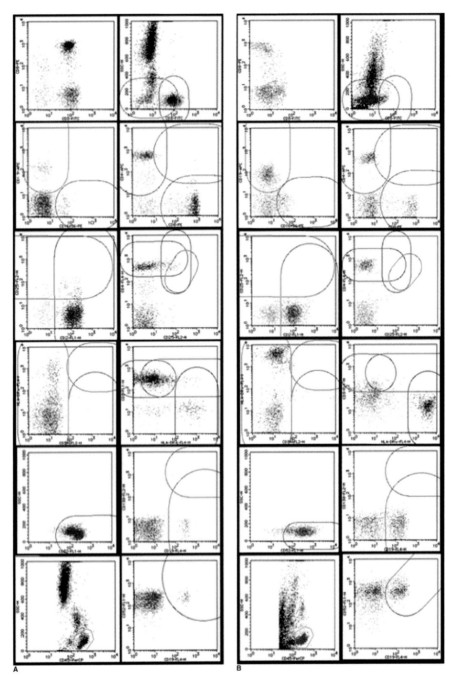

FIGURE 11.10: *(A) Flow cytometry results from peripheral blood of a seven-year-old (female) patient who received a kidney from a living related donor seven months before. The histograms depict the CD45/SSC gating, which is constant in all tubes run, followed by the CD3/CD8 profile used to guide the attractors in the CD3/SSC that picks the cluster of CD3-positive (green/orange) and CD3-negative (blue) lymphocytes. These last CD3 positives are then (bottom histogram) subdivided into CD8/CD4 clusters. Lymphocytes that are clustered into a red CD2-positive attractor are transported to a CD25/CD4 gate that subdivides the CD4 positives into three populations, the CD45/CD2/CD4(dim)/CD25 (bright-blue) "natural" regulatory cells (nTreg), the CD45/CD2/CD4/CD25(dim-red) "activated" T cells, and the CD45/CD2/CD4/CD25(negative-yellow) "naïve" T cells. Lymphocytes are also assessed for the Campath 1-H binding epitope CD52 including the presence on B cells. CD138 identifies plasma cells. (B) Flow cytometry panel used in a transplant patient – OKT3 effect. Patient received a multivisceral transplant, six months before. He developed a steroid-resistant rejection episode. After several days (9/10-day course) of OKT3 therapy, there was (in circulation) an increase in the amount of T cells and NK cells. Abundant (20–30 percent) CD4+ and CD8+ cells are present but due to the lack of CD3 recognition are left as 0.47 and 1.36 percent, respectively, due to CD3 masking by OKT3. The majority of circulating cells are CD52 positive.*

complexity can compromise data comparison between different sites and limit the ability for standardization of immune monitoring assays. The lack of standardization of these assays from lab to lab is reflected in the fact that only a few tests that are commercially available have clearance from the FDA and are offered as clinical tests. There are a variety of reasons for the difficulty in test standardization but among them is the fact that whole cells are used, often with standard numbers versus phenotypically identical populations being used as the starting point in the assay. Thereafter, cells are usually cultured and it can be very difficult to obtain identical conditions between different lab environments; minor changes can profoundly affect the readout of these tests. Finally, the significant number of sequential steps that may be necessary and that can affect the test readout can be difficult to standardize.

Antigen-specific (or nonspecific) T-cell or B-cell responses can be measured by several techniques and each has its own limitations and advantages. *Lymphoid proliferation and cytotoxicity assays* are loosely based on the presumption that naive and/or memory cells present in the patient's fluid or tissue sample will respond with primary or anamnestic (secondary) proliferation upon in vitro exposure to antigen. The antigen may be nonspecific (e.g., mitogens, antibody cross-linking of receptors) or specific according to original immune stimulant within the recipient (e.g., alloantigens of the donor). The level of proliferation or cytotoxicity that subsequently occurs is a reflection of the level of stimulation that ensued following the antigen exposure and this is extrapolated to mirror the level of immune cell activation that occurs in vivo in the host.

The *mixed lymphocyte culture* (MLC) is a test that has been used in transplantation for several decades in multiple configurations (69). The basic principle of the test is that lymphocytes from two different individuals with HLA-mismatched antigens tend to proliferate against each other when placed in culture together within three to seven days. Typically, to single out a single population response from the bidirectional reaction, one population (the donor cell population) is inhibited from proliferating by preculture treatment with irradiation or mitomycin C (and is named the *stimulator* population), while the other untreated population (from the recipient) is named the *responder* population. The degree of genetic disparity between the responder and stimulator as well as the level of memory cells specific to the stimulator will often be proportional to the level of proliferation that ensues. The MLC can be very useful in pretransplant determinations of living donor compatibility and/or sensitization. Among the limitations of this assay is the lack of standardization between institutions, the protracted amount of time for the readout (can be seven days), and the high level of complexity required for its performance. The measurement of proliferation can be performed with radioactive ^{3}H-tritium or with proliferation dyes (e.g., CFSE), which

are nonradioactive and allow for simultaneous determination of the nature of the responding cells by flow cytometry as well as the extent of proliferation. Nevertheless, over the years, the MLC has tended to be replaced by many of the HLA typing techniques mentioned earlier in the chapter.

The *mixed lymphocyte reaction* (MLR) is a test usually run parallel to the MLC and provides a measurement of the response potential of the cells placed in the MLC. The basic principle is to stimulate a single population of cells from the donor or recipient by mitogens (PHA, CoA, LPS, etc.), which do so independently of their genetic markup. Measurement of the response could also be done as in the MLC (with the same advantages and disadvantages). One test that is FDA approved and that measures proliferation of peripheral CD4+ T cells in response to the mitogens PHA is the Cylex ImmuKnow® test. This is a test based on the MLR previously mentioned but with significant changes. It is performed without cell separation (done in whole blood), and after seventeen hours of stimulation with the mitogens, CD4-positive cells are pulled out mechanically and assessed for the amount of ATP generated in relation to the immune cell activity in a luminometer. This test has a clear relationship in many studies with the level of immunosuppression present in the host (70); as such, several studies have demonstrated that monitoring serial levels of ImmuKnow in transplant patients may predict the onset of acute rejection or overimmunosuppression (71).

Cytotoxic T lymphocyte (CTL) measurement is classically performed with a chromium release assay (72). The basic principle of the test starts with generating an MLC as described above. After seven days, the activated responder cells (primed responders) are then exposed to freshly prepared donor cells (same used as stimulator) now tested, not for proliferation but for the ability to kill the targets. Target cells expressing antigen (e.g., alloantigen) on their surface are labeled with a radioactive isotope of chromium (^{51}Cr). The patient's primed cells are mixed with the target cell and incubated for several hours. Lysis of antigen-expressing cells releases ^{51}Cr into the medium. Specific lysis is calculated by comparing lysis of target cells in the presence or absence of patient effector primed cells and is usually expressed as the percent specific lysis (72). CTL response can also be assessed by measuring cytokine production (e.g., IFN-α) by antigen-specific effector cells in an *ELISPOT* (enzyme-linked immunoSpot) assay (73). In this assay, APCs are immobilized on the plastic surface of a microtiter well, and effector cells are added at various effector : target ratios. The binding of APCs by antigen-specific effector cells triggers the production of cytokines by the effector cells. The cells can be stained to detect the presence of the molecule in question (e.g., granzyme) and the number of positively staining foci (spots) is quantitated microscopically (Figure 11.11). Circulating antigen-

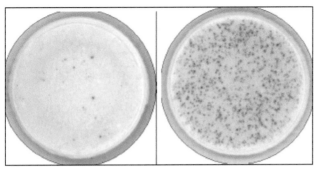

FIGURE 11.11: *ELISPOT assay for granzyme B. Cell-mediated cytotoxicity involves exocytosis of cytoplasmic granules from the effector toward the target cell. The granules contain proteins, including perforin and granzyme B. Granzyme B is present mainly in the granules of CD8+ CTL and NK cells and mediates the lethal hit that kills virus-infected and tumor cells. Measurement of granzyme B release in response to the appropriate target is useful as a valuable nonradioactive alternative to the 51Cr-release assays for measuring antigen-specific CTL cytotoxicity. The well on left shows human peripheral blood cells not stimulated with alloreactive cells, while the well on the right shows granzyme B releasing cells after stimulation with the appropriate targets.*

specific CD8+ T cells (and more recently CD4+ T cells) can also be identified by the *tetramer* assay. In this test, a specific epitope is bound to synthetic tetrameric forms of fluorochrome-labeled MHC class I or class II molecules (74,75). CD8+ T cells recognize antigen in the form of short peptides bound to class I molecules, while CD4+ cells bind peptides on class II molecules; thus, cells with the appropriate T-cell receptor will bind to the labeled tetramers and can be measured by flow cytometry. As compared to the CTL or ELISPOT assays the tetramer assay measures only *binding* to the T-cell receptor, not the functional status of the cells. This remains an important limitation of the tetramer assay since all cells that bind a particular antigen do not necessarily become activated. Another limitation of the tetramer assay is that tetramers of all class I or class II subtypes are not always available, so that some combinations may not be possible to test. Correlation between ELISPOT, tetramer, and cytotoxicity assays has not always been established. Recently, functional activity of cytotoxic lymphocytes measures the secretion or expression of the molecules associated or involved in cell-mediated killing. Among the mechanisms of cell-mediated cytotoxicity is exocytosis of cytoplasmic granules from the effector cell toward the target cell. These membrane-enveloped lysosomes are principally composed of granzymes and perforin. The lipid bilayer surrounding them contains *l*ysosomal-*a*ssociated *mem*brane glyco*p*roteins (LAMPs) including LAMP-1 (CD107a). As part of the fusion of membranes during the degranulation process, CD107a, once exclusive to granule membrane, is now expressed on the surface of effector cells (76,77). Upon induction of apoptosis, phos-

phatidylserine is externalized resulting in its accessibility to the surface. This phospholipid can bind annexin V. Thus, antibodies specific for CD107a and labeled annexin V (78) can be used by flow cytometry to identify effector cells and apoptotic target cells. This assay may ultimately replace the more classical ^{51}CR assay.

Limiting dilution assay (LDA): These assays measure precursor frequencies of different effector populations [e.g., T-helper (Th) cells, T-cytotoxic cells] within a sample to a specific antigen (e.g., alloantigen) and the readout can be proliferation or cytotoxicity. These tests are labor intensive and time consuming to perform and the numbers of donor and recipient cells available are often limited. There are a variety of methods used for LDA analysis with many based on the single-hit Poisson model or double-hit model (79). The LDA is a very useful test in estimating levels of effector cell populations but is rarely used in standard clinical transplantation scenarios.

The measurement of intracellular cytokine along with coexpression of other lineage markers by flow cytometry or fluorescent microscopy has been a very useful tool to identify T-cell subpopulations such as Th1 and Th2 cells. These cells have polarized cytokine gene expression and secretion (e.g., Th1 – IFN-γ; Th2 – IL-4, IL-5, IL-9, and IL-13). Indeed, heightened activity of either Th1 or Th2 cells have been associated with a variety of disease states [e.g., Th1 – sarcoidosis, graft rejection, some autoimmune conditions (80); Th2 – extracellular pathogens, antibody production, asthma] (81), so that measurement of their levels often has some utility in assessing certain disease states. Th1 cell levels vary during transplant rejection or infectious disease in transplant patients (82), and their measurement has generally been performed on the basis of the type of cytokine being expressed. Recently, other markers for Th subset identification have emerged such as GATA3 (83,84) and T bet (85). Future assays may evaluate differential expression of these nuclear factors as a means of measuring these different effector T-cell populations.

REFERENCES

1. Apanius, V., P.D., Slev, P.R., Ruff, L.R., Potts, W.K. 1997. The nature of selection on the major histocompatibility complex. *Crit Rev in Immunol,* 17(2): 179–224.
2. Gorodezky, C., Alaez, C., Murguia, A., Rodriguez, A., Balladares, S., Vazquez, M., Flores, H., Robles, C., Gorodezky, C., Alaez, C., et al. 2006. HLA and autoimmune diseases: type 1 diabetes (T1D) as an example. *Autoimmun Rev,* 5: 187–94.
3. Arnett, F.C., Moulds, J.M. 1991. HLA class III molecules and autoimmune rheumatic diseases. *Clini Exp Rheumatol,* 9: 289–96.
4. Ahmad, T., Marshall, S.E., Jewell, D. 2006. Genetics of inflammatory bowel disease: the role of the HLA complex. *World J Gastroenterol,* 12(23): 3628–35.

5. Afzali, B., Lechler, R.I., Hernandez-Fuentes, M.P. 2007. Allorecognition and the alloresponse: clinical implications. *Tis Ant, 69*: 545–56.

6. Sheldon, S., Poulton, K., Sheldon, S., Poulton, K. 2006. HLA typing and its influence on organ transplantation. *Methods Mol Biol, 333*: 157–74.

7. Bray, R.A. 2001. Flow cytometry in human leukocyte antigen testing. *Semin Hematol, 38*: 194–200.

8. Tambur, A.R., Klein, T. 2000. Flow cytometry application in organ transplantation. *Israel Med Assoc J, 2*: 310–5.

9. Middleton, D. 1999. History of DNA typing for the human MHC. *Rev Immunogenet, 1*: 135–56.

10. *Middleton, D.* 2002. Current and emerging technology for HLA typing. *Int J Hematol, 76 Suppl. 2*: 150–1.

11. Welsh, K., Bunce, M. 1999. Molecular typing for the MHC with PCR-SSP. *Rev Immunogenet, 1*: 157–76.

12. Erlich, H.A., Opelz, G., Hansen, J. 2001. HLA DNA typing and transplantation. *Immunity, 14*: 347–56.

13. Charron, D. 2005. Immunogenetics today: HLA, MHC and much more. *Curr Opin Immunol, 17*: 493–7.

14. Miretti, M.M., Beck, S. 2006. Immunogenomics: molecular hide and seek. *Hum Genom, 2*: 244–51.

15. *ASHI Laboratory Manual*, edition 4.2, 2007, Complement Dependant Cytotoxicity, p. 205.

16. Cao, K., Chopek, M., Fernandez-Vina, M.A. 1999. High and intermediate resolution DNA typing systems for class I HLA-A, B, C genes by hybridization with sequence-specific oligonucleotide probes (SSOP). *Rev Immunogenet, 1*: 177–208.

17. Mwenda, J.M., Shotake, T., Yamamoto, T., Uchihi, R., Bambra, C.S., Katsumata, Y. 1999. DNA typing of primate major histocompatibility complex (Mhc)-DQA1 locus by PCR and dot blot hybridization. *Cell Mol Biol, 45*: 1249–56.

18. Hong, S.-K., Kim, B.-J., Yun, Y.-J., Lee, K.-H., Kim, E.-C., Park, E.-M., Park, Y.-G., Bai, G.-H., Kook, Y.-H. 2004. Identification of Mycobacterium tuberculosis by PCR-linked reverse hybridization using specific rpoB oligonucleotide probes. *J Microbiol Methods, 59*: 71–9.

19. Mantovani, V., Martinelli, G., Bragliani, M., Buzzi, M., Selva, P., Collina, E., Farabegoli, P., Rosti, G.A., Bandini, G., Tura, S. et al. 1995. Molecular analysis of HLA genes for the selection of unrelated bone marrow donor. *Bone Marrow Transplant, 16*: 329–35.

20. Shigenari, A., Ando, A., Renard, C., Chardon, P., Shiina, T., Kulski, J.K., Yasue, H., Inoko, H. 2004. Nucleotide sequencing analysis of the swine 433-kb genomic segment located between the non-classical and classical SLA class I gene clusters. *Immunogenetics, 55*: 695–705.

21. Dorak, M.T., Shao, W., Machulla, H.K.G., Lobashevsky, E.S., Tang, J., Park, M.H., Kaslow, R.A. 2006. Conserved extended haplotypes of the major histocompatibility complex: further characterization. *Gene Immunity, 7*: 450–67.

22. Pena, J.A., Calderon, R., Perez-Miranda, A., Vidales, C., Dugoujon, J.M., Carrion, M., Crouau-Roy, B. 2002. Microsatellite DNA markers from HLA region (D6S105, D6S265 and TNFa) in autochthonous Basques from Northern Navarre (Spain). *Ann Hum Biol, 29*: 176–91.

23. Akalin, E., Watschinger, B. 2007. Antibody-mediated rejection. *Semin Nephrol, 27*: 393–407.

24. Saidman, S. 2007. Significance of anti-HLA and donor-specific antibodies in long-term renal graft survival. *Transplant Proc, 39*: 744–6.

25. Zeevi, A., Girnita, A., Duquesnoy, R., Zeevi, A., Girnita, A., Duquesnoy, R. 2006. HLA antibody analysis: sensitivity, specificity, and clinical significance in solid organ transplantation. *Immunol Res, 36*: 255–64.

26. Altermann, W.W., Seliger, B., Sel, S., Wendt, D., Schlaf, G. 2006. Comparison of the established standard complement-dependent cytotoxicity and flow cytometric crossmatch assays with a novel ELISA-based HLA crossmatch procedure. *Histol Histopathol, 21*: 1115–24.

27. Bray, R.A., Nickerson, P.W., Kerman, R.H., Gebel, H.M. 2004. Evolution of HLA antibody detection: technology emulating biology. *Immunol Res, 29*: 41–54.

28. Watanabe, J., Scornik, J.C. 2006. Measuring human complement activation by HLA antibodies. *Arch Pathol Lab Med, 130*: 368–73.

29. Gebel, H.M., Bray, R.A., Nickerson, P. 2003. Pre-transplant assessment of donor-reactive, HLA-specific antibodies in renal transplantation: contraindication vs. risk. *Am J Transplant, 3*: 1488–500.

30. Piatosa, B., Rubik, J., Grenda, R. 2006. Is positive flow cytometric cross-match a risk factor for early cadaveric kidney graft dysfunction? *Transplant Procs, 38*: 53–5.

31. Gibney, E.M., Cagle, L.R., Freed, B., Warnell, S.E., Chan, L., Wiseman, A.C. 2006. Detection of donor-specific antibodies using HLA-coated microspheres: another tool for kidney transplant risk stratification. *Nephrol Dial Transplant, 21*: 2625–9.

32. Scornik, J.C., Guerra, G., Schold, J.D., Srinivas, T.R., Dragun, D., Meier-Kriesche, H.U. 2007. Value of posttransplant antibody tests in the evaluation of patients with renal graft dysfunction. *Am J Transplant, 7*: 1808–14.

33. Mansour, I., Messaed, C., Azoury, M., Klayme, S., Naaman, R. 2001. Panel-reactive antibodies using complement-dependent cytotoxicity, flow cytometry, and ELISA in patients awaiting renal transplantation or transplanted patients: a comparative study. *Transplant Proc, 33*: 2844–7.

34. Bryan, C.F., McDonald, S.B., Baier, K.A., Luger, A.M., Aeder, M.I., Murillo, D., Muruve, N.A., Nelson, P.W., Shield, C.F., Warady, B.A. et al. 2002. Flow cytometry beads rather than the antihuman globulin method should be used to detect HLA Class I IgG antibody (PRA) in cadaveric renal regraft candidates. *Clin Transplant, 16 Suppl. 7*: 15–23.

35. Susskind, B. 2007. Methods for histocompatibility testing in the early 21st century. *Curr Opin Organ Transplant, 12*: 393–401.

36. Wallemacq, P.E. 2004. Therapeutic monitoring of immunosuppressant drugs. Where are we? *Clin Chem Lab Med, 42*: 1204–11.

37. Lin, S., Cosgrove, C.J. 2006. Perioperative management of immunosuppression. *Surg Clin North Am, 86*: 1167–83.

38. Calne, R.Y. 2007. Transplantation: current developments and future directions. *Front Biosci, 12*: 3727–33.

39. Kirk, A.D. 2006. Induction immunosuppression. *Transplantation, 82*: 593–602.

40. Armstrong, V.W., Schuetz, E., Zhang, Q., Groothuisen, S., Scholz, C., Shipkova, M., Aboleneen, H., Oellerich, M. 1998. Modified pentamer formation assay for measurement of tacrolimus and its active metabolites: comparison with liquid chromatography-tandem mass spectrometry and microparticle enzyme-linked immunoassay (MEIA-II). *Clin Chem*, 44: 2516–23.

41. Murthy, J.N., Davis, D.L., Yatscoff, R.W., Soldin, S.J. 1998. Tacrolimus metabolite cross-reactivity in different tacrolimus assays. *Clin Biochem*, 31: 613–7.

42. Davis, D.L., Murthy, J.N., Gallant-Haidner, H., Yatscoff, R.W., Soldin, S.J. 2000. Minor immunophilin binding of tacrolimus and sirolimus metabolites. *Clin Biochem*, 33: 1–6.

43. Taylor, P.J. 2004. Therapeutic drug monitoring of immunosuppressant drugs by high-performance liquid chromatography-mass spectrometry. *Therapeutic Drug Monitor*, 26: 215–9.

44. Andrews, D.J., Cramb, R. 2002. Cyclosporin: revisions in monitoring guidelines and review of current analytical methods. *Ann of Clin Biochem*, 39: 424–35.

45. Filler, G. 2007. Calcineurin inhibitors in pediatric renal transplant recipients. *Paediat Drugs*, 9: 165–74.

46. Gustafsson, F., Ross, H.J. 2007. Proliferation signal inhibitors in cardiac transplantation. *Curr Opin Cardiol*, 22: 111–6.

47. Powell, J.D., Zheng, Y., Powell, J.D., Zheng, Y. 2006. Dissecting the mechanism of T-cell anergy with immunophilin ligands. *Curr Opin Investig Drugs*, 7: 1002–7.

48. Reichenspurner, H. 2005. Overview of tacrolimus-based immunosuppression after heart or lung transplantation. *J Heart Lung Transplant*, 24: 119–30.

49. Chapman, J.R., Nankivell, B.J. 2006. Nephrotoxicity of ciclosporin A: short-term gain, long-term pain? *Nephrol Dial Transplant*, 21: 2060–3.

50. Hartford, C.M., Ratain, M.J. 2007. Rapamycin: something old, something new, sometimes borrowed and now renewed. *Clin Pharmacol Therap*, 82: 381–8.

51. Allison, A.C., Eugui, E.M. 2005. Mechanisms of action of mycophenolate mofetil in preventing acute and chronic allograft rejection. *Transplantation*, 80: S181–90.

52. Gupta, R.K., Jain, M., Sharma, R.K. 2004. Serum & urinary interleukin-2 levels as predictors in acute renal allograft rejection. *Indi J Med Res*, 119: 24–7.

53. Tilg, H., V.W., Aulitzky, W.E. et al. 1989. Neopterin excretion after liver transplantation and its value in differential diagnosis of complications. *Transplantation*, 48: 594–9.

54. Langan, L.L., Park, L.P., Hughes, T.L., Irish, A., Luxton, G., Witt, C.S., Christiansen, F.T. 2007. Post-transplant HLA class II antibodies and high soluble CD30 levels are independently associated with poor kidney graft survival. *Am J Transplant*, 7: 847–56.

55. Dong, W., Shunliang, Y., Weizhen, W., Qinghua, W., Zhangxin, Z., Jianming, T., He, W. 2006. Prediction of acute renal allograft rejection in early post-transplantation period by soluble CD30. *Transplant Immunol*, 16: 41–5.

56. Oliveira, G., Xavier, P., Murphy, B., Neto, S., Mendes, A., Sayegh, M.H., Guerra, L.E. 1998. Cytokine analysis of human renal allograft aspiration biopsy cultures superna-

tants predicts acute rejection. *Nephrol Dial Transplant*, 13: 417–22.

57. Ghafari, A., Makhdoomi, K., Ahmadpour, P., Afshari, A.T., Lak, S.S., Fakhri, L. 2007. Serum T-lymphocyte cytokines cannot predict early acute rejection in renal transplantation. *Transplant Proc*, 39: 958–61.

58. Rodriguez-Iturbe, B. 1996. Cellular adhesion molecules in transplantation. *Transplant Proc*, 28: 3285–9.

59. Mathew, J.M., Fuller, L., Carreno, M., Garcia-Morales, R., Burke, G.W., 3rd, Ricordi, C., Esquenazi, V., Tzakis, A.G., Miller, J. 2000. Involvement of multiple subpopulations of human bone marrow cells in the regulation of allogeneic cellular immune responses. *Transplantation*, 70: 1752–60.

60. Crellin, N.K., Garcia, R.V., Levings, M.K. 2007. Flow cytometry-based methods for studying signaling in human CD4+CD25+FOXP3+ T regulatory cells. *J Immunol Methods*, 324: 92–104.

61. Setoguchi, R., Hori, S., Takahashi, T., Sakaguchi, S. 2005. Homeostatic maintenance of natural Foxp3+ CD25+ CD4+ regulatory T cells by interleukin (IL)-2 and induction of autoimmune disease by IL-2 neutralization. *J Exp Med*, 201: 723–35.

62. Cox, K., North, M., Burke, M., Singhal, H., Renton, S., Aqel, N., Islam, S., Knight, S.C. 2005. Plasmacytoid dendritic cells (PDC) are the major DC subset innately producing cytokines in human lymph nodes. *J Leukocyte Biol*, 78: 1142–52.

63. Fuller, L., Carreno, M., Zheng, S., Esquenazi, V., Yang, W., Miller, J. 1991. Isolation of anti-OKT3 and anti-(anti-OKT3) from a kidney transplant recipient. *Transplant Proc*, 23: 305–6.

64. Smith, T.F., Espy, M.J., Mandrekar, J., Jones, M.F., Cockerill, F.R., Patel, R. 2007. Quantitative real-time polymerase chain reaction for evaluating DNAemia due to cytomegalovirus, Epstein-Barr virus, and BK virus in solid-organ transplant recipients. *Clin Infect Dis*, 45: 1056–61.

65. Cirocco, R., Markou, M., Rosen, A., Goldsmith, L., Cianco, G., Roth, D., Kupin, W., Burke, G., Esquenazi, V., Tzakis, A. et al. 2001. Polyomavirus PCR monitoring in renal transplant recipients: detection in blood is associated with higher creatinine values. *Transplant Proc*, 33: 1805–7.

66. Everhart, J.E., Wei, Y., Eng, H., Charlton, M.R., Persing, D.H., Wiesner, R.H., Germer, J.J., Lake, J.R., Zetterman, R.K., Hoofnagle, J.H. 1999. Recurrent and new hepatitis C virus infection after liver transplantation. *Hepatology*, 29: 1220–6.

67. Costes, V., Durand, L., Pageaux, G.P., Ducos, J., Mondain, A.M., Picot, M.C., Domergue, J., Larrey, D., Baldet, P. 1999. Hepatitis C virus genotypes and quantification of serum hepatitis C RNA in liver transplant recipients. Relationship with histologic outcome of recurrent hepatitis C. *Am J Clin Pathol*, 111: 252–8.

68. Gane, E.J., Naoumov, N.V., Qian, K.P., Mondelli, M.U., Maertens, G., Portmann, B.C., Lau, J.Y., Williams, R. 1996. A longitudinal analysis of hepatitis C virus replication following liver transplantation. *Gastroenterology*, 110: 167–77.

69. Nicklin, S. 1995. Immune function assays. *Methods Mol Biol*, 43: 245–56.

70. Hooper, E., Hawkins, D.M., Kowalski, R.J., Post, D.R., Britz, J.A., Brooks, K.C., Turman, M.A. 2005. Establishing pediatric immune response zones using the Cylex Immu-Know assay. *Clin Transplant*, *19*: 834–9.

71. Zeevi, A., Britz, J.A., Bentlejewski, C.A., Guaspari, D., Tong, W., Bond, G., Murase, N., Harris, C., Zak, M., Martin, D. et al. 2005. Monitoring immune function during tacrolimus tapering in small bowel transplant recipients. *Transplant Immunol*, *15*: 17–24.

72. Bromelow, K.V., Galea-Lauri, J., O'Brien, M.E., Souberbielle, B.E. 1998. A highly sensitive whole blood natural killer cell assay. *J Immunol Methods*, *217*: 177–84.

73. Malyguine, A., Strobl, S., Zaritskaya, L., Baseler, M., Shafer-Weaver, K. 2007. New approaches for monitoring CTL activity in clinical trials. *Adva Exp Med Biol*, *601*: 273–84.

74. Ramachandiran, V., Grigoriev, V., Lan, L., Ravkov, E., Mertens, S.A., Altman, J.D. 2007. A robust method for production of MHC tetramers with small molecule fluorophores. *J Immunol Methods*, *319*: 13–20.

75. Li, F., Xu, L., Zha, Q., Chi, X., Jia, Q., He, X. 2007. Preparation and identification of HLA-A*1101 tetramer loading with human cytomegalovirus pp65 antigen peptide. *Cell Mol Immunol*, *4*: 141–6.

76. Penack, O., Fischer, L., Stroux, A., Gentilini, C., Nogai, A., Muessig, A., Ganepola, S., Lange, T., Kliem, C., Marinets, O. et al. 2007. A novel method to quantify and characterize leukemia-reactive natural killer cells in patients undergoing allogeneic hematopoietic stem cell transplantation following conventional or reduced-dose conditioning. *Int J Hematol*, *85*: 326–32.

77. Devevre, E., Romero, P., Mahnke, Y.D. 2006. LiveCount assay: concomitant measurement of cytolytic activity and phenotypic characterization of CD8 (+) T-cells by flow cytometry. *J Immunol Methods*, *311*: 31–46.

78. Nopp, A., Stridh, H., Gronneberg, R., Lundahl, J. 2002. Lower apoptosis rate and higher CD69 expression in neutrophils from atopic individuals. *Inflamm Res*, *51*: 532–40.

79. Russell, C.A., B.L., Vindeløv, L.L. 1999. Design of limiting dilution analysis experiments for helper T lymphocyte precursor frequency determination in the context of allogeneic bone marrow transplantation. *J Immunol Methods*, *27*; *225(1–2)*: 113–24.

80. Hemdan, N.Y., Emmrich, F., Faber, S., Lehmann, J., Sack, U. 2007. Alterations of TH1/TH2 reactivity by heavy metals: possible consequences include induction of autoimmune diseases. *Anna New York Acad Sci*, *1109*: 129–37.

81. Epstein, M.M. 2006. Targeting memory Th2 cells for the treatment of allergic asthma. *Pharmacol Therap*, *109*: 107–36.

82. Cervera, C., Filella, X., Linares, L., Pineda, M., Esteva, C., Anton, A., Marcos, M.A., Cofan, F., Navasa, M., Perez-Villa, F. et al. 2007. TH1/TH2 cytokine release pattern during in vivo cytomegalovirus disease in solid organ transplantation. *Transplant Proc*, *39*: 2233–5.

83. Fang, T.C., Yashiro-Ohtani, Y., Del Bianco, C., Knoblock, D.M., Blacklow, S.C., Pear, W.S. 2007. Notch directly regulates Gata3 expression during T helper 2 cell differentiation. *Immunity*, *27*: 100–10.

84. Amsen, D., Antov, A., Jankovic, D., Sher, A., Radtke, F., Souabni, A., Busslinger, M., McCright, B., Gridley, T., Flavell, R.A. 2007. Direct regulation of Gata3 expression determines the T helper differentiation potential of Notch. *Immunity*, *27*: 89–99.

85. Ariga, H., Shimohakamada, Y., Nakada, M., Tokunaga, T., Kikuchi, T., Kariyone, A., Tamura, T., Takatsu, K. 2007. Instruction of naive CD4+ T-cell fate to T-bet expression and T helper 1 development: roles of T-cell receptor-mediated signals. *Immunology*, *122*: 210–21.

Index

WITHDRAWN
FROM STOCK
QMUL LIBRARY